Manual of Obstetrics

Diagnosis and Therapy

Manual of Obstetrics

Diagnosis and Therapy

Fourth Edition

Edited by
Kenneth R. Niswander, M.D.
Professor Emeritus of Obstetrics and Gynecology, University of California, Davis, School of Medicine; Attending Obstetrician and Gynecologist, University of California, Davis, Medical Center, Sacramento

Arthur T. Evans, M.D.
Associate Editor
Assistant Professor of Obstetrics and Gynecology, University of California, Davis, School of Medicine; Director, Division of Maternal-Fetal Medicine, University of California, Davis, Medical Center, Sacramento

Little, Brown and Company
Boston/Toronto/London

Fourth Edition

Library of Congress Catalog Card No. 90-63727

ISBN 0-316-61173-5

Printed in the United States of America

SEM

Contents

Contributing Authors

Leslie Andrews, M.D.	Volunteer Clinical Faculty and Clinical Assistant Professor of Obstetrics and Gynecology, University of California, Davis, School of Medicine, Sacramento
Mahmoud M. Benbarka, M.D.	Assistant Professor of Internal Medicine, University of California, Davis, School of Medicine, Sacramento
Silverio T. Chavez, M.D.	Clinical Faculty, Department of Reproductive Medicine, University of California, San Diego, School of Medicine; Staff, Department of Obstetrics and Gynecology, Kaiser Foundation Hospital, San Diego
Stuart H. Cohen, M.D.	Associate Professor of Medicine, Division of Infectious Diseases, University of California, Davis, School of Medicine; Clinical Director, Department of Epidemiology and Infection Control, University of California, Davis, Medical Center, Sacramento
Stephen D. Collins, M.D., Ph.D.	Assistant Professor of Neurology and Neurosciences, Case Western Reserve University School of Medicine, Cleveland, Ohio
Gary A. Comstock, M.D.	Active Staff, Department of Obstetrics and Gynecology, Santa Rosa Memorial Hospital, Santa Rosa, California
Jeanne Ann Conry, M.D., Ph.D.	Staff, Department of Obstetrics and Gynecology, Kaiser-Permanente Medical Group, Roseville, California
Arthur T. Evans, M.D.	Assistant Professor of Obstetrics and Gynecology, University of California, Davis, School of Medicine; Director, Division of Maternal-Fetal Medicine, University of California, Davis, Medical Center, Sacramento

Katherine M. Gillogley, M.D.	Assistant Professor of Obstetrics and Gynecology, University of California, Davis, School of Medicine; Department of Obstetrics and Gynecology, University of California, Davis, Medical Center, Sacramento
Boyd W. Goetzman, M.D., Ph.D.	Professor of Pediatrics, University of California, Davis, School of Medicine, Sacramento
Elliot Goldstein, M.D.	Professor of Medicine and Microbiology, University of California, Davis, School of Medicine; Chief, Division of Infectious and Immunologic Diseases, University of California, Davis, Medical Center, Sacramento
Debra Ann Horney, M.D.	Assistant Clinical Professor, Department of Dermatology, University of California, Davis, School of Medicine, Sacramento
Arthur C. Huntley, M.D.	Associate Professor, Department of Dermatology, University of California, Davis, School of Medicine, Sacramento
Cynthia G. Kristensen, M.D.	Nephrologist in Private Practice, Denver
Gary S. Leiserowitz, M.D.	Fellow in Gynecologic Oncology, Mayo Clinic, Rochester, Minnesota
Julie A. Lemieux, M.D.	Assistant Clinical Professor of Obstetrics and Gynecology, University of California, Davis, School of Medicine; Staff Physician, Department of Obstetrics and Gynecology, Kaiser Morse Hospital, Sacramento
Carolyn C. LoBue, M.D., Ph.D.	Assistant Clinical Professor of Obstetrics and Gynecology, University of California, Davis, School of Medicine; Staff Obstetrician and Gynecologist, Kaiser Morse Hospital, Sacramento
H. Trent MacKay, M.D., M.P.H.	Assistant Professor, Clinical Obstetrics and Gynecology, University of California, Davis, School of Medicine, Sacramento
Lorraine A. Milio, M.D.	Assistant Professor of Obstetrics and Gynecology, University of California, Davis, School of Medicine; Staff, Department of Obstetrics and Gynecology, University of California, Davis, Medical Center, Sacramento

Jay M. Milstein, M.D.	Associate Professor, Division of Neonatology, Department of Pediatrics, University of California, Davis, School of Medicine; Medical Director, Special Care Nurseries, University of California, Davis, Medical Center, Sacramento
Michael P. Nageotte, M.D.	Assistant Professor of Obstetrics and Gynecology, University of California, Irvine, College of Medicine; Medical Director, Women's Hospital and Long Beach Memorial Medical Center, Long Beach, California
Kenneth R. Niswander, M.D.	Professor Emeritus of Obstetrics and Gynecology, University of California, Davis, School of Medicine; Attending Obstetrician and Gynecologist, University of California, Davis, Medical Center, Sacramento
Richard H. Oi, M.D.	Professor, Clinical Obstetrics-Gynecology and Pathology, University of California, Davis, School of Medicine, Sacramento
Manuel Porto, M.D.	Associate Professor of Obstetrics and Gynecology, University of California, Irvine, College of Medicine; Director, Division of Maternal-Fetal Medicine, University of California, Irvine, Medical Center, Orange
Peter T. Rogge, M.D.	Assistant Clinical Professor of Obstetrics and Gynecology, University of California, Davis, School of Medicine; Chairman of Obstetrics and Gynecology, Sutter Memorial Hospital, Sacramento
Helayne M. Silver, M.D.	Assistant Professor of Obstetrics and Gynecology, University of California, Davis, School of Medicine; Division of Maternal-Fetal Medicine, University of California, Davis, Medical Center, Sacramento
Robert Nathan Slotnick, M.D., Ph.D.	Assistant Professor, University of California, Davis, School of Medicine; Division of Prenatal Diagnosis, University of California, Davis, Medical Center, Sacramento
Lloyd H. Smith, M.D., Ph.D.	Assistant Professor of Obstetrics and Gynecology, University of California, Davis, School of Medicine, Sacramento

Frances R. Tennant, Ph.D.	Co-Director, Prenatal Diagnosis, Department of Obstetrics and Gynecology, University of California, Davis, Medical Center, Sacramento
Mark C. Williams, M.D.	Assistant Professor of Obstetrics and Gynecology, University of California, Davis, School of Medicine; Division of Maternal-Fetal Medicine, University of California, Davis, Medical Center, Sacramento

Preface

The Fourth Edition of *Manual of Obstetrics* has been largely rewritten rather than revised and updated. The decision to invite new authors—most of them senior house officers or young attending physicians—to do the rewriting was based on our belief that these young doctors know better than do more senior people what a house officer or medical student is likely to seek in a manual. House officers and students continue to be our primary intended audience, although we hope the book is complete enough to meet the needs of obstetricians, family physicians who have obstetric patients, and other specialists whose primary focus may not be obstetric but who care for pregnant patients. In this regard the chapters on medical and surgical diseases that complicate pregnancy constitute a large portion of the book. New chapters have been added to this edition on perinatal chemical use, hepatobiliary disease, perinatal ultrasound, premature rupture of membranes, and sexually and socially transmitted diseases of the newborn.

Arthur T. Evans has been added as associate editor of the Fourth Edition. Dr. Evans offers not only obstetric expertise to the project but also a well-developed sense of the needs of young physicians caring for obstetric patients.

We hope this new edition will prove to be as satisfactory and as helpful to readers as the previous editions seem to have been.

K.R.N.

Pregnancy

Notice. The indications and dosages of all drugs in this manual have been recommended in the medical literature and conform to the practices of the general medical community. The medications described do not necessarily have specific approval by the Food and Drug Administration for use in the diseases and dosages for which they are recommended. The package insert for each drug should be consulted for use and dosage as approved by the FDA. Because standards for usage change, it is advisable to keep abreast of revised recommendations. It is especially important to verify, according to the latest information available, the recommended safe dosages to be used for newborn and small infants.

1 Contraception, Abortion, and Sterilization

H. Trent MacKay

Fertility control should be considered an integral part of the provision of health care. Although no perfect contraceptive exists, a fairly wide range of methods are available, and almost every couple should be able to find a method that suits their needs. However, in order to choose a contraception method intelligently, couples need information and advice from their medical care provider. They will want to know the effectiveness, the shortcomings, the dangers, and the expense of the devices or drugs from which they can choose.

I. **Contraceptive failure.** A recent study by Trussel and Kost [46, 47] has provided a comprehensive review of the literature. Unfortunately, there is much conflicting information, and many of the studies of contraceptive efficacy or failure have serious methodologic flaws. However, the authors have used the existing information to develop Table 1-1. The lowest expected rate represents the authors' "best guess" of the failure rate during the first 12 months of use among couples who use the method perfectly. The typical rate is the rate of failure among average users who experience an accidental pregnancy in the first year of use if they do not stop use of the method for any other reason. The lowest reported rates are those reported in the literature. Unfortunately most of the lowest reported rates for periodic abstinence methods are probably too low because they include data for more than one year of use. In counseling patients about contraceptive choice, it is important to recognize one's own biases about the methods. It is fairly common for counselors to quote lowest expected or lowest reported rates for methods that they favor while quoting typical rates for those they disfavor.

II. **Available agents**

A. **Oral contraceptives.** Oral contraceptives are potent steroid medications that prevent pregnancy primarily by inhibiting ovulation. Either an estrogen or a progestin alone in sufficiently large dose will prevent ovulation, but they are usually combined, since the dose of either medication alone that is necessary to prevent ovulation causes an unacceptably high rate of breakthrough bleeding or other undesirable side effects.

With combination therapy, a tablet containing both agents is taken for 21 days, beginning between the first and fifth day of the initial menstrual cycle or on the first Sunday after the menses begin. The primary antifertility effect is mediated by the progestin, which prevents ovulation as well as effecting changes on the endometrium and on the cervical mucus. The estrogen is added principally to decrease the number of days of vaginal bleeding experienced by the patient. Recently, triphasic pills have become available. They contain different doses of progestin, and in some cases estrogen, in each seven-day segment of the cycle and allow a further reduction in hormone dose from the levels found in the monophasic pills. A preparation containing only a progestin is also available. The antifertility effect of this drug is somewhat lower than the combination pills, and the incidence of breakthrough bleeding is substantially higher. The major advantage of this pill is the lack of side effects caused by estrogen.

1. **Effect on various organ systems.** In addition to their infertility activity, oral contraceptives exert effects on many other organ systems. These effects are important for a number of reasons. Certain organ function tests are altered substantially by oral contraceptives, thus complicating the diagnosis of disease

Table 1-1. Contraceptive failure rates

	Percentage of women experiencing an accidental pregnancy in the first year of use		
Method	Lowest expected	Typical	Lowest reported
Chance	85	85	43.1
Spermicides	3	21	0.0
Periodic abstinence		20	
Ovulation method	3		10.5
Sympto-thermal	2		12.6
Calender	9		14.4
Withdrawal	4	18	6.7
Cervical cap	6	18	8.0
Sponge			
Parous women	9	28	7.7
Nulliparous women	6	18	13.9
Diaphragm	6	18	2.1
Condom	2	12	4.2
IUD			
Progestasert	2.0		1.9
Copper T 380A	0.8		0.5
Pill		3	
Combined	0.1		0.0
Progestin only	0.5		1.1
Depo-Provera	0.3	0.3	0.0
Norplant	0.04	0.04	0.0
Female sterilization	0.2	0.4	0.0
Male sterilization	0.1	0.15	0.0

Source: Adapted with permission of the Population Council, from James Trussell et al., Contraceptive failure in the United States: An update. *Stud. Fam. Plann.* 21(1):51–54, 1990.

in these organs during oral contraceptive use. Contraindications to the use of pills frequently are based on the pills' effects on a particular organ system. The side effects of the pills may result from an undesirable action of the drug on certain organs.

a. Effect on reproductive organs. Ovulation is prevented, thus decreasing the number of patients with functional ovarian cysts. Combined therapy usually produces a secretory effect on the endometrium, and this may produce marked glandular suppression and amenorrhea. Although the earlier, high-dose combination pills frequently produced enlargement of leiomyomas, the low-dose pills with less than 50 μg estrogen do not have this effect. The cervix may exhibit a polyploid hyperplasia, and there is some controversy about the relationship of pill use and the development of cervical dysplasia and carcinoma [38]. Breast tenderness is a well-recognized side effect of oral contraceptives, caused primarily by the estrogen in the medication. Oral contraceptives decrease the incidence of benign breast disease. Although there is no evidence of an overall increase in the risk of breast cancer with pill use, the pill may accelerate the development of preexisting breast cancers in young women [43]. If given during the postpartum period, combination, but not progestin-only, pills may decrease milk production. Pill use apparently decreases a woman's risk of developing serious pelvic infection by approximately 50% [28].

b. **Effect on other endocrine organs.** Estrogen increases the amount of circulating binding globulins, thus increasing the total amount of bound circulating hydrocortisone and thyroxine. Since these increases are in the bound fraction of the hormone, no recognized change occurs in either adrenal or thyroid function in patients maintained on the medications. Some patients experience a rise in plasma insulin levels, which is followed soon thereafter by a rise in the fasting blood glucose or by an abnormality in glucose tolerance. In most patients, these levels revert to normal after use of the medication is discontinued. The pill does not cause diabetes, although certain women (those in whom pregnancy-induced diabetes occurred and those with a family history of diabetes) are at an increased risk of conversion to a frank diabetic state. The effects on carbohydrate metabolism apparently are mediated by the progestin content of the pills or by a synergistic action between the estrogen and progestin components. Spellacy [40] has shown that deterioration of glucose tolerance does not occur with pills containing only 35 μg of ethinyl estradiol and only 0.4–0.5 mg of norethindrone.

   Inhibition of ovulation by oral contraceptives is induced primarily by the progestin component of the medication and is mediated apparently by an inhibition of the release of luteinizing hormone releasing factor from the hypothalamus. If the progestin component is too high, either prolonged amenorrhea during medication or postmedication amenorrhea may result. This effect is discussed in sec. **2.a.(4).**

c. **Effect on other organ systems.** A minimal increase in certain blood-clotting factors (factors VII, IX, and X, and fibrinogen) has been reported with oral contraception, but these changes probably are of no clinical importance. The hypertension that occurs in a small number of patients treated with oral contraceptives may be mediated through changes in the renin-angiotensin system. As discussed in sec. **2.a.(3),** discontinuation of the medication usually results in a return of the blood pressure to normal. Some liver function tests may show elevated levels, but this change is of no known clinical significance. Cholestasis may occur with the medication just as it may occur during pregnancy. Certain liver tumors are related to long-term oral contraceptive use and are discussed in sec. **2.a.(2).** Hyperpigmentation of the skin of the face in a butterfly distribution (melasma) is seen in a few patients taking oral contraceptives. This may not disappear completely after discontinuation of pill use.

   Whether certain effects of the medications—nausea and vomiting, depression, loss of libido, and headache—are caused by effects on the central nervous system is not known. Whereas some of the symptoms may be emotionally induced, headache may be a precursor of a cerebrovascular accident (CVA), and persistent, severe headache is a reason to discontinue the medication.

2. **Side effects.** Since oral contraceptives are potent agents capable of exerting effects on virtually all organ systems, it is not surprising that side effects are common. Most are merely annoying, but a few are life-threatening. Counseling of patients who choose oral contraception obviously must include a description of the serious complications of the medication, with an estimation of the risk that is being taken by the patient.

   a. **Major complications**

      (1) **Vascular complications.** An increase of the risk of **superficial and deep venous thrombosis** and **pulmonary embolism** in women on oral contraceptives has been well established by a number of retrospective epidemiologic studies that estimated the risk of venous thromboembolism in oral contraceptive users to be 3–6 times as great as in nonusers [48]. The difference is greatest if only the diagnosis of idiopathic deep venous thrombosis or pulmonary embolism is used. The risk of superficial venous thrombosis seems less affected by the oral contraceptive medication. There

is evidence that the estrogenic component of the oral contraceptives is responsible for this increase in the risk of venous thromboembolism [15]. A dose-effect relationship is evident with a much lower risk of venous thromboembolism with the lower-dose oral contraceptives containing 35 μg or less of estrogen [32]. There seems to be no association between duration of oral contraceptive use and venous thromboembolism, and the increased risk disappears shortly after discontinuation of the medication.

(a) In older studies, the risk of **thrombotic and hemorrhagic stroke** was increased two- to threefold in patients on oral contraception [8, 37, 49]. Two recent studies [31, 33] of healthy women using low-dose oral contraceptives showed no significant increase in the risk of stroke. Because of the association of vascular-type headaches and stroke, women who develop persistent headaches that appear to be of vascular origin should discontinue oral contraceptive use [36].

(b) Myocardial infarction. There is an increased risk of myocardial infarction among oral contraceptive users, but this increased risk appears to be confined to women over the age of 35 who smoke or have other risk factors such as diabetes, hypertension, or hyperlipidemia [37]. The Walnut Creek study [33] and the Puget Sound study [31] found no increased risk of myocardial infarction. It appears that for women who are under the age of 35 or over the age of 35 without risk factors, the risk of myocardial infarction with oral contraceptive use is minimal.

(2) Tumors

(a) Liver tumors. An association exists between oral contraceptive use and the development of a rare liver tumor, hepatocellular adenoma [11]. These tumors appear to be related to the estrogenic component and are related to both the dose and duration of use of oral contraceptives. Although extremely rare, these tumors are difficult to diagnose and potentially fatal because of their vascularity and potential for intraperitoneal hemorrhage. The liver should be routinely palpated at the annual exam of all women on oral contraceptives. If suspicion of such a tumor exists, computed tomography or magnetic resonance imaging (MRI) scanning should be done. Although some of the tumors have been resected successfully, it appears that they will usually regress spontaneously if oral contraceptives are discontinued.

A recent study [27] has suggested an increased risk of hepatocellular carcinoma with oral contraceptive use. However, the impact of this increased risk is small as this is an extremely rare tumor in young women. Furthermore, there has been no increase in the incidence of this tumor in the United States since the introduction of oral contraceptives in 1960.

(b) Breast cancer. One of the most closely examined aspects of oral contraceptives is their possible relation to breast cancer. Although the majority of studies to date, including the large Cancer and Steroid Hormone study [6], show no increase in breast cancer risk, several recent studies have suggested an increased risk of premenopausal breast cancer among oral contraceptive users [18, 26, 43]. Each of these studies found an increased risk in a different subgroup, and such inconsistency is reassuring. However, these studies do suggest the possibility that oral contraceptives may accelerate the development of preexisting breast cancers, even though not actually increasing the total number of cancers.

(c) Endometrial and ovarian cancer. Oral contraceptive use has been shown to decrease the incidence of both endometrial and ovarian cancer [5, 7]. Almost all of the studies on both these cancers and oral contraceptive use have shown a protective effect. For women who have used oral contraceptives for at least one year, the relative risk of endometrial cancer is 0.5. The relative risk of ovarian cancer is 0.6, and a protective effect is seen with as little as three to six months of use. For both cancers, the protective effect continues for at least 15 years after the last use of oral contraceptives.

(d) Cervical cancer. The association of oral contraceptive use and cervical cancer remains controversial. In a recent analysis of 16 epidemiologic studies of oral contraceptive use and the risk of cervical dysplasia, carcinoma in situ, and invasive cancer [38], there is a suggestion of a small increase in risk. Unfortunately, many of the studies have failed to control for at least a few of the known risk factors related to the risk of cervical cancer such as number of sexual partners, age at first intercourse, or smoking history. Nonetheless, there appears to be a consistent trend in the studies that suggests a relationship. Certainly all women using oral contraceptives should have an annual Pap smear.

(3) Hypertension. It seems well established that a slight increase in mean systolic and diastolic pressure occurs in women on oral contraceptives. The increase in blood pressure is rarely severe. Spellacy [41] suggested that the rise in blood pressure is caused by the estrogen component of the pill, but the study of oral contraception by the Royal College of General Practitioners [35] suggested a relationship between the progestin component and hypertension but none with the estrogen component. The hypertension does not seem to be dose-related and may occur as early as one to three months or as late as eight years after initiation of oral contraception. The etiology is unknown, and Weinberger [51] believes that changes in the renin-angiotensin-aldosterone system cannot fully explain the hypertension. Cessation of oral contraceptives results in a decline of blood pressure to normal levels in most patients. Whether oral contraceptive use identifies a group of women likely to develop subsequent hypertension or whether the hypertension is only a drug-related phenomenon is unknown. All women in whom oral contraception is initiated should have their blood pressure checked within three months. If hypertension has developed, oral contraceptive use should probably be discontinued.

(4) Postpill amenorrhea. Amenorrhea of more than six months' duration occurs in 0.2–0.8% of contraceptive pill users after discontinuation of the drug. A diagnostic investigation is indicated if amenorrhea continues for six months or more or is associated with galactorrhea.

b. Minor side effects. Certain minor but troublesome side effects are associated with oral contraceptive use. These symptoms include breakthrough bleeding, nausea, vomiting, weight gain, and other annoyances.

(1) Intermenstrual bleeding is very common during the first three months of oral contraceptive use and will usually abate by the fourth month of use. After the first three months of use, bleeding that occurs early in the cycle may be related to the low estrogen content of the pill, and bleeding that occurs late in the cycle may be the result of a deficient progestin content. Although the bleeding may disappear spontaneously, a switch to a different pill will usually solve the problem. Another recommended approach, based on the concept that most breakthrough bleeding is due to an atrophic, decidualized endometrium, is to add a small dose of estrogen (such as 20 μg of ethinyl estradiol) for one to three cycles [42].

(2) Nausea and vomiting are related to the estrogen content of the pill. They occur most commonly during the first few months of pill use. The symptoms may be eliminated by changing to a pill with a lower estrogen dose or by simply having the patient take the pill consistently with the evening meal or at bedtime [14].

(3) Weight loss is reported as frequently as **weight gain** with oral contraceptives. The cause of weight gain may be fluid retention, related to the estrogen or progestin; increased subcutaneous fat deposition, related to the estrogen; or increased appetite, related to the anabolic effect of some progestins. An appropriate switch in the pill formulation or decreased caloric intake and increased physical activity, or a combination of these, may reduce the symptoms.

3. **Contraindications.** Use of the pill is not recommended if any of the following is present:
   a. History of thrombophlebitis, pulmonary embolus, cerebral hemorrhage, or coronary artery disease
   b. Impaired liver function
   c. Known or suspected carcinoma of the breast or uterus or other estrogen-dependent malignancy
   d. Undiagnosed genital bleeding
   e. Pregnancy
   f. History of cholestasis during pregnancy
   g. History of hepatic adenoma
4. **Caution in the prescription of oral contraceptives** should be exercised in the following circumstances:
   a. Leiomyomas of the uterus
   b. Hypertension
   c. Epilepsy
   d. Diabetes or a strong family history of diabetes
   e. History of migraine headaches
   f. Age 40 or older with the presence of a cardiovascular risk factor including diabetes, hypertension, or hyperlipidemia
   g. Heavy smoking over age 35
   h. Planned elective major surgery
5. **Choice of medication**
   a. **Initial prescription.** When a patient has decided to take oral contraceptives (see sec. **III**), the choice of pill should be made with the following limitations in mind:
      (1) A pill with as low a dose of estrogen as the patient will tolerate should be prescribed, as most of the serious complications are related to the estrogen component.
      (2) A pill containing only a progestin is associated with a higher contraceptive failure rate than are combination pills.
   b. **When prescribing the pill,** first be certain that the patient does not have an absolute contraindication. If a relative contraindication exists, inform the patient and encourage her to consider other contraceptive methods. The initial pill prescribed should contain no more than 35 μg of estrogen. The patient who is just beginning to use oral contraception should be given sufficient medication for a 3-month period, and she should be encouraged to read the package insert. Any symptom of thrombophlebitis, pulmonary embolism, coronary occlusion, CVA, or an eye problem should be reported immediately. If all goes well, the patient should be seen at 3 months, when a history regarding headaches, blurred vision, and leg, chest, or abdominal pain is taken. The blood pressure should be checked. The patient should then be seen at 12-month intervals, at which time a history of possible complications is taken and a brief physical examination—including breast, abdominal, and pelvic examination—and Pap smear are performed.
   c. **Change in medication.** If the patient is experiencing minor complications, a change in medication may be indicated. The physician may change the medication to a more estrogen-dominant or a more progestin-dominant pill, depending on the symptoms experienced by the patient (Table 1-2).
   d. **The mini-pill,** an oral contraceptive preparation containing only a progestin, may be appropriate for a patient who has a contraindication to an estrogen-containing pill. The mini-pill may also be used in those patients who develop estrogen-related side effects on the combined preparations. Because of a relatively high rate of intermenstrual bleeding, frequently irregular menses, and a reduced effectiveness in comparison with the combined oral contra-

Table 1-2. Side effects of oral contraceptive medication

Excess estrogen	Deficient estrogen	Excess progestin	Deficient progestin
Nausea and vomiting Headache Cyclic weight gain Nervousness Heavy withdrawal bleeding	Early-cycle spotting and breakthrough bleeding Amenorrhea	Depression Weight gain Oligomenorrhea or amenorrhea	Late-cycle spotting and breakthrough bleeding Excessive withdrawal bleeding

Source: K. R. Niswander, *Obstetric and Gynecologic Disorders: A Practitioner's Guide.* Flushing, N.Y.: Medical Examination, 1975.

ceptives, the mini-pill has not been popular in the United States. However, it is still a highly effective form of contraception and may be appropriate for selected patients.

B. Other hormonal contraceptives

1. **Norplant** is an implantable hormonal contraceptive system that consists of six 34 mm × 2.4 mm Silastic rods containing levonorgestrel that is slowly released at a rate of 80 μg/day over a five-year period. This system is currently marketed in a number of countries and was approved in 1990 by the Food and Drug Administration (FDA) for use in the United States. The rods are usually implanted into the inner aspect of the upper arm and should be removed at the end of five years. Norplant is very effective, with a pregnancy rate ranging from 0.2 per 100 woman-years in the first year to 1.1 per 100 woman-years in the fifth year of use [39]. Because it does not contain estrogen, Norplant may be suitable for women with some contraindications or side effects from combination oral contraceptives. Women who are seeking long-term contraception but do not desire sterilization are ideal candidates for Norplant. The most common problems leading to the removal of Norplant include irregular bleeding, headache, and weight gain.
2. **Depo-Provera** is an extremely effective injectable progestin contraceptive that is approved for use in over 90 countries. Primarily for political reasons, Depo-Provera has not been approved by the FDA for contraceptive use in the United States, although it is used on a limited basis for contraception in this country. At the standard contraceptive dose of 150 mg IM every 3 months, the failure rate is approximately 0.4 per 100 woman-years [17]. Most women using Depo-Provera experience amenorrhea, and the most common reason for discontinuation is irregular bleeding. Other side effects include weight gain, headache, and mood changes. In spite of the accumulation of a large body of reassuring evidence from worldwide use of Depo-Provera, the FDA has refused approval. The future availability of newer injectable and implantable hormonal contraceptives will diminish the need for Depo-Provera.
3. **Other injectable and implantable hormonal contraceptives** are currently under development. Several monthly injectable contraceptives containing both an estrogen and a progestin are either currently available in other countries or under development. These agents markedly reduce the incidence of irregular bleeding. In addition, under development are several biodegradable progestin-containing implant systems using capsules or pellets that are effective for at least a year, as well as injectable systems using biodegradable progestin-containing microspheres that are effective for three months [17].

C. Intrauterine devices. The exact mechanism of action of the intrauterine device (IUD) is uncertain. Neither ovulation nor steroidogenesis is affected, and tubal peristalsis appears unchanged. Prior to the availability of several recent studies, it was felt that the IUD primarily functioned as an abortifacient, that it prevented implantation of the fertilized egg. However, there is considerable evidence to suggest that the IUD acts prior to fertilization.

1. **Effectiveness.** The lowest expected failure rate with the IUD is approximately 1 to 2 pregnancies per 100 woman-years, and the lowest reported rate is 0.5 to 3.0 pregnancies. Because the method does not depend on the user to any significant degree after placement of the device, the method failures are largely those of unrecognized expulsions or incorrect insertion of the IUD.
2. **Complications.** The only relatively serious complications of the IUD are pregnancy and pelvic inflammatory disease (see **a** and **b**). Minor complications, such as cramps and bleeding, are serious only if they require removal of the device, with subsequent loss of pregnancy protection. Spontaneous expulsion occurs in 1–10% of users during the first year of use. Most expulsions occur during the first year of use and are particularly likely during the first three months [30]. Expulsion is more likely to occur with the nonmedicated devices, none of which are currently marketed in the United States. Unfortunately, expulsion may occur without symptoms, and so the patient must be instructed to palpate the string protruding from the cervix on frequent occasions, especially during the first three months of use and routinely after her menses. Uterine perforation is rare in the hands of an experienced clinician, and the risk can be minimized by (1) determining the position of the uterus by bimanual examination, (2) sounding the uterus before insertion, and (3) exerting traction on the tenaculum attached to the cervix during insertion, since this traction tends to straighten out the long axis of the uterine cavity. Perforation is usually asymptomatic, and the complication is suspected first when the tail of the device cannot be palpated or seen or when pregnancy occurs. If perforation is suspected, the IUD can be located by one of several methods: an ultrasound of the pelvis or an x ray of the pelvis with or without another IUD in the uterus. Although the risk of bowel obstruction is probably minimal, a copper or hormone-containing device should be surgically removed from the peritoneal cavity. The necessity for removing nonmedicated devices is an unsettled issue. The device may be removed either through laparoscopy, through an incision in the posterior cul-de-sac if the device is behind the uterus, or by laparotomy in certain patients.
   - a. **Pregnancy.** Should pregnancy occur with an IUD in place, three major concerns must be explained to the patient:
     - **(1)** Immediate removal of the device reduces the risk of spontaneous abortion from 50% to approximately 25%.
     - **(2)** The pregnancy is more likely to be ectopic than in a patient not using an IUD. The likelihood does not result from an absolute increase in the risk of pregnancy in an ectopic location but rather from the fact that the IUD protects better against intrauterine than against ectopic pregnancies [30].
     - **(3)** Serious life-threatening infection, especially in midpregnancy, may occur if the IUD is not removed. The risk is sufficiently great to encourage removal for this reason alone. If the string is not visible and cannot be grasped within the cervical canal, the woman should be advised about the risks of continuing the pregnancy and offered the option of a therapeutic abortion.
   - b. **Pelvic inflammatory disease.** Women currently using an IUD are more likely to develop pelvic inflammatory disease (PID) than those using either barrier methods, oral contraceptives, or no method of contraception. However, there has been much confusion about the relation of IUD use to PID. In a recent study [23], reanalyzing information from the Women's Health Study, there was no increased risk of PID in women using an IUD who had only one recent sexual partner and who were either married or cohabiting. Among previously married women, the relative risk was slightly elevated at 1.8, and among never-married women the relative risk was significantly

elevated at 2.6. Single women are probably more likely to have multiple sexual partners and to be exposed to the risk of sexually transmitted pelvic infections. The risk of PID with the IUD is also related to the length of time since insertion. Several studies have shown a transient but statistically significant increase in the risk of PID in the first month of use that then falls gradually over the next few months [22]. Although infections that occur at the time of insertion or in the first few months of use may be related to bacterial contamination at the time of IUD insertion, infections occurring after this time are probably due to sexually transmitted organisms. The provision of prophylactic antibiotics at the time of IUD insertion (such as doxycycline 200 mg PO, one hour prior to insertion) appears to be useful in reducing the risk of PID in the first month of use [13]. Consideration of the use of antibiotic prophylaxis is currently recommended by both of the IUD manufacturers in the United States.

Any IUD user who complains of fever, pelvic pain, abdominal tenderness, cramping, or unusual vaginal bleeding should be suspected of harboring a pelvic infection. The patient should be instructed to report to her physician when any of these symptoms appears. If pelvic examination reveals suspected PID, appropriate diagnostic tests should be performed, IUD removal should be recommended, and antibiotics should be started. If the infection appears to be a mild one, the patient need not be hospitalized.

3. **Choice of device.** Two types of IUDs are currently available in the United States: the Progestasert, a progestin-containing IUD, and the Paragard or T-Cu 380A, a copper-containing device. Because of medicolegal and economic considerations, the Lippes Loop, Copper-7, and Copper-T were recently removed from the American market, but you may encounter women still using one of these devices.
   a. **The Progestasert** is a small T-shaped device containing 38 mg of progesterone that is released at a rate of 65 μg/day and maintains its contraceptive efficacy for about one year. The failure rate of the Progestasert is approximately 2.9 pregnancies per 100 woman-years [30].
   b. **The Paragard or T-Cu 380A** is a T-shaped device with copper wire wound around the vertical arm and copper sleeves on the horizontal arms. It is currently approved by the FDA for four years' use, although in clinical trials it has been demonstrated to be effective for at least six years. The Paragard is one of the most effective IUDs ever marketed, with an overall failure rate of 0.5 pregnancies per 100 woman-years.
4. **Intrauterine device insertion.** It is important to obtain informed consent prior to IUD insertion. To facilitate this, both IUD manufacturers include a comprehensive patient information pamphlet with each device. The pamphlets should be read and signed by the patient and clinician and preserved as part of the medical record. The exact method of IUD insertion can be found on the package insert supplied with each device. The inserter mechanism in each case is devised to minimize the risk of perforation of the uterus and to simplify insertion for the clinician. The following are general guidelines for insertion:
   a. Perform a careful bimanual examination to rule out abnormalities of the pelvic organs (especially pregnancy and pelvic infection) and to determine the position of the uterus. An IUD can be inserted into a uterus in virtually any position, but perforation is most likely to occur with an unrecognized retroverted uterus.
   b. With a speculum in the vagina, paint the cervix with an antiseptic solution.
   c. Grasp the anterior lip of the cervix with a tenaculum, and sound the uterus for the direction of the canal and the depth of the cavity. To make the insertion more comfortable, you may wish to inject 1 ml of 1% Xylocaine into the cervix prior to attaching the tenaculum and to inject 5 ml into each paracervical area at 4 and 8 o'clock on either side of the cervix.
   d. Following the manufacturer's instructions, insert the IUD into the introducer under sterile conditions.

e. With steady traction on the tenaculum, pass the IUD introducer through the cervical canal into the fundus of the uterus.
f. Release the IUD string from the introducer, and withdraw the inserter barrel over the plunger, allowing the IUD to remain in the uterus.
g. Clip the string to a length of approximately 1 in.

It is strongly recommended to reserve the IUD for women who have had previous pregnancies because insertion of the device is easier and less painful in these women, expulsion is less likely to occur, and if PID occurs and terminates reproductive capacity, the complication is less tragic in a multipara. The patient should have easy access to her physician so that she can report untoward effects such as bleeding or pelvic pain. If these effects are severe, or the result of a pelvic infection, it may be necessary to remove the device.

5. **Absolute contraindications** to use of the IUD include [18]
   a. Active or recent **pelvic infection** or a history of recurrent pelvic infection.
   b. **Suspected pregnancy.** To avoid inadvertent insertion into a pregnant uterus, it is best to perform insertion during menses or in the first two weeks of the cycle. However, if it is certain that the patient is not pregnant, insertion may be performed at any time in the cycle.
6. **Strong relative contraindications** include
   a. **Undiagnosed abnormal vaginal bleeding,** suspicion of genital malignancy, or an unresolved abnormal Pap smear.
   b. **Risk factors for PID** are exposure to sexually transmitted diseases including a recent postabortal infection or puerperal endometritis, multiple sexual partners, or an impaired response to infection such as occurs with diabetes or steroid treatment.
   c. **History of ectopic pregnancy.**
   d. **Coagulopathy or anticoagulant therapy.**
7. **Other relative contraindications** include valvular heart disease, distortion of the endometrial cavity by a myoma or congenital malformation, and severe menorrhagia or dysmenorrhea.

D. Barrier methods

1. **Diaphragm and spermicide.** The diaphragm is a dome-shaped device that is inserted over the cervix of the woman before coitus. The dome is molded of a thin layer of latex and is surrounded by a firm ring formed by a circular, rubber-covered spring. The device is squeezed to allow insertion through the introitus into the vagina, where it assumes its original shape since it fits the contours of the vagina (Fig. 1-1). The diaphragm is available in diameters from 50–95 mm and must be properly fitted by a health care provider to the individual patient. The device prevents pregnancy by the dual mechanism of a partial physical barrier between the sperm and the cervix and the spermicidal action of the vaginal cream or jelly used with the diaphragm. Use of the diaphragm without the spermicidal agent is associated with a high failure rate. The device has a lowest expected failure rate of 3 pregnancies per 100 woman-years, with a typical failure rate of 18. No serious side effects are definitely associated with diaphragm use, although there have been reports of nonfatal toxic shock syndrome associated with the device [24]. In all cases, the diaphragm had been left in place longer than 36 hours, thus emphasizing the importance of diaphragm removal within no more than 24 hours post insertion. There appears to be approximately a twofold increase in the risk of urinary tract infections among diaphragm users, probably related to changes in vaginal flora and the pressure of the diaphragm on the urethra [12]. Questions of teratogenicity of spermicidal preparations have largely been put to rest by several recent reports [3, 25, 50].
   a. **Method of use.** The clinician estimates the distance from the posterior fornix of the vagina to the posterior surface of the symphysis pubis by careful pelvic examination. The diaphragm prescribed should be the largest one that will fit comfortably between these two landmarks. In the presence of the clinician, the patient is asked to insert the diaphragm, directing it in a posterior direction. If the diaphragm is directed anteriorly, the cervix may be en-

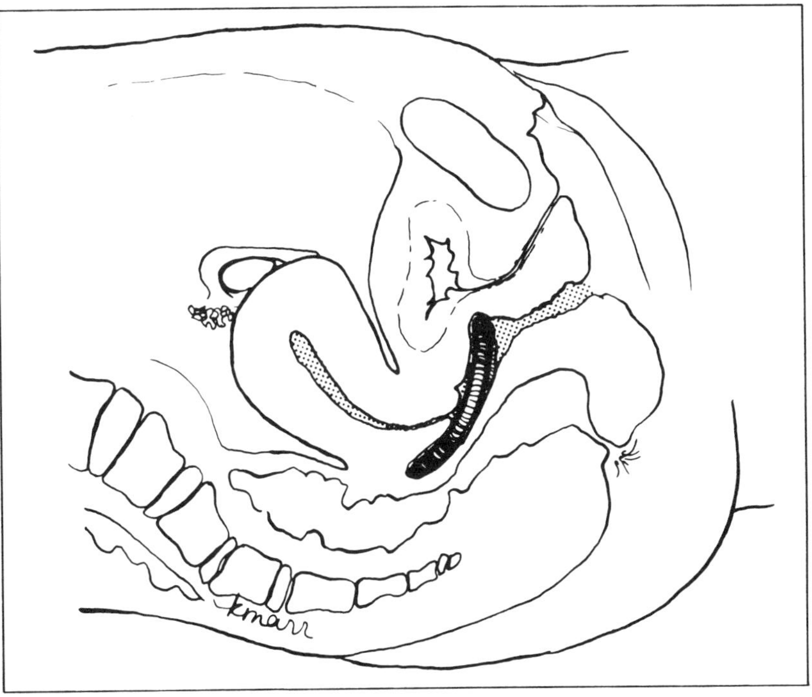

Fig. 1-1. Proper placement of contraceptive diaphragm. (From K. R. Niswander, *Obstetric and Gynecologic Disorders: A Practitioner's Guide*. Flushing, N.Y.: Medical Examination, 1975.)

countered and the diaphragm will not be inserted easily. After insertion into the posterior fornix, the diaphragm rim is tucked snugly behind the symphysis pubis, and the index finger should be used to palpate the cervix to ascertain that it is covered by the soft latex dome. Diaphragms come in several different styles, including flat spring, coil spring, and arcing spring, and it is important to fit the patient with the specific style that you intend to prescribe. Before insertion, an appropriate amount of spermicidal jelly or cream is placed on the surface of the dome that is fitted against the cervix. The diaphragm may be inserted from a few minutes to an hour or more before intercourse and should be removed no sooner than six to eight hours following intercourse. If a second coital episode occurs during the six-hour interval, additional spermicide should be inserted without removing the diaphragm. The patient should be thoroughly instructed in diaphragm use and should demonstrate her ability to both insert and remove the diaphragm prior to leaving the office.

b. Contraindications. Severe vaginal prolapse, cystocele, and urethrocele may interfere with a good fitting of the device, and pelvic relaxation constitutes a relative contraindication. Women who have previously had toxic shock syndrome or who have recurrent urinary tract infections are not good candidates for diaphragm use.

2. Cervical cap. The cervical cap is a cup-shaped device that is inserted directly onto the cervix prior to coitus. The Prentif Cavity Rim cervical cap is currently the only cervical cap marketed in the United States and has been approved by the FDA since February 1988. It is available in four sizes from 22–31 mm in diameter, and proper fitting is critical. However, many women cannot be fitted with the four currently available sizes. Because of the difficulty in learning insertion technique, it may require an hour or more to adequately train a woman to use a cervical cap [9]. The failure rate is approximately the same as the diaphragm.

a. **Method of use.** The cap must be carefully fitted to the cervix, as it maintains its position by suction, and a loose-fitting cap will not stay in place. The cap should be one-third to one-half filled with spermicidal jelly or cream and may be inserted many hours in advance of coitus. It should be checked for dislodgement after intercourse and left in place for at least 6 but no longer than 24 hours after intercourse. The cap should be removed by breaking the suction on the cervix with pressure on one side of the rim [4].

b. **Contraindications** to cap use include the inability to fit a cap or the inability of the woman to properly insert the cap. Significant structural abnormalities of the cervix, recurrent PID, allergy to latex or spermicide, and a past history of toxic shock syndrome are also contraindications. In the original study leading to approval of the cap, a small number of women showed progression of their Pap smears from class I to III. Although the significance of this finding is questionable, it is recommended that women using the cap have an initial Pap smear or a repeat Pap smear within three months.

3. **Condom.** Condoms have a lowest reported failure rate of 4 pregnancies per 100 woman-years. The typical failure rate is 12 pregnancies. A highly motivated couple may be expected to approach the theoretic effectiveness. Because of the growing concern with sexually transmitted diseases including acquired immunodeficiency syndrome (AIDS), there has been increased use of condoms in the United States. The condom is an effective barrier to the transmission of gonorrhea, syphilis, human immunodeficiency virus, human papilloma virus, and herpes simplex virus [44]. Protection may be further enhanced by the use of spermicide with the condom.

a. **Method of use.** Since the condom depends on physical factors for its effectiveness, it is important to discuss the technique of use in some detail with patients who request this form of contraception. The patient should be given the following instructions:

(1) Place the condom on the erect penis before any penile penetration of the vagina is permitted.

(2) Immediately after ejaculation and before the erection is lost, withdraw the penis, taking care to hold the rim of the condom so it cannot slip off the penis.

(3) A contraceptive jelly, cream, or foam may be used to increase the effectiveness of the condom. Some condoms come packaged with spermicidal cream. Do not use petroleum jelly.

b. **Complications and side effects.** No known serious complications are associated with the use of the condom. A few patients will develop an allergy to the rubber. Some patients will complain that use of a condom results in a decrease in sensation during intercourse; these couples should be encouraged to use another method of contraception.

4. **Contraceptive foam.** Because of its dispersal characteristics, contraceptive foam is more effective than either contraceptive jelly or cream and should be the only spermicide used as a separate contraceptive method. Spermicidal foam has a theoretic failure rate of 2 pregnancies per 100 woman-years with an actual use rate as high as 30 pregnancies. The chemical effect of the spermicidal agent is to immobilize and kill the sperm.

a. **Method of use.** Instructions to patients are simple. The can containing the foam should be shaken 20 times before the foam is dispensed, ensuring adequate dispersion of the spermicide. The applicator is inserted with care deeply into the vagina and then is withdrawn ½ in. before releasing the foam. The foam should be inserted very shortly before intercourse. The user should not douche for at least six to eight hours following intercourse.

b. Side effects. Spermicidal foams, jellies, and creams appear to have no major side effects, but a controversial report [16] suggested the possibility of an increase in congenital malformations among infants born to mothers who may have inadvertently used vaginal spermicides in early pregnancy. A number of subsequent studies [3, 50] have shown no evidence of a relation between vaginal spermicide use and fetal anomalies. An occasional allergic reaction is reported. Foam has an unpleasant taste and so may interfere with pleasurable orogenital contact.

c. Other chemical agents. Other vaginal chemical contraceptives are also available. Spermicides are available in the form of suppositories and as a contraceptive film. The effectiveness of these methods is similar to contraceptive foam.

5. Contraceptive sponge. The vaginal contraceptive sponge is a polyurethane foam sponge impregnated with the spermicide nonoxynol-9. It may be placed in the vagina by the user any time up to 24 hours before expected coitus. Its contraceptive effect is mediated in three ways: (1) It releases spermicide to kill sperm, (2) it provides a physical barrier to the sperm, and (3) it absorbs the male ejaculate, thus reducing the number of sperm available for fertilization. It is marketed over the counter, comes in one universal size and so requires no professional fitting, and can be used for multiple acts of coitus within the 24-hour period of its effectiveness. In a study of sponge users and diaphragm users, effectiveness did not appear to differ significantly in the two groups [28]. However, there was a higher failure rate for parous than for nulliparous women in one U.S. study, but this information has not been borne out in other studies around the world [10]. The sponge is a satisfactory method of contraception for women who desire convenience and who are willing to accept a slightly higher pregnancy rate than with many other methods.

E. Natural family planning. Several methods of natural family planning are based on the detection of ovulation with periodic abstinence during the fertile period [20]. Because these methods require abstinence for varying periods during the cycle, they require a high degree of motivation as well as careful training of the users. These methods have the approval of the Roman Catholic Church, a factor that may be of importance to some couples.

1. Calendar method. The calendar method requires that a woman record the length of her menstrual cycle for 6–12 months. Since ovulation occurs 12–16 days before the first day of the next menstrual period, and the lifespan of the ovum is 24 hours and of sperm is 48 hours, the fertile period can be calculated in the following way: The beginning of the fertile period can be estimated by subtracting 18 days (16 days plus 2 days sperm survival) from the shortest cycle, and the end of the fertile period can be estimated by subtracting 11 days (12 days minus 1 day ovum survival) from the length of the longest cycle. For instance, if a woman has cycles varying from 24–34 days in length, she should abstain from day 6 of her cycle ($24 - 18 = 6$) to day 23 ($34 - 11 = 23$), a total of 17 days of abstinence in each cycle. These dates theoretically should encompass all possible pregnancy exposure dates. The more irregular the cycles are, the longer the period of abstinence should be. There are widely varying reports of efficacy with this method, but a recent study [21] showed a failure rate of approximately 40 per 100 woman-years. Because of the long period of abstinence required for many women and the relatively low efficacy, the calendar method is not the natural family planning method of choice.

2. Basal body temperature method. If a woman takes her body temperature under the same conditions and at the same time every morning, i.e., under basal conditions, a biphasic curve will be recognized if she is menstruating normally. Shortly after ovulation, the basal temperature rises 0.6–0.8°F, and when the temperature rise has been sustained for three days, this is good evidence that ovulation has occurred and the remainder of the month is a "safe" period. Though it may be used alone as a method of contraception, it is frequently used in conjunction with the following method.

3. **Mucous method.** If a woman can recognize changes in her vaginal secretions from the thick, tenacious cervical secretions of the preovulatory and postovulatory periods to the thin, watery secretions of the ovulatory period, it is safe to have intercourse when the ovulatory mucus is no longer present. Confusion can result from the presence of vaginal discharge resulting from infection or from the use of intravaginal medications.
4. **Sympto-thermal method.** The sympto-thermal method combines several of the aforementioned methods and adds some additional factors. In general, both the basal body temperature and cervical mucus are monitored. With this method, the first day of mucus change would indicate the need for abstinence until three days after the rise in basal body temperature or four days after the peak mucus. In addition, women may watch for symptoms that precede or accompany ovulation such as mittelschmerz, spotting, vulvar swelling, or breast tenderness. Softening and dilatation of the cervix and movement of the cervix to a position higher or deeper in the vagina may also be detected.

F. **Miscellaneous methods**

1. **Withdrawal** as a method of contraception is very old but unreliable. The method has a typical failure rate of 18 pregnancies per 100 woman-years. The risks of the method are that (1) preejaculatory secretions of the male frequently contain sperm, (2) precise male control is difficult to achieve, and (3) the method may exert an adverse emotional impact on one or both partners. The only advantage of the method is that it is available under all circumstances and at no cost.
2. **Postcoital douching** with various substances is another very old and very unreliable method of contraception. Since sperm appear in the cervical mucus within 90 seconds of ejaculation in some cases, the method yields extremely poor results.
3. **Lactation** provides some pregnancy protection in the postpartum period. Breast-feeding women may not ovulate for as long as 24 months after delivery, although lactational amenorrhea depends on the pattern of breast-feeding. Frequent suckling of short duration or fewer episodes of longer duration may maintain lactational amenorrhea [14]. In one study from Rwanda [1], 50% of nonlactating women were found to have conceived by four months post partum, whereas 50% of lactating women still had not conceived at just over 18 months post partum. The method cannot be recommended for the individual patient, although it may have some effectiveness in population control.

G. **Postcoital contraception.** Some patients will present in the physician's office with a history of unprotected intercourse at midcycle and will request a contraceptive method that will ensure protection from pregnancy. Several choices are available to the physician under these circumstances, but no method is completely satisfactory or always effective.

1. **Hormonal postcoital contraception** has been used with a high degree of effectiveness. Combination oral contraceptives, specifically two pills of 50 μg ethinyl estradiol with 0.5 mg norgestrel (Ovral) taken within 72 hours of unprotected intercourse and repeated 12 hours later, have a failure rate of less than 1.5% [52]. Other methods employing high-dose estrogens are undesirable because of frequent severe nausea and vomiting.
2. **Copper intrauterine device.** Copper-bearing IUDs have been shown to be effective postcoital contraceptives if inserted within five days of unprotected intercourse. Because of the risk of pelvic infection, the IUD should not be used as a postcoital contraceptive for rape victims unless accompanied by prophylactic antibiotic therapy [29].
3. **Immediate menstrual extraction or a dilatation and curettage** to disrupt

the endometrium before implantation can occur is an effective method of preventing pregnancy.

III. Helping the patient choose the best contraceptive method. A very important factor in the choice of a contraceptive is the motivation of the patient. Some contraceptive users simply cannot be bothered with remembering to take a pill or insert a diaphragm. The IUD may be an appropriate method for this individual. Another patient may wish a method that carries virtually no risk of complications or death—probably a barrier method backed up by abortion for the occasional failure. Contraceptive methods vary in their degree of effectiveness, safety, and convenience. Whereas one patient may want the most effective method at any cost, another may prefer convenience at the cost of safety or effectiveness. Thus, the first step in helping a patient choose a contraceptive method is to learn what is most important to that patient.

A. Safety. The safety of a particular contraceptive method can be assessed only by recognizing the inherent risk of morbidity or mortality associated with the method itself and adding to that risk the danger associated with pregnancy carried to term or terminated with abortion should the device fail to prevent conception. Tietze and Lewit [45] made this calculation for all of the commonly used methods, and their conclusions are illustrated in Fig. 1-2. Up to the age of 30, oral contraception, the IUD, and barrier methods are approximately equally safe, and all are much safer than the risk of unintended pregnancy if no contraception is used. Between the ages of 30 and 35, a similar relationship is noted, but an additional mortality risk associated with smoking in oral contraceptive users is evident. Beyond the age of 35, the pill is associated with a higher mortality risk than the IUD,

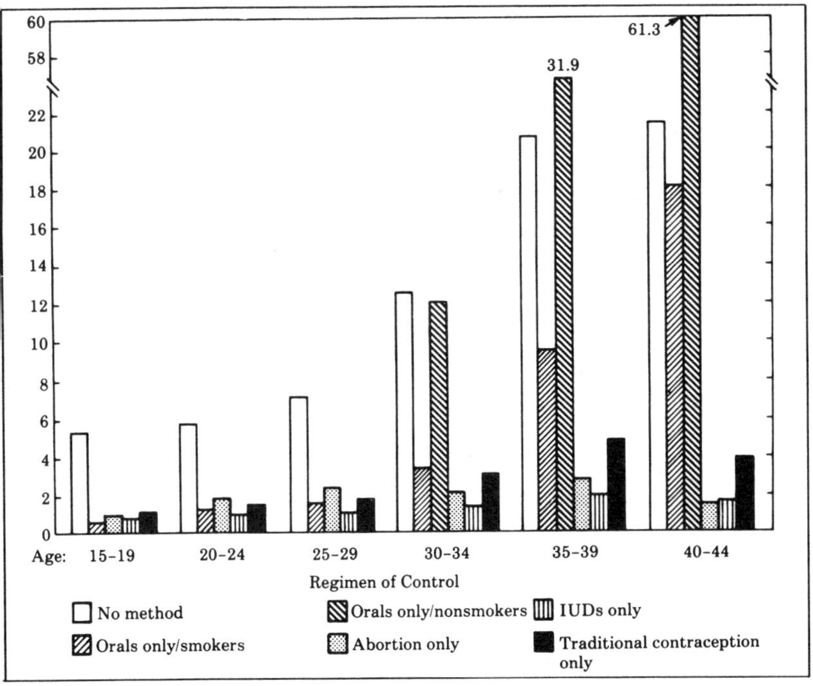

Fig. 1-2. Estimated annual deaths per 100,000 nonsterile women. (Modified from C. Tietze and S. Lewit, Life risks associated with reversible methods of fertility regulation. *Int. J. Gynaecol. Obstet.* 16:456, 1979. Reprinted with permission.)

especially in a smoker. **Of great importance to some patients is the fact that a barrier method of contraception backed up by early abortion provides the very safest method of contraception at any age, with 100% effectiveness.** Some patients, of course, will not and cannot accept abortion as a contraceptive backup.

B. **Effectiveness** depends very heavily on the motivation of the individual patient, perhaps even more than on the effectiveness of the device itself. Oral contraception provides nearly 100% protection **if used perfectly.** Barrier methods, **if used perfectly,** provide better protection than oral contraception carelessly used. The counselor therefore must assess the motivation of the patient. If a couple cannot remember to use a method when it is needed, they may do better with a method that requires no action (e.g., an IUD). Convenience may be of utmost importance to such a patient. Some patients will not be bothered with a coitally related method such as a diaphragm. The safety of a barrier method is lost in a patient who cannot remember to use the device.

C. **Sterilization** may be the method of choice for some couples, especially those who are old enough to be certain that they want to terminate their childbearing capability permanently. Patients who desire sterilization must be reminded that the operation is irreversible. Operations to restore fertility are expensive and may be associated with a high failure rate. The patient should also be reminded that any operation carries a certain risk of mortality, even if it is a small one.

IV. Legal abortion

A. Definitions

1. **Legal abortion** is the intentional termination of pregnancy before viability, in a manner consistent with current law or custom. At the present time in the United States, the law, established by an opinion of the United States Supreme Court in 1973, essentially sanctions abortion on demand through the second trimester of pregnancy [34]. Thus, abortion is a legal method of terminating an unwanted pregnancy of 26 weeks or less for any patient who desires it. The recent Webster decision has introduced the possibility of state-legislated restrictions on abortion, and the Supreme Court is continuing to review cases that could result in further restrictions.

2. **Therapeutic abortion** is a term that should be reserved for those few instances when abortion is indicated for medical reasons. Few of these medical indications are absolute, and the decision to terminate a pregnancy frequently is based not only on the risk to the gravida's health or to the fetus but also on such factors as the patient's ability to care for a child after birth. In deciding on therapeutic abortion, a couple may not wish to assume certain risks such as those involved in pregnancy or in the child care required thereafter. A few women with severe heart disease or severe hypertension, especially if the disease has affected the myocardium, retina, or kidneys, or severe renal disease may require abortion. Incapacitating disease of the lungs, unremitting ulcerative colitis, or cancer of the breast are other examples of diseases requiring abortion in certain instances. Similarly, some patients with emotional illness are best managed with abortion. Most abortions, however, are performed for elective reasons.

B. **Criteria for selection of technique.** When the decision for abortion has been made, the best technique must be selected from the variety available. The choice will depend primarily on (1) the length of gestation, (2) whether an accompanying sterilization procedure is to be performed, (3) the presence or absence of a pathologic condition in the uterus, and (4) a diagnosis that contraindicates a particular technique. The earlier an abortion is performed, the safer the procedure.

1. **The techniques currently available** to effect abortion include (1) suction, (2) dilatation and evacuation (D and E), and (3) intravaginal or intraam-

niotic use of various agents. Hysterotomy may be indicated under certain very rare circumstances but is almost never performed at the current time because of a markedly increased risk of morbidity and mortality. Hysterectomy is performed only when necessitated by a pathologic condition of the uterus.

2. **The length of gestation** is the major factor in the choice of technique. Suction abortion is indicated up through the fifteenth week, depending on the experience of the clinician. The later the abortion is performed, the greater the risk of excessive blood loss or uterine perforation. D and E, requiring instrumental removal of the products of conception, is recommended between 16 and 24 weeks and in the hands of experienced clinicians may be safer than other techniques. However, some physicians continue to prefer other methods for late abortion, notably vaginal prostaglandins.

C. **Rh_0 (D) immune globulin.** Whenever an abortion is performed on an Rh-negative patient whose blood is not sensitized to the Rh factor, Rh_O (D) immune globulin (RhoGAM) should be given. If the pregnancy is 12 gestational weeks or less, a dose of 50 μg within 72 hours of the procedure is sufficient. With later abortion, 300 μg is used.

V. **Sterilization.** Surgical sterilization has become the most common method of contraception for married women in the United States. Approximately 1 million sterilization procedures are performed annually in the United States, with about 60% of the procedures being performed on women [4]. The perceived risks of other highly effective methods of contraception, such as oral contraceptives or the IUD, often lead couples or individuals to choose sterilization when childbearing has been completed.

A. **Legal requirements** for sterilization have been introduced by many states, and stringent requirements were introduced by the federal government in 1979 for patients whose medical care is funded by the government. Physicians performing sterilization procedures should be aware of the applicable legal requirements.

The **federal requirements** are rigid and include the following restrictions:

1. The individual to be sterilized must be at least 21 years old at the time the consent is obtained.
2. The individual must be mentally competent.
3. A 30-day waiting period must expire between the time of consent and surgical procedure. A reduction in this waiting period to 72 hours is allowed in the case of an individual who consents to be sterilized preceding premature delivery or an emergency abdominal operation. In no case can the 72-hour delay be reduced further.
4. The consent cannot be obtained during labor or when a patient is seeking to obtain an abortion.

B. **Procedures**

1. **Female sterilization.** Nearly all operations intended to sterilize the female interrupt the continuity of the fallopian tubes. An exception occurs when a significant pathologic condition of the uterus coexists with an indication for sterilization. Hysterectomy in such a patient may be good practice. Sterilization of the female may be done in the immediate postpartum period or as an interval procedure. During the postpartum period, the Pomeroy tubal ligation is the most widely used procedure.

   a. **Sterilization regret** is a relatively common occurrence, with an incidence up to 20% in some studies [2]. However, a much smaller number of women actually seek reversal procedures. Successful reversal has been reported in 51–73% of cases, but only 20–30% of women are candidates for this attempted reversal [19].

2. **Male sterilization.** Approximately 40% of the sterilization procedures in the United States are performed on males. The procedure usually is done in the physician's office, under local anesthesia. Through small scrotal incisions, each vas deferens is identified and ligated at two points with

transection between the points of ligature. The cut ends usually are cauterized. The mortality associated with the operation is virtually zero although a few complications such as hematoma formation can occur. The failure rate is less than 1%. Although operative reversibility frequently is successful, the patient should regard the procedure as permanent.

References

1. Bonte, M., and Van Balen, H. Prolonged lactation and family spacing in Rwanda. *J. Biosoc. Sci.* 1:97, 1969.
2. Boring, C. C., Rochat, R. W., and Becerra, J. Sterilization regret in Puerto Rican women. *Fertil. Steril.* 49:973, 1988.
3. Bracken, M. B. Spermicidal contraceptives and poor reproductive outcomes: the epidemiologic evidence against an association. *Am. J. Obstet. Gynecol.* 151:552, 1985.
4. Burkman, R. T. *Handbook of Contraception and Abortion.* Boston: Little, Brown, 1989.
5. Cancer and Steroid Hormone Study, CDC and NICHD. Combination oral contraceptive use and the risk of endometrial cancer. *J.A.M.A.* 257:796, 1987.
6. Cancer and Steroid Hormone Study, CDC and NICHD. Oral contraceptive use and the risk of breast cancer. *N. Engl. J. Med.* 315:405, 1986.
7. Cancer and Steroid Hormone Study, CDC and NICHD. The reduction in risk of ovarian cancer associated with oral contraceptive use. *N. Engl. J. Med.* 316:650, 1987.
8. Collaborative Group for the Study of Stroke in Young Women. Oral contraception and stroke in young women. *J.A.M.A.* 231:718, 1975.
9. Connell, E. B. Barrier contraceptives. *Clin. Obstet. Gynecol.* 32:377, 1989.
10. Edelman, D. A., McIntyre, S. L., and Harper, J. A. A comparative trial of the Today contraceptive sponge and diaphragm. *Am. J. Obstet. Gynecol.* 150:869, 1984.
11. Edmondson, H. A., Henderson, B., and Benton, B. Liver cell adenomas associated with the use of oral contraceptives. *N. Engl. J. Med.* 294:470, 1976.
12. Fihn, S. D., et al. Association between diaphragm use and urinary tract infection. *J.A.M.A.* 254:240, 1985.
13. Grimes, D. A. Whither the intrauterine device? *Clin. Obstet. Gynecol.* 32:369, 1989.
14. Hatcher, R. A., Kowal, D., and Guest, F. *Contraceptive Technology: International Edition.* Atlanta: Printed Matter, 1989.
15. Inman, W. H., et al. Thromboembolic disease and the steroidal content of oral contraceptives: A report to the Committee on Safety of Drugs. *Br. Med. J.* 2:203, 1970.
16. Jick, H., et al. Vaginal spermicides and congenital disorders. *J.A.M.A.* 245:1329, 1981.
17. Kaunitz, A. M. Injectable contraceptives. *Clin. Obstet. Gynecol.* 32:356, 1989.
18. Kay, C. R., and Hannaford, P. C. Breast cancer and the pill: A further report from the Royal College of General Practitioners' oral contraceptive study. *Br. J. Cancer* 58:675, 1988.
19. King, T. M., and Zabin, L. S. Sterilization: Efficacy, safety, regret and reversal. *Female Patient [Suppl.]* 1:3, 1981.
20. Labbok, M. H., and Queenan, J. T. The use of periodic abstinence for family planning. *Clin. Obstet. Gynecol.* 32:387, 1989.
21. Laing, J. G. Natural family planning in the Philippines. *Stud. Fam. Plann.* 15:49, 1984.
22. Lee, N. C., et al. Type of intrauterine device and the risk of pelvic inflammatory disease. *Obstet. Gynecol.* 62:1, 1983.
23. Lee, N. C., et al. Type of intrauterine device and the risk of pelvic inflammatory disease revisited: new results from the Women's Health Study. *Obstet. Gynecol.* 72:1, 1988.

24. Lee, R., Dillon, M. P., and Bashler, E. Barrier contraceptives and toxic shock syndrome (letter to the editor). *Lancet* 2:21, 1982.
25. Louik, C., et al. Maternal exposure to spermicides in relation to certain birth defects. *N. Engl. J. Med.* 317:474, 1987.
26. Miller, D. R., et al. Breast cancer before age 45 and oral contraceptive use: New findings. *Am. J. Epidemiol.* 129:269, 1989.
27. Neuberger, J., et al. Oral contraceptives and hepatocellular carcinoma. *Br. Med. J.* 292:1355, 1986.
28. Ory, H. W. The contraceptive health benefits from oral contraceptive use. *Fam. Plann. Perspect.* 14:182, 1982.
29. Osathanondh, R. Conception Control. In K. J. Ryan, R. Berkowitz, and R. L. Barbieri (eds.), *Kistner's Gynecology*. Chicago: Year Book, 1990.
30. Population Information Program. IUDs—A new look. *Popul. Rep.* Series B, no. 5, March 1988.
31. Porter, J. B., Hershel, J., and Walker, A. M. Mortality among oral contraceptive users. *Obstet. Gynecol.* 70:29, 1987.
32. Porter, J. B., et al. Oral contraceptives and nonfatal cardiovascular disease. *Obstet. Gynecol.* 66:1, 1985.
33. Ramcharan, S., et al. The Walnut Creek Contraceptive Drug Study. A prospective study of the side effects of oral contraceptives. *J. Reprod. Med.* 25:360, 1980.
34. *Roe v. Wade,* 93 United States Supreme Court 705 (1973).
35. Royal College of General Practitioners. *Oral Contraception.* New York: Pitman, 1974.
36. Royal College of General Practitioners. Oral contraception study. Further analyses of mortality in oral contraceptive users. *Lancet* 1:541, 1981.
37. Royal College of General Practitioners. Oral Contraceptive Study. Incidence of arterial disease among oral contraceptive users. *J. R. Coll. Gen. Pract.* 33:75, 1983.
38. Schlesselman, J. J. Cancer of the breast and reproductive tract in relation to the use of oral contraceptives. *Contraception* 40:1, 1989.
39. Sivin, I. International experience with Norplant and Norplant-2 contraceptives. *Stud. Fam. Plann.* 19:81, 1988.
40. Spellacy, W. N. Carbohydrate metabolism during treatment with estrogen, progestogen and low dose oral contraceptives. *Am. J. Obstet. Gynecol.* 6:732, 1982.
41. Spellacy, W. N. The effect of intrauterine devices, oral contraceptives, estrogens and progestogens on blood pressure. *Am. J. Obstet. Gynecol.* 112:912, 1972.
42. Speroff, L., Glass, R. H., and Kase, N. G. *Clinical Gynecologic Endocrinology and Infertility* (4th ed.). Baltimore: Williams & Wilkins, 1989.
43. Stadel, B. V., et al. Oral contraceptives and premenopausal breast cancer in nulliparous women. *Contraception* 38:287, 1988.
44. Stone, K. M., Grimes, D. A., and Magder, L. S. Primary prevention of sexually transmitted diseases: A primer for clinicians. *J.A.M.A.* 255:1763, 1986.
45. Tietze, C., and Lewit, S. Life risks associated with reversible methods of fertility regulation. *Int. J. Gynaecol Obstet.* 16:469, 1979.
46. Trussell, J., et al. Contraceptive failure in the United States: an update. *Stud. Fam. Plann.* 21:51, 1990.
47. Trussell, J., and Kost, K. Contraceptive failure in the United States: a critical review of the literature. *Stud. Fam. Plann.* 18:237, 1987.
48. Vessey, M., et al. A long-term follow-up study of women using different methods of contraception: An interim report. *J. Biosoc. Sci.* 8:373, 1976.
49. Vessey, M. P., Lawless, M., and Yeates, D. Oral contraceptives and stroke: Findings in a large prospective study. *Br. Med. J.* 289:530, 1984.
50. Warburton, D., et al. Lack of association between spermicide use and trisomy. *N. Engl. J. Med.* 317:478, 1987.
51. Weinberger, M. H. The Blood Pressure Effects of Oral Contraceptives. In

J. Sciarra, G. Zatuchni, and J. Speidel (eds.), *Risks, Benefits and Controversies in Fertility Control.* Hagerstown, MD: Harper & Row, 1978.
52. Yupze, A., Smith, P., and Rademaker, A. A multi-center clinical investigation employing ethinyl estradiol combined with dl norgestrel as a postcoital contraceptive agent. *Fertil. Steril.* 37:508, 1982.

2 Prenatal Care

Julie A. Lemieux

Care designed to optimize the health of two interdependent patients is a special challenge—one enhanced by many factors. Rapid advances in technology continue to improve our ability to assess fetal development and well-being. Women today desire more information, and many desire more control of the birthing process. Social issues require careful attention. The woman's personal situation and support systems must be explored as the family prepares for a new member. Chemical use, legal and illicit, is a frequent problem and must be considered a potential complication in all pregnancies. And at the same time, prenatal care must be accomplished in a cost-effective manner and within the present medicolegal climate.

Prenatal care has many components. Initially, confirmation of the diagnosis of pregnancy and the estimated gestational age must be established. This allows accurate assignment of the estimated date of confinement. Next is a full history and physical exam with laboratory evaluation. Regular periodic visits follow, with ongoing patient education. All information obtained should be recorded in a concise manner that is accessible to other members of the health care team. It is helpful to use a standardized format for charting so that important factors are not overlooked.

I. **Diagnosis of pregnancy and accurate dating** are essential for avoiding risks in the first weeks of gestation and for handling possible medical complications, premature labor, or postdates pregnancy.

A. **Presumptive signs.** Amenorrhea is often the first sign of possible conception. It must be regarded with caution, however, as lack of menses may be due to other factors such as anovulation, stress, chronic disease, or lactation. Other early pregnancy subjective signs and symptoms perceived by the woman include breast fullness/tenderness, skin changes, nausea, vomiting, urinary frequency, and fatigue. Between 12 and 20 weeks' gestation, the woman will note an enlarging abdomen and the perception of fetal movement.

B. **Probable signs** are highly suggestive of the diagnosis of pregnancy. Presumptive and probable signs do not differentiate between an ectopic and an intrauterine pregnancy.

1. **Uterine enlargement, softening of the uterine isthmus** (Hegar's sign), **and vaginal and cervical cyanosis** (Chadwick's sign) are probable signs of pregnancy.
2. **Pregnancy tests.** Common urine pregnancy tests used today are very sensitive and may be positive up to one week following implantation or within days of the first missed menstrual period. The first-voided morning urine is the most concentrated specimen for analysis. Radioimmunoassay for serum testing of the beta subunit or human chorionic gonadotropin (HCG) may be accurate a few days after implantation (or even before the first missed period). HCG production is maximum at 60–70 days of gestation and thereafter declines. These tests do not differentiate between trophoblastic disease (molar pregnancy or choriocarcinoma, for example) and normal pregnancy.

   Other bioassay techniques employed in the past, such as progesterone withdrawal, are of historical interest only. Progestin should not be given to a women presumed to be pregnant because of potential fetal anomalies (especially limb defects), although this effect is rare.

C. **Positive diagnostic signs**

1. **Fetal heart tones** can be detected as early as 9—10 weeks from the last menstrual period (LMP) by Doppler technology. The DeLee fetoscope detects fetal

heart tones at 18–20 weeks from the LMP, depending on the hearing acuity of the individual, fetal positions, and thickness of tissue layers. Normal fetal heart rate is between 120 and 160 beats per minute.

2. Presence of active **fetal movements** palpated by the observer is diagnostic of pregnancy. Bowel activity often simulates fetal movements and may be confusing to the patient. Fetal activity ("quickening") is first felt by the patient at approximately 16–18 weeks and thereafter is a valuable indication of fetal well-being.

3. **Ultrasonic and radiologic examination.** An intrauterine gestational sac can be identified by ultrasound at five to six weeks, and by seven to eight weeks a fetal pole with movement and cardiac activity is seen. Vaginal probe ultrasound has made these early measurements even more accurate. Fetal age can be estimated by crown-rump length, and the number of fetuses may be identified. Between 10 and 14 weeks' gestation, the fetal measurements including biparietal diameter and femur length may be used to estimate fetal age accurately. Further into the second trimester it is possible to evaluate fetal anatomy and possible fetal anomalies. Placental location and amniotic fluid volume may also be noted as the pregnancy continues. To date, there is no proof that diagnostic ultrasonic exposure has adverse effects on the developing human fetus.

   Fetal skeletal clarification can usually be demonstrated by roentgenography at approximately 16 weeks' gestation. Radiation, however, should be avoided during the first trimester and used thereafter only as absolutely indicated. With the common availability of ultrasound, roentgenographic diagnosis of pregnancy is no longer indicated.

D. **Estimated date of confinement.** The mean duration of pregnancy as calculated from the LMP has been found to be 280 days or 40 weeks. The estimated date of confinement (EDC) can be calculated by Nägele's rule: To the first day of the LMP add seven days and then subtract three months. Deviations from this calculation may be made for various reasons (e.g., irregular or prolonged menstrual cycles, or a known single sexual exposure). If the date of the LMP is unknown or does not correlate with the uterine size at the first visit, ultrasonography may be used to establish the EDC.

II. **Complete history and physical examination** are performed after the diagnosis of pregnancy is established. An important goal is to develop a trusting, working relationship between the patient and the health care team.

A. **Historical information** assists in the assessment of risk status.

1. **Menstrual and contraceptive history.** A known menstrual history is usually the most reliable predictor of delivery date. It should be remembered that women with recent birth control pill usage may have post-pill amenorrhea and, therefore, pregnancy dating may be in error. The intrauterine device (IUD) use should be noted and its presence, absence, or removal carefully documented.

2. **Gynecologic and obstetric history.** Previous gynecologic infections or problems should be recorded. The obstetric history is recorded as the gravidity and parity. **Gravidity** is the total number of pregnancies. **Parity** is expressed as four serial numbers: term deliveries, premature deliveries, abortions (spontaneous and elective), living children. Details of past pregnancies such as character and length of labor, type of delivery, complications, infant status, and birth weight should be noted. Recurrent first-trimester losses or history of second trimester losses may suggest genetic problems or an incompetent cervix.

3. **Medical and surgical history, prior hospitalizations.**

4. **Environmental exposures, medications** taken in early pregnancy, **drug reactions** and allergic history, diethylstilbesterol (DES) exposure.

5. **Family history** of medical illnesses, hereditary illness, multiple gestation.

6. **Social factors.** Home situation, family and social support, and possible physical or mental abuse history should be assessed and appropriate referral made. Accurate history of chemical use is not always easily obtained. Use of legal substances such as cigarettes and alcohol, as well as illicit chemical use, is

pervasive in all social and racial groups. All of these chemicals have serious ramifications for fetal development and pregnancy outcome.

7. **Review of systems,** conventional and specific as related to pregnancy: nausea, vomiting, abdominal pain, constipation, headaches, syncopal episodes, vaginal bleeding or discharge, dysuria or urinary frequency, swelling, varicosities, hemorrhoids.

B. Physical exam

1. **Complete physical examination** with attention directed to specific organ systems as a positive history is elicited. This should include height, weight, funduscopic exam, thyroid and breast, lymph nodes, lungs, heart, abdomen with fundal height and presence of fetal heart tones, extremities, and a basic neurologic screening. The examiner must be aware of the normal changes found in pregnancy.

2. **Pelvic exam**
   - a. **External genitalia.** Evidence of previous obstetric injury should be noted.
   - b. **Vagina.** Under hormonal influence of pregnancy, cervical secretions are increased, thus raising the vaginal pH, which may cause a change in the bacteriologic flora of the vagina. No treatment is necessary unless diagnosis of a specific infection is made (see sec. **B.3).**
   - c. **Cervix** is routinely evaluated with a Pap smear and culture for gonorrhea. *Chlamydia* culture should also be done in high-risk populations.
     - **(1)** Cervical eversion is normal.
     - **(2)** Softening of the cervix is normal and nabothian cysts are of no consequence. Effacement or dilatation of the internal os is abnormal except near term and may indicate premature labor or incompetent cervix.
     - **(3)** Morphologic cervical changes (ridges, hood, or collar) or vaginal adenosis may indicate DES exposure in utero. These women have a higher incidence of incompetent cervix and premature delivery and should be evaluated accordingly.
   - d. **Uterus.** Estimation of gestational age by uterine size is one of the most important elements of the first examination. A normal nongravid uterus is firm, smooth, and approximately 3 × 4 × 7 cm. The uterus will not change noticeably in consistency or size until five to six weeks after the LMP, or four weeks from conception. Gestational age is estimated by uterine size in volume from the LMP (i.e., 8 weeks = 2 times normal size, 10 weeks = 3 times normal, and 12 weeks = 4 times normal). At 12 weeks, the uterus fills the pelvis so that the fundus of the uterus is palpable at the symphysis pubis. By 16 weeks, the uterus is midway between the symphysis pubis and the umbilicus. At 20 weeks, it reaches the umbilicus. Thereafter, there is a rough correlation between weeks of gestation and height of the fundus when measured in centimeters from the top of the symphysis pubis to the top of the uterine fundus (MacDonald's measurement).

     After correcting for minor discrepancies resulting from adiposity and variation in body shape, a uterine size that exceeds the anticipated gestation by three or more weeks as calculated from the last normal menstrual period suggests multiple gestation, molar pregnancy, leiomyomas, uterine anomalies, adnexal masses, or simply an inaccurate date for the LMP. Ultrasonography is the best diagnostic tool for this situation. The finding that uterine size is less than expected may indicate inaccurate dating or intrauterine growth failure.
   - e. **Adnexa** are difficult to evaluate as the fallopian tubes and ovaries are lifted out of the pelvis by the enlarging uterus. Any questionable masses should be confirmed by ultrasound.
   - f. **Clinical pelvimetry.** Evaluation of the bony pelvis to predict adequacy for labor has been a traditional component of the initial obstetric visit. This method yields too many falsely positive and falsely negative results to be of predictive clinical usefulness. There may be situations when x-ray or computed tomography pelvimetry may provide some useful information in later stages of pregnancy (e.g., evaluation for vaginal breech delivery).

3. **Common lesions and infections** that may be encountered on pelvic exam.
   a. **Bartholin's gland abscess.** A painful, erythematous, cystic enlargement on either side of the lateral vaginal introitus indicates obstruction and infection of Bartholin's gland. Treatment includes sitz baths, analgesic, and when fluctuant, incision and drainage. Cyst formation may result from incomplete resolution of an abscess. Marsupialization after the puerperium may be advisable for recurrent problems.
   b. ***Condylomata acuminata.*** Venereal warts are hyperkeratotic, flat, or polypoid lesions found in the vulvar or perineal areas, vagina, or cervix and caused by infection with the human papilloma virus. (Certain viral types have been shown to be associated with the development of dysplasia and ultimately with epithelial carcinoma.) Pregnancy may stimulate proliferation of these lesions, which may become friable. Rarely, cesarean delivery is necessary to prevent extensive vaginal damage at delivery. There is also an ill-defined risk of transmission of human papilloma virus to the infant with development of laryngeal papillomata. The mode of transmission is unknown and currently no consensus exists regarding the protective benefit to the neonate of cesarean versus vaginal delivery.
      Treatment of the lesions is more difficult in pregnancy. Podophyllin resin, trichloroacetic acid, 5-fluorouracil, and immunotherapy should be avoided. However, cryotherapy, electrocauterization, or laser may be used on external lesions.
   c. **Herpes simplex viral infection.** Characteristic lesions are small, painful, superficial, erythematous vesicles that ulcerate. Treatment is symptomatic only, as acyclovir cream or tablets are contraindicated in pregnancy. Fetal infection may be fatal and must be avoided.
   d. **Monilial vulvovaginitis.** Monilial (also called candidal or yeast) infection with the characteristic curdy, white, itchy discharge is common. This can be treated safely during pregnancy with nystatin or miconazole nitrate creams or suppositories in the usual dose regimens.
   e. ***Trichomonas vaginalis.*** Vulvar or vaginal burning or itching with a frothy, malodorous discharge is a frequent finding with this infection. Metronidazole (Flagyl) is the treatment of choice but is contraindicated during the first trimester because of possible teratogenicity. Clotrimazole suppositories (one nightly for one week) have been used with an improvement in symptoms and a 70% cure rate. For severe cases, metronidazole may be used during the second and third trimesters, but the 2-gm dose should be avoided. The sexual partner should also be treated.
   f. ***Gardnerella vaginalis.*** Infection with *Gardnerella vaginalis,* also referred to as bacterial vaginosis or *Haemophilus vaginalis* vaginitis, produces a white to gray malodorous discharge that is usually nonirritating. The current drug of choice is metronidazole, but it is restricted in pregnancy, as mentioned above. Ampicillin 500 mg PO qid for 7 days may be used, and the partner treated with metronidazole 500 mg PO bid for 5–7 days.
   g. ***Neisseria gonorrhoeae.*** Symptoms may include dysuria, burning, or only vaginal or cervical discharge. Many patients are asymptomatic. Microscopically, gram-negative intracellular diplococci are seen in the discharge, but culture confirmation is imperative. Usual treatment regimens may be administered; however, tetracycline is contraindicated in pregnancy. Due to the high rate of coexistent infection, it is recommended that women with gonorrheal infection be treated for *Chlamydia* (see the following). Sexual partners should be treated, and a test of cure culture should be obtained after treatment.
   h. ***Chlamydia trachomatis.*** Symptoms of the infection from this obligatory intracellular parasite range from asymptomatic to cervicitis, discharge, and discomfort. Diagnosis is made by special culture, or in some areas more rapid tests are available. The infection can be passed to the neonate in the form of conjunctivitis or pneumonia. Treatment is erythromycin 250–500 mg qid PO for 10–14 days. Tetracycline is effective but is contraindicated

in pregnancy. The sexual partner must be treated, and a test of cure culture should be obtained following treatment.

i. Laboratory evaluation

(1) Routine initial screen. Complete blood count, ABO blood typing and Rh factor, antibody screen, urine analysis and culture, serologic test for syphilis, rubella titer, Pap smear, cervical culture for gonorrhea, tuberculosis skin testing. Hepatitis B surface antigen screen and cervical culture for *Chlamydia* are indicated in high-risk groups.

4. Specialized screening test

a. Hemoglobin electrophoresis is indicated in some groups: in those of black ancestry for sickle hemoglobin, in Mediterranean couples for beta-thalassemia, and in Asians for alpha-thalassemia.

b. Tay-Sachs carrier status analysis is indicated in Jewish couples.

c. A screen for the **human immunodeficiency virus** should be encouraged in high-risk populations and offered to all women, with consent.

d. A history positive for a certain illness, or abnormalities in other screening labs should be investigated with further tests as indicated.

e. Herpes cultures are valuable in confirming the diagnosis but have little value in predicting the fetus at risk. Therefore, screening cultures are not recommended.

f. Routine screening ultrasound has been suggested. Due to its high cost and uncertain benefit in cases without other indications for a sonogram, it is not currently considered a standard of care in uncomplicated pregnancies.

g. Urine or blood toxicology screens may be indicated for the evaluation of illicit chemical use.

5. Midtrimester screening tests

a. The couple should be counseled regarding **maternal serum alpha fetoprotein** testing for birth defects, to be completed between the fifteenth and twentieth weeks of gestation. Although there are numerous causes for an abnormal alpha-fetoprotein value, its primary purpose is to screen for neural tube defects. Abnormal results are further evaluated by ultrasound and amniocentesis.

b. At 26–30 weeks a **one-hour glucola** (blood glucose measurement one hour after a 50-gm oral glucose load) and **repeat hemoglobin and hematocrit** are obtained. The glucola measurement has become a valuable test for gestational diabetes in all pregnant patients. Those with a particular risk (e.g., previous gestational diabetes or fetal macrosomia) may warrant earlier testing. Abnormal results are evaluated with a three-hour oral glucose tolerance test.

c. At 28–30 weeks an **antibody screen** is obtained in Rh-negative women and RH_0 (D) immune globulin is administered if the screen is negative.

III. Risk assessment. Information gathered must be evaluated to assess the risk for the outcome of the present developing pregnancy. Designation of a pregnancy as **high risk** implies a need for special care or appropriate referrals. Major categories for increased risk should be identified antepartum and given appropriate consideration in subsequent pregnancy management: (1) preexisting medical illness, (2) previous pregnancy complications such as perinatal mortality, prematurity, fetal growth retardation, malformations, placental accidents, and maternal hemorrhage, and (3) evidence of poor maternal nutrition. Also, the health care team must be able to recognize the appearance of complicating events that may transform a low-risk pregnancy into a high-risk pregnancy.

IV. Genetics referral. Congenital disease is a major cause of infant morbidity and mortality. Indications for genetic referral include (1) maternal age of more than 35 years at the time of the birth; (2) family history of congenital anomalies or inherited disorders; (3) abnormal development or mental retardation of a previous child; (4) ethnic background associated with inheritable diseases; (5) chemical use or exposure to teratogens; and (6) three or more consecutive spontaneous abortions.

V. Subsequent prenatal care. Regular periodic visits with a methodic approach allow ongoing evaluation of the fetal-maternal unit and reassurance of the normal progress of the pregnancy. For low-risk pregnancies, the recommended frequency of prenatal visits is monthly up to 28 weeks, every 2 weeks up to 36 weeks, and weekly until delivery. Standard assessment at each prenatal visit includes maternal weight, blood pressure, uterine size, auscultation of fetal heart tones, and evaluation for edema, proteinuria, and glucosuria. All information is recorded on a standardized form.

VI. Patient education

A. Nutrition. A commonsense approach is necessary, as many gaps exist in our knowledge in this area. Suggestions include eating food from each of the major food groups, taking adequate liquids (especially water), adding fiber, and ensuring adequate calcium intake. For a woman whose weight is normal before pregnancy, a normal weight gain is 20–30 lb, or 12–15 kg (Table 2-1). This is usually achieved by eating a well-balanced diet containing 60–80 gm of protein, 2300 or more calories, low sugars and fats, high fiber, and at least three glasses of milk or other dairy equivalents daily. An underweight woman is at increased risk for a growth-retarded infant. Excessive weight gain or preexisting maternal obesity (more than 200 lb or 90 kg) may, in some cases, may be associated with increased risk of fetal macrosomia. This may create a significant risk factor for birth trauma and delivery by cesarean section.

B. Working during pregnancy. Most women can safely work until term without complications. A flexible approach must be taken. Pregnant women may have less tolerance to heat, humidity, environmental pollutants, prolonged standing, or heavy lifting. Pregnant women who should probably not work include those with a history of two premature deliveries, incompetent cervix, fetal loss secondary to uterine abnormalities, cardiac disease greater than class II, Marfan's syndrome, hemoglobinopathies, diabetes with retinopathy or renal involvement, third-trimester bleeding, premature rupture of the membranes, or multiple gestation after 28 weeks.

C. Exercise. Women should be encouraged to exercise if they have no complicating factors. Recommendations should be tailored to the individual patient by differentiating between a trained athlete and a sedentary woman. The trained athlete can continue rigorous training during pregnancy but should avoid raising her core temperature or becoming dehydrated. Exercise should be varied during the third trimester to avoid too much stress on knee and ankle joints. Walking, swimming, and prenatal aerobic classes can be adapted to the needs of most women.

D. Smoking should be discontinued during pregnancy. It is important to counsel patients about this and record their compliance. The potentially harmful effects of cigarette smoke during pregnancy include low birth weight, premature labor, miscarriage, stillbirth, crib death, birth defects, and increased respiratory problems in neonates. More than 10 cigarettes a day can have a pronounced effect on birth weight. Many women do not realize the severity of the risks. Patient education is important, with counseling and referral to appropriate community groups.

E. Seat belt use. The proper technique is the same as for the nonpregnant automobile passenger: The lap belt is worn low and snugly across the hip bones; the shoulder harness is worn over one shoulder and under the opposite arm, loosely enough to place a clenched fist between the sternum and the belt.

Table 2-1. Weight gain in pregnancy

Prepregnancy weight (PPW)	Suggested weight gain (lb)
< 90% of ideal PPW	30
90–135% of ideal PPW	20
> 135% of ideal PPW	16

Source: R. L. Naeye, et al. Weight gain and the outcome of pregnancy. *Am. J. Obstet. Gynecol.* 135:3–9, 1979.

F. Sexual relations. There are no sexual restrictions for the uncomplicated patient. Whatever is comfortable and pleasurable may be continued unless and until a pregnancy complication occurs (e.g., undiagnosed bleeding, preterm labor, known placenta previa, rupture of the membranes). The forcing of air into the vagina during orogenital sex should be warned against, specifically because of reports of sudden maternal death or stroke.

G. Fetal movements. Fetal activity is usually of cyclic frequency and may vary throughout pregnancy. Lack of fetal movement or a marked decrease in frequency may be a warning signal of fetal distress.

H. Warning signs of preterm labor. Studies have suggested improved rates of early diagnosis and treatment of preterm labor with education of the patient and delivery room staff. The following list is modified from Creasy and colleagues [2].

1. A feeling that the baby is "balling up" that lasts more than 30 seconds and occurs more than 4 times/hour.
2. Contractions or intermittent pains or sensations between nipples and knees lasting over 30 seconds and recurring 4 or more times/hour.
3. Menstrual-like sensations, occurring intermittently.
4. Change in vaginal discharge, including bleeding.
5. Indigestion or diarrhea.

I. Common complaints. Many discomforts are expected in pregnancy, and these are related to cardiovascular changes, hormonal effects, uterine growth, and change in body posture. After investigation to rule out a serious pathologic condition, treatment may be directed to symptomatic relief.

1. **Headache and backache.** Acetaminophen (Tylenol) 325–650 mg q3–4h should be sufficient. For severe headache or migraine, codeine or other related narcotic may be used. Aspirin should be avoided [1].
2. **Nausea and vomiting.** No antinausea medication is being marketed as safe in pregnancy. First-trimester "morning sickness" may be relieved by eating frequent small meals, getting out of bed slowly after eating a few crackers, and avoiding spicy or greasy foods. If symptoms are severe and persistent, hospitalization and intravenous fluids may be needed. In patients who require antiemetics, there is no known association of birth defects with the use of promethazine (Phenergan), diphenhydramine (Benadryl), and several other antihistamines [1].
3. **Constipation.** A high-fiber diet, increased fluid intake, and regular exercise are recommended. Stool softeners such as docusate sodium (Colace) or psyllium hydrophilic mucilloid (Metamucil) may help. Mild laxatives should be used sparingly, and only if the aforementioned measures fail.
4. **Varicosities.** Support stockings and leg elevation are recommended.

J. Other important information to be presented to the patient includes when and where to call for questions and problems, childbirth classes, signs of the onset of labor, obstetric analgesic options, indications for cesarean section, home safety, infant care and feeding, access to consumer information (e.g., infant safety products, furniture, car seats) and birth control counseling.

References

1. Briggs, G. G., et al. *Drugs in Pregnancy and Lactation.* Baltimore: Williams & Wilkins, 1983.
2. Creasy, R. K., et al. System for predicting spontaneous preterm birth. *Obstet. Gynecol.* 55:692–695, 1980.

Selected Reading

Pritchard, J. A., and MacDonald, P. C. (eds.). *Williams' Obstetrics* (17th ed.). New York: Appleton-Century-Crofts, 1985.

3 Perinatal Chemical Use

Arthur T. Evans

Chemical use is reaching epidemic proportions in the United States. Clearly, a significant number of women are using chemicals during pregnancy. While it is apparent that chemical use is related to a number of perinatal complications, such as spontaneous abortion, premature birth, fetal growth retardation, and the neonatal withdrawal syndrome, it is not known to what extent chemical use is the etiology of these events as opposed to other perinatal factors.

I. Definition. The difficulties encountered in the terminology of chemical use emphasize the complex nature of the problem. The term **chemical** is used rather than **drug** or **substance** because it is descriptive of the use to obtain a chemical effect. Many forms of chemical use exist and virtually any compound can be considered a source for chemical use. In this chapter, **chemical use** refers to the nonmedicinal use of regulated or controlled chemicals. This does not include over-the-counter, nonprescription medications.

II. Extent of use. The total number of women using chemicals during pregnancy is unknown. Few comprehensive population-based studies have been conducted. The 1985 *Household Survey on Drug Abuse* by the National Institute on Drug Abuse [5] estimated that 15% of reproductive-age women were "substance abusers." An informal survey in 1988 of 36 hospitals across the United States asked the rate of perinatal chemical use [1]. With a variety of screening protocols, the incidence of positive toxicology tests was 11%. The range was 0.4–27%, with the rate proportional to the thoroughness of the screening protocol and not related to the percentage of public and private patients screened. A county-based study in Florida with public and private patients found that 14.8% of all women entering perinatal care were positive for alcohol, marijuana, cocaine, or opiates. No difference was found between public (16.3%) and private (13.7%) patients [2]. At the University of California, Davis (UCD), all women admitted to the obstetrics service have a urine toxicology screen performed for cocaine, amphetamines, and opiates. In UCD's predominantly urban pregnant population, the prevalence rate for cocaine, amphetamines, and opiates at the time of admission was 20.5% in 1988 [3]. The incidence of use throughout pregnancy is unknown. Because most chemicals (except marijuana) are detectable in the blood or urine for only one to five days after use, the incidence of use is much more difficult to ascertain than prevalence.

III. Complications. Although many of the perinatal complications associated with chemical use are chemical specific, some risks and complications are commonly encountered.

A. Multiple chemical use. Many individuals, whether pregnant or not, engage in multiple rather than single chemical use. Alcohol and cigarettes are the most commonly used chemicals and they also are frequently used in conjunction with other chemicals. Individuals will often move from one chemical to another depending on what is most obtainable. This presents a particular problem when attempting to discontinue a chemical, as the patient may merely substitute the use of another chemical. Addictive behavior is difficult to treat, and resumption of chemical use after pregnancy is common even in highly motivated patients. Control or cessation of use during pregnancy requires extensive counseling and long-term supportive therapy.

B. Infectious diseases. Chemical use places women at particular risk for contracting specific infectious diseases.

1. **Sexually transmitted diseases.** Women engaged in chemical use frequently use sexual activity as a means to obtain chemicals. This may involve prostitution; trading sex for chemicals, food, or shelter; or simply having multiple sexual partners. This places them at risk for syphilis, gonorrhea, and chlamydia as well as acquired immunodeficiency syndrome (AIDS) and hepatitis B. All women who use chemicals must be considered at risk for sexually acquired human immunodeficiency virus (HIV) and hepatitis B whether or not they use needles. Appropriate screening for all these infections should be done with the initial prenatal visit and consideration given to repeat testing at 36–40 weeks' gestation.
2. **Parenterally transmitted diseases.** The use of needles with chemical use presents particular risks for the individual. Needle sharing is common and sterilization of needles using agents such as bleach is sporadic. HIV and hepatitis B are specific risks to these individuals. There is also the risk of injecting bacteria with contaminated needles and causing cellulitis, abscesses, thrombophlebitis, and other infectious complications.

C. Aberrant social behavior. Criminal activities often accompany chemical use. The social dysfunction that disrupts many of these individuals' lives is just as detrimental as the chemicals themselves. This extends into difficulties with personal and family relationships and can ultimately interfere with parenting abilities. Every effort should be made to enlist the available social and support services for these women during pregnancy. Pregnancy is often a time when women involved in chemical use are particularly receptive to intervention.

D. Poor general health. The activities of chemical use often lead to disregard for personal health, hygiene, and nutrition. In extreme cases, diseases of debilitation are seen, including malnutrition, tuberculosis, and unattended infections. A careful evaluation should be performed for medical problems not directly related to pregnancy. Pregnancy is often one of the few times that chemical-using women come in contact with the medical care system.

IV. Methods of detection

A. Measurable amounts of a chemical are detectable in blood, urine, saliva, hair [4], amniotic fluid, and neonatal meconium [6] following use. Only hair is able to detect prior past use. Chemicals (except marijuana) are detectable in maternal body fluids for only one to five days following use (Table 3-1). Fetal presence of a chemical can be significantly longer due to slower drug metabolism with fetal hepatic immaturity and sequestration in the amniotic fluid. In particular, amniotic fluid and neonatal meconium may retain chemicals longer and indicate prior use. Maternal urine is usually the easiest and most readily available fluid to analyze, since pregnant women provide urine specimens with each office and hospital visit for protein and glucose determinations.

B. The most common technique for initial identification of chemicals in the clinical setting is **immunoassay,** usually with an enzyme-linked system specific for each chemical or class of chemical either gas-liquid chromatography or thin-layer chromatography. This reliably eliminates cross-reactivity with other chemicals.

Table 3-1. Length of time chemicals are measurable in biologic fluids

Alcohol	3–16 hr
Amphetamines	24–72 hr
Cocaine	24–60 hr
Opiates	36–72 hr
Marijuana	2–8 wk
PCP	7 days
LSD	2 hr–2 wk

Without confirmatory testing, identification problems can occur such as ephedrines that may be taken in cold medicines being identified as amphetamines or confusion of the various types of opiates. Care must be taken to document situations where a patient may have received a prescribed medication such as Demerol or morphine prior to collection of a urine sample for toxicology testing and therefore may have a positive result. This is seldom a problem with cocaine or amphetamine testing.

C. The decision on how to conduct chemical screening during pregnancy is based on the options of **selective versus universal toxicology screening.** With selective screening, individuals are chosen for testing on the basis of specific criteria. These are usually characteristics or behavioral markers that are felt to be associated with a greater probability of chemical use. These typically include low socioeconomic status, ethnicity, lack of prenatal care or poor compliance with care, presence of needle marks, a history of chemical use, or a history of criminal activity. With universal screening, all individuals are tested with the only inclusion criteria being pregnancy. Selective screening has the advantage of being less costly. Its advantage is that chemical use cannot be uniformly defined by historical or demographic factors. Universal screening has the advantage of identifying the greatest possible number of chemical-use pregnancies while avoiding discriminatory biases; however, it is more expensive and only identifies use within a specific time period. The selection of which type of screening to use ultimately depends on the institution, local patterns of chemical use, and the availability of counseling and intervention services.

V. Alcohol

A. Patterns of use. It is estimated that 11% of pregnant women have an alcohol consumption problem [9]. Although there is now a greater social awareness that any amount of alcohol use during pregnancy is undesirable, it remains legal for pregnant women to purchase and consume alcoholic beverages.

B. Perinatal effects

1. Fetal alcohol syndrome (FAS) is the most dramatic expression of the harmful effects of perinatal alcohol consumption. FAS affects 1–2 of every 1000 pregnancies [7]. The key features of FAS are

a. Intrauterine growth retardation

b. Microcephaly

c. Microphthalmia

d. Abnormal central nervous system (CNS) development (mental retardation, developmental delay, and other neurologic abnormalities)

e. Abnormal midline facial features (flattened nasal bridge and philtrum, thin upper lip, and short palpebral fissures)

2. Fetal alcohol effect (FAE) is the incomplete expression of the FAS features. It is not yet known to what extent even lesser expressions of alcohol effect are exhibited in the fetus.

The amount of alcohol required to produce FAS or FAE has not been precisely defined. Studies have demonstrated a "threshold effect" at the level of five or more drinks/day, throughout pregnancy, resulting in 32% of infants with anomalies and 12% with microcephaly [8] (versus rates of 9% and 0.4%, respectively, in controls). The level of alcohol consumption at which the risk becomes negligible is unknown; however, it appears that levels of less than one to two drinks/day are not associated with FAS findings. "Binge" drinking or single episodes of ingestion of large quantities of alcohol may also place the fetus at risk for FAS. For estimation of alcohol consumption by source, one glass of wine = one glass of beer = one ounce of hard liquor.

3. Additional problems that may be related to perinatal alcohol consumption are second-trimester abortions, fetal distress, and low Apgar scores.

4. Alcohol and cigarette smoking are frequently associated with each other as well as with the use of other chemicals. Alcohol and smoking have an additive risk for adverse perinatal effects such as intrauterine growth retardation [10].

C. Summary. Women should be advised not to consume alcohol in any amount during pregnancy. If alcohol use occurs, it should be limited to less than two drinks/day on an irregular basis, and binge drinking should be avoided.

VI. Tobacco

A. Patterns of use. Cigarette smoking is the most common form of chemical use during pregnancy. At UCD 31.7% of all pregnant women reported smoking cigarettes during their pregnancy. Among toxicology-positive women, this increased to 77.7%. Tobacco use during pregnancy should be considered a risk factor for the use of other chemicals.

B. Perinatal effects

1. **Increased mortality.** There is little dispute that smoking is detrimental to pregnancy outcome. In the Ontario Perinatal Mortality Study [11], perinatal mortality was increased by 27% with smoking.
2. Smoking is associated with an increase in
   a. Spontaneous abortion
   b. Placenta previa
   c. Premature rupture of the membranes
   c. Placental abruption
   d. Intrauterine growth retardation
   e. Sudden infant death syndrome (SIDS)
3. **Intrauterine growth retardation** is the most significant and consistent fetal effect of cigarette smoking. The mean reduction in birth weight is 200 gm [12]. A symmetric reduction in growth begins early and involves all fetal systems.
4. A direct relationship exists between **the number of cigarettes smoked and the magnitude of toxic effect** on the pregnancy. The Ontario study [11] reported an increase in perinatal mortality of 20% in women smoking less than one pack of cigarettes/day versus 35% with more than one pack/day. The level of smoking at which no reduction in fetal growth and birth weight occurs has not been determined.

C. Summary. Pregnant women should be questioned about tobacco use and should be advised to stop smoking. Failing that, reduction to as few cigarettes/day as possible is beneficial.

VII. Marijuana. Marijuana (cannabis) is used for the hallucinogenic effect of its psychoactive ingredient, tetrahydrocannabinol (THC). It also has antiemetic properties, and an oral form of THC, dronabinol, is available for prescription use to treat nausea.

A. Patterns of use

1. Marijuana is the most frequently used of the illicit chemicals. It is estimated that 10–37% of all adults use or have used marijuana.
2. A study of urban, indigent women reported that 28% either admitted using marijuana or tested positive by urine toxicology prenatally or immediately post partum [14].

B. Perinatal effects

1. **Placental transfer of THC** to the fetus is slow, resulting in fetal levels that are several times lower than maternal [13].
2. **Intrauterine growth retardation** is the primary effect on the fetus. It is a dose-dependent effect with a mean decrease in weight of 105 gm [17]. With more than five marijuana cigarettes/week, the mean weight reduction increases to 130 gm. Head circumference and fetal length are also decreased [19].
3. Marijuana use during pregnancy **may shorten gestation** [15, 16, 18]. The effect may be dose related. It is unclear whether or not the effect on length of gestation is independent of concomitant alcohol and tobacco use.
4. No evidence shows that marijuana use is associated with fetal distress or congenital anomalies.

C. Summary. Pregnant women should be advised to not use marijuana because of its ability to interfere with fetal growth. Excluding abstinence, reduction in the amount used will likely lessen the impact on fetal growth.

VIII. Cocaine. Cocaine (benzoylmethylecgnine) acts to block uptake of norepinephrine and dopamine at the presynaptic site, resulting in an excess of these at the postsynaptic receptor with consequent exaggerated sympathetic activity. Its systemic effects are due to excess sympathetic stimulation, while its euphoria effect results from excess dopamine in the CNS. Once ingested, cocaine is metabolized and detoxified in both the blood and the liver by cholinesterases. Its two primary metabolites, benzoylecgonine and ecgonine methyl ester, are then excreted in the urine. Benzoylecgonine is the primary metabolite that is measured in either blood or urine toxicology testing.

A. Patterns of use

1. It was estimated in 1985 that 30 million people in the United States had used cocaine and that 5 million were regular users [29].
2. The true incidence of perinatal cocaine use is unknown. Cocaine is only detectable by toxicology testing for up to three days after use. The two studies that have reported on the prevalence of use with universal toxicology screening found that 8.5% and 8.0% of women were positive for cocaine at the time of admission to the labor unit [3, 33]. The data in these studies were derived from indigent, urban populations. It remains to be determined if the same rates of positivity exist in other patient populations.

B. Toxicity

1. Cocaine can be injected intravenously, snorted into the nose, or smoked and inhaled into the lungs where it is rapidly absorbed through the respiratory epithelium. Inhalation has become popular with the availability of "crack," the crystalline form of cocaine alkaloid. Crack is cheap and produces a more intense effect because of its rapid absorption. Its onset of effect is almost immediate but lasts only 5–20 minutes (Table 3-2), creating a desire to have more frequent use to maintain the euphoric effect.
2. Cocaine toxicity results from its **intense activation of the sympathetic nervous system,** producing vasoconstriction and hypertension. This alters tissue perfusion and oxygen availability.
3. **Plasma cholinesterase activity is reduced in pregnant women, fetuses, and newborn infants, placing them at greater risk for cocaine toxicity.** Individuals, whether pregnant or not, with plasma pseudocholinesterase deficiency are at risk for sudden death with cocaine use because of limited cocaine metabolism and consequent high cocaine levels.
4. The clinical manifestations of cocaine toxicity are
   a. Hypertension
   b. Tachycardia
   c. Hyperpyrexia
   d. Seizures
   e. Cardiac arrhythmias
   f. Myocardial infarction
   g. Cerebrovascular accidents
   h. Pulmonary edema
   i. Intestinal ischemia
5. No effective chemical detoxification or replacement therapy is available for cocaine addiction. Treatment centers on abstinence and psychosocial counseling.

C. Perinatal effects

1. Maternal cocaine use produces both **maternal and fetal vasoconstriction, tach-**

Table 3-2. Cocaine: Onset and duration of effect

Route	Onset effect	Peak effect	Duration (min)
Nasal	1–5 min	20–60 min	60–75
PO	Delayed	30–90 min	60–75
IV	2–3 min	30–60 min	60–75
Smoked ("crack")	4–6 sec	8–16 sec	5–20

ycardia, and hypertension. Uterine blood flow is decreased, placental perfusion is reduced, and uteroplacental insufficiency may result.

2. Most studies have demonstrated that perinatal cocaine use is associated with increases in the following complications [23, 26–28, 31–33]:
   a. Multiple chemical use
   b. Spontaneous abortion
   c. Preterm birth
   d. Preterm labor
   e. Premature rupture of the membranes
   f. Fetal distress
   g. Fetal growth retardation manifested by reduction in birth weight, head circumference, and length
   h. Intrauterine fetal death
   i. Multiple chemical use
   j. Neonatal toxicity
   k. Infant toxicity via breast milk containing cocaine
   l. Interference with childhood growth and development
3. Several complications have been inconsistently reported to be increased with perinatal cocaine use and remain controversial.
   a. **Placental abruption** has been increased in studies where identification of cocaine use was by selective toxicology screening [20, 23, 31]. Studies that have used universal toxicology screening have not found a statistical increase in placental abruption in cocaine-positive women [3, 33]. This suggests that the association is not strong or that it may depend on other factors.
   b. **SIDS** was initially reported to occur in 15% of infants of maternal cocaine users [25]. Bauchner and colleagues [21], however, were not able to find the same effect.
   c. **Congenital anomalies** have been reported to be increased in cocaine-exposed infants [22, 30, 34]. Those most commonly reported have been gastrointestinal and urinary tract anomalies. Neither of the universal toxicology screening studies was able to demonstrate a statistically significant increase in anomalies in cocaine-exposed infants [3, 33].
   d. **Fetal cerebral infarction** has been reported in an infant exposed to a large amount of cocaine for three days prior to delivery. The etiology was presumed to be fetal cocaine effects. The frequency with which this occurs is unknown [24].

D. **Summary.** Cocaine use during pregnancy has a profound effect on perinatal outcome. The risk of prematurity is significantly increased, and fetal growth and development are compromised. The possibility of cocaine use should not be ignored in any pregnancy.

VIII. Amphetamines

A. Patterns of use

1. Amphetamines and methamphetamines are used in much the same way as cocaine. They activate the sympathetic nervous system and produce a similar type of euphoria.
2. Amphetamines are no longer used for weight control during pregnancy and as such have no prescribed indication during pregnancy.
3. There appears to be significant variation in the amount of amphetamine use throughout the United States, with greater use in the western United States. In the UCD study, it was found through universal toxicology screening that among toxicology-positive women the distribution of cocaine (45.6%) and amphetamine (35.4%) use prior to labor was essentially the same. However, amphetamine use was limited almost exclusively to white and, to a lesser extent, Hispanic women [3].

B. Toxicity

1. Amphetamine use results in **hyperactivity, insomnia, loss of appetite, and malnutrition** with prolonged use [40].
2. Significant maternal complications include **cardiac arrhythmias** and a rela-

tively rare **vasculitis** involving the cerebral, pulmonary, and renal vascular trees [38, 39].

3. **Hallucinations** may occur with high blood levels.

C. **Perinatal effects**

1. Amphetamines traverse the placenta and directly affect the fetus.
2. **Reduction in birth weight** and **growth retardation** have been reported [35–37]. The UCD study demonstrated a significant reduction in the mean birth weight (225 gm) and mean head circumference (0.8 cm) in infants of amphetamine-positive women [3].
3. Congenital anomalies, abruptio placenta, and fetal distress have not been reported as significant risks with amphetamine use.
4. **Neonatal withdrawal** occurs when there has been regular maternal use and is usually manifested as lethargy and poor feeding.

D. **Summary.** Amphetamine use presents significant maternal and fetal risks. Regular users are likely to be malnourished and have poor health care habits. The fetus is at risk for growth retardation and neonatal withdrawal. Antenatal intervention, cessation of use, and optimization of nutrition and prenatal care is the ideal treatment.

X. **Opiates.** Opiates are used because of their euphoric and sedative effects. When used on a regular basis, opiates induce an intense addiction in both mother and fetus.

A. **Patterns of use**

1. **Opiate addiction** does not appear to be increasing significantly. In the UCD study, only 6.3% of the toxicology-positive pregnancies were due to opiates [3].
2. Opiate addiction typically occurs at the end of a progression from other chemicals, such as alcohol, marijuana, cocaine, and amphetamines, which may seem more benign. Opiate addiction is also seen in conjunction with chronic illness or pain where indiscriminate prescription of narcotics can lead to dependence.
3. **Heroin** is the opiate of greatest concern. It is a street drug that is sold in uncertain concentrations, mixed with a variety of impure "cutting" agents.
4. **Methadone** is the legally available opiate that is used for treating heroin addiction either by detoxification or long-term maintenance. It is a long-acting narcotic that is taken orally once each day.
   a. **Pregnant heroin users** should be placed on methadone maintenance during pregnancy.
   b. There is no single regimen for **methadone dosing during pregnancy.** A dose of methadone is usually selected that will prevent withdrawal symptoms. That dose is either maintained for the duration of the pregnancy or it is gradually decreased to a dose of 20–40 mg/day. Daily doses of less than 30 mg are considered to be "low" doses [44].
   c. It remains controversial whether methadone detoxification is safe during pregnancy because of reports of associated premature labor and fetal distress. However, the experience with **methadone withdrawal during pregnancy** is extremely limited, and much of the information has come from uncontrolled withdrawal situations.
   d. An additional concern about antenatal detoxification has been the **high rate of recidivism** (relapse) and the use of other chemicals as withdrawal occurs.
5. **Nonheroin narcotic addiction** should be managed by detoxification or discontinuation of the narcotic during the second trimester, if possible.

B. **Toxicity**

1. **Maternal overdose** is always a possibility because of the variable concentration of heroin as it is purchased on the street. The symptoms of narcotic overdose are obtundation, respiratory depression, and pinpoint pupils. Pulmonary edema may also occur. The treatment is reversal with naloxone, a narcotic antagonist, at a dose of 0.01 mg/kg.
2. The **narcotic withdrawal or abstinence syndrome** occurs with reduction in narcotic doses sufficient to lower tissue levels and to produce withdrawal symptoms. In the milder form, these symptoms include agitation, sweating, runny nose, and tearing; in the more severe form, abdominal pain, diarrhea, uterine

contractions, and muscle pains and cramps. Although the syndrome is not life-threatening in adults, it is uncomfortable.

3. **Narcotic antagonists,** such as naloxone, and narcotics with a partial antagonist effect, such as pentazocine or Stadol and Nubaine, can precipitate withdrawal symptoms.

C. **Perinatal effects**

1. **Growth retardation** occurs in 12–45% of heroin pregnancies. It is symmetric, early-onset intrauterine growth retardation [43]. Methadone also produces growth retardation but to a lesser degree [47]. Longer periods of methadone maintenance have been associated with longer gestation and increased birth weight [43]. Higher doses of methadone have also been associated with increased head circumference. However, methadone-exposed fetuses may continue to have development problems and delays throughout childhood [46]. In the UCD study, the mean birth weight of infants of opiate-positive pregnancies (primarily heroin users) was reduced by 139 gm while the head circumference was essentially unaffected. Because the sample size was only 19 opiate-using women, this did not reach statistical significance [3].
2. **Preterm labor** has been reported to occur in 20–35% of these pregnancies. The UCD study demonstrated a preterm labor rate of 10.5% with opiate use versus 12.6% in control patients [3].
3. **SIDS** occurs with greater frequency in opiate-exposed infants. The risk is 2–4% versus 0.25% for the general population [41].
4. Opiate use has not been linked to congenital anomalies.
5. **Neonatal withdrawal syndrome** occurs in up to 95% of these infants, with 12–25% experiencing severe symptoms [42]. It is controversial whether methadone improves management of neonatal withdrawal. With methadone the symptoms appear later and may be less severe than with heroin, but the symptoms also tend to persist longer [45].

D. **Summary.** Opiate use during pregnancy carries increased risks for growth retardation, preterm labor, and neonatal withdrawal syndrome. Opiate use complicating pregnancy should be treated with referral to an appropriate chemical treatment program. For regular heroin use, methadone treatment should be started at a dose sufficient to eliminate heroin use as well as other chemicals. Discontinuation of methadone during pregnancy is controversial and potentially dangerous without experienced monitoring.

XI. **LSD.** Lysergic acid diethylamide (LSD) is a chemical hallucinogen. It does not have any conventional medical indications for use in the United States, although it has been used experimentally to treat psychiatric disorders.

A. **Patterns of use**

1. In the 1960s and 1970s, LSD was used in relatively large doses to obtain maximum hallucinogenic effects. It is now being used at smaller doses that produce less intense CNS effects.
2. LSD is ingested orally and is colorless, odorless, and tasteless. It is now commonly applied to media such as filter paper or the back of stamps, where it is both transported and ingested easily. This format makes it particularly difficult to detect, and particularly dangerous because unsuspecting individuals, particularly children, can ingest it.
3. The number or percentage of women who use LSD during pregnancy is unknown. The fact that there are few reported hallucinogenic LSD crises in pregnant women suggests that perinatal LSD use is uncommon.
4. Almost never is LSD the sole chemical used by an individual. It is most frequently used with alcohol, cigarettes, marijuana, cocaine, and amphetamines.

B. **Perinatal effects**

1. The primary maternal effect of LSD is **hallucinations.**
2. It has not been linked to complications such as preterm labor, placental abruption, or preeclampsia.
3. Chromosome damage and breakage were initially reported with LSD use [48]. A matched, controlled study of psychiatric patients treated with LSD did not

demonstrate any significant difference in chromosome abnormalities [53]. When viewed with the rest of the literature, little convincing data exist that LSD itself causes chromosome damage that has any clinical relevance [49–51].

4. Spontaneous abortion is not increased in pregnancies exposed to LSD alone [52].
5. **Congenital anomalies** have been reported from pregnancies with LSD exposure. No studies document congenital anomalies with controlled use of LSD alone. No specific pattern of distribution or type of anomalies has been described.
6. The long-term effects of perinatal LSD exposure on infant and child development are unknown.

C. Summary. The available information on the impact of perinatal LSD exposure suggests that its effects are limited. It does not appear to produce significant chromosome damage, spontaneous abortion, or congenital anomalies. However, its use during pregnancy should be discouraged.

XII. PCP. Pencyclidine (PCP) is used for its hallucinogenic properties. It is not considered to be a physically addicting chemical, but it can produce extremely dramatic psychiatric effects. In these respects it is similar to LSD.

A. Patterns of use. Few statistics are available on the use of PCP during pregnancy. It is generally not considered to be widely used among pregnant women. Golden and colleagues [54], however, reported that 0.8% of 2327 pregnant women were positive for PCP in 1984 by either testing or history, and 7.3% admitted to past use. Another study analyzed 200 cord blood samples for PCP and found that 12% were positive [56].

B. Perinatal effects

1. In adults PCP produces **perceptual changes** along with incoordination. It also blunts one's sense of pain.
2. The effect of PCP on the fetus is unknown. Its primary impact is on the **neonatal neurobehavioral status,** when it produces what appear to be similar changes to those seen in adults.
3. Pencyclidine is not generally considered to be responsible for congenital anomalies, although they have been reported [55].

C. Summary. Although PCP has not been conclusively demonstrated to be linked to fetal structural anomalies, it has been linked with abnormal infant neurologic development and function. The use of PCP should be avoided throughout pregnancy.

XIII. Organic solvents. The aromatic hydrocarbons (ARHs), a group of organic solvents, have wide industrial use. They are present as solvents or thinners in paints, glue, varnish, enamel, lacquer, and resins. They are rapidly absorbed through the skin, lungs, and gastrointestinal tract. Placental transport to the fetus occurs because of their high lipid solubility.

Toluene is the primary ARH of abuse. It conjugates to hippurate in the liver and then excretes in the urine. Confirmation of toluene use is by blood toluene or urinary hippurate levels. Toluene is detectable up to five days after use, whereas hippurate is only present for up to two days [57]. Neither is measured by standard toxicology screens.

A. Patterns of use

1. Exposure during pregnancy may occur inadvertently in the work setting by handling or inhaling ARHs. Voluntary exposure has become popular due to the psychotropic effects.
2. **Toluene** is the primary ARH for recreational use, with spray paint and glue being the most common sources. It is typically either applied to a rag and placed over the nose and mouth for inhalation or sprayed into an empty "pop top" can and inhaled [58]. This often produces a tell-tale sign of paint around the nose or mouth.
3. Toluene use has been reported to occur most commonly among Hispanics and Native Americans. The majority of toluene users are female and from very low socioeconomic levels [58, 59]. An absence of multiple chemical use may be another unique feature of toluene use [59].
4. The extent of toluene use overall and in pregnancy is unknown. Goodwin [58]

reported a total of 12 cases identified from 15,000 deliveries over a three-year period at Maricopa Medical Center in Phoenix. It is likely that voluntary toluene use is more of a regional phenomenon than other chemicals, predominating in areas with large Hispanic and Native American populations.

B. Toxicity

1. The predominant maternal effect of toluene is on the CNS, producing an **intoxication** or "high" sensation.
2. **Cardiac arrhythmias** and sudden death may occur.
3. Chronic use may result in impaired mental capabilities and ultimately **cortical atrophy and cerebellar degeneration** [62].
4. **Renal tubular acidosis** is the most dramatic component of acute maternal toluene toxicity. It is a frequent finding in toluene users [63].
   - **a.** The characteristic findings are hyperchloremic acidosis with a decreased serum bicarbonate, acidotic pH, hyperchloremia, hypokalemia, a normal anion gap, and a urine pH of 6.0 or greater.
   - **b.** This form of renal tubular acidosis is reversible with return to normal acid-base status in two to three days, although renal function may remain abnormal for several weeks.

C. Perinatal effects

1. A spectrum of fetal effects is emerging that encompasses features similar to fetal alcohol syndrome [58, 60, 61]. Specific abnormalities that have been reported include
   - **a.** Intrauterine growth retardation
   - **b.** Craniofacial abnormalities typical of FAS
   - **c.** Microcephaly
   - **d.** Hydrocephalus
   - **e.** Limb anomalies

   Goodwin and colleagues [59] described 23 children born to 10 toluene-using women with no observed congenital anomalies.
2. **Neonatal hyperchloremic metabolic acidosis,** similar to the maternal condition, occurs in infants born to women with toluene toxicity.
3. Fetal distress has not been reported with toluene toxicity despite its associated maternal and fetal metabolic acidosis.

D. Summary. Toluene exposure is a risk to both mother and fetus. Hyperchloremic metabolic acidosis occurs with toxicity in the mother, the fetus, and the newborn. It is likely that a fairly typical "fetal toluene or solvent syndrome" will emerge similar to FAS. Pregnant women should be advised to avoid organic solvents. If they must use them, it should be with good ventilation to prevent inhalation and with protection to prevent skin or mucous membrane contact.

References

1. Chasnoff, I. J. National Association for Perinatal Addiction, Research and Education press release. September, 1988.
2. Chasnoff, I. J., Landress, H. J., and Barrett, M. E. The prevalence of illicit-drug or alcohol use during pregnancy and discrepancies in mandatory reporting in Pinella County, Florida. *N. Engl. J. Med.* 322:1202, 1990.
3. Gillogley, K. M., et al. The perinatal impact of cocaine, amphetamine and opiate use detected by universal intrapartum screening. *Amer. J. Obstet. Gynecol.* 163(5):1535–1543, 1990.
4. Graham, K., et al. Determination of gestational cocaine exposure by hair analysis. *J.A.M.A.* 262:3328, 1989.
5. National Institute on Drug Abuse. *National Household Survey: 1985 Population Estimates by National Institute on Drug Abuse.* Rockville, MD: Division of Epidemiology and Statistical Analysis, U.S. Department of Health and Human Services, 1987.
6. Ostrea, E. M., et al. Drug screening of meconium in infants of drug-dependent mothers: an alternative to urine testing. *J. Pediatr.* 115(3):474, 1989.

ALCOHOL

7. Jones, K. L., Smith, D. W., and Ulleland, C. N. Patterns of malformation in offspring of alcoholic mothers. *Lancet* 1:1267–1271, 1973.
8. Ouellette, E. M., et al. Adverse effects on offspring of maternal alcohol abuse during pregnancy. *N. Engl. J. Med.* 297:528, 1977.
9. Sokol, R. J., et al. The Cleveland NIAA perspective alcohol-in-pregnancy study: The first year. *Neurobehav. Toxicol. Teratol.* 3:203, 1981.
10. Streissguth, A. P., Barr, H. M., and Martin, D. C. The effects of maternal alcohol, nicotine and caffeine use. *Alcoholism-NY* 4:152, 1980.

TOBACCO

11. Ontario Perinatal Study Committee. *Second Report of the Perinatal Mortality Study in Ten University Teaching Hospitals* (Vol. 1.) Toronto: Ontario Department of Health, 1967.
12. Simpson, W. J. A. A preliminary report on cigarette smoking and the incidence of prematurity. *Am. J. Obstet. Gynecol.* 73:808, 1957.

MARIJUANA

13. Blackard, C, and Tennes, K. Human placental transfer of cannabinoids. *N. Engl. J. Med.* 311(12):797, 1984.
14. Frank, D. A., and Zuckerman, B. S. Cocaine use during pregnancy: Prevalence and correlates. *Pediatrics* 82:888, 1988.
15. Fried, P. A., Watkinson, B., and William, A. Marijuana use during pregnancy and decreased length of gestation. *Am. J. Obstet. Gynecol.* 150:23, 1984.
16. Gibson, G. T., Baghurst, P. A., and Colley, D. P. Maternal alcohol, tobacco and cannabis consumption and the outcome of pregnancy. *Aust. N.Z. J. Obstet. Gynecol.* 23:15, 1983.
17. Hingson, R., et al. Effects of maternal drinking and marijuana use on fetal growth and development. *Pediatrics* 70:539, 1982.
18. Linn, S., et al. The association of marijuana with outcome of pregnancy. *Am. J. Public Health* 73:1161, 1983.
19. Zuckerman, B., et al. Effects of maternal marijuana and cocaine use on fetal growth. *N. Engl. J. Med.* 320:762, 1989.

COCAINE

20. Acker, D., et al. Abruptio placentae associated with cocaine use. *Am. J. Obstet. Gynecol.* 146:220, 1983.
21. Bauchner, H., et al. Risk of sudden infant death syndrome among infants with in utero exposure to cocaine. *J. Pediatr.* 113:831, 1988.
22. Chasnoff, I. J., Chisum, G. M., and Kaplan, W. E. Maternal cocaine use and genitourinary malformations. *Teratology* 37:201, 1988.
23. Chasnoff, I. J., et al. Cocaine use in pregnancy. *N. Engl. J. Med.* 313(11):666–669, 1985.
24. Chasnoff, I. J., et al. Perinatal cerebral infarction and maternal cocaine use. *J. Pediatr.* 108:456, 1986.
25. Chasnoff, I. J., et al. Prenatal cocaine exposure is associated with respiratory pattern abnormalities. *Am. J. Dis. Child.* 143:583, 1989.
26. Chasnoff, I. J., et al. Temporal patterns of cocaine use in pregnancy. *J.A.M.A.* 261:1741, 1989.
27. Chasnoff, I. J., Lewis, D. E., and Squires, L. Cocaine intoxication in a breast-fed infant. *Pediatrics* 80:836, 1987.
28. Cherukuri, R., et al. A cohort study of alkaloidal cocaine ("crack") in pregnancy. *Obstet. Gynecol.* 72:147, 1988.
29. Cregler, L. L., and Mark, H. Medical complications of cocaine abuse. *N. Engl. J. Med.* 315:1495, 1986.
30. Griffith, D. R. The Effects of Perinatal Cocaine Exposure on Infant Neurobehavior and Early Maternal-Infant Interactions. In I. J. Chasnoff (ed.), *Drugs, Alcohol, Pregnancy and Parenting*. Boston: Kluwer, 1988. Pp. 105–113.

31. Keith, L. G., et al. Substance abuse in pregnant women: Recent experience at the Perinatal Center for Chemical Dependency of Northwestern Memorial Hospital. *Obstet. Gynecol.* 73:7151, 1989.
32. MacGregor, S. N., et al. Cocaine use during pregnancy: Adverse perinatal outcome. *Am. J. Obstet. Gynecol.* 157:686, 1987.
33. Neerhof, M. G., et al. Cocaine abuse during pregnancy: Peripartum prevalence and perinatal outcome. *Am. J. Obstet. Gynecol.* 161:633, 1989.
34. Urogenital anomalies in the offspring of women using cocaine during early pregnancy—Atlanta, 1968–80. *M.M.W.R.* 38(31):536, 1989.

AMPHETAMINES

35. Ericksson, M., Larsson, G., and Zetterstrom, R. Amphetamine addiction and pregnancy. *Acta Obstet. Gynecol. Scand.* 60:253, 1981.
36. Larrson, G. The amphetamine addicted mother and her child. *Acta Paediatr. Scand.* [Suppl.]278:6, 1980.
37. Naeye, R. L. Maternal use of dextroamphetamine and growth of the fetus. *Pharmacology* 129:637, 1977.
38. Rodger, B. D., and Lee, R. V. Drug Abuse. In G. N. Burrows and T. F. Ferris (eds.), *Medical Complications During Pregnancy.* Philadelphia: Saunders, 1988. P. 570.
39. Samuels, S. I., Maze, A., and Albright, G. Cardiac arrest during cesarean section in a chronic amphetamine abuser. *Anesth. Analg.* 58:528, 1979.
40. Sussman, S. Narcotic and methamphetamine use during pregnancy. *Am. J. Dis. Child.* 106:457, 1973.

OPIATES

41. Chavez, C. J., et al. Sudden infant death syndrome among infants of drug-dependent mothers. *J. Pediatr.* 95:407, 1979.
42. Connaughton, J. F., et al. Perinatal addiction: Outcome and management. *Am. J. Obstet. Gynecol.* 129:679, 1977.
43. Doberczak, T. M., et al. Impact of maternal drug dependency on birth weight and head circumference of offspring. *Am. J. Dis. Child.* 141:1163, 1987.
44. Finnegan, L. P. (ed.). *Drug Dependence in Pregnancy: Clinical Management of Mother and Child.* National Institute on Drug Abuse, Services Research Monograph Series. Rockville, Md.: U.S. Government Printing Office, 1980. P. 37.
45. Kandall, S. R., and Gartner, L. M. Late presentation of drug withdrawal symptoms in newborns. *Am. J. Dis. Child.* 127:58, 1974.
46. Rosen, T. S., and Johnson, H. L. Children of methadone maintained mother. Follow-up to 18 months of age. *J. Pediatr.* 101:192, 1982.
47. Zelson, C., Lee, S. J., and Casalino, M. Neonatal narcotic addiction. *N. Engl. J. Med.* 289:1216, 1973.

LSD

48. Cohen, M. M., Marinello, M. J., and Back, N. Chromosomal damage in human leukocytes induced by lysergic acid diethylamide. *Science* 155:1417–1419, 1967.
49. Dishotsky, N. I., et al. LSD and genetic damage: Is LSD chromosome damaging, carcinogenic, mutagenic, or teratogenic? *Science* 172:431–440, 1971.
50. Long, S. Y. Does LSD induce chromosomal damage and malformations? A review of the literature. *Teratology* 6:75–90, 1972.
51. Matsuyama, S. S., and Jarvik, L. F. Cytogenetic effects of psychoactive drugs. *Mod. Probl. Pharmacopsychiatry* 10:99–132, 1975.
52. McGlothlin, W. H., Sparkes, R. S., and Arnold, D. O. Effect of LSD on human pregnancy. *J.A.M.A.* 212:1483–1487, 1970.
53. Robinson, J. T., et al. Chromosome aberrations and LSD: A controlled study in 50 psychiatric patients. *Br. J. Psychiatry* 125:238–244, 1974.

PCP

54. Golden, N. L., et al. Pencyclidine use during pregnancy. *Am. J. Obstet. Gynecol.* 148:254, 1984.

55. Golden, N. L., Sokol, R. J., and Rubin, I. L. Angel dust: possible effects on the fetus. *Pediatrics* 65:18, 1980.
56. Kautman, K. R., et al. Pencyclidine in umbilical cord blood: preliminary data. *Am. J. Psychiatry* 140:450, 1983.

ORGANIC SOLVENTS

57. Brugone, F., et al. Decline of blood and alveolar toluene concentration following two accidental human poisonings. *Int. Arch. Occup. Environ. Health* 53:157, 1983.
58. Goodwin, T. M. Toluene abuse and renal tubular acidosis in pregnancy. *Obstet. Gynecol.* 71:715, 1988.
59. Goodwin, J. M., et al. Inhalant abuse, pregnancy and neglected children. *Am. J. Psychiatry* 138:1126, 1981.
60. Hersh, J. H., et al. Toluene embryopathy. *J. Pediatr.* 106:922, 1985.
61. Holmberg, P. C. Central nervous system defects in children born to mothers exposed to organic solvents during pregnancy. *Lancet* 2(8135):177, 1979.
62. King, M. D. Neurological sequelae of toluene abuse. *Hum. Toxicol.* 1:281, 1982.
63. Taher, M. B., et al. Renal tubular acidosis associated with toluene "sniffing." *N. Engl. J. Med.* 290:104, 1974.

4 Cardiovascular Complications

Michael P. Nageotte

Pregnancy is normally accompanied by several significant physiologic changes in the maternal cardiovascular system. These include changes in blood volume, cardiac output, pulse, blood pressure, and peripheral vascular resistance. In the vast majority of pregnancies, these changes pose no significant threat and are well tolerated. Even in women with preexisting rheumatic heart disease and most forms of congenital heart disease, the attendant physiologic changes of pregnancy do not result in a significant threat to maternal or fetal well-being. However, certain patients will experience a sudden decompensation of cardiac function during pregnancy. Included in this group are patients with well-diagnosed cardiac dysfunction as well as patients who demonstrate for the first time during pregnancy decompensation owing to underlying cardiac problems. It is very important for those rendering care to pregnant women to have a clear understanding of the normal changes in pregnancy, so that the care givers can correctly manage normal complaints as well as recognize, as early as possible, those symptoms that suggest significant underlying cardiac dysfunction.

I. Physiologic changes during pregnancy

A. Blood volume. A dramatic increase in maternal circulating blood volume occurs during pregnancy. The average increase is between 40 and 50% above the nonpregnant state, with the alterations in blood volume beginning as early as the sixth week of gestation. The rise in blood flow/volume occurs at a rapid rate until approximately the twentieth to the twenty-fourth week of gestation, with a subsequent slower but steady rise until a plateau is reached late in the third trimester. Some controversy remains as to whether blood flow continues to rise until term. Most recent investigations would suggest that, in fact, a leveling off occurs prior to 40 weeks' gestation [24]. Changes in blood volume appear to be of a greater magnitude in multigravida patients as well as in women with multiple gestations. Because plasma volume increases more than red blood cell mass, a relative hemodilution normally occurs during the pregnant state. This results in a fall in hematocrit despite an absolute increase in red blood cell mass.

B. Cardiac output. Cardiac output increases during pregnancy, with a maximum rise of approximately 40% above the nonpregnant level, slightly less than the increase in blood volume. This change in cardiac output begins very early in pregnancy, possibly as early as the tenth week of gestation. Cardiac output appears to continue to rise, at least until the thirty-eighth gestational week, with a subsequent fall that is not positionally related. Maternal position directly influences cardiac output, with maximum output being observed in the left lateral decubitus position. With the patient in the supine position, the enlarging uterus can completely occlude the inferior vena cava, particularly in the third trimester. This results in a fall in cardiac output owing to decreased venous return. Cardiac output is the product of heart rate times the stroke volume, and both of these components have been studied to assess their relative contributions to the observed rise in cardiac output.

1. Heart rate. The heart rate rises progressively during pregnancy and appears to be more responsible than stroke volume for maintaining cardiac output. As the heart rate increases, the stroke volume decreases to nonpregnant values [24].

2. **Stroke volume.** The stroke volume usually rises approximately 30–40% until the end of the second trimester. A fall in stroke volume is normally observed during the third trimester.

C. **Blood pressure and systemic vascular resistance.** Both maternal blood pressure and systemic vascular resistance decrease during normal pregnancy. Mean arterial blood pressure declines until midpregnancy, and then, during the third trimester, it rises toward prepregnancy levels. The decrease in peripheral vascular resistance is the major cause for this observed drop in blood pressure, with a diastolic pressure showing the more marked change. During pregnancy, there appears to be a decreased sensitivity of vascular responsiveness to angiotensin II [10], which may be a leading reason for these observed changes in blood pressure. Renin and angiotensin levels are increased during pregnancy.

II. Diagnostic tests

A. **Chest roentgenography.** No characteristic roentgenographic changes can be attributed solely to pregnancy, and each "abnormality" must be viewed on an individual basis. These include straightening of the left heart border, which can be noted during normal pregnancy but may also indicate left atrial enlargement. Pulmonary artery prominence may be due to lordotic posturing during normal pregnancy or it may be secondary to pulmonary hypertension. Azygous vein enlargement may be normal or may be secondary to central venous pressure elevation. Screening chest roentgenograms are of no value as a routine procedure in pregnancy. When indicated, it is important to use appropriate abdominal shielding to minimize the risks of radiation exposure to the fetus.

B. **Electrocardiography.** Although a useful tool in the evaluation of suspected cardiac disease, the electrocardiogram (ECG) may be misleading during pregnancy. Transient ST segment and T wave changes are of no apparent significance; neither is the left axis shift of the QRS complex, with all of these changes having been frequently described in pregnancy. Several different kinds of arrhythmias have been described during pregnancy, including paroxysmal supraventricular tachycardia, premature atrial and ventricular beats, sinus bradycardia, sinus tachycardia, and wandering atrial pacemaker [14, 26]. In an asymptomatic patient there is usually no need to treat these findings.

C. **Echocardiography.** A noninvasive test, echocardiography represents the single most significant advance in recent years for the evaluation of heart disease in pregnancy. The different types used are the basic M-mode, two-dimensional echocardiography, and the Doppler technique using color-flow. The M-mode (motion-mode) technique displays the intensity of reflected ultrasonic beams versus time on an oscilloscope. Two-dimensional echocardiography adds the ability of detecting spacial anatomy. The Doppler principle is applied in the third technique in which ultrasound reflected from a moving target will have frequency shifts directly related to the velocity of red blood cell movement. This allows for visualization of cardiac anatomy as well as measurement of flow velocity. Use of the echocardiogram has revolutionized our ability to detect anatomic abnormalities within the heart as well as to obtain reliable assessments of cardiac performance. The addition of color-flow Doppler has further improved the accuracy of this modality.

III. Intrapartum cardiovascular changes

A. **Cardiac output.** Cardiac output increases during labor, particularly during the second stage and immediately post partum. These changes are exacerbated in the absence of adequate analgesia or anesthesia. Presumably due to catecholamine release, increased mean arterial blood pressure is noted intrapartum in these patients. Changes in vital signs can be minimized by placing the patient in the left lateral decubitus position and, particularly in the cardiac patient, by appropriate use of conduction anesthesia.

In the immediate postpartum period, cardiac output has been observed to double secondary to removal of venal caval compression and autotransfusion resulting from the decrease in uterine size [13]. This lasts for varying lengths of time, but there is usually rapid return to a minimally increased cardiac output in the days that follow delivery. A decreased heart rate is noted in many patients intrapartum. This is believed to be a reflex bradycardia secondary to the elevations in blood pressure. In a patient who has persistent tachycardia, particularly after delivery, or in a patient who is already known to be volume depleted, as in preeclampsia, tachycardia is most likely to result if fluid or blood is lost. Careful monitoring of patients with these changes by invasive cardiovascular techniques may be indicated, particularly in a patient with underlying cardiac disease. In parallel with the increases in cardiac output during labor and immediately post partum, the stroke volume usually increases.

B. **Blood volume.** Secondary to the normal blood loss of delivery, blood volume decreases immediately post partum. This does not usually pose a problem to the patient as there is an increased blood volume during pregnancy as well as a discontinued significant arteriovenous shunt following delivery of the placenta. Venous return is increased as a result of removal of obstruction from the large uterus and autotransfusion from uterine contraction.

IV. **Management of cardiac disease**

A. **Diagnosis**

1. **Symptoms.** In many pregnant patients who are free of any underlying cardiac abnormalities, shortness of breath, lightheadedness, syncope, chest pains, and palpitations are common complaints. Abnormalities may be noted in the ECG and chest roentgenogram. It is important to have a high level of suspicion when these complaints are heard from patients with known or suspected underlying cardiac disease as they may reflect heart failure. Symptoms of particular note include worsening shortness of breath, postural syncope, and chest pain, all of which must be specifically elevated.
2. **Signs.** Signs that are suggestive of underlying cardiac disease include jugular venous distention, peripheral cyanosis, clubbing, a harsh systolic flow murmur, or any diastolic murmur.

B. **Management**

1. **Appropriate evaluation** is of significant importance as early as possible during the pregnant state. This includes referral to a tertiary care center where specific diagnostic or therapeutic procedures are more readily available.
2. A team including a perinatologist in close consultation with a cardiologist, pediatrician, nursing personnel, and an anesthesiologist interested and experienced in the management of heart disease in pregnancy is of crucial importance.
3. **Counseling and education** of a highly motivated patient make for easier management and decision making, especially in those cases where life-threatening decisions must be made.
4. **Minimization of cardiac work** in patients with underlying heart disease is particularly important in the pregnant state. Maternal anxiety must be alleviated with constant reassurance and understanding of maternal status. Protracted periods of relative or absolute bed rest may also be necessary for many pregnant patients with underlying heart disease. Especially in patients with mitral stenosis, strict bed rest should be the rule.
5. As in any patient who is pregnant, **diet** plays an important role in the management scheme of the pregnant cardiac patient. A weight gain of 20–25 lb is thought to be a reasonable goal, and a well-balanced diet is encouraged. The only adjustment specific to the cardiac patient would be limiting the sodium intake to 2 gm/day. Positive sodium balance is necessary for both the patient and her growing fetal-placental unit, and, therefore, restricting sodium intake further is not recommended. However, in a patient with congestive heart failure, significant salt restriction is indicated. As in normal pregnancy, iron and calcium supplementation along with folic acid replacement is necessary, particularly after the first trimester.
6. Although rare, **infective endocarditis** in pregnancy imposes important management problems. Usually owing to the existence of underlying cardiac abnormality, most often secondary to rheumatic heart disease, endocarditis may lead to rapid deterioration of clinical status during pregnancy as a result of the increased demands on previously damaged cardiac valves. Aggressive med-

ical and surgical management is crucial in patients with infective endocarditis during pregnancy; maternal mortality has been cited to be between 15 and 30% [9, 18, 28].

The appropriate use of prophylactic antibiotics is imperative to avoid this complication. Although the efficacy of antibiotic prophylaxis against bacterial endocarditis has not been proved in pregnancy, the recommendation of the American Heart Association should be followed in the pregnant as well as in the nonpregnant patient. To prevent the recurrence of endocarditis, women with a history of at least one attack of rheumatic fever should maintain an antibiotic dosage schedule as in the nonpregnant state. During periods of potential bacteremia, patients with increased susceptibility to bacterial endocarditis should receive antibiotic prophylaxis [32]. Among these would be patients with underlying cardiac lesions who are undergoing dental extractions and urologic procedures. With respect to uncomplicated vaginal delivery, the issue of bacteremia leading to endocarditis is debated. The reported incidence of bacteremia leading to endocarditis is exceedingly low [1]. Routine use of antibiotic prophylaxis is recommended only for uncomplicated vaginal deliveries in patients with prosthetic heart valves. For complicated deliveries or cesarean sections, antibiotics should be instituted after the active phase of labor has begun. The recommended treatment is ampicillin, 2 gm IV, in addition to gentamicin, 1.5 mg/kg IV or IM, given 1 hour before delivery and repeated once 8 hours post partum [19]. For the patient who is allergic to penicillin, 1 gm of vancomycin is infused over 30–60 minutes along with the gentamicin schedule.

7. Prior to conception, **rubella immunization** should be sought in all women. In women with heart disease, immunization against influenza and pneumococcal infections should be considered also.
8. As in any patient at risk for intrauterine growth retardation, patients with certain cardiac lesions should undergo **routine antepartum monitoring** in the form of nonstress tests or contraction stress tests or biophysical profile. These patients would include those with uncorrected cyanotic congenital heart disease or class III or IV cardiac status. Additionally, serial ultrasonography to follow growth parameters is indicated.
9. **Intrapartum monitoring** is extremely important, since during this period the patient with underlying cardiac disease is at her greatest risk. Approximately two-thirds of recorded maternal deaths in patients with heart disease occur intrapartum or immediately post partum, presumably owing to the changes in cardiac parameters previously described [23]. Coordination of the obstetric, medical, and anesthesia personnel on the management team is vital to maximize outcome.

V. Medical management of cardiac disease during pregnancy

A. Digitalis preparations. Digitalis glycosides are steroid compounds used extensively for the treatment of congestive heart failure as well as various supraventricular arrhythmias. As a result of their positive inotropic and chronotropic effects and their antiarrhythmic properties resulting from slowing of conduction through the atrioventricular node, digitalis preparations have many indications for use. Digoxin is the most commonly used preparation. Accumulated experience over many years has provided evidence that digitalis preparations are very safe for use in pregnancy [6]. Although there is much controversy as to how much digitalis crosses the placenta, no evidence exists of any harmful fetal effects. It should be kept in mind that because of the expansion of maternal blood volume and the increased glomerular filtration rate during pregnancy, an increased dosage of digoxin often will be necessary to maintain therapeutic serum levels as pregnancy progresses. This can be accomplished by dosage adjustment, with the desired therapeutic concentration in maternal serum being between 1 and 2 μg/ml. Daily doses between 0.5 and 1.0 mg are not unusual.

B. Beta-agonists. Both the myocardium and the myometrium possess alpha-adrenergic and beta-adrenergic receptors. The smooth muscle of the uterus contracts in response to the alpha-adrenergic stimulation and relaxes with beta-adrenergic stimulation. Secondary uterine effects should be considered in patients treated with cardiac medications that result in either type of stimulation. Likewise, women taking beta-agonists for complications of pregnancy such as premature labor may experience secondary but significant cardiac effects. The myocardium is believed to have primarily beta-1-receptors, whereas the myometrium has primarily beta-2-receptors. Stimulation of beta-1-receptors results in increased heart rate, whereas stimulation of beta-2-receptors results in myometrial relaxation. Additional side effects noted with beta-1-receptor stimulation are widening of pulse pressure and a decrease in serum potassium, with an influx of potassium into the cell from the serum. Complications including pulmonary edema, myocardial ischemia, and maternal death have been reported in mothers exposed to beta-agonists for treatment of premature labor. Women with underlying heart disease possess an absolute contraindication to treatment with beta-agonists for tocolysis.

C. **Beta-antagonists.** Beta-blockers are widely used in medicine for treatment of migraine headaches, hyperthyroidism, various arrhythmias, and systemic hypertension. There is controversy regarding the safety of beta-blockers in pregnancy. Propranolol has been demonstrated in animal models to lower umbilical blood flow [4]. Reports of an increased incidence of growth retardation, delayed neonatal respirations, bradycardia, hypoglycemia, and blunting of accelerations of the fetal heart rate intrapartum have all been described in patients receiving beta-blocker therapy for various indications during pregnancy [20]. Whether this phenomenon is dose related or caused by the underlying disease for which the therapy is indicated is unclear. No evidence exists to suggest that beta-blockers are teratogenic, and recent reports support their use for pregnant patients with hypertension [3].

D. **Anticoagulants.** Patients requiring anticoagulation during pregnancy because of underlying cardiac abnormalities or concurrent thromboembolic phenomena pose a particular problem. A number of complications in both mother and fetus have been demonstrated with warfarin derivatives, and particularly in the first and third trimesters of pregnancy, coumarin derivatives are contraindicated. Heparin has been shown to be an effective prophylactic as well as therapeutic agent, and because of its molecular weight and large anionic charge, it does not cross the placenta in any measurable amount. Consequently, it is the drug of choice during pregnancy when anticoagulation is indicated.

E. **Diuretics.** Diuretic therapy should be avoided during pregnancy unless treatment of congestive heart failure is necessary. Studies suggest that maternal plasma volume depletion will result in impaired fetal growth. In addition, there have been reports of fetal hyponatremia, hypokalemia, jaundice, thrombocytopenia, and acute maternal hemorrhagic pancreatitis associated with the maternal ingestion of thiazide diuretics during pregnancy [5].

F. **Antiarrhythmic drugs.** Arrhythmias otherwise treated with atropine, quinidine, or procainamide should be so treated during pregnancy without fear of adverse reaction to the fetus or newborn. Phenytoin should be avoided whenever possible, particularly in early pregnancy, because of the reported fetal hydantoin syndrome that occurs in approximately 10% of fetuses chronically exposed to this drug [16]. Lidocaine readily crosses the placenta and has been reported to increase uterine tone and decrease uterine blood flow when used as an anesthetic agent in a paracervical block. Fetal bradycardia, either secondary to direct myocardial suppression or secondary to changes in uterine perfusion and tone, has also been reported acutely [17]. There is no evidence of a teratogenic potential with lidocaine, and so it can be safely administered in pregnancy as the drug of choice for certain acute ventricular tachyarrhythmias.

G. **Calcium channel blockers.** Calcium channel blockers are newer agents with demonstrated efficacy in the treatment of hypertension, angina pectoris, and tachyarrhythmias. There is a paucity of large controlled studies on the use of these agents in pregnancy, and so many practitioners are reluctant to use them because of possible side effects on mother and fetus. Verapamil has been reported to be successful in the transplacental cardioversion of fetal paroxysmal atrial tachycardia.

H. Electrical cardioversion. Although experience with this technique is limited, transthoracic electrical cardioversion has been reported to have been successfully and safely performed in all three trimesters of pregnancy [27]. The issue of potential fetal complications must be considered, however. One concern is the possible provocation of fetal ventricular fibrillation, since the current discharge on the cardioverter is synchronized to the R wave of the ECG of the mother and not of the fetus. The risk of this complication is believed to be small, because the amount of energy reaching the fetal heart is minuscule and the fetal heart appears to have a higher threshold for fibrillation.

VI. Cardiac surgery. Cardiac surgery during pregnancy rarely is indicated and, other than as a lifesaving measure, should be avoided if possible. Aggressive medical management is preferable; the vast majority of pregnant women with rheumatic heart disease, coronary artery insufficiency, or congenital heart lesions can be managed medically. Although maternal mortality does not appear to be significantly increased with surgical procedures during pregnancy, there does appear to be an increase in fetal mortality, particularly if cardiopulmonary bypass is required [2].

A. Mitral stenosis. Extensive experience has been gained with closed cardiac surgery of the mitral valve (mitral valvotomy) in all stages of pregnancy. This operative procedure does not appear to increase the risk of fetal loss, and the indications for it are the same as in the nonpregnant state, including sudden intractable pulmonary edema resistant to aggressive medical therapy. Profuse uncontrollable hemoptysis is another indication for emergency mitral valvotomy. However, it is best to perform valvular surgery, either closed or open, as an elective procedure in the nonpregnant patient. Careful management of women with a history of cardiac or pulmonary failure, thromboembolism or atrial fibrillation, and fixed valvular stenosis can prevent the need for surgery during the pregnant state. Fetal mortality as a complication of open heart surgery has been reported to be between 30 and 50%.

B. Coronary artery bypass surgery. Coronary artery bypass surgery has been performed during pregnancy but rarely is necessary in women who are pregnant. In most reports, pregnant women who were operated on for coronary artery bypass were not known to be pregnant at the time of surgery.

VII. Intrapartum and postpartum management

A. Premature intervention for patients with underlying cardiac disease is rarely necessary in the absence of clinical decompensation. Spontaneous labor at term in a controlled setting is preferable, and elective cesarean section is rarely indicated other than for obstetric indications. However, patients with severe aortic stenosis, complicated coarctation of the aorta with hypertension, pulmonary hypertension secondary to Eisenmenger's complex, primary pulmonary hypertension, severe mitral stenosis, or patients with congestive heart failure and an uninducible cervix are ones for whom primary cesarean section should be strongly considered.

B. Choice of anesthesia depends on the underlying cardiac lesion and the skill and experience of the anesthesiologist involved in the patient's care. Balanced general anesthesia or epidural anesthesia is best tolerated, but a clear understanding of the physiology of the specific cardiac abnormality is crucially important [31]. The avoidance of hypertension with induction of general anesthesia and the avoidance of hypotension with activation of a conduction anesthetic are goals that must be considered in the selection of anesthesia. Patient comfort during labor is important so that catecholamine release and increased demands on the heart intrapartum can be minimized. Shortening the second stage of labor by employing forceps deliveries when it is obstetrically safe is to be considered. This allows for avoidance of the maternal Valsalva maneuver, which results in major cardiovascular changes.

C. Monitoring of both fetus and mother during labor and delivery is vital. As already discussed, intrapartum monitoring in the form of an internal electrode and uterine pressure catheter is indicated during labor. In addition, pulmonary artery catheterization to allow for measurement of pulmonary artery wedge pressure, cardiac output, and central venous pressure is strongly encouraged. Placement of an arterial line should also be considered, particularly in the patient undergoing a surgical delivery.

D. **Careful monitoring in the postpartum state** is also important, as marked changes in cardiac output occur during this time. Indeed, this is a high-risk period in the case of many cardiac lesions, and an increased incidence of maternal deaths have been reported post partum. This is particularly true in patients with pulmonary hypertension who can suddenly decompensate owing to an increase in right-to-left shunt with resultant hypoxia and cardiac arrhythmia.

E. **Early ambulation and breast-feeding** should be encouraged unless otherwise contraindicated. Close monitoring for a longer period of time in the postpartum state is indicated for cardiac patients as opposed to the uncomplicated parturient, owing to the increased risk of cardiac failure, endocarditis, and thromboembolism.

VIII. **Cardiac lesions associated with significant risk of maternal-fetal mortality.** In discussing risks of maternal intolerance to pregnancy, it is helpful to have a knowledge not only of the specific cardiac lesions present but also of the functional classification of the patient. Although the latter is not entirely predictive, the intrinsic risk to the patient depends on the functional impairment as reflected by the New York Heart Association's classification. Patients in classes III and IV are at particularly high risk for complications during pregnancy. The classifications are as follows:

Class I Asymptomatic
Class II Symptomatic with heavy exercise
Class III Symptomatic with light exercise
Class IV Symptomatic at rest

A. **Eisenmenger's complex.** Defined as pulmonary hypertension at systemic levels owing to high pulmonary vascular resistance and a reversal of bidirectional shunt at the aortopulmonary, ventricular, or atrial level, Eisenmenger's complex poses a particular risk during pregnancy. Maternal mortality approaching 50% has been reported with this disorder during pregnancy, the presumable causes being pulmonary infarction, brain abscess, congestive heart failure, and a sudden arrhythmia [11]. Frequently, the terminal event is irreversible cardiopulmonary collapse during labor and delivery or immediately post partum. Believed to be caused by the alteration of the delicate balance between the pulmonary and systemic vascular compartments, the blood loss associated with delivery may result in an acute reversal of left-to-right shunt. Hypoxia rapidly results in further pulmonary vasoconstriction in response to this change. This in turn worsens the shunt from right to left, with an irreversible vicious cycle leading ultimately and unavoidably to death. Additionally, these patients appear to be at increased risk for pulmonary embolism, which could result in an increased pulmonary vascular resistance. Pregnancy is strongly contraindicated in these patients. However, early elective pregnancy termination has reported maternal morbidity and mortality [11]. Management of these patients includes protracted hospitalization, supplemental oxygen therapy, and prophylactic anticoagulation in the antepartum period. Skilled aggressive cardiovascular monitoring is crucially important throughout the intrapartum and postpartum periods, and therapeutic anticoagulation should be strongly considered after delivery.

B. **Primary pulmonary hypertension.** The exact etiology of primary pulmonary hypertension, which predominantly affects young women, is unclear. It is probably not entirely accurate to consider this disorder in the general category of congenital heart disease, but the natural course of the disease terminates either by sudden death or by the development of intractable congestive heart failure resistant to therapy. Maternal mortality with primary pulmonary hypertension approaches 50%. The underlying physiologic alteration is elevated pulmonary vascular resistance secondary to thickening of the walls of the pulmonary arteries, with fibrosis of the intima and fibroelastosis. There is no underlying congenital heart defect, although an enlarged right ventricle and normal to small left ventricle are often discovered. This disease is reported in increased numbers in patients with Raynaud's phenomenon and as a reaction to certain drugs, as well as in familial patterns suggestive of autosomal dominant inheritance [12, 29]. Pregnancy is contraindicated in patients with this disease, and pregnancy termination should be strongly encouraged as early as possible. Patients who refuse therapeutic abortion should be hospitalized by no later than 20 weeks' gestation and aggressively managed. Employment of bed rest, anticoagulation, and supplemental oxygen therapy is also recommended.

C. **Coarctation of the aorta.** Although rarely seen because of aggressive early surgical intervention by pediatric cardiologists and cardiovascular surgeons, coarctation of the aorta can pose an increased risk of maternal mortality during pregnancy. Secondary to the narrowing of lumina of the aorta, usually just distal to the origin of the left subclavian artery near the insertion of the ligamentum arteriosum, an increased resistance to left ventricular outflow causes a decrease of blood flow to the lower extremities. Hypertension in the upper extremities with absence or near-absence of pulse of the lower extremities is a classic sign. Concerns during pregnancy include long-standing hypertension, aortic rupture secondary to dissection, central nervous system bleeding secondary to rupture of berry aneurysms, and congestive heart failure secondary to left ventricular dysfunction. Surprisingly, fetal growth and outcome as well as the incidence of preeclampsia do not appear to be worsened in patients with coarctation of the aorta. Early reports suggest that pregnancy is particularly high risk for the patients, with cesarean section being the recommended delivery route, but no effort was made to separate complicated from uncomplicated coarctation [15]. A complicated coarctation occurs when the aortic narrowing is associated with other congenital cardiac anomalies. These include bicuspid aortic valve, abnormalities of the mitral valve, patent ductus arteriosus, ventricular septal defect, and mitral insufficiency. Overall, patients with complicated coarctation have a significantly shorter life expectancy and poorer pregnancy outcome than those patients with uncomplicated or surgically repaired lesions. However, even in patients with uncomplicated coarctation, long-standing hypertension may lead to left ventricular dysfunction and cardiac failure during pregnancy. Additionally, the unresolved issue remains of whether the risk of aortic dissection is increased during pregnancy owing to the reported changes in the vessel walls that naturally occur in the pregnant state.

D. **Marfan's syndrome.** An autosomal dominant condition in which an error in protein metabolism results in abnormalities in the structure of collagen and elastin, Marfan's syndrome has been associated with increased maternal mortality. Although any organ may be involved, death usually results from cardiac or great vessel complications. Mitral valve prolapse is the most common cardiac lesion, but dilatation of the ascending aorta with involvement of the aortic root sinuses probably is more important with respect to maternal mortality. The underlying defect appears to be cystic degeneration of the media of the vessel walls, and this process may be accelerated during pregnancy by estrogen-induced changes. Additionally, increased cardiac output and widened pulse pressure normally occur during pregnancy. Although maternal mortality as high as 50% has been reported in women with Marfan's syndrome, more recent reports suggest that the outcome of pregnancy is not so grim [21]. It is suggested that aortic dilatation greater than 40 mm, demonstrated by echocardiogram, would indicate a patient in a high-risk category for aortic dissection, one for whom pregnancy termination is indicated. Management of Marfan's syndrome during pregnancy involves controlling cardiac output with the use of beta-blockers. Initially during the intrapartum period, the patient should be kept in the left lateral decubitus position, and conduction anesthesia should be employed. Avoidance of a bearing-down effort and the use of forceps in the second stage of labor are also indicated. Prophylactic antibiotics are definitely indicated.

E. **Tetralogy of Fallot.** The tetralogy of Fallot represents 5% of cardiac malformations present at birth and is the most common cyanotic condition to extend beyond infancy. It is a combination of pulmonary stenosis with a large ventricular septal defect, dextroposition of the aorta, and right ventricular hypertrophy. The basic physiologic lesion is pulmonary stenosis with right-to-left shunt at the ventricular level that results in cyanosis. Mean age at death is 12–15 years without surgical correction. However, corrected tetralogy of Fallot has resulted in a substantial proportion of these patients surviving to childbearing age. In patients in whom tetralogy of Fallot has not been corrected and who successfully conceive, further cyanosis results from an increase in the right-to-left shunt through the ventricular septal defect as a consequence of the decreased peripheral vascular resistance during pregnancy. The major prognostic factor in relating to pregnancy outcome is the degree of cyanosis. The prognosis is much poorer in patients with recurring syncopal episodes, a hematocrit elevated above 60%, right ventricular hypertrophy, or arterial oxygen saturation of less than 80%. However, patients in whom tetralogy of Fallot has been corrected and who no longer have any cyanosis have very successful outcomes. In patients with persistent cyanosis, intrauterine growth retardation is also a concern, with fetal survival only approximately 40% if the mother has had no prior surgery.

F. Hypertrophic cardiomyopathy. Also known as *asymmetric septal hypertrophy* or *idiopathic hypertrophic subaortic stenosis,* hypertrophic cardiomyopathy is a condition in which hypertrophy of the left ventricle and, occasionally, of the right ventricle, is unexplained. Typically, it involves the septum more than the free wall of the left ventricle, and left ventricular outflow is impeded. Inherited usually as an autosomal dominant gene, this disease has a very wide degree of penetrance, and indeed, seemingly sporadic cases occur. Death is usually sudden and may occur at a young age. It is believed to be secondary to a sudden arrhythmia or tachycardia, but no specific symptomatology precedes death. Pregnancy is usually well tolerated in patients with this abnormality, although fatalities have been reported [22]. Diagnosis can be well established using echocardiography; more invasive studies such as cardiac catheterization are not recommended. All dyspnea-related symptoms in pregnancy must be carefully evaluated, and beta-blocker therapy should be used for relief of obstruction. Arrhythmia, if present, should be appropriately treated, and fetal assessment should be followed with serial echograms, particularly in patients on beta-blocker therapy. Beta-mimetic tocolytic therapy in these patients is absolutely contraindicated. This is because use of these agents further aggravates ventricular outflow obstruction. Magnesium sulfate is probably a safer drug. The use of epidural anesthesia is believed to be inadvisable owing to the risk of a sudden decrease in afterload and venous return to the heart if hypotension inadvertently occurs. In this situation, sudden decompensation of the cardiac condition is possible.

G. Mitral stenosis. Rheumatic heart disease in general has been decreasing in both incidence and frequency over the past few decades. This changing trend has correlated best with the widespread use of antibiotics that are effective against streptococcus, along with improved rheumatic fever prophylaxis. Despite this change, however, rheumatic heart disease remains the predominant form of cardiac disease in pregnant women, accounting for 75–80% of all cases. Of the cases of rheumatic heart disease in pregnancy, close to 70% are mitral stenosis. Patients with mitral stenosis are at risk for developing complications during pregnancy. Those who are at highest risk have New York Heart Association class III or IV impairment. However, maternal deaths have also been reported in patients with mitral stenosis who had prepregnancy New York Heart Association class I or II impairment. The danger is secondary to the physiologic changes that normally occur during pregnancy. These include a rise in heart rate and a general increased demand on the heart. The rate of flow across the mitral valve must be increased to accommodate the increased cardiac output; this is accomplished by a rise in pressure of the left atrium. Depending on the degree of obstruction of blood flow from the left atrium to the left ventricle during diastole, increased pressure in the left atrium and pulmonary vessels will vary. Acute pulmonary edema will result when this pressure exceeds 25 mm Hg. Indeed, pulmonary edema will often occur for the first time during pregnancy at the peak of cardiac demand or during a time of stress from anxiety, labor, exercise, or infection. Atrial fibrillation is another complication of mitral stenosis, which results in the inefficient movement of blood across the mitral valve during diastole in addition to the increased risk for arterial embolization. Aggressive management of pulmonary edema includes the use of diuretics, intravenous morphine sulfate, rotating tourniquets, and the control of heart rate with digitalis. Atrial fibrillation occurring during pregnancy is a poor prognostic sign. Control with digitalis, quinidine, or electrical cardioversion, and appropriate employment of anticoagulant prophylaxis with heparin are indicated for both acute and chronic management of atrial fibrillation in pregnancy. Intrapartum management includes use of conduction anesthesia with delivery in the Sims' position to maintain cardiac output and attempt to minimize added stresses on the heart. Surgical correction of mitral stenosis, including mitral valve commissurotomy and mitral valve replacement, has been reported during pregnancy. Mitral valve replacement should be employed only in the patient in whom medical management is unsuccessful, and every consideration should be given to closed mitral valve commissurotomy. As in any patient with valvular disease, the appropriate use of prophylactic antibiotics at the time of delivery is indicated.

H. Peripartal cardiomyopathy. Characterized by its occurrence during the peripartal period in women with no previous history of heart disease and in whom no specific etiology of heart failure can be found, peripartal cardiomyopathy is a distinct, well-described syndrome of cardiac failure in late pregnancy or in the postpartum period. Presenting as myocardial failure, often with frank pulmonary edema, the specific etiology of this syndrome has yet to be clearly elucidated. Associations with hypertension, multiparity, multiple gestation, preeclampsia, and lower socioeconomic status (particularly black patients) have all been suggested, but the findings are not consistent. More recent proposed etiologies include viral myocarditis and hypersensitivity reactions [17]. Maternal mortality has been reported to be between 30 and 60%, with a perinatal mortality of at least 10% [17]. However, many reports suffer from a lack of neonatal statistics. Therapeutic modalities include strict bed rest, diuretics, digitalis glycosides, sodium restriction, and prophylactic heparin for the period that cardiomegaly persists. Additionally, steroids and immunosuppressive agents may play a role in the treatment of peripartal cardiomyopathy. In a certain group of patients with this disease, cardiomegaly does not resolve, and these patients have a much poorer prognosis. In women whose heart size returns to normal, maternal mortality is 10–15%, whereas in those whose heart size does not return to normal, maternal mortality has been reported to be as high as 85% [7]. Patients seem to tolerate subsequent pregnancies fairly well if cardiomegaly resolves, although there is a high incidence of recurrence of peripartal cardiomyopathy in subsequent pregnancies. In patients in whom cardiomegaly persists, subsequent pregnancies carry an unacceptably high maternal death rate. Most cardiologists consider this form of cardiomyopathy to be a medical contraindication to future pregnancies, and permanent sterilization is strongly recommended.

I. Myocardial infarction. Because of its low incidence in young women, coronary artery disease, specifically myocardial infarction, is rarely seen during pregnancy. Since its first description in 1922, 68 cases have been in the literature [30]. Not surprisingly, pregnancy is poorly tolerated in patients who suffer myocardial infarction, with overall mortality rates ranging between 30 and 40%. Note that this rate increases the later in pregnancy that the infarction occurs. Patients with a history consistent with angina or previous myocardial infarction should have an extensive evaluation performed prior to pursuing pregnancy.

J. Prosthetic heart valves. Since the first human implantation of a valvular prosthesis in 1952, over 200,000 valve replacements have been done throughout the world. Over 200 pregnancies have been reported in women with such valves, and although maternal mortality has been surprisingly low, the patient with a prosthetic valve poses a myriad of management problems during pregnancy. Maternal and fetal risks depend on the valve that has been replaced, the type of prosthesis itself, and the need for therapeutic continuous anticoagulation. Glutaraldehyde preserved porcine heart valves offer a major advantage over other valvular prostheses. Most patients with porcine valves do not require continuous anticoagulation. To avoid the well-described maternal and fetal risks associated with oral anticoagulation as well as the risks associated with heparin therapy (e.g., osteoporosis, thrombocytopenia), young women who require valvular replacement should strongly consider these xenografts. The long-term survival of these prostheses is unclear, and the possibility of a second surgical procedure 10–15 years later may be necessary.

1. **Aortic valve replacement.** Patients with aortic valve prosthesis have different hemodynamics and pregnancy performance than patients with a mitral valve prosthesis. The ability to adjust cardiac output for both exercise and pregnancy requirements has been demonstrated in patients with aortic valve replacement. Because of this, pregnancy is not contraindicated from a hemodynamic standpoint. Furthermore, patients who have no history of previous thromboembolism and who have not required anticoagulant management before pregnancy have been reported to negotiate pregnancy very safely. Nonetheless, after delivery, anticoagulation is recommended for a period of 10–14 days [25].
2. **Mitral valve prosthesis.** Fetal mortality has been reported to be increased among mothers with a mitral valve prosthesis [23], in contrast to aortic valve replacement. The reasons for this include the required use of anticoagulants, presence of a low fixed cardiac output at rest, and inability of patients with mitral valve replacement to adjust appropriately to exercise and pregnancy demands. Patients with rigid prostheses are managed during pregnancy in a manner similar to patients with mitral stenosis, with the additional requirement of anticoagulation therapy. Oral anticoagulants are contraindicated during pregnancy, particularly in the first and third trimesters, and very little information is available on the use of continuous or depo-heparin therapy for anticoagulation in these patients. Consequently, termination of pregnancy should be strongly suggested to the patient with mitral valve prosthesis who requires continuous anticoagulation. With the use of porcine xenografts in young women with mitral stenosis who require valve replacement, the prognosis is at least theoretically improved.

IX. Pregnancy termination and contraception for cardiac patients

A. Abortion. With improvements of both medical and surgical management of heart disease in pregnancy, the specific disease entities for which pregnancy is a clear maternal risk have decreased in numbers. However, patients with cyanotic heart disease, pulmonary hypertension, Marfan's syndrome with dilatation of the aortic root, persistent cardiomegaly following peripartal cardiomyopathy, and prosthetic heart valves requiring continuous anticoagulation should strongly consider pregnancy termination. Abortion has risks though, and maternal deaths have been reported with elective termination of pregnancy in patients with these underlying lesions [11]. For patients desiring pregnancy termination, early intervention with appropriate antibiotic prophylaxis and a procedure that is performed in a hospital setting where skilled anesthesiologists and cardiologists are available is strongly encouraged.

B. Contraception. Although the perfect birth control method for any woman, with or without heart disease does not exist, certain forms of contraception are not appropriate for a patient with underlying heart disease. Because of the increased incidence of thromboembolic phenomena associated with the use of oral contraception, patients at increased risk for this complication are not candidates for the contraceptive pill. The intrauterine device, although a very effective means of contraception, carries the risk of bacteremia, both at the time of insertion and throughout its term within the uterine cavity. Bacteremia and endocarditis have been reported after insertion of the intrauterine device, but the actual risk of this complication is not known [8]. If this contraceptive method is chosen by the patient, then informed consent should be obtained and prophylactic antibiotics should be used at the time of insertion. Barrier contraception offers women the safest form of birth control but is less reliable than intrauterine devices or oral contraceptives. The newer contraceptive mini-pill might be used in certain patients. Additionally, progesterone-only pills may be considered, although they are not as reliable as other oral contraceptives and are associated with a high incidence of breakthrough bleeding. Medroxyprogesterone acetate (Depo-Provera), 150 mg q4mo IM, should also be considered.

References

1. Baker, T. H., Machikaua, J. H., and Stapelton, J. J. Asymptomatic puerperal bacteremia. *Am. J. Obstet. Gynecol.* 94:903, 1966.
2. Becker, R. M. Intracardiac surgery in pregnant women. *Ann. Thorac. Surg* 36(4):453, 1983.
3. Bott-Kanner, G., et al. Propranolol and hydralazine in the management of essential hypertension in pregnancy. *Br. J. Obstet. Gynaecol.* 87:110, 1980.
4. Chez, R. A., et al. Effects of Adrenergic Agents on Ovine Umbilical and Uterine Blood Flows. In L. D. Longo and D. D. Reneau (eds.), *Fetal and Newborn Circulation* (Vol. 2): *Fetal and Newborn Cardiovascular Physiology*. New York Garland STPM, 1978. P. 1.
5. Christianson, R., and Page, E. W. Diuretic drugs and pregnancy. *Obstet. Gynecol.* 48:647, 1976.
6. Conradsson, T. B., and Werklo, L. Management of heart disease in pregnancy *Prog. Cardiovasc. Dis.* 16:407, 1974.
7. Demakis, J. B., et al. Natural course of peripartal cardiomyopathy. *Circulation* 44:1053, 1971.
8. DeSwiet, M., Ramsey, E. D., and Rees, G. M. Bacterial endocarditis after insertion of intrauterine device. *Br. Med. J:* 2:76, 1975.
9. Deviri, E., et al. Pregnancy after valve replacement with porcine xenograft prosthesis. *Surg. Gynecol. Obstet.* 160:437, 1985.
10. Gant, N. F., et al. A study of angiotensin II pressor response throughout primigravida pregnancy. *J. Clin. Invest.* 52:2682, 1973.
11. Gleicher, N., et al. Eisenmenger's syndrome and pregnancy. *Obstet. Gynecol Surv.* 34:721, 1979.
12. Kingdon, H. S., et al. Familial occurrence of primary pulmonary hypertension *Arch. Intern. Med.* 118:422, 1966.
13. Kjeldsen, J. Hemodynamic investigations during labor and delivery. *Acta Obstet. Gynecol. Scand.* [Suppl.] 89, 1979.
14. Klein, V., and Repke, J. T. Supraventricular tachycardia in pregnancy: Cardioversion with verapamil. *Obstet. Gynecol.* 63:165, 1984.
15. Mendelson, C. L. Pregnancy and coarctation of the aorta. *Am. J. Obstet. Gynecol.* 39:1014–1017, 1940.
16. Monson, R. R., et al. Diphenylhydantoin and selected congenital malformations. *N. Engl. J. Med.* 289:1049, 1973.
17. Paul, R. H., and Freeman, R. K. Fetal cardiac response to paracervical block anesthesia. Part II. *Am. J. Obstet. Gynecol.* 113:595, 1972.
18. Pedowitz, P., and Hellman, L. M. Pregnancy and healed subacute bacterial endocarditis. *Am. J. Obstet. Gynecol.* 66:294, 1953.
19. Prevention of bacterial endocarditis. *Med. Lett.* 4:91–92, 1984.
20. Pruyn, S. C., Phelan, J. P., and Buchanan, G. C. Long-term propranolol therapy in pregnancy, maternal and fetal outcome. *Am. J. Obstet. Gynecol.* 135:485, 1979.
21. Pyeritz, R. E. Maternal and fetal complications of pregnancy in Marfan syndrome. *Am. J. Med.* 71:784, 1981.
22. Shah, D. M., and Sundeiji, S. G. Hypertrophic cardiomyopathy and pregnancy: Report of a maternal mortality and review of the literature. *Obstet. Gynecol. Surv.* 40:444, 1985.
23. Szekely, P., and Julian, D. G. Heart disease and pregnancy. *Curr. Probl. Cardiol.* 4:1, 1979.
24. Ueland, K., et al. Maternal cardiovascular dynamics: IV. The influence of gestational age on the maternal cardiovascular response to posture and exercise. *Am. J. Obstet. Gynecol.* 104:856, 1969.

25. Ueland, K., Tatum, H. J., and Metcalfe, J. Pregnancy and prosthetic heart valves. *Obstet. Gynecol.* 27:257, 1966.
26. Upshaw, C. B. A study of maternal electrocardiograms recorded during labor and delivery. *Am. J. Obstet. Gynecol.* 107:17, 1970.
27. Veille, J. C. Peripartum cardiomyopathies: A review. *Am. J. Obstet. Gynecol.* 148:805, 1984.
28. Vogel, J. H. K., Pryor, R., and Blount, S. G. Direct current defibrillation during pregnancy. *J.A.M.A.* 193:970, 1965.
29. Von Reyn, C. F., et al. Infective endocarditis: An analysis based on strict care definitions. *Ann. Intern. Med.* 94:501, 1981.
30. Walcott, G., Burcell, H. B., and Brown, A. L. Primary pulmonary hypertension. *Am. J. Med.* 49:70, 1970.
31. Wolf, M. G., and Braunwald, E. General Anesthesia and Noncardiac Surgery in Patients with Heart Disease. In E. Braunwald (ed.), *Heart Disease.* Philadelphia: Saunders, 1980. Pp. 1911–1922.
32. Wynne, J. Mitral valve prolapse (editorial). *N. Engl. J. Med.* 314:577, 1986.

5

Renal Complications

Cynthia G. Kristensen

Pregnancy is accompanied by a number of physiologic alterations of the urinar tract, renal function, and hemodynamics, and what may be normal in the nongravi state may be distinctly abnormal in the pregnant woman.

I. Renal alterations in pregnancy

A. Anatomic alterations. Kidney size increases by 1.0–1.5 cm, and the renal pelve calyces, and ureters are dilated, especially on the right side. Dilatation begin in the first trimester and usually resolves within a few weeks post partum bu may persist for up to three months. It is mediated by both mechanical and hor monal influences and is accompanied by decreased peristalsis of the entire col lecting system. The large resultant dead space leads to errors in timed urin collections and may predispose to pyelonephritis in women with bacteriuria.

B. Functional changes. Renal plasma flow increases by 50–80% in the first tw trimesters and falls slightly in the third [9]. The glomerular filtration rate (GFR increases by approximately 50% by the tenth week, remains elevated until th thirty-sixth week, then falls slightly, and returns to nonpregnant levels a fe weeks post partum [41]. As a result, normal serum creatinine and blood ure nitrogen (BUN) concentrations in pregnancy are 0.5–0.7 mg/dl and 8–10 mg/d respectively, compared with nongravid values of 0.8 mg/dl and 10–15 mg/dl [13 Uric acid clearance also increases in pregnancy [9], so that serum uric aci concentration averages 3.0 mg/dl, compared to 4.2 mg/dl in nongravidas, and a elevated value is a clue to hemoconcentration or a decreased GFR.

Given the large increment in GFR, renal tubular adaptations occur that com pensate for the massively increased filtered load of electrolytes, glucose, an amino acids. The greatest adaptation is in the reabsorption of sodium, which i conserved normally, though subtle salt-wasting may occur in the presence c marked sodium restriction [2, 32]. Glycosuria occurs at normal blood sugar con centrations and may vary from day to day [9]. Aminoaciduria and proteinuri also increase, though a urine protein excretion above 300 mg/24 hours is abnor mal. The ability to concentrate and dilute the urine is unimpaired.

Serum electrolytes reflect renal compensation for a mild respiratory alkalosi [30], with a normal bicarbonate of 18–20 mEq/liter in pregnancy. Plasma os molality averages 5–10 mOsm/liter lower than in nongravid women, such tha plasma sodium is 135–136 mEq/liter. Osmolar regulation behaves as thoug there is a "reset osmostat" [10]; importantly, a plasma sodium of 140 mEq/lite indicates hemoconcentration.

C. Volume and hemodynamic alterations. Plasma volume increases markedly be ginning early in pregnancy, prior to the development of a significant uteropla cental shunt [6]. Total body water is increased by 7–9 liters in the absence c edema. Concomitantly, blood pressure falls as a result of vasodilatation, and th cardiac output rises 30–40% by the twenty-fourth week. Normal blood pressur averages 103 ± 11/56 ± 10 mm Hg midpregnancy, 109 ± 12/69 ± 9 mm Hg i the third trimester, and rises toward nonpregnant levels near term. Pregnan women excrete an acute sodium load similar to nongravid women, indicatin that the increased plasma volume and decreased blood pressure are sensed a normal [4].

II. General guidelines. A urinalysis, a urine culture, and serial blood pressure deter minations are adequate screens for renal disease in pregnancy. An abnormal uri nalysis or elevated blood pressure should be investigated by serum electrolytes, creatinine, and BUN. Proteinuria should be quantitated with a 24-hour urine collection for creatinine and protein. The urinary creatinine is useful as a gauge of the completeness of the urine collection, i.e., creatinine excretion is approximately 15–20 mg/24 hours/kg lean body weight. Newly discovered proteinuria or hematuria should prompt an investigation for underlying renal disease, especially one that requires treatment, such as systemic lupus erythematosus (SLE). Hypertension in the first half of pregnancy should raise suspicion of underlying hypertensive or renal disease.

III. Renal complications in pregnancy

A. Urinary tract infections. Asymptomatic bacteriuria occurs in 4–7% of women, and 1–2% develop symptomatic cystitis with dysuria and frequency. Pyelonephritis supervenes in 25–30% of women with untreated bacteriuria and can be prevented in 90% by antibiotic treatment [36].

1. **Asymptomatic bacteriuria** is generally defined as a colony count of greater than or equal to 10^5 organisms/ml, though a pure growth of greater than or equal to 10^4 gram-negative organisms/ml should probably be treated as well [29]. **Symptomatic cystitis,** even with fewer organisms, should be treated in the same manner, and antibiotics should begin prior to obtaining culture results.
2. **Pyelonephritis** in pregnancy, unlike in nongravid women, may be complicated by a reversible decrement in GFR [43], and patients can quickly develop septic shock. The most common pathogens are *Escherichia coli* and *Klebsiella pneumoniae*. Patients should be hospitalized for intravenous antibiotics and fluids. If fever and pain continue for more than 48–72 hours, the possibility of a resistant organism, obstruction, perinephric abscess, or an infected calculus or cyst should be considered. Oral antibiotics may be employed once fever and pain have resolved for at least 24 hours. Upper tract urinary infections may be associated with an increased incidence of fetal prematurity [17].
3. **Antibiotic therapy** should be given for 10–14 days for cystitis or asymptomatic bacteriuria, and for 4–6 weeks for pyelonephritis. Antibiotic choice should be guided by sensitivity testing and considerations of maternal and fetal toxicity. Effective oral regimens include ampicillin, 0.25 gm qid; amoxicillin, 0.25 gm tid; sulfisoxazole, 0.5 gm qid; nitrofurantoin, 100 mg qid; and cephalexin, 0.25 gm qid. Intravenous cephalosporins in usual doses, or ampicillin plus an aminoglycoside, are effective for pyelonephritis [5]. Ampicillin resistance is common, so it should not be used alone as initial therapy for pyelonephritis.
   a. **Contraindicated antibiotics.** Sulfonamides should not be used within four weeks of delivery due to the risk of kernicterus, and trimethoprim is contraindicated because it may be associated with teratogenicity. Aminoglycosides should be used with caution and for only short periods because of fetal oto- and nephrotoxicity. Tetracyclines cause fetal bone and teeth abnormalities. Nitrofurantoin and sulfonamides may cause hemolysis in patients with glucose 6-phosphate dehydrogenase deficiency.
4. Following successful therapy, surveillance cultures are important, and subsequent infections should be treated. Some authorities recommend antibiotic prophylaxis for women with two or more infections during pregnancy; others rely on biweekly cultures and retreatment as needed [29]. Effective prophylactic therapy includes nitrofurantoin 100 mg hs or sulfisoxazole 0.5 gm bid. Although postpartum urologic investigation is often recommended for women with recurrent urinary tract infections, the actual yield of significant, treatable anomalies is 5% or less [15]. The indications for such testing include chronic hypertension, renal insufficiency, hematuria, a family history of polycystic renal disease, or if infection does not respond to appropriate antibiotics or recurs with the same organism immediately following treatment.

B. Urinary calculi. Calculi are not more common in pregnancy, despite increased urinary calcium concentrations. They can cause pain, urinary tract obstruction, or bleeding, or a combination, and may cause poor response to therapy of urine infections [7]. Unilateral flank pain and microscopic hematuria provide clues to the diagnosis. Diagnostic ultrasonography has the advantage of avoiding radiation but may be difficult to interpret due to the normal dilatation of the collecting system. A modified intravenous pyelogram with a scout and a 20-minute film generally will be positive. Treatment of renal colic consists of analgesia and hydration, and the urine should be strained. If a stone is collected it should be analyzed. Operative intervention is reserved for persistent obstruction or infection. Patients with struvite (magnesium-ammonium-phosphate) calculi, usually associated with *Proteus* or *Pseudomonas* infection, are candidates for suppressive antibiotic therapy throughout gestation. Metabolic investigation should be deferred until the postpartum period.

C. **Urinary tract malformations.** Urinary tract malformations, such as a pelvic kidney, may coexist with other congenital anomalies of the genitourinary tract that are associated with poor obstetric outcome. Some structural lesions cause increased susceptibility to infection or hypertension.

D. **Underlying renal disease in pregnancy**

1. **Primary renal disease.** Conception and successful pregnancy are uncommon in patients with a serum creatinine greater than or equal to 2 mg/dl. The prognosis for a successful pregnancy in women with primary renal disease depends largely on adequate and early hypertensive control, on the absence of severe prolonged nephrotic syndrome, and on reasonably well preserved renal function [20, 25]; it depends less on the particular disease. The risk of hypertensive complications, including prematurity, intrauterine growth retardation, and neonatal mortality, is greatly enhanced, particularly if blood pressure is elevated in the first half of gestation. Nephrotic syndrome with severe hypoproteinemia in early pregnancy is associated with poor fetal outcome [35].

   Although the most common cause of nephrotic-range proteinuria (> 3 gm/24 hours) in pregnancy is **preeclampsia** [14], worsening of proteinuria in patients with preexisting renal disease is common and does not necessarily imply worsening of the disease [27]. Membranous nephropathy deserves special consideration because of its association with venous thrombosis and pulmonary emboli. Prophylactic subcutaneous heparin should be considered in patients who are at bed rest or have a history of thrombosis. Patients with interstitial nephritis, vesicouretheral reflux, or polycystic kidney disease are at particular risk of infection, and cultures should be monitored biweekly.

   The diagnosis of superimposed preeclampsia is difficult in patients with renal disease who may already have hypertension and proteinuria. Preeclampsia often occurs early and with increased severity. Deterioration of maternal renal function or uncontrolled hypertension is an indication for pregnancy termination. As long as blood pressure is controlled, pregnancy does not appear to adversely affect renal function in women with mild to moderate renal insufficiency (serum creatinine < 2 mg/dl) [1, 26, 27]. However, women with more advanced renal dysfunction may experience irreversible deterioration [24].

   Renal biopsy is rarely necessary during pregnancy and is associated with increased risk of bleeding complications.

2. **Systemic disease involving the kidneys.** Patients with systemic disease involving the kidney are at risk due to complications of the primary disease and the renal and hypertensive complications.

   a. **Collagen disease, especially systemic lupus erythematosus.** Patients with SLE who are in remission for at least six months prior to conception and have a serum creatinine less than or equal to 1.5 mg/dl tend to have successful pregnancies [22]. Active disease at the time of conception, or presentation during pregnancy, is associated with a stormy course and frequent maternal and fetal complications [3]. Antecedent proteinuria may increase without an exacerbation of SLE, but new-onset proteinuria or hematuria indicates active disease. The SLE should be treated aggressively in pregnancy and renal function should be monitored carefully. Corticosteroids and azathioprine should be used as needed [12], but cyclophosphamide should be avoided if possible. Other autoimmune diseases are less common, and patients with renal involvement often have hypertensive complications.

b. Diabetic nephropathy. The coexistence of retinopathy and proteinuria in a diabetic almost certainly indicates diabetic nephropathy. Hypertension and hypertensive complications are common, and renal function may deteriorate reversibly late in gestation. However, no evidence shows that pregnancy has an adverse effect on the overall course of diabetic renal disease [28]. Control of hypertension is essential to preserve kidney function and to prevent retinal hemorrhage. Urinary tract infections and papillary necrosis are frequent.

c. Chronic hypertension and nephrosclerosis. Severe hypertensive complications are greatly increased [27] and may occur early in gestation [42]. Inadequate blood pressure control in the first half of gestation is associated with a dismal prognosis [33]. Preeclampsia may not be prevented by early blood pressure control, but maternal and fetal outcomes are greatly improved [33, 40].

d. Sickle cell anemia. Patients with sickle cell disease (Hb-SS or -SC) or trait (Hb-SA) are prone to papillary necrosis, gross hematuria, and urinary infections even in the absence of a sickle crisis [36]. A sloughed renal papilla may cause hematuria, obstruction, and pain and predisposes to infection. Adequate hydration and antibiotic therapy are essential.

E. Acute renal failure. Acute renal failure (ARF) is a syndrome of rapid onset of impaired renal function, characterized by progressive azotemia, i.e., the inability to excrete creatinine and other products of daily metabolism. Oliguria or anuria is present if urine volume is less than 400–500 ml/24 hours or 50–100 ml/24 hours, respectively. The differential diagnosis is broad, and one must consider the clinical setting; the clinical features such as intravascular volume, blood pressure, and urine volume; and the laboratory findings. Table 5-1 shows some of these factors.

1. **Septic abortion** as a cause of ARF is usually due to *Clostridium welchii* or *Streptococcus pyogenes* and has a mortality of about 30% [18]. Aggressive treatment with intravenous fluids, antibiotics, and often surgery is necessary. Patients usually recover renal function, though cortical necrosis may occur.
2. **Prerenal renal failure.** Hyperemesis gravidarum causes fluid loss and electrolyte imbalance, and ARF can generally be avoided by volume repletion. Blood loss associated with abruptio placentae or uterine hemorrhage is an example of absolute volume loss, whereas "relative" volume loss occurs with the vasodilatation of sepsis. Volume should be provided quickly in the form of blood, colloid, or crystalloid.
3. **Preeclampsia and eclampsia.** The sensitivity of the kidney to insults is greatly enhanced in preeclampsia, presumably due to relative deficiency of vasodilatory prostaglandins. Renal blood flow and vascular volume are decreased [16, 19], vascular responsiveness to endogenous vasoconstrictors is increased, and often evidence exists of intravascular coagulation. Older patients, who often have underlying hypertensive renal disease, have a higher incidence of ARF associated with preeclampsia [18]. Treatment consists of delivery and judicious use of intravenous fluids and antihypertensives.
4. **Acute fatty liver of pregnancy and the HELLP syndrome** (hemolysis, elevated liver enzymes, low platelets) are frequently accompanied by renal failure [38]. The prognosis of the patients is largely determined by the liver disease, rather than the renal disease. Patients who survive acute fatty liver often have residual renal dysfunction.
5. **Acute tubular necrosis** (ATN) is a syndrome rather than a specific pathologic diagnosis and generally has multiple contributing factors, including hypotension, vasoconstriction, intravascular coagulation, incompatible blood transfusion, or infection, or a combination of these [34]. Frequently, no single insult seems to have been severe enough to cause renal failure. Renal function generally recovers more quickly in ATN associated with pregnancy than in ATN from other causes, and the prognosis is better. Management of ATN is supportive, with dietary and fluid restrictions and dialysis as needed.
6. **Bilateral cortical necrosis** is much rarer today than several decades ago and

Table 5-1. Acute renal failure in pregnancy

Etiology	Urine output	Urinalysis	Urine sodium (mEq/liter)	FE_{Na} (%)	Urine osmolality (mOsm/liter)	Urine-specific gravity
Prerenal	Oliguric	Bland or scant, with hyaline casts	< 20	< 1	> 500	> 1.020
ATN	Nonoliguric or oliguric	Renal tubular epithelial cells, coarsely granular tubular casts	> 40	> 3	< 350	1.010
Preeclampsia, eclampsia	Oliguric	Proteinuria; features may be those of prerenal ARF or of ATN				
Cortical necrosis	Oliguric or anuric	2 − 3 + protein, RBC, WBC, granular casts, ± RBC casts	> 40	> 3	< 350	1.010
Obstruction	Anuric to polyuric; may fluctuate	Depends on cause: bland, RBCs, or crystalluria	Depends on acuity: like prerenal if very acute, like ATN if > few hours			
Acute glomerulonephritis	Oliguric or nonoliguric	Hematuria, RBC casts, variable proteinuria				
Pyelonephritis	Nonoliguric: often oliguric if septic	WBC, WBC casts, bacteriuria				
Postpartum renal failure	Often oliguric or anuric	May be bland: look for evidence of intravascular hemolysis or consumption coagulopathy on blood tests				

FE_{Na} = [(urine Na/plasma Na)/(urine creatinine/plasma creatinine)] × 100; ATN = acute tubular necrosis; ARF = acute renal failure; RBC = red blood cell; WBC = white blood cell.

is generally associated with abruptio placentae, intrauterine hemorrhage, amniotic fluid embolism, prolonged intrauterine fetal death, and less frequently with preeclampsia [18]. The diagnosis should be suspected when oliguric or anuric ARF is prolonged more than 10 days, and is confirmed by renal biopsy or arteriography [14]. Cortical calcifications may be apparent on x ray after several weeks. Renal function may recover, often incompletely. Management is the same as in ATN. Why cortical necrosis is largely a disease of pregnancy is unknown and may be related to intravascular coagulation disturbances and altered sensitivity of the vascular endothelium to damage in pregnancy.

7. **Idiopathic postpartum ARF** occurs from a few days to 10 weeks post partum, generally following an uneventful pregnancy. It often has the features of hemolytic uremic syndrome, i.e., microangiopathic hemolytic anemia and severe oliguric or anuric renal failure [21, 31]. Extrarenal manifestations may occur, including central nervous system involvement, as seen in thrombotic thrombocytopenic purpura. Treatment is supportive, and dialysis is usually required. Renal prognosis is poor, though patient survival has improved due to dialysis and the management of bleeding complications.

F. **Pregnancy in women on dialysis.** Conception is uncommon, and most pregnancies end in abortion. However, several successful pregnancies have occurred, though with a high incidence of hypertensive complications, vaginal bleeding, and low-birth-weight babies [39]. Hemodialysis may precipitate labor, and patients have been treated prophylactically with magnesium during dialysis. Increased dialysis frequency is recommended to minimize fluid and electrolyte shifts and to avoid either hypertension or hypotension. Alternatively, continuous ambulatory peritoneal dialysis may be used, with adjustments in dialysate volume as needed. Most physicians recommend against pregnancy until the patient has a functioning transplant.

G. **Pregnancy in renal transplant patients** is usually well tolerated and successful if these preconception criteria are met: (1) stable renal function with a serum creatinine less than 2 mg/dl and no evidence of rejection; (2) no hypertension; (3) no significant proteinuria; (4) no evidence of pelvocalyceal distention on a recent pyelogram; (5) treatment with less than or equal to 15 mg/day prednisone and less than or equal to 2 mg/kg/day azathioprine or less than 5 mg/kg/day cyclosporine; and (6) good general health for at least two years following transplantation [11, 23]. Patients require close monitoring by the nephrologist and obstetrician, with frequent determinations of blood pressure, renal function, protein excretion, and urine cultures. Prednisone, cyclosporine, and azathioprine are not associated with significantly increased fetal anomalies and should be maintained in usual doses [23].

The better the preconception renal function, the better the obstetric outcome. In patients with normal serum creatinine, GFR increases during pregnancy, similar to normals. Near term, GFR falls approximately 35% from its peak level during gestation, compared to a fall of 17–20% in normal gravidas [8]. Proteinuria more than 0.5 gm/24 hours is usual. Patients with even mild elevation of serum creatinine are at greater risk for hypertensive complications, prematurity, and deterioration of renal function [37]. Renal functional deterioration in the first two trimesters, or greater than expected in the third, requires immediate hospitalization and evaluation for rejection, cyclosporine toxicity, superimposed preeclampsia, infection, or obstruction [23]. Renal biopsy should be performed if necessary, and termination of pregnancy is recommended if renal functional deterioration is not quickly reversed by such measures as reduction of the cyclosporine dose or treatment of rejection or infection [37].

References

1. Barcelo, P., et al. Successful pregnancy in primary glomerular disease. *Kidney Int.* 30:914, 1986.
2. Bay, W. H., and Ferris, T. F. Factors controlling plasma renin and aldosterone during pregnancy. *Hypertension* 1:410, 1979.

3. Bobrie, G., et al. Pregnancy in lupus nephritis and related disorders. *Am. J. Kidney Dis.* 9(4):339, 1987.
4. Brown, M. A., et al. Sodium excretion in normal and hypertensive pregnancy: a prospective study. *Am. J. Obstet. Gynecol.* 159:297, 1988.
5. Chapman, S. T. Bacterial infections in pregnancy. *Clin. Obstet. Gynecol.* 13(2):397, 1986.
6. Clapp, J. F., III, et al. Maternal physiologic adaptations to early human pregnancy. *Am. J. Obstet. Gynecol.* 159:1456, 1988.
7. Coe, F. L., Parks, J. H., and Lindheimer, M. D. Nephrolithiasis during pregnancy. *N. Engl. J. Med.* 298:324, 1978.
8. Davison, J. M. The effect of pregnancy on kidney function in renal allograft recipients. *Kidney Int.* 27:74, 1985.
9. Davison, J. M., and Dunlop, W. Renal hemodynamics and tubular function in normal human pregnancy. *Kidney Int.* 18:152, 1980.
10. Davison, J. M., et al. Altered osmotic thresholds for vasopressin secretion and thirst in human pregnancy. *Am. J. Physiol.* 246:F105, 1984.
11. Davison, J. M., and Lindheimer, M. D. Pregnancy in renal transplant recipients. *J. Reprod. Med.* 27:613, 1982.
12. Fine, L. G., et al. Systemic lupus erythematosus in pregnancy. *Ann. Intern. Med.* 94:667, 1981.
13. First, M. R., and Pollack, V. E. Pregnancy and Renal Disease. In R. W. Schrier and C. W. Gottschalk (eds.), *Diseases of the Kidney*. Boston: Little, Brown, 1988.
14. Fisher, K. A., et al. Nephrotic proteinuria with pre-eclampsia. *Am. J. Obstet. Gynecol.* 129:643, 1977.
15. Fowler, J. E., Jr., and Pulaski, E. T. Excretory urography, cystography, and cystoscopy in the evaluation of women with urinary-tract infection. *N. Engl. J. Med.* 304(8):462, 1981.
16. Gallery, E. D. M., Hunyor, S. N., and Gyory, A. A. Plasma volume contraction: a significant factor in both pregnancy-associated hypertension (preeclampsia) and chronic hypertension in pregnancy. *Q. J. Med.* 48(192):593, 1979.
17. Gilstrap, L. C., et al. Renal infection and pregnancy outcome. *Am. J. Obstet. Gynecol.* 141:709, 1981.
18. Grunfeld, J. P., Ganeval, D., and Bournerias, F. Acute renal failure in pregnancy. *Kidney Int.* 18:179, 1980.
19. Hankins, G. D. V., et al. Longitudinal evaluation of hemodynamic changes in eclampsia. *Am. J. Obstet. Gynecol.* 150:506, 1984.
20. Hayslett, J. P. Interaction of renal disease and pregnancy. *Kidney Int.* 25:579, 1984.
21. Hayslett, J. P. Postpartum renal failure. *N. Engl. J. Med.* 312:1556, 1985.
22. Hayslett, J. P., and Lynn, R. I. Effect of pregnancy in patients with lupus nephropathy. *Kidney Int.* 18:207, 1980.
23. Hou, S. Pregnancy in organ transplant recipients. *Med. Clin. North Am.* 73(3):667, 1989.
24. Hou, S. H., Grossman, S. D., and Madias, N. E. Pregnancy in women with renal disease and moderate renal insufficiency. *Am. J. Med.* 78:185, 1985.
25. Jungers, P., et al. Chronic kidney disease and pregnancy. *Adv. Nephrol.* 15:103, 1986.
26. Katz, A. I., et al. Effect of pregnancy on the natural history of kidney disease. *Contrib. Nephrol.* 25:53, 1981.
27. Katz, A. I., et al. Pregnancy in women with kidney disease. *Kidney Int.* 18:192, 1980.
28. Kitzmiller, J. L., et al. Diabetic nephropathy and perinatal outcome. *Am. J. Obstet. Gynecol.* 141:741, 1981.
29. Lenke, R. R., VanDorsten, J. P., and Schifrin, B. S. Pyelonephritis in pregnancy: a prospective randomized trial to prevent recurrent disease evaluating suppressive therapy with nitrofurantoin and close surveillance. *Am. J. Obstet. Gynecol.* 146:953, 1983.

30. Lim, V. S., Katz, A. I., and Lindheimer, M. D. Acid-base regulation in pregnancy. *Am. J. Physiol.* 231(6):1764, 1976.
31. Lindheimer, M. D., et al. Acute Renal Failure in Pregnancy. In B. M. Brenner and J. M. Lazarus (eds.), *Acute Renal Failure* (2nd ed.). New York: Churchill-Livingstone, 1988.
32. Lindheimer, M. D., and Katz, A. I. The Renal Response to Pregnancy. In B. M. Brenner and R. C. Recotr, Jr. (eds.), *The Kidney* (2nd ed.). Philadelphia: Saunders, 1981.
33. Mabie, W. C., Pernoll, M. O., and Biswas, M. K. Chronic hypertension in pregnancy. *Obstet. Gynecol.* 67:197, 1986.
34. Madias, N. E., Donohoe, J. F., and Harrington, J. T. Postischemic Acute Renal Failure. In B. M. Brenner and J. M. Lazarus (eds.), New York: Churchill-Livingstone, 1988.
35. Packham, D. K., et al. Membranous glomerulonephritis and pregnancy. *Clin. Nephrol.* 28(2):56, 1987.
36. Pathak, U. N., et al. Bacteriuria of pregnancy: results of treatment. *J. Infect. Dis.* 120(1):91, 1969.
37. Penn, I., Makowski, E. L., and Harris, P. Parenthood following renal transplantation. *Kidney Int.* 18:221, 1980.
38. Pockros, P. J., Peters, R. L., and Reynolds, T. B. Idiopathic fatty liver of pregnancy: findings in ten cases. *Medicine* (Baltimore) 63(1):1, 1984.
39. Redrow, M., et al. Dialysis in the management of pregnant patients with renal insufficiency. *Medicine* (Baltimore) 67:199, 1988.
40. Sibai, B. M., and Anderson, G. D. Pregnancy outcome of intensive therapy in severe hypertension in first trimester. *Obstet. Gynecol.* 67:517, 1986.
41. Sims, E. A. H., and Krantz, K. E. Serial studies of renal function during pregnancy and the puerperium in normal women. *J. Clin. Invest.* 37:1764, 1958.
42. Uhle, B. U., Long, P., and Oats, J. Early onset pre-eclampsia: recognition of underlying renal disease. *Br. Med. J.* 294:79, 1987.
43. Whalley, P. J., Cunningham, F. G., and Martin, F. G. Transient renal dysfunction associated with acute pyelonephritis of pregnancy. *Obstet. Gynecol.* 46(2):174, 1975.

6 Hematologic Complications

Gary S. Leiserowitz

This chapter discusses a variety of hematologic disorders that complicate pregnancy. These problems range from the most common ("physiologic anemia of pregnancy") to the uncommon but serious (leukemia in pregnancy). Any pertinent discussion is based on appreciating the normal physiology prior to looking at pathologic conditions.

I. Normal physiology. Changes occur in the plasma volume, the numbers of formed elements, and the levels of coagulation factors during pregnancy (Table 6-1). The upper and lower limits of these changes in the hematologic elements are somewhat variably defined, but general ranges can be appreciated [1, 18].

A. Red blood cells. Increases in both the number of red blood cells (RBCs) and plasma volume occur. Plasma volume increases 3 times that of red cell volume. Multiple-gestation pregnancy is associated with an even greater increase. The increases occur gradually in early pregnancy, becoming more pronounced in the second trimester, and plateauing in late pregnancy. The greater increase in plasma volume than red cell volume leads to a decrease in the hemoglobin/hematocrit, resulting in the "physiologic anemia" of pregnancy. This does not represent a disorder. Although disagreement persists, an acceptable lower limit for hemoglobin is 10 gm/dl or 30% for hematocrit. This increase in red cell and plasma volume provides for the increased perfusion needs of the fetal-placental unit and gives a margin of safety associated with blood loss during delivery.

B. White blood cells. An increase in the total white cell count is frequently noted during pregnancy, with counts between 9 and 15 $\times$ 10^9 cells/liter. A left shift (i.e., the presence of immature white cells such as bands) is also commonly present. A much greater increase in the white blood cell (WBC) count is seen with infection. Slighter increases can be difficult to interpret when trying to determine if infection is present.

C. Platelets. Whether a change in the platelet count can be expected in pregnancy is not agreed on. An acceptable range is 140–400 $\times$ 10^9 cells/liter.

D. Coagulation factors. Coagulation factors are noted to increase in pregnancy, of which factor VIII and fibrinogen increase the most, and factors XI and XIII change the least. The presence of activated clotting factors during pregnancy suggests activation of the coagulation system. Fibrinolytic activity is also decreased. This leads to the "hypercoagulability" of pregnancy, which increases the risk of venous thrombosis [33].

II. Anemia. Anemia is the most common medical complication in pregnancy. As many as 56% of pregnant women are anemic, depending on the geographic and socioeconomic group studied [18]. The signs and symptoms range from subclinical with mild anemia to the presence of pallor, fatigue, anorexia, weakness, lassitude, dyspnea, and edema in severe anemia. A discussion of etiologies follows.

A. Evaluation. At the first prenatal visit, questions relating to a history of anemia, bleeding diathesis, and other blood disorders should be obtained. Routine laboratory studies should include a complete blood count (CBC). It is important to note that the hemoglobin/hematocrit tend to be low in pregnancy normally. The RBC indices may be more helpful in deciding if abnormalities such as iron deficiency (low mean corpuscular volume [MCV]) or megaloblastosis (high MCV) are present. The hemoglobin/hematocrit should be repeated during the third trimester (around 32 weeks), and more frequently if indicated. Certain ethnicities

Table 6-1. Normal pregnancy values of the different blood elements

Blood element	Pregnancy values
Red blood cell	
Hematocrit (2nd trimester)	31.2–35.5%
(3rd trimester)	31.9–36.5%
White blood cell	9–15 × 10^9 cells/liter
Platelets	140–400 × 10^9 cells/liter
Coagulation factors	
Fibrinogen	Increased up to 200%
Prothrombin	No change
V	No change
VII	Increased up to 200%
VIII	Increased up to 300%
IX	Slight increase
X	Increased up to 200%
XI	Slight decrease
XIII	Slight decrease

Source: Adapted from H. M. Anderson, Maternal Hematologic Disorders. In R. K. Creasy and R. Resnik (eds.), *Maternal-Fetal Medicine* (2nd ed.). Philadelphia: Saunders, 1989.

should have screening tests for specific conditions. Black patients should have a Sickledex test or a hemoglobin electrophoresis to check for sickle cell trait/disease and a determination for glucose 6-phosphate dehydrogenase deficiency. Patients from the Mediterranean, the Middle East, India, and Southeast Asia are at risk for thalassemia, which also can be picked up on hemoglobin electrophoresis. Further studies include urine analysis, iron studies, reticulocyte count, peripheral blood smear, plus others as indicated. Bone marrow studies are rarely indicated in pregnancy.

B. Maternal prognosis. Severe anemia can increase the risk of morbidity and mortality. Blood loss during delivery ranges from 500 ml for a vaginal delivery to 1000 ml or more for cesarean section or delivery complications. The anemic patient has a decreased margin of safety against these blood losses.

C. Fetal prognosis. Severe maternal anemia (below 6 gm/dl) has been associated with poor pregnancy outcomes such as prematurity, low birth weight, abortion, and fetal death. The effects of mild and moderate anemia on pregnancy outcome are less clear. They are occasionally associated with poor fetal outcome, although this is confounded by the concomitant presence of maternal disease, malnutrition, and low socioeconomic status [22].

III. Specific anemias

A. Anemias resulting from inadequate production of hemoglobin are seen in nutritional deficiencies (e.g., iron deficiency) or inadequate production of hemoglobin chains (e.g., thalassemia).

1. Iron-deficiency anemia. This is the most common cause of anemia in pregnancy. Oral iron intake may be inadequate to maintain iron stores due to menstrual blood loss during reproductive life. Pregnancy will exacerbate the loss of iron stores due to increased maternal blood production and fetal growth needs. The average menstruating woman requires between 10 and 13 mg of available iron in her daily diet to compensate for an average daily loss of about 2 mg. Because of pregnancy, an increase to 15–18 mg/day of elemental iron is required [1]. Pregnancy costs the woman about 1220 mg of elemental iron (500 for RBC expansion, 300 for fetus/placenta, 190 for basal loss, 230 for delivery loss). That is balanced by maternal gain of 760 mg (490 from diet, 270 returned to storage after delivery), leaving a deficit of 460 mg that is borrowed from maternal stores or must come from iron supplementation [22].

a. Causes. Factors contributing to iron deficiency include the following:
  (1) Inadequate iron intake due to dietary insufficiency or inability to tolerate iron supplements.
  (2) Bleeding during pregnancy, vaginally or from another source.
  (3) Multiple gestation, which may increase the iron requirement and may be responsible for a greater blood loss at delivery.
  (4) Iron malabsorption.
  (5) Concurrent antacid use, which may prevent iron absorption.
  (6) Poor dietary habits or pica.

b. Diagnosis. The symptoms are nonspecific and diagnosis depends on laboratory evaluation. Mild iron deficiency anemia may not be manifested on the CBC until maternal iron stores are significantly depleted. Thereafter, the following changes may be noted:
  (1) Initially a normochromic, normocytic anemia is seen.
  (2) A microcytic, hypochromic anemia then occurs. The MCV falls to a level of 70–80 fL (normal, 90 ± 10 fL).
  (3) Serum iron falls below 60 μg/dl.
  (4) Unsaturated iron-binding capacity rises above 350 μg/dl.
  (5) Serum ferritin correlates well with bone marrow stores, making a bone marrow examination rarely necessary. Levels below 30 μg/l are diagnostic of iron deficiency.

c. Differential diagnosis will include consideration of anemia of chronic disease and heterozygous thalassemia. The finding of thalassemia minor that produces a mild anemia with a borderline low MCV should not exclude the diagnosis of iron-deficiency anemia. If suspected, serum ferritin should help differentiate between the two.

d. Management
  (1) Prophylaxis. Thirty to 60 mg/day of elemental iron is sufficient, but more may be needed to treat iron deficiency [15]. Many different iron preparations are available, but ferrous sulfate is the least expensive. Ferrous sulfate, 300 mg, provides 60 mg of elemental iron.
  (2) Treatment. Ferrous sulfate, 300 mg tid or bid, will treat iron deficiency.
  (3) Side effects. The ability to treat iron-deficiency anemia with oral iron is limited by the gastrointestinal side effects of nausea, diarrhea, or constipation. Alternatives include ferrous sulfate liquid diluted in water or juice (to prevent staining of the teeth) or slow-release iron tablets.
  (4) Cautions. Lack of response to oral iron therapy requires a reevaluation of the patient. Considerations for lack of response include patient noncompliance, inaccurate diagnosis of iron deficiency, occurrence of complicating illness, unrecognized blood loss, and malabsorption of iron. In the case of malabsorption, use of parenteral iron may be necessary. If severe iron-deficiency anemia is present late in pregnancy, blood transfusion may be necessary.

2. Anemia of chronic illness includes intestinal disease, parasitic disease (e.g., malaria), chronic or subclinical infection (e.g., urinary tract infection [UTI]), peptic ulcer disease, and neoplasia. These will present as a normochromic, normocytic anemia unresponsive to iron therapy. The diagnosis of a specific condition requires a high index of suspicion followed by careful history and physical examination. The treatment is determined by the specific etiology.

3. Anemia resulting from folic acid deficiency. Folic acid deficiency is common in pregnancy. In the nonpregnant woman, the recommended daily requirement for folic acid is 0.4 mg; this increases to 0.8–1.0 mg during pregnancy. Folate stores are limited and easily depleted within a few months in times of increased demand (e.g., pregnancy). All supplies of folate must come from external sources: Prime dietary sources are fruits and vegetables, of which the best are spinach, lettuce, asparagus, broccoli, lima beans, lemons, melons, and bananas. Folic acid deficiency is the most common cause of megaloblastic anemia. The consequence of folic acid deficiency in the absence of anemia on pregnancy is unclear, but associations have been made with prematurity, intrauterine growth retardation, and abruptio placentae. Therefore folic acid supplementation is recommended.

a. **Diagnosis.** The symptoms of anemia associated with folic acid deficiency are nonspecific. Deficiencies in either folic acid or B_{12} can present with glossitis and roughness of skin. However, the concomitant presence of neurologic symptoms is diagnostic of B_{12} deficiency and is almost never seen with folic acid. The anemia of folic acid deficiency is megaloblastic with an MCV usually greater than 110. The macrocytosis can be masked by concomitant iron deficiency or thalassemia. Neutropenia, thrombocytopenia, and hypersegmented granulocytes are usually present on the peripheral blood smear. The presence of an elevated serum iron and transferrin saturation also differentiates this from iron deficiency anemia. B_{12} deficiency is extremely rare in pregnancy, and therefore megaloblastic anemia is almost always due to folic acid deficiency [1].

b. **Prognosis for the fetus.** Folic acid deficiency has been associated with such pregnancy complications as low-birth-weight infants, smaller maternal blood volume, abruptio placentae, prematurity, and other maternal-fetal complications. These may also be explained, however, by the presence of other factors such as low socioeconomic status and malnutrition.

c. **Management.** The daily dose of folic acid is 1.0 mg, whether for prophylaxis or treatment. If given for megaloblastic anemia, an increased reticulocyte count should be seen with three to four days. If neurologic symptoms are present, a B_{12} level should be drawn, since folic acid will correct the anemia but not the neurologic symptoms. Oral folic acid is sufficient for treatment unless folic acid antagonists are being used, at which time parenteral folic acid is indicated.

4. **Anemia from B_{12} deficiency.** B_{12} is absorbed in the ileum, bound to intrinsic factor. Intrinsic factor is secreted in the stomach by the fundic parietal cells. These same cells are responsible for hydrochloric acid secretion. B_{12} deficiency is rarely due to inadequate ingestion, except in strict vegetarians. Inadequate synthesis and production of intrinsic factor, or malabsorption syndromes are common causes. Illustrations of these problems include pernicious anemia (rare in this age group), previous gastric or intestinal surgery, and tapeworm infestations. These are uncommon in most pregnant women in the United States, making B_{12} deficiency a much less common etiology for megaloblastic anemia than is folic acid deficiency. In addition, neurologic symptoms are common in B_{12} deficiency and rare in folic acid deficiency.

a. **Diagnosis.** Laboratory evaluation is necessary to establish the diagnosis. A radioimmunoassay is used to measure B_{12} serum levels. Vitamin B_{12} levels may fall to 80–120 pg/ml during pregnancy; levels below 50 pg/ml are indicative of B_{12} deficiency. The Schilling test is used to measure B_{12} absorption but is contraindicated in pregnancy because of use of radioactive cobalt. However, if vitamin B_{12} deficiency is present, then a Schilling test must be done at a safe time after delivery. In addition, neurologic abnormalities are seen, as well as elevated serum bilirubin and lactic dehydrogenase levels. Serum folate is frequently elevated unless there is an associated folic acid deficiency [14].

b. **Management.** If a deficiency is documented, 1 mg B_{12} is given parenterally weekly for 5–6 weeks. Serum levels should respond within six weeks. A brisk reticulocytosis should manifest within three to five days.

5. **Thalassemias.** Thalassemia results from inadequate synthesis of one or both α and β hemoglobin chains. The clinical variability is great, from subclinical to lethal. Thalassemia is found throughout the world but is concentrated in the Mediterranean areas, the Middle East, India, and Southeast Asia. α-Thalassemia is usually seen in the Mediterranean, Southeast Asian, and Indian populations. β-Thalassemia is more common in blacks and Mediterraneans. The genetic heritability is passed as an autosomal recessive trait. In β-thal-

assemia, the β-chains are absent or inadequately produced. In α-thalassemia the α-chains are synthesized in less than normal amounts, due to deletion of α-chain genes. The α- and β-chains that are present are structurally normal.

a. α-Thalassemia. The α-gene locus contains two structural genes. The genotype of normal individuals is aa/aa. The clinical severity increases as each allele is deleted.

(1) **The carrier state** is represented by -a/aa and is clinically silent. The heterozygous state is seen with -a/-a or --/aa and is called **α-thalassemia minor.** It is clinically asymptomatic, except during great stress. A mild microcytic, hypochromic anemia with poikilocytosis and anisocytosis is seen. Newborns carry 2–10% of **Bart's hemoglobin** (a tetramer of γ-chains).

(2) **Hemoglobin H disease** is seen with a deletion of three α-chains (--/-a). Splenomegaly and occasionally hepatomegaly are seen. Chronic moderate hemolytic anemia is present with a reticulocytosis, microcytosis, hypochromasia, and poikilocytosis. Both hemoglobin H (a tetramer of β-chains) and Bart's hemoglobin are seen. Hemoglobin H disease occurs mostly in Southeast Asians and is unusual in blacks.

(3) **The absence of all four α-chains** is incompatible with extrauterine life; the fetus will have hydrops or will abort early in pregnancy. A large amount of **Bart's hemoglobin** will be present. These pregnancies are notable for a high incidence of toxemia [1].

(4) **Treatment.** In α-thalassemia minor, folate may need to be supplemented. Iron-deficiency anemia must be ruled out as a cause of microcytic, hypochromic anemia. In severe cases, transfusion may be required.

(5) **Prognosis for the mother and infant.** In α-thalassemia minor, the pregnancy may be complicated by anemia. In silent carriers, no complications are seen. In hemoglobin H disease, a more severe anemia can be seen, and transfusions are more often needed.

b. β-Thalassemia. In the United States, most β-thalassemia is present in the black population.

(1) **β-Thalassemia minor.** β-Thalassemia minor is the heterozygous state. Variable clinical severity is seen in β-thalassemia minor. The condition is suspected when a patient is treated for iron-deficiency anemia and fails to respond. A moderate to severe microcytic, hypochromic anemia is seen associated with a relatively high red cell count. Hemoglobin A_2 is elevated above 3.5%. Serum iron and ferritin concentrations are elevated. Mild to moderate splenomegaly may be present. Except for mild anemia, most pregnancies are uncomplicated. Folic acid supplementation may be necessary. Transfusions are occasionally needed for the more severe anemia.

(2) **β-Thalassemia major.** β-Thalassemia major is the homozygous state. This more severe disease is also known as **Cooley's anemia.** Pregnancy rarely occurs, as individuals are severely affected. If they survive, their course is marked by profound, transfusion-dependent anemia, growth retardation, and heart failure.

c. Genetic considerations. Improvements in **prenatal diagnosis** of the hemoglobinopathies and the thalassemias allow for early in utero identification of the severely affected fetus. Termination can then be offered for the severely affected fetus, or reassurance if the fetus is unaffected or mildly affected. Those couples at risk must be identified early and offered genetic counseling. Techniques for prenatal diagnosis include **genetic counseling** with a determination of risk based on mendelian inheritance patterns, and direct determination of the fetal genotype by tissue sampling early in pregnancy. Fetal tissue is obtained by placentocentesis or fetoscopy for fetal blood, amniocentesis performed in the early second trimester for fetal amniocytes, or chorionic villus sampling performed between 7 and 11 weeks of gestation.

B. Excessive destruction of erythrocytes (hemolytic anemias). Anemia results from an inability of the bone marrow to keep up with the destruction of RBCs. Folic acid deficiency also can accompany hemolytic anemia due to increased erythrocyte synthesis.

1. **Sickle cell anemia.** This group of diseases is caused by a hemoglobinopathy due to abnormal β hemoglobin chains. The substitution of glutamic acid to valine at the sixth position causes hemoglobin S. Other single amino acid substitutions also can cause abnormal hemoglobins that lead to instability, reduced solubility, RBC cell wall rigidity, and a changed oxygen affinity. The homozygous individual will have both abnormal β-chains; the heterozygote will have one abnormal and one normal β-chain. The homozygote generally has severe disease. If the patient is heterozygous for more than one trait, the combination may be worse than either one separately (e.g., hemoglobin sickle cell disease). The rigid RBC will not pass easily through the microcirculation, causing vasoocclusions that lead to infarction.

   a. **Trait.** The frequency of sickle cell trait (hemoglobin SA) is 1 in 12 in the U.S. black population, whereas sickle cell disease (hemoglobin SS) is 1 in 708. Although classically considered a disease of blacks, other ethnicities including Italians, Turks, Greeks, and Caribbean natives also are at risk. Individuals with sickle cell trait are normally asymptomatic. Only the presence of severe stresses (such as decreased oxygen tension in very high elevations) or illness will cause the trait to manifest clinically.

   b. **Disease.** β-Chain synthesis does not reach sufficient levels to cause symptoms until about 6 months of age. Thereafter, the increased concentration of hemoglobin S makes the cells susceptible to sickling and hemolysis, causing anemia and splenomegaly. Major problems are infections and vaso-occlusive episodes. Children are at increased risk for certain infections including sepsis, meningitis, pneumonia, osteomyelitis, and UTIs. The functional asplenia following vaso-occlusive microinfarctions compromises the immune system leading to infections caused by encapsulated organisms. Vaso-occulsive crises occur because rigid RBCs are unable to pass in the microcirculation causing infarctions. Target areas include the extremities, lungs, spleen, splanchnic bed, brain, and eyes. Pain resulting from these infarctions can mimic other conditions (e.g., pulmonary crises with fever mimic pneumonia) and are a source of clinical confusion. The diagnosis is made by the presence of irreversibly sickled RBCs on peripheral smear with normal, target, fragmented, and nucleated cells. The abnormal hemoglobin electrophoresis shows greater than 80% hemoglobin S and F. The family history and family studies are also important [30].

   c. **Other abnormal hemoglobins** are sometimes implicated in hemolytic anemias. Hemoglobin sickle cell disease usually is mild but can be subject to painful crises. The clinical syndrome, although milder, is similar to sickle cell anemia. Hemoglobin S/β-thalassemia is similar in presentation.

   d. **Risk to mother and fetus.** The course of hemoglobin S disease prior to pregnancy frequently predicts how the woman will do during the pregnancy. The spontaneous abortion rate does not appear to be increased. There is an increased incidence of perinatal mortality and low-birth-weight infants, but recent studies have shown generally good results [5, 21]. Termination of the pregnancy because of maternal sickle cell anemia is largely unwarranted and should be decided on an individual basis. Generally pregnancy proceeds normally except for an increased incidence of UTIs. Occasionally, an inability to concentrate urine (hyposthenuria) occurs due to renal papillary necrosis and loss of deep medullary nephrons. Hematuria is uncommon, and other potential causes must be ruled out first prior to attributing it only to sickle cell trait.

   e. **Management.** The pregnant woman with sickle cell anemia should be followed by physicians comfortable with high-risk pregnancies. They require careful obstetric care to improve perinatal outcome. No medication will prevent sickling.

(1) Blood transfusions are needed to treat vaso-occlusive crises and anemia. Partial exchange transfusions will increase the concentration of hemoglobin A. This will decrease sickling and improve oxygen delivery to the fetus providing an improved perinatal outcome. The target is a concentration of hemoglobin A greater than 25% and a hematocrit between 25 and 30%. Transfusion therapy, however, can be complicated by fluid overload, iron overload, hepatitis, and human immunodeficiency virus (HIV) infection and therefore must be used judiciously.

(2) Iron supplementation is not necessary because of the increased iron stores secondary to the frequent transfusions.

(3) Folic acid supplementation of 1 mg/day is recommended.

(4) Urinary tract infections occur more frequently. Careful monitoring for asymptomatic bacteriuria and UTIs is necessary.

(5) Sickle cell crises must be treated with generous fluid support and blood transfusions as necessary.

(6) Fetal surveillance should be started late in the third trimester by either a nonstress test or a contraction stress test.

(7) Labor and delivery are managed based on obstetric principles. Cesarean section should only be performed for obstetric indications. If abdominal delivery is necessary, regional anesthesia is preferred to general anesthesia. If possible, a partial exchange transfusion is recommended prior to induction of general anesthesia to get the concentration of hemoglobin A to about 50%. This should decrease the risk of pulmonary and systemic vaso-occlusive crises.

(8) Genetic counseling is important. See sec. **A.5.c.**

(9) Contraception is problematic in patients with severe hemoglobinopathies. They are at increased risk for thromboembolic disorders, and therefore oral contraception may be relatively contraindicated. Similarly, they are also at increased risk for infection, and so the intrauterine device also may not be a good choice. Permanent sterilization should be considered when the patient is finished with childbearing.

2. Hereditary spherocytosis. Among whites, this autosomal dominant disease is the most common cause of a hemolytic anemia. The incidence of the disease is estimated at 1 per 5000. The expression of the disorder is variable; mild cases frequently go undetected [1].

a. Diagnosis. The presence of anemia, jaundice, and splenomegaly is noted clinically in childhood. The diagnosis is made by the presence of microspherocytes on peripheral smear, increased erythrocyte fragility in hypotonic saline, and the identification of other affected family members.

b. Management. Most affected patients will already have had a splenectomy, and so the pregnancy is generally unaffected.

(1) If a splenectomy has not been previously done, the treatment of the anemia should be supportive with transfusion as necessary.

(2) Folic acid supplementation is given.

(3) Splenectomy should be avoided in pregnancy if possible.

(4) These patients are also at risk for cholelithiasis due to pigmentary gallstones from the chronic hemolysis.

(5) Splenectomized individuals are at risk for sepsis, especially from pneumococcus. Pneumococcal vaccine should be given prior to the pregnancy, as its use in pregnancy is not approved.

(6) Genetic counseling is important for affected individuals.

3. Glucose 6-phosphate dehydrogenase deficiency is the most common form of inherited hemolytic anemia, with more than 100 million cases in the world. The enzyme is necessary to protect the erythrocyte from oxidation. Its absence makes the RBC susceptible to a variety of oxidizing agents, including analgesics, sulfa drugs, antimalarials, quinines, some nonsulfa antibiotics (e.g., nitrofurantoin, nalidixic acid), and many others. It is inherited as a X-linked trait. The condition can be identified in 10% of the American black male population but only in 3% of the black female population. It causes a mild chronic hemolysis in this group. Greek, Sardinians, and Sephardic Jews have a more severe hemolysis, which is characterized by hemolysis precipitated by eating fava beans.

a. Effect on pregnancy. Pregnant women may be predisposed to hemolytic episodes in the third trimester. The hematocrit may be below 30%. The use of antimicrobial agents may precipitate further hemolysis. Urinary tract infections may be more common, and it may be prudent to screen patients at risk for the disorder prior to treatment. The affected fetus is at risk for neonatal jaundice from chronic hemolytic anemia. If the anemia is severe enough, hydrops may result. Even breast-fed infants may be at risk if exposed to oxidants or fava beans ingested by the mother.

b. Management

(1) Hemolytic episodes during pregnancy require a prompt discontinuation of the causative medication.

(2) Infections should be sought out and treated.

(3) Transfusion support may be necessary.

(4) Screening for the defect should be considered prior to treating the patient at risk.

(5) Screening for the newborn infant at risk should be considered.

(6) Genetic counseling should be offered.

C. Bone marrow failure (aplastic anemia). Bone marrow failure is uncommon and occurs rarely in pregnancy. Several agents are well associated with aplastic anemia (e.g., chloramphenicol, phenylbutazone, gold salts), but hundreds of others have also been implicated. Withdrawal of the agents will often, but not always, lead to resolution.

1. Diagnosis. Clinical presentations include profound anemia, bleeding, and infection. Pancytopenia is found on the CBC. A bone marrow aspirate and biopsy are necessary to make the diagnosis and to exclude other causes for pancytopenia [20].

2. Prognosis for the mother. Mortality rate is very high. There are only a few reported cases of aplastic anemia in pregnancy. It is not clear if the pregnancy was a causative factor. In some cases, the aplastic anemia resolved after delivery. Fetal wastage is very high. In addition, maternal mortality is 15%.

3. Management. Treatment involves supportive care, stimulation of hematopoiesis, and consideration of bone marrow transplant.

a. Supportive care includes blood transfusions and treatment of infections. In rare cases, this might be sufficient to allow the pregnancy to continue.

b. Androgen therapy has been found to stimulate bone marrow in some patients. Unfortunately, this is contraindicated in pregnancy, especially if the fetus is female.

c. The role of pregnancy termination is unclear. Therapeutic abortion is inconsistently associated with remission. It may be necessary, however, in order to treat the patient with anabolic steroids.

d. Occasionally immunosuppressive agents such as antithymocyte globulin, steroids such as prednisone, or monoclonal antibody therapy directed against T helper cells will bring about improvement.

e. Bone marrow transplant has become the treatment of choice. It is most successful when instituted early in the course of the disease. Finding a suitable donor that is a twin or HLA compatible is difficult. Termination of the pregnancy would be necessary if a suitable donor could not be found.

IV. Hematologic malignancies

A. Leukemia. Leukemia is a rare event in pregnancy. The incidence is not known but is estimated not to exceed 0.9–1.2 cases per 100,000 women per year [4]. The leukemias are divided into chronic and acute, and then subdivided into histologic categories. Use of cell surface markers and histochemical staining, plus careful examination of the leukemic cells in peripheral blood and bone marrow allow for a precise determination of category.

1. **Acute leukemia.** Hematologic malignancies are usually either acute lymphocytic leukemia (ALL) or acute nonlymphocytic leukemia (ANLL) when seen in pregnancy. Usually ALL is seen in childhood and is less common in the reproductive years. Therefore, these pregnancies occur more often in women who have been treated for ALL, survived, and remained fertile. If ALL presents during the adult years, it usually has a worse prognosis. An ANLL is uncommonly seen in childhood. Its prognosis is worse. Though remission can be achieved with chemotherapy, only a small percentage (10–20%) have prolonged remissions. Pregnancy associated with ANLL is rare because ANLL is rare in reproductive-age women, and ANLL patients rarely conceive.
   a. **Risk in pregnancy.** The presence of leukemia during pregnancy raises several concerns: (1) the effect of pregnancy on the prognosis of leukemia, (2) the effect of leukemia on the prognosis for the pregnancy, (3) the effect of treatment for leukemia on the pregnancy, and (4) fertility prognosis following treatment.
      (1) Studies have not shown a worse prognosis for leukemic patients during pregnancy. There is concern that the immunosuppressive effect of pregnancy (as illustrated by the immunotolerance of fetal tissue by the mother) might increase the risk of cancer developing in pregnancy or allow a more fulminant course. This effect has not been demonstrated, and the immunotolerance appears to be specific for the fetus only, since cell-mediated immunocompetence is intact [28].
      (2) The pregnancy is at risk in leukemic patients, with increased rates of abortion, fetal wastage, preterm delivery, and perinatal mortality (usually related to preterm delivery), even in the face of treatment. In untreated leukemia, maternal mortality is the most significant cause of perinatal mortality. Good pregnancy outcomes have been obtained when patients are treated for leukemia but are largely influenced by maternal response to therapy. Metastasis of maternal leukemia to the placenta or fetus is a concern. Although rare cases of metastasis to the placenta have been reported, metastasis to the fetus is even rarer [8, 32].
      (3) Great concerns remain about the teratogenic and mutagenic effects of **radiation and chemotherapy** on the fetus. It is clear from animal models that the first trimester (during organogenesis) is the time of greatest risk. The data are less clear for later in pregnancy. It is surprising, therefore, that the literature shows such a little risk of teratogenesis in surviving pregnancies, even in the first trimester [4, 23, 32]. In contrast, intrauterine growth retardation is commonly seen in the pregnancies of leukemia survivors. There has been inadequate study of follow-up of these children after delivery, so their long-term development, both physically and intellectually, is yet to be determined. Given the clearly dismal prognosis of leukemia in the absence of therapy, and the lack of documented side effects of chemotherapy in utero, it seems that chemotherapy should not be withheld or significantly delayed, especially if the mother is acutely ill.
      (4) The **fertility of female leukemia patients** appears to be diminished during acute disease. For patients treated for ALL in childhood and in remission, fertility rates are diminished compared to normal, but remain good. The older the patient is when she is treated for leukemia (or lymphoma), the less likely that she will maintain or have return of ovarian function. Prepubertal women have the best fertility rates following chemotherapy or radiation therapy, or both.
   b. **Management.** Management is based on the stage of pregnancy at the time of diagnosis of leukemia. In the first trimester, the patient should be offered termination given the concerns about the potential fetal consequences of chemotherapy or radiation therapy, and the maternal complications of leukemia. If abortion is refused, the patient should be treated with chemotherapy since the maternal prognosis is dismal without treatment. Late in pregnancy, consideration can be given to a slight delay in treatment to allow

for delivery prior to institution of chemotherapy. If the patient is acute, or the possibility of a viable fetus is remote, then therapy should be offered promptly. During the pregnancy, the fetus should be monitored for adequate growth, since intrauterine growth retardation is common. Adequate nutrition is another serious problem, both for the mother and the fetus. The mother can be compromised by the disease or the chemotherapy. Nutritional support including total parenteral nutrition is indicated for the compromised patient. For the patient with ALL in remission, it is reasonable to allow pregnancy. In ANLL, pregnancy should be delayed to see if remission will be of lasting duration since relapse is common. Oral contraception is the method of choice, since ovulation is suppressed and menstrual flow is diminished, thus preventing menorrhagia in patients both with acute disease and in remission.

2. **Chronic leukemia.** In the vast majority of cases, only chronic myelogenous leukemia (CML) is seen associated with pregnancy, since chronic lymphocytic leukemia is a disease of persons older than 50 years. CML is characterized by a chronic phase and an acute phase (blast crisis). During the chronic phase, the pregnant patient can be treated expectantly without chemotherapy as long as the white cell count is not too elevated and the patient is not thrombocytopenic. Generally CML can be treated with a single agent, busulfan, to control the WBC count. There is evidence that this can increase the risk of low-birth-weight infants, and so the risks should be carefully weighed [23]. If the patient suffers a blast crisis, chemotherapy is necessary, and management of the pregnancy should be similar to that of acute leukemia (see sec. **A.1.b**).

B. Lymphomas. Lymphomas can be divided into Hodgkin's and non-Hodgkin's lymphomas (NHLs).

1. **Hodgkin's lymphoma.** Hodgkin's lymphoma is seen in young people, and so intercurrent pregnancy is not as rare as with the leukemias. Prognosis and treatment are largely based on the stage at the time of presentation. Patients with localized disease are treated with radiation therapy, whereas disseminated disease is treated with chemotherapy. Patients with disease on both sides of the diaphragm, large mediastinal or abdominal masses, or multiple splenic nodules are treated with a combination of both, or chemotherapy alone. Staging procedures are done to determine who needs radiation for localized disease and who will need chemotherapy for regional or disseminated disease. The more localized the disease, the more important thorough staging is. If disseminated, the patient will receive chemotherapy anyway, and so fewer staging procedures are necessary. If the patient is pregnant, staging procedures such as exploratory laparotomy, splenectomy, and liver biopsy are contraindicated, making the decision about extent of disease difficult. However, other than for localized disease above the diaphragm, radiation therapy even with shielding is contraindicated because of the risk to the fetus. Therefore, chemotherapy will be chosen unless the stage is confidently determined to be localized.
2. **Non-Hodgkin's lymphoma.** Non-Hodgkin's lymphoma (NHL) is a heterogeneous group of lymphomas whose therapy and prognosis are dependent on histology. They are roughly classified into three groups by prognosis: high grade, intermediate grade, and low grade. Staging is less critical in Hodgkin's disease but remains a useful tool for oncologists. Low-grade lymphomas are usually seen in older age groups and are very rare in the childbearing years. High-grade and intermediate-grade lymphomas are frequently seen in women of childbearing age. The cure rate for these lymphomas is 50–60% given appropriate therapy. Radiation therapy can be used for localized disease, but this is rare. Chemotherapy is generally the therapy of choice for this broad group of diseases.
3. **Risk in pregnancy.** Lymphoma does not affect the course of pregnancy and the pregnancy does not affect the course of the lymphoma. If the disease is indolent, consideration can be given to postponing treatment until after the pregnancy. However, Hodgkin's lymphoma, in particular, is potentially curable in most of cases, and so treatment should not be necessarily delayed. High-grade NHL

is a rapidly progressive disease with a median survival of six months. Since cure rates approach 50%, it is imperative therapy not be delayed. Radiation therapy during pregnancy carries defined risks to the fetus. The fetus must be protected against radiation. Chemotherapy has unknown risks, as noted in the discussion on leukemia. Generally, the prognosis for the fetus depends on the maternal status. Maintenance of good nutrition and good health should allow for a good outcome. With indolent disease, this can occur without therapeutic intervention.

4. **Management.** Both Hodgkin's lymphoma and NHL are usually treated with radiation or chemotherapy depending on the stage. Early gestations should be considered for termination because of the risks to the fetus from treatment, as discussed with leukemia. Radiation therapy is only reasonable during early pregnancy and for localized disease, because otherwise the teratogenic and mutagenic risks become too great. Chemotherapy is used otherwise. Indolent disease late in gestation may be observed until completion of the pregnancy, but the potential opportunity to cure the mother may be lost in an attempt to protect the fetus from potential risk.

V. **Disorders of hemostasis.** The ability of the patient to maintain hemostasis when challenged by vaginal delivery or cesarean section is generally assumed by her caretakers. However, when these mechanisms fail to stem bleeding, the patient will be faced with a potential life-threatening hemorrhage. An assessment of the patient's experience with hemostatic challenges should be obtained during the initial **prenatal evaluation.** The patient should be asked about bleeding following surgery or injuries. Abnormal bleeding following a dental extraction, for example, especially if delayed or if a blood transfusion was required, suggests the presence of a bleeding disorder. Many bleeding disorders are mild until challenged, and so such a history may be the opportunity to make the diagnosis prior to a major hemostatic challenge. The pattern of bleeding problems will suggest the appropriate investigation. **Platelet deficiency,** either in number or function, will frequently manifest by mucosal bleeding either spontaneously or with minor challenges. Examples include epistaxis, gingival bleeding, gastrointestinal bleeding, or menorrhagia. Patients may have an exaggerated response to aspirin or other nonsteroidal anti-inflammatory drugs. Bleeding problems may be immediate or delayed even if adequate hemostasis was obtained at the time of surgery. **Deficiencies in coagulation factors** may result in either immediate or delayed bleeding. Hemarthrosis or deep muscle hematomas are characteristic. **Disorders of fibrinolysis** are suggested in situations of delayed bleeding or poor wound healing. A laboratory evaluation should be triggered by an abnormal bleeding history and focused on those hemostatic elements most likely to be abnormal. Routine lab studies beyond prothrombin time/partial thromboplastin time (PT/PTT) and platelet count have a very low yield in the absence of an abnormal history. They are not necessary prior to routine procedures. In contrast, the evaluation of a patient with an abnormal history prior to a bleeding challenge may save unnecessary blood loss.

A. **Mechanisms of normal hemostasis.** A brief review of the mechanisms of normal hemostasis is necessary prior to a discussion of specific bleeding disorders. Hemostasis is a complex process involving three interacting systems: platelet function, coagulation factors, and fibrinolysis. Regulation of the process involves both promotion and inhibition. Abnormalities in either can lead to a bleeding diathesis [2, 7].

1. **Platelets.** Vascular damage leads to exposure of thromboplastic elements that cause platelets to adhere to the endothelial surface. Once adherent to the damaged vasculature, the platelets change configuration and release chemical mediators that induce aggregation of other platelets. This forms a platelet plug that is the first step in obtaining hemostasis. Simultaneously, these platelets become activated and initiate the coagulation cascade.

2. **Coagulation factors.** Soluble plasma proteins interact to provide deposition of fibrin in areas of vascular damage where the platelet plug is present. The coagulation enzymes exist in proenzymes forms. They are then cleaved to

activated forms that catalyze and amplify activation of other enzymes. This leads to a cascade effect that ultimately leads to formation of thrombin (Fig. 6-1). Thrombin subsequently converts fibrinogen to fibrin. The soluble fibrin monomers then stabilize by cross-linking into fibrin polymers that adhere to the platelet plugs. The coagulation cascade can be initiated by an intrinsic or extrinsic pathway. The intrinsic pathway is so named because all necessary elements exist in the plasma. The extrinsic system is activated by tissue factors extrinsic to the plasma. Main screening tests of the coagulation cascade reflect these pathways: the PT reflects the extrinsic system, and the PTT reflects the intrinsic system. The actual process is less separate than implied, and so the elements of the extrinsic pathway can lead to activation of the intrinsic pathway. The intrinsic pathway contains factors XII, XI, IX, and VIII. The extrinsic pathway contains tissue thromboplastin and factor VII. The common pathway contains factors X, V, PT, and fibrinogen. Regulation of the system involves a delicate balance of activation and inhibition. Antithrombin III is the best known of several known inhibitory proteins because of its potentiating interaction with heparin.

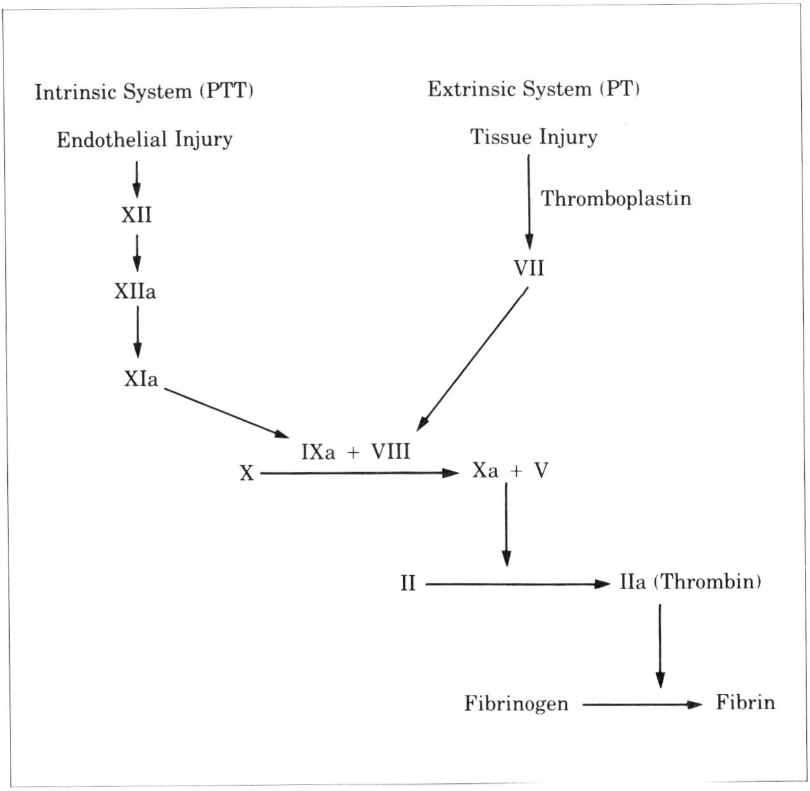

Fig. 6-1. The classic coagulation cascade. The intrinsic system is activated by endothelial damage and is reflected by measurement of the partial thromboplastin time (PTT). The extrinsic system is activated by tissue damage and is reflected by measurement of the prothrombin time (PT). Proenzymes are generally cleaved to make the activated form (e.g., II $\rightarrow$ IIa), and these often catalyze the conversion of other proenzymes.

3. **Fibrinolysis.** This system exists to lyse the fibrin clot and thus limit the size of the fibrin clot formed. Tissue plasminogen activator is released by several stimuli, and in the presence of fibrin, it converts plasminogen to plasmin. Plasmin then will lyse the fibrin clot. Defects in this system can lead to thrombotic complications or premature clot dissolution causing delayed bleeding.

B. **Congenital disorders of hemostasis** are uncommon, but important disorders that can have clinical variability from mild (subclinical) to severe. Patients afflicted with these conditions are often affected prior to pregnancy. If the manifestation is mild, the bleeding diathesis may not be apparent until challenged by delivery or surgery. Screening tests for these defects include platelet count, PT, PTT, and bleeding time. Although the bleeding time is more sensitive to platelet abnormalities, it is a good in vivo test of the effectiveness of the entire coagulation system. It will not elucidate the specific defect. The bleeding history and the results of the aforementioned screening tests will decide the need for more detailed evaluation.

1. **Von Willebrand's disease,** an autosomal dominant condition, is the most common congenital bleeding disorder. The defect involves von Willebrand's factor, which is responsible for platelet adhesion to the damaged endothelial surface. A defect in this system will lead to a bleeding diathesis due to platelet dysfunction. The condition varies from subclinical to severe. The condition may not become apparent until surgery or the patient ingests aspirin. The von Willebrand's factor is complexed with factor VIII procoagulant into a large multimer. Because factor VIII is carried with von Willebrand's factor, a deficiency in the von Willebrand's factor will lead to a deficiency in factor VIII (similar to hemophilia). There are several subtypes of the disease. Type I, a quantitative deficiency of normal factor, is the most common type, accounting for about 80% of cases. Type IIA is also autosomal dominant. In this form the von Willebrand's factor is made but is abnormal and functions poorly if at all. Type IIB is autosomal dominant and is characterized by a normal protein that is too rapidly cleared from the plasma, leading to a deficiency of the factor. Type III is a rare autosomal recessive disease characterized by absent von Willebrand's factor.

   a. **Diagnosis.** Classically, the factors that lead to the diagnosis of von Willebrand's disease include positive family history, positive bleeding history, prolonged bleeding time, and prolonged PTT [24]. However, many patients will not present with all the elements noted. Only if the factor VIII level is below 25–30% will the PTT be prolonged. Similarly, the von Willebrand's factor must be below 30% to cause a prolonged bleeding time. The most important assay for the functional activity of von Willebrand's factor is based on the influence of an antibiotic, ristocetin, to cause formalinized platelets to agglutinate. This in vitro test best approximates the level and function of von Willebrand's factor to cause platelet adhesion in vivo to the damaged endothelial surface. It also correlates well with clinical bleeding and a prolonged bleeding time. Abnormalities in the von Willebrand's factor protein can be detected on electrophoresis. To make the diagnosis of von Willebrand's disease in the suspected patient with a bleeding disorder, a screening PTT and bleeding time can be obtained. If both are normal and suspicion continues, then one can check the PTT and bleeding time twice more. Alternatively, a ristocetin cofactor assay is done to establish the diagnosis.

   b. **Management.** As noted at the beginning of the chapter, the coagulation factors are frequently elevated in pregnancy. Patients with von Willebrand's disease will often experience an amelioration in their condition because of an elevation in the factor. If the disease is mild, then the elevation may be sufficient to raise both ristocetin cofactor and factor VIII to normal or supranormal levels. As the disease becomes more severe, this elevation in the factors may not be sufficient to provide normal hemostasis. Patients with von Willebrand's disease can be followed with serial bleeding times. If at term the bleeding time is normal, and the factor VIII coagulant activity is at least 50%, then no special treatment is required [3]. If the bleeding time is elevated to greater than 20 minutes, then therapy should be initiated in the expectation of delivery (or cesarean section).

Current therapy involves transfusion of cryoprecipitate that contains ristocetin cofactor, factor VIII, fibrinogen, and other coagulation factors. Prophylactic treatment at the onset of labor is an initial dose of 0.24 bags/kg and then 0.12 bags/kg every 12 hours for a total of 7 days. This will equal about 15–25 bags initially, followed by 7–12 bags tid thereafter [24]. After delivery, the vasopressin analog, desmopressin (DDAVP) can be given in lieu of cryoprecipitate. The DDAVP causes release of stored von Willebrand's factor from the endothelial cells and often is sufficient to bring the bleeding under control. Experience in pregnancy is minimal, with only a few reports [6]. Caution during pregnancy is advised, since the neonatal effects are not known, and maternal water intoxication has been seen. Patients with von Willebrand's disease are candidates for the hepatitis B vaccine, since they are at risk for substantial transfusions of blood products.

2. **Hemophilia A.** Hemophilia A is due to a deficiency of factor VIII. It is a sex-linked recessive condition that usually affects males. It is rarely seen in females but can occur if the X chromosome carrying the defective gene is expressed while the normal gene is not. Carriers of the gene will have factor VIII levels of about 50%, which is sufficient to provide normal hemostasis. If that level is less than 25%, then a bleeding disorder can manifest. In pregnancy, the factor VIII levels will rise. If the level remains below 25%, then treatment will be necessary. Cryoprecipitate or factor VIII transfusions are used to replenish the levels to at least 60%. Cryoprecipitate was preferred to factor VIII transfusions to decrease the risks of hepatitis and human immunodeficiency virus (HIV). Recombinant human factor VIII is now available without the risk of HIV or hepatitis. Mild conditions can be treated with DDAVP, but cautions on use in pregnancy should be taken as noted before. Prenatal diagnosis is important since the mothers are obligate carriers, and the male fetus has a 50% risk of inheritance. Fetal blood can be tested for factor VIII procoagulant activity and compared to the amount of the multimeric form (the complex of von Willebrand's factor and factor VIII procoagulant). Very low or absent amounts of factor VIII coagulant activity are consistent with severe hemophilia. In the near future, prenatal diagnosis will be made by direct assays for the abnormal gene on the X chromosome by restriction endonuclease analysis.
3. **Hemophilia B.** Hemophilia B, an uncommon sex-linked recessive disorder, is due to a deficiency of factor IX. Its presentation is indistinguishable from hemophilia A. The diagnosis is made by an assay specifically for factor IX. Similar to hemophilia A, mild afflictions may not require treatment. However, if the levels of factor IX fall below 25%, then treatment is warranted with factor IX, since neither factor VIII concentrate nor cryoprecipitate contains sufficient amounts to correct the deficiency. Prenatal diagnosis is similarly important in hemophilia A. A DNA analysis of cultured fetal fibroblasts will be used to establish the diagnosis in the future.
4. **Other congenital disorders of hemostasis.** These other conditions can involve problems with fibrinolysis or platelet function, and, generally, all are rare. It is important to mention factor XIII deficiency since it can present with delayed bleeding problems. Factor XIII is responsible for establishing cross-links between fibrin monomers and thus stabilizing the fibrin clot. Deficiency of this factor leads to a bleeding diathesis and poor wound healing. The affected neonate characteristically will have bleeding from the umbilical cord stump.

C. **Acquired disorders of hemostasis** stem from various problems, including hepatic dysfunction, vitamin K deficiency, anticoagulant medications, antibodies to coagulation factors, hematologic malignancies, platelet disorders, and disseminated intravascular coagulation [19]. Many of these problems are distinctly uncommon, and so attention will be paid to the more important conditions seen in association with pregnancy.

1. **Anticoagulant medications** include heparin and coumarin. The pregnant patient may be taking these drugs for a preexisting condition, such as a prosthetic heart valve, or for a problem presenting in pregnancy, such as a deep venous thrombosis. These medications can be dangerous in pregnancy and their use must be carefully regulated. Coumarin is largely contraindicated in pregnancy, especially in the first trimester, because of its teratogenic effects. Its use should be restricted to those situations where long-term therapy with heparin is not possible or has significant deleterious consequences. Coumarin does pass the placenta, and so the fetus is also anticoagulated, and thus at risk for bleeding complications. Coumarin has been found not to pass into breast milk in nursing mothers, and so it can be used safely post partum [13]. Heparin does not pass the placenta, and so the risk of fetal hemorrhage is not increased. Long-term therapy with heparin can cause osteoporosis as well as increase the risk of maternal hemorrhage. So the decision to commit a patient to long-term anticoagulation should not be undertaken lightly. Heparin does have the advantage of easy reversibility. In four hours, the anticoagulation effect is nearly absent just by stopping the medication, and a more rapid reversal can be obtained by use of protamine sulfate.
2. **Lupus anticoagulant,** an acquired immunoglobulin, is seen in association with systemic lupus erythematosus, other autoimmune diseases, pregnancy, and occasionally in association with drugs. It is directed against platelet phospholipid [26]. It is called an anticoagulant because the PTT is prolonged and this abnormality is not corrected by addition of normal plasma. Nevertheless, a bleeding diathesis is not seen, but rather venous or arterial thromboses. Recurrent spontaneous abortions are common in women with the lupus anticoagulant. Placental infarctions have been seen in association with fetal loss. Thrombocytopenia also can be present and can be a cause of bleeding problems rather than the presence of the anticoagulant. Use of steroids or aspirin (or both) has been reported to improve pregnancy outcome.
3. **Thrombocytopenia.** Many causes can result in thrombocytopenia. They are usually the result of inadequate production, increased consumption, or increased destruction of platelets. Nutritional deficiencies, aplastic anemia, and infiltrative bone marrow malignancies are examples of inadequate production. Increased consumption occurs in disseminated intravascular coagulation (DIC). Increased destruction can occur due to antibodies directed against the platelets, microangiopathic hemolytic anemia, certain drugs, and thrombotic disorders. Major causes are considered in sec. **6.a.**
4. **Idiopathic or immunologic thrombocytopenic purpura** (see Chap. 14).
5. **Thrombotic thrombocytopenic purpura** (see Chap. 14).
6. **Disseminated intravascular coagulation** has a large variety of causes. Many different terms have been used to describe the hemostatic disorder that results from abnormalities in the coagulation, platelet, and fibrinolytic systems. A more general term, **consumptive thrombohemorrhagic disorders,** better describes the group of hemostatic and thrombotic conditions [27]. DIC implies a general intravascular activation of the coagulation, platelet, and fibrinolytic systems. Several obstetric problems associated with bleeding diathesis do not involve all these systems (such as preeclampsia and saline-induced abortion). The range of presentations is highly variable, such as acute versus chronic, mild versus severe, and localized versus disseminated.
   a. Causes
      (1) Abruptio placentae occurs when a normally implanted placenta separates from the uterus prior to the birth of the fetus. Vaginal bleeding is present 80% of the time but may be concealed. Significant blood loss can result but may be concealed in the retroplacental clot. The bleeding diathesis results from consumption of fibrinogen and platelets in the retroplacental clot, as well as activation of the fibrinolytic system. Decreased coagulation factors, especially factors V, VII, VIII, and fibrinogen are seen, as well as a decreased platelet count. Fibrin(ogen) degradation products (FDP) may be increased from lysis of fibrinogen and fibrin. An

improvement in the diagnosis of fibrinolysis has recently appeared with an assay for d-dimers, a major component of the breakdown of cross-linked fibrin clot by plasmin. This very sensitive test is positive in almost all patients with DIC [11, 16].

(a) Diagnosis. In severe placental abruption the patient classically presents with tetanic, painful uterine contractions, vaginal bleeding, and a dead fetus. Less extreme presentations are common, and all the aforementioned elements may not be present. Depending on the severity of the abruption, any of the following can be seen: decreased hemoglobin/hematocrit, decreased platelet count, prolonged PTT, prolonged bleeding time, decreased fibrinogen, and elevated FDPs. The degree of laboratory abnormalities does not always correlate with the clinical picture.

(b) Management. The definitive management requires evacuation of the uterus. This allows for effective cessation of bleeding from the placental bed and stems the further uncontrolled consumption of coagulation elements. Whether the evacuation should be done by augmented vaginal delivery or by cesarean section depends on whether the fetus is alive or stillborn, the degree of hemorrhage, and the degree of the hemostatic disorder. In situations of thrombocytopenia (platelets below 50,000/ml), platelet transfusions are indicated. Hypofibrinogenemia is managed by transfusions of fresh-frozen plasma or cryoprecipitate. Note that fibrinogen concentrate carries an unacceptably high risk of hepatitis and HIV transmission. Human recombinant clotting factors including fibrinogen will likely obviate this complication in the near future. Heparin is contraindicated because of the risk of worsening the hemostatic disorder.

(2) Retained dead fetus. The consumptive coagulopathy seen with a fetal demise occurs after five weeks and is chronic in nature. Hemorrhagic consequences are far less common. Decomposition of the fetus and placenta causes passage of thromboplastic material into the maternal circulation. A low-grade consumption of coagulation factors and platelets can follow. Induced vaginal delivery will usually suffice to stop the release of tissue thromboplastin and DIC. In cases of multiple gestation where one fetus is demised and the other(s) alive, persistent DIC may be a problem, and so use of heparin can prevent further consumptive coagulation. Heparin must be stopped prior to labor and delivery. Platelet and coagulation factor transfusions are usually not required.

(3) Amniotic fluid embolism, an unusually catastrophic condition, results from a bolus of amniotic fluid into the maternal circulation. This foreign material lodges in the pulmonary circulation and leads to respiratory failure and circulatory collapse. Maternal mortality has been reported as high as 80%. If the patient survives the initial insult, DIC is invariably seen a short time later due to the release of thromboplastic material from the amniotic fluid into the maternal circulation. No specific treatment is available. Supportive therapy involves ventilatory support, circulatory support with vasopressors, and replacement of coagulation factors as needed.

(4) Saline induction of abortion. Hypertonic saline is used in some areas of the United States for induction of second-trimester abortion. Less than 1 in 1000 procedures are complicated by a mild DIC. The cause is unclear but felt to be due to destruction of fetus and placenta, releasing thromboplastic materials into the maternal circulation.

(5) Septic abortion and intrauterine infection. Severe intrauterine infection due to gram-negative and anaerobic bacteria can be associated with a fulminant DIC. The endotoxins present in the gram-negative bacteria are responsible for the myriad of pathologic disturbances. These include sepsis, shock, endothelial wall damage, activation of the coagulation system, and the release of microthrombi that can cause end organ ischemia.

Clinical manifestations are also myriad and include the potential for circulatory collapse, respiratory and renal failure, central nervous system disturbances, and DIC in the most extreme cases. Use of broad-spectrum antibiotics and control of the nidus of infection are of primary importance. Evacuation of uterine contents is mandatory. Heparin use is controversial.

(6) **Preeclampsia.** In severe cases of preeclampsia/eclampsia, thrombocytopenia can be seen as part of the HELLP syndrome (hemolysis, elevated liver functions, and low platelets). It is postulated to be caused by a microangiopathic hemolytic anemia. Endothelial wall damage with subsequent deposition of fibrin (especially in the glomerular capillaries of the kidneys) with arteriolar spasm causes platelet adhesion and consumption, and hemolytic anemia. Generally, consumption of coagulation factors is not seen, and in fact there is evidence of a hypercoagulable state as manifested by increased fibrinogen level, decreased fibrinolysis, and elevated FDPs [33]. Antithrombin III can be decreased secondary to the proteinuria commonly seen in preeclampsia. The patient may be at risk for thrombotic complications if the proteinuria is severe, as indicated by proteinuria greater than 10 gm/24 hour or a serum albumin less than 2 gm/dl [25, 34]. Heparin may be indicated for venous thrombosis prophylaxis but does not ameliorate the course of preeclampsia. The treatment for preeclampsia/eclampsia is expedited delivery of the baby and removal of the placenta. The thrombocytopenia will spontaneously resolve, and rarely are platelet transfusions indicated.

VI. **Blood transfusion therapy.** Teleologically, the increased RBC mass and plasma volume not only allow for adequate perfusion of the utero-placental-fetal unit during the developing pregnancy, but also act as a buffer against the blood loss of delivery. Average blood loss for vaginal delivery is 300–500 ml, and it is 800–1000 ml for a cesarean section. Blood loss can be excessive during delivery, because of obstetric complications (e.g., placenta previa, placental abruption), or medical/surgical complications (bleeding diathesis, severe anemia, maternal trauma). Indications for transfusion therapy in pregnancy include maintaining circulatory volume for perfusion, providing adequate oxygen delivery to maternal and fetal tissues, and providing coagulation factors necessary to maintain hemostasis.

A. **Transfusion screening.** To avoid mismatch of blood components, donor blood is subject to testing to ensure that a major hemolytic transfusion reaction will not occur. Donor and recipient blood is screened for the following antigen/antibodies:

1. **ABO**
2. **$Rh_o(D)$**
3. **Irregular antibodies**

In emergent situations, there may not be time for a full cross-match, which generally takes 45 minutes. Use of type-specific blood is associated with a low risk of **transfusion reactions** (about 0.03%) [29]. Other than emergencies, only fully cross-matched blood should be used, to avoid transfusion reactions. Type-specific blood is preferred to O-negative donor blood, since transfusion reactions can still occur due to irregular antibodies in patient serum.

B. **Component therapy.** Use of blood components provides specific components for specific needs and stretches the usefulness of a single blood donation. The use of whole blood has diminished because of component therapy. Also, unless the whole blood is less than 24–48 hours old, it will lose greater than 50% of the activity of its platelets and coagulation factors, greatly diminishing its usefulness.

1. **Red blood cells.** In most cases packed red cells suffice for blood replacement. It is unusual that whole blood must be used. Isotonic saline must be used as a dilutant for transfusion, as neither lactated Ringer's solution nor 5% dextrose in water is acceptable. Given the risks of transmissible disease, the indications for transfusion should be certain. It is not necessary routinely to transfuse for a given level of hemoglobin/hematocrit. In pregnancy, the increased plasma to RBC mass may lead to "physiologic anemia." The red cell mass is increased, and so the patient will tolerate lower hematocrits than the nonpregnant pa-

tient. In our institution, unless the blood loss is acute, we do not transfuse for hematocrits above 20%, unless the patient is symptomatic. We offer transfusion to patients with hematocrits below 20%, unless chronic anemia has been present.

a. **Frozen red cells** can be used instead of packed red cells but obviously must be thawed prior to use and therefore are of limited value in an emergency. Their best use is for those patients with unusual antibodies where other blood is difficult to obtain, or for storage of autologous blood for an operation anticipated in the future.

b. **Leukocyte-poor cells** are indicated for patients who have previously experienced febrile reactions from previous transfusions. In some patients, donor leukocyte antigens are responsible for these reactions. Washed red cells have greatly diminished leukocytes. Blood filters are now available that eliminate most of these unwanted cells and cell debris.

c. **Autologous blood.** Autologous blood can be donated ahead from patients for whom major surgery is planned. In pregnant patients, the most common anticipated major surgeries would be cesarean section or cesarean hysterectomy for cervical or ovarian cancer. A hemoglobin above 11 gm/dl is necessary for consideration of autologous donation. A mechanical cell saver can be used to salvage autologous blood but requires set-up and experienced personnel. Its usefulness in obstetric surgery is questionable.

2. **Platelet transfusion.** In situations of massive transfusion (> 8–10 units of blood), the platelet count may decrease secondary to dilution. In a surgical setting, consideration should be given to transfusion of platelets when the platelet count falls below 70,000–80,000 [10]. Preexisting thrombocytopenia may be another indication for platelet transfusion, but the cause must be determined first. Platelet transfusion for idiopathic thrombocytopenic purpura is usually of little benefit. Thrombocytopenia associated with DIC may resolve without therapy, and platelet transfusions are only necessary in the face of a documented bleeding disorder. If the patient develops DIC during surgery, and the patient has received a transfusion, a major transfusion reaction must be ruled out. Type-specific platelets should be used if available. A female patient who is Rh negative and receives Rh-positive platelets should receive RhoGAM 300 μg to prevent isoimmunization [29].

3. **Plasma components**

a. **Fresh-frozen plasma.** Fresh-frozen plasma is best used to replace coagulation factors that have been depleted due to dilution, consumption, or a congenital bleeding disorder. This contains factors V and VIII, and fibrinogen. It also provides colloid support for hypovolemic patients and is least likely to be infectious.

b. **Cryoprecipitate.** Cryoprecipitate contains factor VIII and fibrinogen and is best used where coagulation factors must be replaced in as small of a volume as possible. Patients who receive platelet transfusions may not need coagulation factor replacement since there is some plasma in the platelet transfusions. Since cryoprecipitate is a pooled plasma product, it carries a much higher rate of transfusion-related infection than single donor plasma.

c. **Albumin** is used as colloid support to maintain circulatory volume. It is used when crystalloid solutions are not sufficient because of loss of oncotic pressure due to increased capillary permeability. In contrast to the above components, it is pasteurized and therefore does not carry the risk of transmissible disease such as HIV or hepatitis.

C. **Complications of transfusion therapy.** Despite careful testing, transfusion of blood components still carries the risk of transfusion reactions, transmissible disease, and metabolic changes.

1. **Transfusion reactions**

a. **Hemolytic reactions.** Hemolytic reactions occur due to mismatch of donor and recipient blood, usually from an ABO mismatch. The cause is generally human error, such as a failure to follow matching and identification procedures. The presence of antibody in the patient's serum can cause immediate hemolytic destruction of the donor cells. Typical symptoms include a burning sensation in the arm, chills, fever, shortness of breath, chest pain or tightness, back pain, and diaphoresis. Tachycardia, tachypnea, and hypotension also may be present. A DIC with clinical bleeding problems can occur and may be the only sign in an anesthetized patient [29]. The blood transfusion must be stopped immediately. The donor blood and a sample of patient blood must be sent to the lab for repeat cross-match. Treatment includes general circulatory support and prevention of DIC and acute renal failure.

b. **Febrile reactions** are common during transfusion therapy. They are usually due to allergic reaction to donor leukocyte antigens. It is acceptable to pretreat patients with 650 mg of acetaminophen and 50 mg of diphenhydramine. If the patient then develops a fever and chill, the transfusion should be stopped and evaluated for a hemolytic transfusion reaction. The donor blood and patient blood should be subjected to a repeat cross-match. If recurrent febrile reactions persist, use of leukocyte-poor blood may be necessary.

c. **Allergic reactions** are also common and are usually due to histamine release. Antihistamines are used to treat the urticaria. Severe reactions may require more intense treatment.

2. **Transmissible disease**

   a. **Hepatitis.** Ever since the universal screening of donor blood for hepatitis B, this has been almost completely eliminated as a cause of posttransfusion hepatitis. Rarely, seronegative but infectious blood can cause hepatitis B in susceptible patients. Ninety-five percent of posttransfusion hepatitis is now felt to be due to non-A, non-B (NANB) hepatitis. Until recently, the cause was unknown but felt to be due to a transmissible agent that was an as yet uncharacterized virus. This virus has recently been characterized and is now called **hepatitis C** [17]. Currently, blood banks use surrogate testing for the unknown virus that includes an elevated alanine aminotransferase and the presence of anti-hepatitis B core antigen. Hepatitis C is felt to be the major cause of posttransfusion hepatitis—up to 85% in one study [12]. The risk of NANB hepatitis is unknown, since most patients remain asymptomatic, but is felt to occur in 7–10% of blood recipients [31]. The use of an assay for the presence of hepatitis C to eliminate infected donor blood will increase the safety of transfusion therapy.

   b. **Human immunodeficiency virus infection.** Since the acquired immunodeficiency syndrome became recognized in 1981, use of blood products has been identified as a risk factor for its transmission, especially factor VIII transfusions for hemophiliacs. Later, HIV transmission from blood transfusions was identified and efforts made to decrease that risk. The development of the enzyme-linked immunoassay, backed up by the western blot assay, has allowed for testing of the presence of HIV in donated blood products. This testing is preceded by donor screening procedures designed to eliminate those donors who are in high-risk categories. However, some persons with latent HIV infection are not recognized by any screening procedure. The culmination of these procedures has greatly decreased the actual risk of HIV transmission from blood products. It is currently felt to be no higher than 1 in 40,000 blood products [9]. **The key to minimizing the risk of any transfusion-related illness is not to transfuse patients unnecessarily.**

References

1. Anderson, H. M. Maternal Hematologic Disorders. In R. K. Creasy and R. Resnik (eds.), *Maternal-Fetal Medicine* (2d ed.). Philadelphia: Saunders, 1989.
2. Brandt, J. T. Current concepts of coagulation. *Clin. Obstet. Gynecol.* 28:3, 1985.
3. Caldwell, D. C., Williamson, R. A., and Goldsmith, J. C. Hereditary coagulopathies in pregnancy. *Clin. Obstet. Gynecol.* 28:53, 1985.
4. Catanzarite, V. A., and Ferguson, J. E., II. Acute leukemia and pregnancy: A

review of management and outcome, 1972–1982. *Obstet. Gynecol. Sur.* 39:663, 1984.
5. Charache, S., et al. Management of sickle cell disease in pregnant patients. *Obstet. Gynecol.* 55:407, 1980.
6. Chediak, J. R., Alban, G. M., and Maxey, B. Von Willebrand's disease and pregnancy: Management during delivery and outcome of offspring. *Am. J. Obstet. Gynecol.* 155:618, 1986.
7. Corash, L. Laboratory Evaluation of Hemostasis. In R. K. Laros, Jr. (ed.), *Blood Disorders in Pregnancy*. Philadelphia: Lea & Febiger, 1986.
8. Dildy, G. A., III, et al. Maternal malignancy metastatic to the products of conception: A review. *Obstet. Gynecol. Sur.* 44:535, 1989.
9. Dodd, R. Y. Transfusion and AIDS. *International Ophthalmol. Clin.* 29:83, 1989.
10. Edmunds, L. H., Jr., and Addonizio, V. P., Jr. Massive Transfusion. In R. W. Colman, et al. *Hemostasis and Thrombosis—Basic Principles and Clinical Practice*. Philadelphia: Lippincott, 1987.
11. Elms, M. J., et al. Measurements of crosslinked fibrin degradation products—An immunoassay using monoclonal antibodies. *Thromb. and Haemost.* 50:591, 1983.
12. Esteban, J. I., et al. Hepatitis C virus antibodies among risk groups in Spain. *Lancet* 2:294, 1989.
13. Ginsberg, J. S., and Hirsh, J. Anticoagulants during pregnancy. *Am. Rev. Med.* 40:79, 1989.
14. Gookin, K., and Morrison, J. C. Anemia Associated with Pregnancy. In J. J. Sciarra (ed.), *Gynecology and Obstetrics,* Vol. 3 (rev. ed.). Philadelphia: Harper & Row, 1987.
15. Gookin, K., and Morrison, J. C. Nutritional Anemias Complicating Pregnancy. In R. K. Laros, Jr. (ed.), *Blood Disorders in Pregnancy*. Philadelphia: Lea & Febiger, 1986.
16. Greenberg, C. S., Devine, D. V., and McCrae, K. M. Measurement of plasma fibrin D-dimer levels with the use of a monoclonal antibody coupled to Latex beads. *Am. J. Clin. Pathol.* 87:94, 1987.
17. Kuo, G., et al. An assay for circulating antibodies to a major etiologic virus of human non-A, non-B hepatitis. *Science* 244:362, 1989.
18. Lange, R. D., and Dynesius, R. Blood volume changes during normal pregnancy. *Clin. Haematol.* 2:433, 1973.
19. Laros, R. K. Acquired Coagulation Disorders. In R. K. Laros, Jr. (ed.), *Blood Disorders in Pregnancy*. Philadelphia: Lea & Febiger, 1986.
20. Laros, R. K. Aplastic Anemia. In R. K. Laros, Jr. (ed.), *Blood Disorders in Pregnancy*. Philadelphia: Lea & Febiger, 1986.
21. Laros, R. K., Jr. The Hemoglobinopathies. In R. K. Laros, Jr. (ed.), *Blood Disorders in Pregnancy*. Philadelphia: Lea & Febiger, 1986.
22. Levin, J. Hematologic Disorders of Pregnancy. In G. N. Burrow and T. F. Ferris (eds.), *Medical Complications During Pregnancy* (2d ed.). Philadelphia: Saunders, 1982.
23. Lewis, B. J., and Laros, R. K., Jr. Leukemia and Lymphoma. In R. K. Laros, Jr. (ed.), *Blood Disorders in Pregnancy*. Philadelphia: Lea & Febiger, 1986.
24. Linker, C. Congenital Disorders of Hemostasis. In R. K. Laros, Jr. (ed.), *Blood Disorders in Pregnancy*. Philadelphia: Lea & Febiger, 1986.
25. Llach, F. Hypercoagulability and thrombotic complications of nephrotic syndrome. *Kidney Int.* 28:429, 1985.
26. Lubbe, W. F., et al. Lupus anticoagulant in pregnancy. *Br. J. Obstet. Gynecol.* 91:357, 1984.
27. Marder, V. J., et al. Consumptive Thrombohemorrhagic Disorders. In R. W. Colman, et al. (eds.), *Hemostasis and Thrombosis—Basic Principles and Clinical Practice*. Philadelphia: Lippincott, 1987.
28. Mills, G. B. Immunology of Cancer in Pregnancy. In H. H. Allen and J. A. Nisker (eds.), *Cancer in Pregnancy*. Mt. Kisco, N.Y.: Futura, 1986.

29. Oberman, H. A. Transfusion Therapy. In R. K. Laros, Jr. (ed.), *Blood Disorder in Pregnancy*. Philadelphia: Lea & Febiger, 1986.
30. Phillips, F. A., and Kazazian, H. H. Haemoglobinopathies and Thalassemias In A. E. H. Emery and D. L. Rimoin (eds.), *Principles and Practice of Medica Genetics*. London: Churchill-Livingstone, 1983.
31. Seeff, L. B., and Dienstag, J. L. Transfusion-associated non-A, non-B hepati tis—Where do we go from here? *Gastroenterology* 95:530, 1988.
32. Sutcliffe, S. B., and Chapman, R. M. Lymphomas and Leukemias. In H. H Allen and J. A. Nisker (eds.), *Cancer in Pregnancy*. Mt. Kisco, N.Y.: Futura 1986.
33. Von Hugo, R., and Graeff, H. Thrombohemorrhagic Complications in the Ob stetric Patient. In R. W. Colman et al. (eds.), *Hemostasis and Thrombosis— Basic Principles and Clinical Practice*. Philadelphia: Lippincott, 1987.
34. Weiner, C. P., et al. Antithrombin III activity in women with hypertensior during pregnancy. *Obstet. Gynecol.* 65:301, 1985.

7 Respiratory Complications

Katherine M. Gillogley

I. Pulmonary physiology. During pregnancy, several changes in pulmonary physiology affect the evaluation and management of women presenting with respiratory complaints. These changes are necessary to meet the increased metabolic and circulatory demands of the growing fetus, placenta, and uterus as well as anatomically accommodating this growth (Figure 7-1).

In pregnancy, the oxygen requirement increases by 20%. The pO_2 remains the same. Tidal volume is increased 40%, while the residual volume is decreased 20%. The respiratory rate remains unchanged, but because of the increased tidal volume, the minute ventilation increases. With the increased ventilation, the pCO_2 decreases to 28–32 mm Hg. The pH of the blood is unchanged, with a compensatory decrease in HCO_3. It is postulated that progesterone is responsible for this increase in ventilation via an increased sensitivity of the respiratory center to carbon dioxide [2]. Anatomically the subcostal angle increases approximately 35 degrees and the transthoracic diameter is also increased. On chest x ray, there are often increased vascular markings in normal pregnancy and the diaphragm is elevated.

II. Dyspnea. The perception of shortness of breath may be experienced by as many as 76% of women at some time during pregnancy but generally stabilizes closer to term [14]. This phenomenon is thought to be secondary to the increased sensitivity to carbon dioxide and the sensation of the increase in ventilation. Tachypnea in the nonlaboring pregnant woman is abnormal and pathology must be ruled out.

III. Asthma. Asthma may complicate 0.4–1.3% of pregnancies. The severity of the disease remains unchanged in approximately one-half of women, is improved in 29%, and is worse in 22% [24]. This effect may vary between pregnancies of an individual woman.

A. Perinatal outcome. Perinatal morbidity and mortality may depend on the level of control of disease. In the Collaborative Perinatal study [6], a perinatal mortality twice that of controls for women with asthma was noted. More recent studies have indicated that with good control of the disease, perinatal morbidity and mortality approximate that of the general population [19, 23].

B. Antepartum management

1. Initial evaluation. At the initial prenatal visit, a history of frequency and severity of exacerbations, hospitalizations, and current and past medications should be obtained from the patient with asthma. Physical examination may indicate the level of control of disease and suggest a need for improving the medication regimen. Baseline spirometry may be useful in the patient with recent or currently active disease.

2. Initial management. It appears that the risks of uncontrolled asthma are of more concern than the risks of medication used to treat asthma. The pregnant asthmatic should be counseled about the importance of this. Women using inhaled bronchodilators or corticosteroids in asthma appear to have no greater risks of congenital anomalies or adverse perinatal outcomes than the general population [18, 19]. The use of theophylline and cromolyn sodium in pregnancy is also considered safe. The theophylline dosage may require reduction during the third trimester because of a decrease in clearance [3]. Theophylline levels should be monitored closely. The therapeutic range is 10–20 μg/ml.

C. Acute exacerbations

1. Evaluation. A careful history and physical examination should be performed, with particular attention to past history of exacerbations, heart rate, respiratory rate, and how well the patient is moving air. An arterial blood gas should be obtained. If the pH is acidotic or the pCO_2 is elevated, present or impending respiratory failure is likely. A shielded chest x ray should be obtained if respiratory infection is suspected.

2. **Management.** The initial management of the acute attack includes administering oxygen by face mask, intravenous hydration, and inhaled or subcutaneously injected bronchodilators. Metaproterenol (Alupent) by inhalation and terbutaline, 0.25 mg SC, both beta-2 selective agents, have had extensive use in pregnancy. Suspected bronchitis should be treated with erythromycin or ampicillin since tetracycline is contraindicated in pregnancy. If no satisfactory response results from the initial bronchodilators, intravenous aminophylline should be given, with an initial loading dose of 6 mg/kg if the patient is not already taking a theophylline preparation. A maintenance dose of 0.5–0.7 mg/kg/hour is then administered. Theophylline levels are to be followed closely. Atropine given by inhalation may also be useful. Recently magnesium sulfate, 1.2 gm IV over 20 minutes, has been used in nonpregnant adults for acute asthma refractory to beta-agonists [21].

   Corticosteroids should be used with **severe exacerbations** or those not responding to the aforementioned therapy. Methylprednisolone (Solu-Medrol), 125 mg every 6 hours given IV, may be given acutely. An oral prednisone taper should follow intravenous steroid therapy. Placement in an intensive care setting with capabilities for mechanical ventilation is suggested for patients with minimal improvement of a severe exacerbation. Pulse oximetry is useful for monitoring oxygen saturation prior to resolution of the severe asthmatic attack.

3. **Labor management.** Symptoms of asthma rarely increase during labor [23]. Asthma medications used in the prenatal period should be continued. Women on corticosteroid therapy prior to labor should receive additional corticosteroids during the labor. Regional anesthesia is preferred if a cesarean section is performed for obstetric reasons.

IV. Cystic fibrosis

A. Incidence. As improved treatment for cystic fibrosis has lengthened survivals, more women with cystic fibrosis are entering the reproductive years. The incidence of cystic fibrosis is 1 in 2000 births. It is estimated that 30% live more than 30 years [13]. Cystic fibrosis may be first diagnosed during pregnancy, as 2–3% of patients may not be recognized until early adulthood [10].

B. Pathology. Cystic fibrosis patients exhibit a mixed obstructive/restrictive pattern of pulmonary disease, have pancreatic insufficiency, and may have cirrhosis.

C. Complications. In one series of 97 completed pregnancies with cystic fibrosis complications included congestive heart failure in 13%, prematurity in 27%, and perinatal death in 11%. Surprisingly the maternal mortality remained similar to that of nonpregnant cystic fibrosis patients [5].

D. Management. The pregnant cystic fibrosis patient is managed similarly to the nonpregnant patient, except that tetracycline is not used. Pulmonary function studies, sputum cultures, and weight gain should be followed closely. A baseline electrocardiogram and echocardiogram may be useful. Fetal growth should be assessed by ultrasound, along with antepartum fetal heart rate monitoring begun in the third trimester.

Because the disease involves an abnormality in exocrine gland secretions, the sodium level of the breast milk of the mother with cystic fibrosis should be checked before breast-feeding is initiated.

Preconceptual counseling concerning maternal risk is based on prepregnancy status of disease. The risk of disease in the infant is 2.5%; however, all will be carriers.

V. Sarcoidosis

A. Incidence. It affects 0.05% of pregnancies.

B. Pathology. Sarcoidosis, though most commonly presenting with pulmonary in-

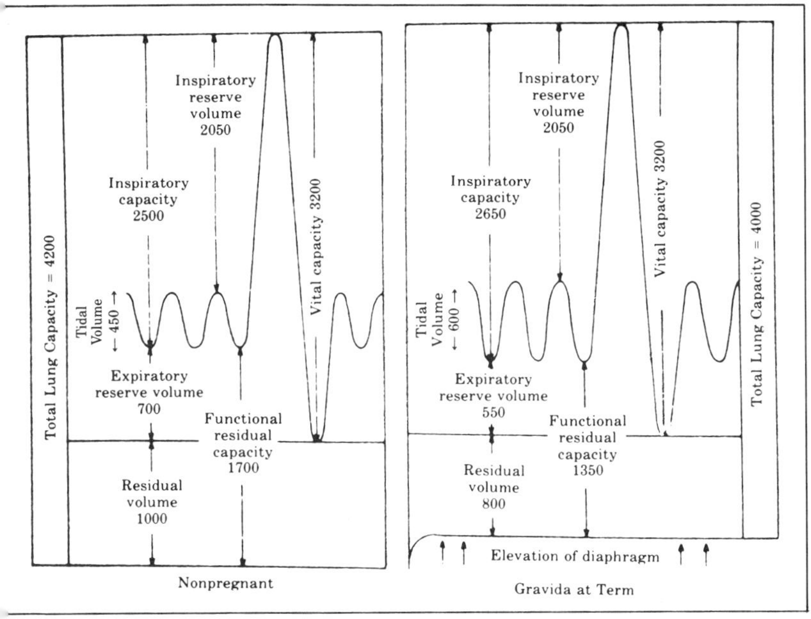

Fig. 7-1. Pulmonary volumes and capacities of the nonpregnant woman and the gravida at term. (From E. A. Leontic, Respiratory disease in pregnancy. *Med. Clin. North Am.* 61:111, 1977.)

volvement, is a granulomatous disease of unknown etiology that may affect multiple systems.

C. Prognosis. Sarcoidosis, in the majority of nonpregnant patients, improves or resolves over several years. In most patients with sarcoidosis, the disease is unchanged or improved during pregnancy. No adverse fetal effects have been reported. Patients with active disease may experience a postpartum exacerbation of symptoms.

D. Management. If sarcoidosis is inactive, the pregnancy is managed in the routine fashion. If active disease is present, corticosteroids may be used to control symptoms.

VI. Infections

A. Antepartum pneumonia

1. **Etiology.** The most common organism isolated is *Streptococcus pneumoniae*. Bacteremia was not found in one recent series of antepartum pneumonias [1] but is commonly reported to be present in pneumonias outside of pregnancy. *Mycoplasma* must also be considered as it is a common cause of community-acquired pneumonias. Other medical complications are frequently present such as asthma, anemia, heart disease, and sickle cell disease [1]. Viral infection, including varicella and influenza, may cause a primary pneumonia or result in a pneumonia that is secondary to a bacterial superinfection.
2. **Diagnosis.** Common symptoms at presentation include fever, chills, cough, sputum production, dyspnea, and pleuritic chest pain. The patient with mycoplasma pneumonia will frequently also report symptoms of sore throat, headache, malaise, or earache. On physical examination, tachypnea, fever, rales, dullness to percussion, and bronchial breath sounds may be found. Significant leukocytosis is common with bacterial pneumonias, whereas no or mild leukocytosis is found with mycoplasma or viral pneumonias. Arterial blood gases may indicate hypoxemia. A shielded chest x ray should be obtained. A single

lobar infiltrate will be commonly found with bacterial pneumonias; patchy multilobar infiltrates are seen more frequently with mycoplasma or viral pneumonias. Viral pneumonias may also reveal interstitial involvement or complete "white out" on chest x ray. Sputum cultures are obtained, checking the Gram's stain for adequacy of the specimen. If mycoplasma is suspected, cold agglutinins or serial complement-fixing antibody titers may be obtained.

3. **Management.** The patient is admitted to the hospital, and intravenous fluids and oxygen are administered. Ampicillin or penicillin is given if pneumococcal disease is strongly suspected; erythromycin is used if mycoplasma is suspected as it will also cover pneumococcus. Fetal monitoring is performed initially in gestations of 26 weeks or longer, until the respiratory status is stabilized. Monitoring for uterine contractions may be useful in any gestation over 20 weeks to rule out preterm labor. A tuberculin skin test should be placed during the hospitalization. Pulse oximetry may be useful in the patient with hypoxemia.

4. **Outcome.** With antibiotic therapy, maternal or fetal mortality or fetal morbidity is now rare with bacterial or mycoplasma pneumonias, unless secondary to a coexisting medical complication [1]. Older reports indicated a high incidence of preterm labor and maternal and fetal mortality [8, 16]. Fulminant varicella or influenza pneumonia, although uncommon, has a high mortality rate in pregnancy.

B. **Bronchitis.** Bronchitis in pregnancy is important because it is common and must be distinguished from pneumonia. Therapy is similar to that used with nonpregnant adults except that tetracycline is not used.

C. **Tuberculosis**

1. **Diagnosis.** Screening for tuberculosis using the Mantoux test (0.1 ml of purified protein derivative [PPD]) should be performed prenatally on all women without a history of a prior positive test in areas with moderate or high rates of disease. In areas with low rates of disease, selective screening of patients with risk factors such as immigration from endemic area, positive household contact, or health care workers is often used. Pregnancy does not affect the reactivity of the tuberculin skin test [17]. All patients with a positive skin test should have a chest x ray with shielding. With an abnormal chest x ray, sputum for acid-fast bacilli on smear and culture should be obtained.

2. **Morbidity.** Pregnancy does not seem to have an adverse effect on the disease. Rather, active tuberculosis that is treated during pregnancy has a good prognosis. If active tuberculosis is untreated, there is a risk as high as 50% of transmission to the newborn during early infancy [9]. Congenital tuberculosis (primary complex in fetal liver) is usually associated with miliary involvement and is rare.

3. **Treatment.** For the pregnant woman with active tuberculosis, a two-drug regimen is given over nine months. Isoniazid (INH) and rifampin are used in doses similar to the nonpregnant adult. Pyridoxine, 50 mg/day should be given whenever INH is used. Ethambutol should be added if INH resistance is suspected. There has been extensive experience with INH and ethambutol in pregnancy without evidence of teratogenicity. There has been some concern over rifampin because of its inhibition of RNA polymerase and also reports of limb reduction defects. Overall, however, congenital anomalies do not appear to be increased with rifampin [22]. Streptomycin should not be used in pregnancy because of a high rate of fetal eighth nerve damage.

For the woman with a recent conversion to a positive PPD and a negative chest x ray, INH prophylaxis may be started in the second trimester. With a positive PPD over a longer or unknown time course, prophylaxis may be started post partum.

D. ***Pneumocystis carinii.*** As the human immunodeficiency virus (HIV) becomes more prevalent is women, there will be a greater incidence of *Pneumocystis* in pregnancy. Cases of *Pneumocystis* in pregnancy described thus far have also reported maternal death [11, 15]. Death from acquired immunodeficiency syndrome in pregnancy is most often from *Pneumocystis* [15].

1. **Diagnosis.** Symptoms include dyspnea, cough, fever, and respiratory failure. Chest x ray reveals bilateral diffuse or patchy infiltrates. The diagnosis is confirmed by identification of *Pneumocystis carinii* in lung biopsy tissue or a bronchoalveolar lavage specimen.
2. **Management.** Intravenous trimethoprim-sulfamethoxazole is the treatment of choice. Pentamidine may be used if trimethoprim-sulfamethoxazole is not tolerated. Oxygen therapy is administered and mechanical ventilation is often required.
3. **Prophylaxis.** The current guidelines from the Centers for Disease Control do not recommend aerosolized pentamidine or oral trimethoprim-sulfamethoxazole in pregnancy for prophylaxis. Close observation of the HIV-infected patient for signs and symptoms of *Pneumocystis* is recommended [7].

VII. Emergencies

A. Pulmonary embolus (see Chap. 15)

B. Amniotic fluid embolus. Amniotic fluid embolus is a rare but catastrophic condition associated with pregnancy. Most cases are associated with labor or cesarean section. The maternal mortality rate is as high as 80%.

1. **Pathophysiology.** The exact mechanism of injury in humans is not clear. Clark and colleagues [4] proposed a model in which the embolization of amniotic fluid causes transient pulmonary arterial spasm producing hypoxia with left ventricular and pulmonary capillary injury in the first phase, followed by left ventricular failure and adult respiratory distress syndrome (ARDS) in the second phase. The etiology of the coagulopathy is unclear.
2. **Diagnosis.** Classic symptoms of amniotic fluid embolus are sudden cardiopulmonary collapse, with severe dyspnea and hypotension. Seizures or hemorrhage may also be presenting symptoms. Pulmonary edema may develop and somewhat later disseminated intravascular coagulation. The diagnosis may be made by aspiration of blood containing fetal squamous cells from a pulmonary artery catheter; however, these have also been found in pregnant patients undergoing the procedure for an entirely different clinical picture [12]. At autopsy the diagnosis is made by finding fetal squamous cells in the pulmonary vessels.
3. **Management.** Immediate, intensive response is necessary. High flow rates of oxygen should be administered by mask. Personnel skilled in intubation and placement of central hemodynamic monitoring lines should be summoned. Cardiopulmonary resuscitation with intubation is frequently necessary within the first hour of symptoms. The fetal heart rate should be continuously monitored. Large-bore intravenous catheters should be placed. A bolus of crystalloid (lactated Ringer's or normal saline) is given for initial treatment of hypotension. If the hypotension persists, dopamine infusion is started. As heart failure is common, central hemodynamic monitoring with a pulmonary artery (Swan-Ganz) catheter is useful in guiding the administration of fluids. Dobutamine is used if an inotropic agent is necessary. Mechanical ventilation with positive end-expiratory pressure (PEEP) is often needed to maintain adequate oxygenation.

   If the patient survives the initial cardiopulmonary collapse, coagulation studies need to be followed closely. Packed red blood cells, fresh-frozen plasma, and platelets are given as needed. Fresh whole blood is a good alternative but is often not available. Cryoprecipitate may be necessary for a fulminant coagulopathy. The use of heparin in this setting is controversial.

C. Pulmonary edema

1. **Etiology.** Pulmonary edema in pregnancy is usually secondary to another condition such as preeclampsia, tocolytic therapy, amniotic fluid embolism, cardiac disease, septic shock, aspiration, or massive fluid resuscitation. It may be of cardiac origin as with decreased ventricular function or fluid overload, involve increased permeability of the pulmonary capillaries, or be secondary to reduced colloid osmotic pressure.
2. **Diagnosis.** Dyspnea, orthopnea, rales, and hypoxemia are the common clinical

symptoms or findings. Fluffy infiltrates or Kerley's B lines will be seen o chest x ray.

3. **Management.** Ultimately treatment is aimed at the underlying disorder. Place ment of a Swan-Ganz (pulmonary artery) catheter may be necessary to asses cardiac function and fluid volume status. Oxygen is administered. If the pu monary edema is secondary to fluid overload, fluid restriction and furosemid therapy are initiated. If the etiology is left ventricular failure, hydralazine o nitroprusside is used for afterload reduction as well as fluid restriction. Wit noncardiogenic pulmonary edema, management is mainly supportive, with us of PEEP if mechanical ventilation is necessary and fluid restricted. The mar agement of noncardiogenic pulmonary edema is discussed in further detail subsequently.

D. Adult respiratory distress syndrome

1. **Diagnosis.** The diagnosis of ARDS is made when there is evidence of diffus alveolar damage with noncardiogenic pulmonary edema [20]. The onset of th disease is acute. Severe hypoxia, decreased pulmonary compliance, increase shunting, and on x ray diffuse pulmonary infiltrates are present.
2. **Etiology.** Etiologies for ARDS include amniotic fluid embolism, preeclampsia eclampsia, trauma, sepsis, aspiration of gastric contents, inhalation injuries overdose or toxicity from various medications or chemicals, pancreatitis, dis seminated intravascular coagulation, blood transfusions, and near-drownin [20].
3. **Management.** The current therapy of ARDS is mainly supportive beyond di agnosing and treating the underlying cause. Careful titration of fluids to main tain perfusion but avoid volume overload is important as failure of other orga systems is often the cause of mortality in ARDS. Mechanical ventilation wit PEEP is used to keep alveoli open and decrease shunting. No evidence show that corticosteroids improve outcome.
4. **Prognosis.** The outcome for pregnant patients with ARDS is similar to th nonpregnant state and depends on the underlying etiology and the extent c involvement of other organ systems.

References

1. Benedetti, T. J., Valle, R., and Ledger, W. J. Antepartum pneumonia in preg nancy. *Obstet. Gynecol.* 144:413, 1982.
2. Burrow, G. N., and Ferris, T. F. *Medical Complications During Pregnancy* Philadelphia: Saunders, 1988.
3. Carter, B. L., Driscoll, C. E., and Smith, G. D. Theophylline clearance during pregnancy. *Obstet. Gynecol.* 68:555, 1986.
4. Clark, S. L., Phelan, J. P., and Cotton, D. B. *Critical Care Obstetrics.* Oradell NJ: Medical Economics, 1987. Pp. 315–331.
5. Cohen, L. F., Di Sant'Agnese, P. A., and Freidlander, J. Cystic fibrosis and pregnancy—a national survey. *Lancet* 2:842, 1980.
6. Gordon, M., et al. Fetal morbidity following potentially anoxigenic obstetri conditions. VII. Bronchial asthma. *Am. J. Obstet. Gynecol.* 106:421, 1970.
7. Guidelines for prophylaxis against *Pneumocystis carinii* pneumonia for person infected with human immunodeficiency virus. *J.A.M.A.* 262:335, 1989.
8. Hopwood, H. G. Pneumonia in pregnancy. *Obstet. Gynecol.* 25:875, 1965.
9. Jacobs, R. F., and Abernathy, R. S. Management of tuberculosis in pregnancy and the newborn. *Clin. Perinatol.* 15:305, 1988.
10. Johnson, S. R., et al. Diagnosis of maternal cystic fibrosis during pregnancy *Obstet. Gynecol.* 61:2S, 1983.
11. Koonin, L. M., et al. Pregnancy-associated deaths due to AIDS in the United States. *J.A.M.A.* 261:1306, 1989.
12. Lee, W., et al. Squamous and trophoblastic cells in the maternal pulmonary circulation identified by invasive hemodynamic monitoring during the peri partum period. *Am. J. Obstet. Gynecol.* 155:999, 1986.

13. Matthews, L. W., and Drotar, D. Cystic fibrosis—A challenging long-term chronic disease. *Pediatr. Clin. North Am.* 31:133, 1984.
14. Milne, J. A., Howie, A. D., and Pack, A. I. Dyspnoea during normal pregnancy. *Br. J. Obstet. Gynaecol.* 85:260, 1978.
15. Minkoff, H., et al. *Pneumocystis carinii* pneumonia associated with acquired immunodeficiency syndrome in pregnancy: A report of three maternal deaths. *Obstet. Gynecol.* 67:284, 1986.
16. Oxorn, H. The changing aspects of pneumonia complicating pregnancy. *Am. J. Obstet. Gynecol.* 70:1057, 1955.
17. Present, P. A., and Comstock, G. W. Tuberculin sensitivity in pregnancy. *Am. Rev. Respir. Dis.* 112:413, 1975.
18. Schatz, M., et al. Corticosteroid therapy for the pregnant asthmatic patient. *J.A.M.A.* 233:804, 1975.
19. Schatz, M., et al. The safety of inhaled B-agonist bronchodilators during pregnancy. *J. Allergy Clin. Immunol.* 82:686, 1988.
20. Shoemaker, W. C., et al. (eds.) *Textbook of Critical Care.* Philadelphia: Saunders, 1989. Pp. 484–490, 500–504.
21. Skobeloff, E. M., et al. Intravenous magnesium sulfate for the treatment of acute asthma in the emergency department. *J.A.M.A.* 262:1210, 1989.
22. Snider, D. E., et al. Treatment of tuberculosis during pregnancy. *Am. Rev. Respir. Dis.* 122:65, 1980.
23. Stenius-Aarniala, B., Piirila, P., and Teramo, K. Asthma and pregnancy: a prospective study of 198 pregnancies. *Thorax* 43:12, 1988.
24. Turner, E. S., Greenberger, P. A., and Patterson, R. Management of the pregnant asthmatic patient. *Ann. Intern. Med.* 93:905, 1980.

8 Gastrointestinal Complications

Mark C. Williams

I. Heartburn or gastric reflux

A. Natural history. Heartburn, or a mediastinal "burning" sensation noted after meals, is seen in up to 70% of pregnant patients. This complaint is most often due to gastroesophageal reflux (GER). GER involves the retrograde passage of (acidic) stomach contents into the distal esophagus.

B. Management. Patients should be instructed to eat small, frequent meals and to avoid large meals and fatty foods in order to promote more rapid gastric emptying. Several hours should be allowed to pass between eating and going to sleep, in order to allow adequate gastric emptying prior to lying down.

Antacid preparations are often useful in decreasing the acidity of gastric contents, and thereby lowering their potential for esophageal irritation should GER occur. Although histamine (H_2) receptor antagonists are useful in the treatment of GER in nonpregnant patients, their use in pregnancy on a chronic basis should be avoided. In animal studies these agents have occasionally been thought to inhibit fetal masculinization by opposing androgens [10] (see sec. **III**).

II. Nausea and vomiting in pregnancy. Nausea and vomiting in pregnancy (NVP) is a clinical entity with a wide range of presentations, varying from mild "morning sickness" to severe symptomatology requiring hospitalization (hyperemesis gravidarum). As many as 85% of patients may experience NVP, and most progress in pregnancy to normal outcomes. The exact etiology of NVP remains obscure.

Pregnancy-related nausea and vomiting most often occur between 6 and 16 weeks of gestation; a small proportion of patients will experience persistent symptoms until delivery has been accomplished. There does not appear to be any associated fetal teratogenesis, even in particularly severe cases of hyperemesis.

A. Differential diagnoses. A wide variety of illnesses may present with severe nausea and vomiting. A thorough history and physical examination, followed by appropriate laboratory evaluations, will exclude most competing diagnoses and confirm the probable etiology. A list of such conditions is provided here (Table 8-1).

B. Initial management. Initial management of NVP includes the avoidance of fatty foods and alcohol. Patients should be encouraged to eat frequent small meals that are high in simple carbohydrates (e.g., crackers, toast). Some patients find that even the smell of certain foods or the act of cooking regular meals is noxious. Efforts should be made to limit the exposure of the patient to such stimuli. If these simple measures are not successful, antiemetic therapy should be considered.

1. Antiemetic therapy. Historically, many medications with antihistaminic or sedative-hypnotic properties, or both, have been used to alleviate NVP, and their safety has been the subject of extensive investigation for more than 20 years.

a. Bendectin, a combination of pyridoxine (vitamin B_6) and doxylamine, was the most widely prescribed such medication in the United States prior to its withdrawal from the market in 1983. In spite of no positive proof of teratogenicity, the medication was withdrawn from the market due to legal concerns. The individual components of Bendectin remain available without prescription.

b. Tables 8-2 and 8-3 detail the antiemetic agents available for use during pregnancy and the classification scheme for potential teratogenicity.

c. The best scheme for managing NVP with antiemetics is to **become familiar**

Table 8-1. Differential diagnosis for nausea and vomiting in pregnancy

Acute appendicitis	Molar pregnancy
Bowel obstruction	Pancreatitis
Food poisoning	Peptic ulcer disease
Hepatitis	Pyelonephritis
Hiatal hernia	Renal colic
Hyperthyroidism	

Table 8-2. Classification of medications in pregnancy

Category A	There is no evidence of risk to fetus in controlled first-trimester studies or in later trimesters. The possibility of risk to fetus appears remote.
Category B	Either of two characterizations apply: (1) Controlled studies in humans fail to demonstrate potentially adverse fetal effects previously uncovered in animal studies, *or*, (2) Studies in animals fail to document fetal risk and controlled human trials are not available.
Category C	Either of two characterizations apply: (1) Studies in animals document potentially adverse fetal effects but controlled human studies are not available, *or* (2) No studies in animals or humans are available. Category C medications should be given only if the anticipated benefit outweighs the potential risk to the fetus.
Category D	There is demonstrated risk to the human fetus, but the risk may be justified under certain extreme circumstances (i.e., life-threatening illness).
Category X	Studies in animals or humans demonstrate fetal risk, and the risks of such medications to the fetus outweigh any possible benefit. These medications are contraindicated in pregnancy and should not be used in patients who may become pregnant.

with two or three agents. Promethazine and prochlorperazine are often used, as both are available in oral and rectal suppository forms. Rectal suppositories are recommended when frequent emesis limits gastric absorption. Metoclopramide has been available for several years and seems to be an excellent agent, but it should be reserved for particularly difficult cases until more experience has been obtained with it in pregnancy. Droperidol has proved very effective in alleviating intractable vomiting in the acute setting.

d. In prescribing these medications, it should be remembered that most have the potential for extrapyramidal (and other) **side effects.** The potential risk to patient and fetus should always be measured against the probable benefit expected.

C. Hyperemesis gravidarum. The term hyperemesis gravidarum (HG) should be reserved for patients with significant metabolic disarrangements attributable to nausea and vomiting, often requiring hospitalization. The etiology of HG is unclear. Parity, psychological stress, and personality types have all been thought to be associated, but most such associations do not remain constant across cultural boundaries.

1. Incidence. The incidence of HG has been reported to vary among populations. Increased rates are noted among whites (16 per 1000 live births), with lower

Table 8-3. Commonly used antiemetics in pregnancy

Class	Generic	Proprietary name	FDA rating	Dose
Piperazine antihistamine derivatives	Buclizine	Bucladin	C[a]	50 mg PO q12h
	Cyclizine	Marezine	B	IM only: 50 mg q6h prn
	Meclizine	Antivert	B[b]	25–50 mg PO q24h
Phenothiazine antihistamine derivatives	Chlorpromazine	Thorazine	C	PO: 10–25 mg q6h IM: 25 mg q4–6h Suppository: 50–100 mg q8h
	Prochlorperazine	Compazine	C	PO: 5–10 mg q8h IM: 5–10 mg q4h, *maximum 40 mg/24 h* Suppository: 25 mg q12h
	Promethazine	Phenergan	C[b]	PO: 25 mg q6h IM or suppository: 12.5–25.0 mg q6h
Antihistamine	Diphenhydramine	Benadryl	B[b]	PO: 25–50 mg q6h
	Doxylamine	Unisom	B[c]	Manufacturer recommends against use in pregnancy.
	Benzquinamide	Emete-con	B[c]	Manufacturer recommends against use in pregnancy.
Dopamine antagonist	Metoclopramide	Reglan	B[b]	PO: 10–15 mg q6h IM: 10 mg q6h IV: 10 mg q6h, given slowly over 1–2 min.
Apomorphine antagonist	Droperidol	Inapsine	C[b]	IM or slow IV: 2.5–5.0 mg. Use in intractable vomiting.

[a]Manufacturer recommends against use in early pregnancy.
[b]Category supplied by manufacturer.
[c]Medications contraindicated in pregnancy by manufacturer.
See Table 8-2.

rates among blacks (7 per 1000 live births). The illness is only infrequently noted in third-world populations.

2. **Evaluation.** Patients presenting with HG will often be suffering from severe dehydration and electrolyte disturbances. They should be thoroughly evaluated for other possible causes of NVP, as listed before.

   Initial evaluation should include taking a complete history and performing a thorough physical examination, with particular attention paid to evaluating the patient's sclera, thyroid gland, abdomen, costovertebral areas, and reflexes. Initial laboratory evaluations should include the following:

   a. Urine analysis
   b. Complete blood count
   c. Basic serum chemistries (sodium, potassium, chlorine, carbon dioxide, glucose, creatinine, and uric acid)
   d. Hepatic enzymes (serum glutamic-oxaloacetic transaminase, serum glutamic pyruvic transaminase, alkaline phosphatase)
   e. Fetal ultrasound evaluation to exclude the possibility of molar pregnancy

3. **Management.** If emesis has persisted for some time, patients may have developed hypochloremia, hyponatremia, and metabolic acidosis. Thiamine (vitamin B_{12}) deficiency presenting as Wernicke's encephalopathy [1–3] has been noted to develop in particularly severe cases of HG. If a significant period of starvation has occurred, supplementation with thiamine (100 mg IM or IV daily) and other B vitamins (added as multivitamins to IV solutions) is recommended until resumption of normal dietary intake.

   a. **Hospitalization.** If hospitalization is required, the patient should be allowed nothing by mouth for 24–48 hours. Adequate hydration and short-term caloric needs should be provided by infusions of intravenous solutions such as 5% dextrose in lactated Ringer's solution at rates appropriate to correct dehydration and maintain daily needs. Antiemetic therapy administered as suppositories or IM medications on a regular (not prn) schedule are recommended. After the patient has begun to experience some resumption of appetite, small amounts of carbohydrate-rich foods such as dry toast and crackers and sips of clear liquids may be allowed, the diet gradually advanced, and oral antiemetics begun.

   b. In **refractory cases,** or where significant intervals of inadequate nutrition and emesis have occurred, some form of hyperalimentation should be considered. Although hyperalimentation in pregnancy was initially viewed with some concern, excellent success with this therapy has been reported in a wide variety of complicated obstetric cases [20–30].

III. **Peptic ulcer disease.** Peptic ulcer disease (PUD) comprises both gastric and duodenal ulcer disorders. Pregnancy complicated by PUD is uncommon, with an incidence estimated at 1 in 4000 pregnancies. The actual incidence may be higher, as diagnosis is difficult in pregnancy and ulcer disease may be attributed to other etiologies. For example, gastric ulcer symptoms are similar to those of reflux esophagitis. It is thought that the pregnant state is protective from PUD [5]. Baird [4] reviewed 233,650 pregnancies and found evidence of ulceration in only 11 cases.

A. **Diagnosis.** Symptoms suggestive of gastric ulcer disease include a dull, nagging epigastric pain with some radiation to the back. Pain will frequently improve after eating or with antacids. In some cases, hematemesis will occur. Diagnostic evaluation in pregnancy is difficult, as radiographic upper GI series are generally contraindicated in pregnancy. An excellent alternative test is endoscopic gastroscopy, which can be safely performed in pregnancy and will often confirm the diagnosis [9]. In selected patients, endoscopy is definitely indicated. Perforating peptic ulcers are associated with a high rate of morbidity and mortality [5, 6, 8], and a thorough endoscopic evaluation may exclude PUD and identify a disease process requiring alternate therapy. Upper gastrointestinal bleeding in pregnancy is much more often due to reflux esophagitis or Mallory-Weiss esophageal tears [7].

B. **Management.** As in the nonpregnant population, most PUD responds to such simple measures as avoidance of alcohol and cigarettes, and frequently administered oral antacid preparations.

Oral antacid preparations (1 oz q2–3 h) will prove adequate therapy in most cases of PUD. Alternate therapy is available in the form of **sucralfate and histamine (H_2) receptor antagonists.** If alternate therapy is required, the previous diagnostic evaluation should be reviewed, and endoscopy, if not already performed, should be considered. Sucralfate and H_2 receptor antagonists are excellent therapeutic modalities among nonpregnant patients, but their safety in human pregnancy is not yet well established.

1. Sucralfate should be reserved for patients with documented PUD that is nonresponsive to vigorous antacid therapy. The recommended dosing schedule is 1 gm PO taken 1 hour prior to meals and at bedtime. Antacid therapy may be combined with sucralfate, but antacids should not be taken within one hour of sucralfate administration. The principal side effect of this medication is constipation.
2. The H_2 receptor antagonists such as cimetidine (Tagamet) and ranitidine (Zantac) are competitive, reversible antagonists for gastric cellular H_2 receptors. By blocking the action of histamine on gastric parietal cells, gastric acid production is inhibited and gastric pH effectively raised. Both medications are FDA class B medications, but they cannot be recommended for extended use in pregnancy at this time.

C. Complications. If significant ongoing bleeding occurs from a gastric ulcer, immediate surgery should be considered. This recommendation varies from the vigorous medical therapy often advised for nonpregnant patients and is based on significant fetal mortality and maternal morbidity reported in such cases [6]. Perforation of a gastric ulcer in pregnancy is an exceptionally dangerous event [8]. There is a very high attendant case fatality rate, possibly due to delay in diagnosis caused by incorrectly ascribing premonitory symptoms to "pregnancy" and deferring vigorous diagnostic evaluation.

IV. Bowel disease. Intestinal disorders in pregnancy mirror the range of gastrointestinal disease in the normal population. Common etiologies include the following: (1) antibiotic-induced disorders (related to overgrowth of *Clostridium difficile* after antibiotic therapy); (2) functional bowel disorders; (3) infectious gastroenteritis (bacterial, parasitic, and viral); and (4) inflammatory bowel disorders (regional enteritis and ulcerative colitis).

A. Gastroenteritis. Acute-onset diarrhea is most often associated with viral or bacterial infection. Enteric pathogens act by either infecting the bowel mucosa, or by producing toxins that cause diarrheal symptomatology. In addition to the aforementioned pathogens, parasitic infections are common causes of diarrhea in areas where public sanitation measures are either inadequate or rendered ineffective by natural catastrophe (Table 8-4).

1. **Natural history.** Diarrheal syndromes associated with local infection usually manifest with fever, abdominal cramping, bloody or mucoid stooling, and often tenesmus. Although diarrhea is present, it is usually not of a voluminous nature.
   a. Patients suffering **bacterial enteritis** caused by *Salmonella, Shigella, Yersinia,* and *Campylobacter* suffer subsequent arthritis in up to 50% of cases. Many patients so affected have the HLA-B27 histocompatibility antigen present.
   b. Certain bacteria, viruses, and parasites (such as *Giardia lamblia*) produce toxins that can cause profound, watery diarrhea. **Toxin-induced gastroenteritis** is usually characterized by voluminous watery stools. A low-grade fever and vomiting are sometimes present, and occasionally there is evidence of blood in the stool.
   c. Generally, **gastroenteritis in pregnancy** does not pose significant risk to the fetus **if** maternal hydration can be maintained. Most infections tend to be localized to the bowel mucosa and do not present a risk for infection of the fetus.
2. **Diagnosis.** Patients presenting with diarrhea persisting more than 24–48 hours should be evaluated as follows:

Table 8-4. Acute gastroenteritis pathogens

Bacterial infections	*Campylobacter jejuni, Escherichia coli, Listeria, Salmonella* sp., *Shigella* sp., *Yersinia enterocolitica, Vibrio parahaemolyticus*
Bacterial toxins	*Bacillus cereus, Clostridium difficile, Vibrio cholera, E. coli, Staphylococcus aureus*
Protozoans	*Entamoeba histolytica, Giardia lamblia,* malaria sp., *Toxoplasma gondii*
Helminths	Cestodes (hydatid, *Taenia*) Nematodes *(Ancylostoma, Ascaris, Enterobius, Strongyloides)* Trematodes *(Schistosoma)*
Viruses	Cytomegalovirus, herpes, polio, others

a. Stool smear for fecal leukocytes

b. Stool cultures for common enteric pathogens such as *Campylobacter, Salmonella, Shigella,* and enterotoxigenic *Escherichia coli*

c. Stool smears, obtained on at least three separate occasions, evaluated for common enteric parasites such as helminthic parasites, *Giardia,* and *Amoeba.* These samples must be examined within several hours of being obtained.

If no leukocytes are present, it is unlikely that a bacterial infection is present.

3. General management considerations. With mild diarrhea, it is usually adequate to encourage oral intake of dilute glucose/electrolyte preparations. Commercial preparations (such as Pedialyte) and beverages such as Gatoraid, 7up, and Kool-Aid are useful. If significant dehydration is present, or if ongoing fluid losses cannot be matched by oral intake, intravenous hydration is indicated. Severe diarrhea is associated with significant fluid balance disturbances. Skin turgor and the urine specific gravity are sensitive indicators of hydration state, with dilute urine of specific gravity less than 1.010 indicating adequate hydration.

4. Therapy. Most cases of infectious bacterial diarrhea will resolve without antibiotic therapy in several days, and inadequate antibiotic therapy may even predispose to chronic carrier states. Most protozoal infections require vigorous antibiotic therapy.

Under most circumstances, medications that act to paralyze bowel motility, such as diphenoxylate (in Lomotil), should be avoided. It is preferable to have the stool exit the bowel rather than to remain in paralyzed bowel segments. If access to sanitary facilities will be temporarily restricted, or in the case of severe abdominal cramping, these medications are acceptable.

B. Bacterial gastroenteritides (infectious and toxin induced). The pathogenesis and treatment options for several common infectious causes of gastroenteritis are discussed in this section. For more information regarding these infections and others, the reader is urged to consult appropriate reference texts. It is important to ascertain the safety in pregnancy of any antimicrobial agent prior to its usage.

1. *Campylobacter.* In the United States, *Campylobacter jejuni* is the second most common cause of infectious diarrhea (*G. lamblia* is most often causative) and is the most commonly isolated bacterial enteric pathogen.

a. Diagnosis. *C. jejuni* enteritis characteristically presents with bloody diarrhea accompanied by fever, abdominal pain, and tenesmus. Symptoms usually resolve within five days; however, on rare occasions they may continue for up to four weeks.

b. Therapy. *C. jejuni* enteritis usually resolves spontaneously without antibiotic therapy, although antibiotic therapy may decrease the length of symptoms and the duration of infectious shedding in the stools. If antibiotics are judged necessary, erythromycin is the antibiotic of choice. Erythromycin estolate should not be given in pregnancy. Other antibiotics effective against *Campylobacter* include aminoglycosides (such as gentamicin) and chloramphenicol.

2. Cholera. *Vibrio cholerae* is a gram-negative aerobe that is usually spread via contaminated water supplies. Poor hygiene may result in fecal-oral transmission as well.

a. **Diagnosis.** The diagnosis of cholera can usually be confirmed by culture of *V. cholerae* from the stool on appropriate culture media.
The principal mechanism of injury in cholera diarrhea is dehydration. Fluid losses with cholera may be massive, often with diarrheal volumes in excess of 3 liters/day. If adequate hydration can be maintained, the infection will eventually subside with time or in response to antibiotic therapy.

b. **Therapy.** Cholera is usually self-limited and often requires no antibiotic therapy. If severe symptomatology persists, antibiotic therapy with chloramphenicol should be considered. Alternate antibiotics include gentamicin and erythromycin. Among nonpregnant patients, tetracycline is the drug of choice.

3. ***Clostridium difficile* enteritis.** Patients receiving antibiotic therapy occasionally experience overgrowth of *Clostridium difficile,* and the onset of pseudomembranous enterocolitis. *C. difficile,* an anaerobic bacillus, is present as normal bowel flora in up to 5% of healthy adults. When the microbiologic environment is altered by antibiotic therapy, *C. difficile* will sometimes be noted to overgrow other competing flora and produce an enterotoxin. Symptoms are usually observed within four to nine days of antibiotic administration but may occur as many as six weeks later. This toxin has a cytopathic effect on bowel mucosa and causes a watery diarrhea usually characterized by fecal leukocytosis and occasionally by blood in the stools as well.

   a. **Diagnosis.** The diagnosis of pseudomembranous enterocolitis is best made by the demonstration of *C. difficile* enterotoxin in the stool. Stool cultures revealing the presence of *C. difficile* are not as helpful, as *C. difficile* is normally found in small numbers of otherwise healthy patients.

   b. **Therapy.** Therapy centers on the use of appropriate antibiotics. Vancomycin is the drug of choice, given at a dosage of 125 mg q6h for 5–10 days. Alternately, metronidazole may be administered 500 mg q8h for a similar time interval. Metronidazole should not be administered in the first 12–16 weeks of pregnancy.

4. **Enterotoxigenic and enteropathogenic *E. coli.*** *E. coli* has recently been found to cause a significant amount of gastrointestinal disease. Infections are caused by ingestion of food or water contaminated with fecal material. Gastrointestinal disease may be caused either by bacterial enterotoxin production, or by local invasion of the bowel mucosa. This family of bacteria is responsible for most cases of traveler's diarrhea (e.g., "turista").

   a. **Therapy.** Diarrhea caused by these enterotoxins is usually self-limited and requires no treatment. As always, hydration should be supported. If oral rehydration proves inadequate, intravenous rehydration is recommended. If the patient shows signs of severe infection, or bacteremia is suspected, parenteral antibiotic therapy is recommended. Aminoglycosides such as gentamicin should be considered as initial therapy, until microbial antibiotic sensitivities become available.

5. ***Salmonella.*** Salmonella gastroenteritis is caused by the ingestion of contaminated food. Typhoid fever, caused by *Salmonella typhi,* is rare in the United States but endemic in other parts of the world. Salmonella gastroenteritis affects pregnancy indirectly. If adequate maternal hydration can be maintained, fetal effects are generally prevented.
Similar syndromes are caused by other *Salmonella* species, such as *S. paratyphi* A and B. These infections are commonly referred to as **paratyphoid fever.** They share many of the features of typhoid fever but often have a milder clinical course.

   a. **Differential diagnoses.** The differential diagnoses for the aforementioned symptoms include brucellosis, leptospirosis, malaria, miliary tuberculosis, psittacosis, the rickettsioses, tularemia, as well as infectious hepatitis, rheumatic fever, and lymphoma.

b. Therapy. Treatment is directed toward the diarrheal illnesses. Supportive care is usually adequate, and antibiotic therapy is often unnecessary. When moderate to severe disease is present, antibiotic therapy should be initiated with either chloramphenicol, ampicillin, trimethoprim/sulfamethoxazole, or certain third-generation cephalosporins, such as ceftriaxone (Rocephin).

(1) Among nonpregnant patients, chloramphenicol and ampicillin are both felt to have significant clinical utility. Often chloramphenicol is advised if severe infections present, as a four- to five-day delay in recovery is seen in 1% of chloramphenicol-treated patients, but among 5–10% of patients treated with ampicillin.

(2) **In pregnancy** complicated by severe typhoid fever, chloramphenicol may be the antibiotic of choice among sensitive strains of *Salmonella.* Within several hours of its administration, *S. typhi* will usually be cleared from the circulation. Although less effective for acute disease, ampicillin is preferred for treatment of chronic carriers. It should be administered at doses of 100 mg/kg/day on a q6h schedule (i.e., 25 mg/kg q6h).

(3) **Chronic carriers** should be evaluated for evidence of cholelithiasis. Patients with cholelithiasis will most often be refractory to antibiotic therapy and will require cholecystectomy. Cholecystectomy is curative in 85% of patients. Patients without evidence of disease may respond to a two- to three-week course of ampicillin and probenecid. These therapies should be considered after delivery, unless persistent symptoms relating to *Salmonella* infection continue to complicate the pregnancy.

6. ***Shigella.*** The *Shigella* genus comprises gram-negative organisms that cause a bloody, mucoid diarrhea that is often referred to as **bacterial dysentery.** Four species of *Shigella* have been identified including *S. dysenteriae, S. boydii, S. flexneri,* and *S. sonnei.* Shigellae both invade the colonic mucosa and produce an enterotoxin, which causes the small bowel to produce a secretory diarrhea. The minimum inoculum of bacteria necessary to cause infection is 100. After an initial incubation period of one to four days, shigellosis will present with high fevers (to 39–40°C), tenesmus, and explosive diarrhea. The stools will often appear to contain moderate amounts of bloody, mucoid matter. Laboratory evaluations will often reveal a leukocytosis, and stool smears will show a predominance of fecal leukocytes. Shigellae may produce superficial mucosal ulceration within the colon, but these ulcers do not tend to rupture (as they do with salmonella infections).

a. Therapy. Specific therapeutic measures for *Shigella* infections include rehydration and avoidance of medications that paralyze normal bowel motility. Preparations such as kaolin/pectin (Kaopectate) and bismuth subsalicylate (Pepto-Bismol) have been found to alleviate symptoms or hasten recovery after the infection has presented. Antibiotic therapy has been shown to shorten the clinical course of infection but does not affect the elimination of bacteria from the stools.

Antibiotic therapy should be considered for severe infections. The antibiotic of choice is ampicillin, but ampicillin-resistant strains are commonly isolated. For moderate disease, ampicillin in doses of 500 mg q6h PO should be given; a dose of 1 gm q6h IV is more appropriate for severe disease. If ampicillin resistance is present in severe disease, chloramphenicol should be considered. Another therapeutic option for this infection is trimethoprim-sulfamethoxazole.

7. **Staphylococcal food poisoning.** *Staphylococcus aureus* occasionally is responsible for epidemics of staphylococcal food poisoning (SFP). When allowed to incubate with unrefrigerated dairy products for one to six hours, it can produce a characteristic group of enterotoxins. These toxins, labeled A–F, cause an explosive secretory diarrhea accompanied by nausea and vomiting. The nausea and vomiting associated with SFP are often quite severe, possibly due to a direct central nervous system action of the enterotoxin(s).

Stool samples in SFP will show no evidence of leukocytosis or blood, as it is a purely toxin-induced diarrhea. The diagnosis should be considered by a history of very recent ingestion of dairy products in combination with unrevealing stool evaluation. The incubation interval for SFP is usually on the order of several hours.

C. Protozoal enteritis

1. ***Giardia lamblia.*** Giardiasis is the most commonly diagnosed protozoal infection in the United States. It is found in 4% of stool samples submitted for parasite evaluation. *G. lamblia* is a multiflagellar protozoan with a two-stage life cycle: trophozoite and cyst. Both trophozoites and cysts are infectious, but most infectious outbreaks are due to contamination of water supplies with cysts, as trophozoites do not survive well outside the bowel. Cysts have been shown to remain viable for more than two months in cold water and are capable of resisting chlorine concentrations usually found in community water supplies (i.e., 0.4 mg/liter). Outbreaks are usually seen among those drinking untreated water from lakes, wells, or streams. Although sewage contamination is the usual infectious reservoir, beavers have been found infected with *Giardia* and may be an alternate infectious reservoir. Direct fecal-oral transmission is possible if careful hand-washing procedures are not followed when dealing with the stool of infected patients (or carriers). Patients may present with symptoms of acute gastroenteritis or may develop a chronic carrier state. The carrier state is best characterized by intermittent bouts of flatulence, epigastric pain, and loose stools.
   a. **Etiology.** The etiology for diarrheal symptoms associated with giardiasis is unknown. Postulated mechanisms include mechanical obstruction of the bowel by proliferating trophozoites, obstruction of bowel mucosal membranes by confluently attached trophozoites, and hepatobiliary dysfunction. The diagnosis can be confirmed by weekly examination of stool samples for cysts and trophozoites, or by evaluation of duodenal fluids. Duodenal sampling can be performed with an oral-enteral catheter or by use of a nylon string (Enterotest) for retrieval. Rarely, a direct jejunal biopsy will be required to confirm the diagnosis.
   b. **Therapy.** In pregnancy, giardiasis is best treated with metronidazole (Flagyl), given either 2 gm/day for 3 days, or 750 mg/day for 5 days. Use of metronidazole should be limited to after the first trimester of pregnancy. Metronidazole at this time is not approved by the FDA for use in treating giardiasis.

      Other medications that may be useful among nonpregnant patients include quinacrine and furazolidone. Quinacrine, an acridine-type dye, is contraindicated in pregnancy. Furazolidone has been shown teratogenic in several species, may potentiate a hemolytic reaction among patients deficient in glucose 6-phosphate dehydrogenase (G-6-PD), and has not been evaluated in human pregnancy.
2. ***Entamoeba histolytica.*** Infection by *Entamoeba histolytica* causes an acute infectious enteritis termed **amebiasis.** Its clinical course ranges from a benign carrier state to severe diarrhea.
   a. **Natural history.** Of seven species of amoeba known to parasitize the human bowel, only *E. histolytica* is known to cause disease in humans. Approximately 10% of the world's population are thought to be chronic carriers, but these rates vary from 1% in developed countries to 50% or more in underdeveloped countries. Postinfectious complications, such as hepatic abscess formation and pleuropulmonary involvement, are most often caused by several virulent strains of *E. histolytica*. These strains are most commonly found in Mexico, western South America, southern Asia, and southeastern Africa. Although it is possible to transmit the infection via intimate contact, within the general population it is most often transmitted via infected water and foodstuffs.
   b. **Diagnosis.** Diagnosis is best made by examination of a fresh stool specimen for cysts or trophozoites. If stool evaluation is not diagnostic, serologic testing for *E. histolytica* is also possible by indirect hemagglutination and immunodiffusion.

c. **Therapy.** In pregnancy, few medications are available to treat amebiasis. Metronidazole (Flagyl or Protostat, 750 mg tid PO for 5–10 days) may potentially be used in pregnancy. Unfortunately, few other agents are available for use in pregnancy. Two possible medications are paromomycin (Humatin) and chloroquine (Aralen).

V. **Helminthic infection.** For disease-specific natural histories, the reader is referred to texts specializing in general internal medicine or tropical medicine. Therapeutic options for these infections in pregnancy are discussed subsequently. The FDA pregnancy categorizations for the most commonly used antihelminthic medications are also discussed here (Table 8-5).

A. **Antihelminthic medications: special considerations**

1. **Mebendazole.** Mebendazole (Vermox) has been shown to have embryocidal and teratogenic effects in pregnant rats at dosages of 10 mg/kg. Incidental exposure during pregnancy among humans has not been found to be associated with an increased rate of fetal waste or teratogenicity. **Its use in pregnancy is not generally recommended.** If alternate therapy is unavailable and the potential risk to the patient is significant, it may be considered for use in the second and third trimesters of pregnancy.

   Among nonpregnant patients, mebendazole is indicated for therapy against *Ancylostoma duodenale, Ascaris lumbricoides, Enterobius vermicularis, Necator americanus,* and *Trichuris trichiura.*

2. **Niclosamide.** Niclosamide (Niclocide) is classed as FDA pregnancy category B, based on the absence of effects on fertility or fetuses in doses 12–25 times greater than equivalent human dosages. No adequate controlled human studies in pregnancy have been done yet. The safety of niclosamide in breast-feeding has not been established. Niclosamide has been found effective against most

Table 8-5. Antihelminthic medications in pregnancy

Cestodes (tapeworms)
- *Diphyllobothrium latum*
  - Niclosamide (single dose of 2 gm PO), praziquantel, paromomycin
- *Echinococcus* species
  - Mebendazole
- *Taenia saginata*
  - Niclosamide (single dose of 2 gm PO), praziquantel
- *Taenia solium*
  - Niclosamide, paromomycin
  - Praziquantel for cerebral cysts. (Mebendazole may be used if absolutely necessary)

Nematodes (roundworms)
- *Ascaris lumbricoides* (roundworm)
  - Mebendazole (pyrantel pamoate if nonpregnant)
- *Ancylostoma duodenale* (hookworm)
  - Mebendazole (pyrantel pamoate if nonpregnant)
- *Enterobius vermicularis* (pinworm)
  - Pyrvinium pamoate (5 mg/kg), mebendazole (thiabendazole possibly useful in special circumstances)
- *Filaria* species
  - Mebendazole
- *Necator americanus* (hookworm)
  - Mebendazole (pyrantel pamoate if nonpregnant)
- *Trichuris spiralis, T. trichura* (whipworm)
  - Mebendazole (pyrantel pamoate if nonpregnant)

Trematodes (flatworms)
- *Clonorchis sinensis; Fasciola hepatica; Fasciolopsis buski; Opisthorchis viverrini, O. felineus; Schistosoma haematobium, S. mansoni, S. japonicum*
  - Praziquantel

cestodes, including *Diphyllobothrium latum, Taenia saginata, Taenia solium,* and *Hymenolepis nana.*

3. **Paromomycin.** Paromomycin (Humatin), an aminoglycoside antibiotic, is very poorly absorbed from the gastrointestinal tract after oral administration. For this reason, relatively high local concentrations can be attained within the bowel lumen without the attendant risks of systemic toxicity usually present with the use of other aminoglycosides. It has been found effective in infections by *T. solium, D. latum,* and *E. histolytica.*
4. **Praziquantel.** Praziquantel (Biltricide) acts against helminths by altering cell membrane permeability and causing rapid contraction of susceptible organisms. It is classed as FDA pregnancy category B, based on the absence of effects on reproduction or fetal development. An increased abortion rate was seen in rats at 3 times the usual human dose. Adequately controlled studies in human pregnancy are not yet available. **Praziquantel should only be used in pregnancy if clearly indicated.** It is secreted in breast milk at concentrations 25% of those found in maternal serum. Breast milk should be discarded for 72 hours after its administration.

   Praziquantel is indicated for treatment of infections by all *Schistosoma* species (i.e., *S. haematobium, S. japonicum, S. mansoni,* and *S. mekongi*), and by the liver flukes *Clonarchis sinensis* and *Opisthorchis viverrini.* Schistosomal infections should be treated by a dose of 20 mg/kg tid PO for 1 day; infections by *Clonarchis* and *Opisthorchis* should be treated by doses of 25 mg/kg tid PO taken for 1 day.
5. **Pyrantel pamoate.** Pyrantel pamoate was first found to be an effective antihelminthic in humans in 1969. This depolarizing neuromuscular blocking agent induces spastic paralysis of susceptible worms by activation of nicotinic receptors. It also inhibits cholinesterase. No information is available on the effects of pyrantel in pregnancy, and for this reason, **it should not be used in pregnancy.**

   Among nonpregnant patients, pyrantel has been found to have activity against *Ancylostoma duodenale, Ascaris lumbricoides, Enterobius vermicularis,* and *N. americanus.* Its antihelminthic activity is antagonistic to that of piperazine, another antihelminthic agent with activity against *Ascaris.* The two medications should not be used concurrently.
6. **Pyrvinium pamoate.** Pyrvinium pamoate (Povan, Vanquin) is the pamoate salt of a cyanine dye. The medication is not commonly used, as newer agents with superior antihelminthic activity against *Enterobius* (pinworm), such as mebendazole and pyrantel, have become available. In pregnancy, however, some authors feel pyrvinium may be somewhat safer than either mebendazole or pyrantel.

   Pyrvinium has activity against *Enterobius* and *Strongyloides.* Doses of 5 mg/kg given once with a second dose after 14 days are often effective in *Enterobius;* administration of 5–6 mg/kg (maximum 350 mg/day) for 7 days has been found effective against *Strongyloides.* No more than 350 mg/day should be given. Because pyrvinium is a dye, it has a propensity to stain underclothes and bedding.
7. **Thiabendazole.** Thiabendazole (Mintezol) is classed as FDA pregnancy category C, based on the absence of harmful effects in reproductive and teratologic studies among rabbits, rats, and mice. Cleft palate and axial skeletal anomalies were found when thiabendazole was administered as an olive oil suspension to pregnant mice. No well-controlled studies have been done on humans. Its mechanism of action has not been ascertained but may involve inhibition of helminth-specific fumarate reductase.

   Thiabendazole is indicated for treatment of strongyloidiasis, trichinosis, and both cutaneous and visceral larva migrans. It may also be considered as therapy for ascariasis, trichuriasis (whipworm), and uncinariasis (i.e., hookworm: infection by *A. duodenale* and *N. americanus*). It has also been found to have activity against *E. vermicularis.* The safety of this medication in breast-feeding patients is uncertain. The maximum daily dose is 3 gm/day.

VI. Inflammatory bowel disease. Inflammatory bowel disease (IBD) such as regional enteritis (Crohn's disease) and ulcerative colitis occasionally complicate pregnancy. Regional enteritis and ulcerative colitis are examples of two similar but distinct disorders that in fact may represent varied expression of a similar disease process. Inflammatory bowel disease affects approximately 1 in 1000 pregnancies. The peak years of disease onset are ages 15–35 for both diseases.

Certain generalizations may be made about these disorders: (1) **Regional enteritis,** or Crohn's disease, often shows transmural involvement of the bowel and usually involves the colon and small bowel. Fistula formation is common. Patches of diseased bowel may be found at varying locations throughout the gastrointestinal tract; and (2) **ulcerative colitis** most commonly involves the rectum and colon. It tends to cause confluent disease, with no "skip" areas.

Both diseases are associated with frequent rectal bleeding and diarrhea. Fertility does not appear impaired in patients suffering from IBD. Similarly, once pregnant, IBD patients do not appear to suffer increased pregnancy complications (premature birth, miscarriage, or congenital anomalies)[14]. Patients approximately have a 30% chance of experiencing recurrent disease sometime during pregnancy. This rate is comparable to the rate observed among nonpregnant populations. If an exacerbation of IBD complicates a pregnancy, there is an increased likelihood of miscarriage or preterm labor [11, 13, 15–17].

A. Management. Always evaluate the patient for other causes of diarrhea or rectal bleeding, or both.

B. Therapy. Therapy for acute exacerbation includes the following:

1. Rest the gastrointestinal tract. Nothing should be administered PO for several days, except medications.
2. Corticosteroid therapy should be initiated. Prednisolone PO in doses of 20–60 mg/day is commonly used.
3. Sulfasalazine PO should be begun at doses of 3–4 gm/day.
4. IV hydration with isotonic solutions of dextrose and electrolytes should be administered.
5. Enemas with sulfasalazine or corticosteroids may be helpful.
6. **Corticosteroid medications** are commonly used, and the possibility of parasitic infection should be excluded prior to their administration. Although relatively large doses of sulfasalazine and corticosteroids are commonly used in managing IBD exacerbations during pregnancy, there does not appear to be any associated increase in teratogenesis. With severe IBD, parenteral hyperalimentation may be necessary [20, 22].
7. Patients with IBD often require **bowel surgery.** Although pregnancy is not a contraindication for such surgery, in later stages of pregnancy it may not be possible to perform otherwise indicated surgical procedures [12, 14, 18, 19].

VII. Functional bowel disorders. Functional bowel disorder (FBD) is characterized by bowel function abnormalities related to psychological rather than physical abnormalities. An FBD should be suspected if complaints pertaining to bowel function seem to worsen during times of high stress or anxiety. A finding that helps to confirm the diagnosis of FBD is the absence of any bowel symptomatology during the hours of sleep, as most organic bowel pathology is not limited to the waking hours. Care should be exercised in assigning this diagnosis, as underlying pathology may eventually present in patients with FBD. If worsening symptoms occur in a patient with FBD, it is best to evaluate the patient appropriately before ascribing worsening symptoms to FBD.

VIII. Lactose intolerance. It is currently recommended that calcium intake during pregnancy and lactation be increased from 800 mg/day to 1200 mg/day. Patients are often advised to increase their dietary intake of milk products to achieve this goal. Women suffering from lactose intolerance may have difficulty following these instructions. On a worldwide basis, intolerance of dietary lactose is a very common phenomenon [31].

True lactose intolerance is evidenced by gastrointestinal discomfort with increased peristalsis and watery diarrhea. Studies indicate that even with documented lactase deficiency, patients may be able to ingest small amounts of lactose-containing products without significant discomfort [32, 33]. Also, Villar has reported an apparent increase in intestinal lactase activity during pregnancy. In the study group, 44% of lactase maldigesters developed the ability to digest lactose by 36 weeks' gestation [34].

Patients experiencing increased symptoms with augmented dietary milk intake should supplement dietary calcium from other sources, while maintaining a symptom-free daily intake of dietary milk.

IX. Summary. Gastrointestinal diseases (GID) are among the most common intercurrent diseases complicating pregnancy. In general, pregnancy does not alter the incidence or risks of GIDs. The significant exception to this is inflammatory bowel disease, in which up to one-third of patients will experience activation or worsening of the disease. The detrimental perinatal effects of GIDs generally result from their impact on maternal nutrition. GIDs, particularly those that are chronic, have the potential for hindering maternal intake of calories and nutrients, thereby interfering with maternal and fetal weight gain. Therapy should be directed toward achieving adequate maternal weight gain and appropriate fetal growth. Direct fetal infection from maternal gastrointestinal organisms is rare. Instead, with maternal GI infection, adverse perinatal effects usually result from the maternal disease itself, chorioamnionitis, or preterm labor or delivery. Control of the maternal disease provides the best opportunity for achieving a favorable outcome.

References

HYPEREMESIS

1. Lavin, P. J., et al. Wernicke's encephalopathy: a predictable complication of hyperemesis gravidarum. *Obstet. Gynecol.* 62(3 Suppl.):13s–15s, 1983.
2. Watanabe, K., Tanaka, K., and Masuda, J. Wernicke's encephalopathy in early pregnancy complicated by disseminated intravascular coagulation. *Virchows Arch* 400(2):213–218, 1983.
3. Wood, P., et al. Wernicke's encephalopathy induced by hyperemesis gravidarum. Case reports. *Br. J. Obstet. Gynaecol.* 90(6):583–586, 1983.

PEPTIC ULCER DISEASE

4. Baird, R. M. Peptic ulceration in pregnancy. Report of a case with perforation. *Can. Med. Assoc. J.* 94:861–862, 1966.
5. Clark, D. H. Pregnancy and peptic ulcer in women. *Br. Med. J.* 1:1254–1257, 1953.
6. Jones, P. F., McEwan, A. B., and Bernard, R. M. Hemorrhage and perforation complicating peptic ulcer in pregnancy. *Lancet* 2:350, 1969.
7. Palmer, E. D. Upper gastrointestinal disease in pregnancy. *Am. J. Med. Sci.* 242:223, 1961.
8. Parry, G. K. Perforated duodenal ulcer in the puerperium. *N.Z. Med. J.* 80:448, 1974.
9. Rustgi, V. K., et al. Endoscopy in the Pregnant Patient. In V. K. Rustig and J. N. Cooper (eds.), *Gastrointestinal and Hepatic Complications in Pregnancy.* New York: Wiley, 1986. Pp. 104–123.

CIMETIDINE

10. McGivern, R. F. Influence of prenatal exposure to cimetidine and alcohol on selected morphological parameters of sexual differentiation: a preliminary report. *Neurotoxicol. Teratol.* 9(1):23–26, 1987.

INFLAMMATORY BOWEL DISEASE

11. Baiocco, P. J., and Korelitz, B. I. The influence of inflammatory bowel disease and its treatment on pregnancy and fetal outcome. *J. Clin. Gastroenterol.* 6(3):211–216, 1984.
12. Cooksey, G., Gunn, A., and Wotherspoon, W. C. Surgery for acute ulcerative colitis and toxic megacolon during pregnancy. *Br. J. Surg.* 72(7):547, 1985.

13. Fedorkow, D. M., Persaud, D., and Nimrod, C. A. Inflammatory bowel disease: a controlled study of late pregnancy outcome. *Am. J. Obstet. Gynecol.* 160(4):998–1001, 1989.
14. Lindhagen, T., et al. Fertility and outcome of pregnancy in patients operated on for Crohn's disease. *Int. J. Colon Dis.* 1(1):25–27, 1986.
15. Mayberry, J. F., and Weterman, I. T. European survey of fertility and pregnancy in women with Crohn's disease: a case control study by European collaborative group. *Gut* 27(7):821–825, 1986.
16. Nielsen, O. H., et al. Pregnancy in Crohn's disease. *Scand. J. Gastroenterol.* 19(6):724–732, 1984.
17. Nielsen, O. H., et al. Pregnancy in ulcerative colitis. *Scand. J. Gastroenterol.* 18(6):735–742, 1983.
18. Warsof, S. L. Medical and surgical treatment of inflammatory bowel disease in pregnancy. *Clin. Obstet. Gynecol.* 26(4):822–831, 1983.
19. Watson, W. J., and Gaines, T. E. Third-trimester colectomy for severe ulcerative colitis. A case report. *J. Reprod. Med.* 32(11):869–872, 1987.

PARENTERAL NUTRITION

20. Gatenby, S. J. Maintenance of pregnancy in Crohn's disease by parenteral nutrition: a case study. *Hum. Nutr. Appl. Nutr.* 41(5):345–349, 1987.
21. Gray, D. S., and Cabaniss, M. L. Home total parenteral nutrition in a pregnant diabetic after jejunoileal bypass for obesity. *J. Parenter. Enteral Nutr.* 13(2):214–217, 1989.
22. Jacobson, L. B., and Clapp, D. H. Total parenteral nutrition in pregnancy complicated by Crohn's disease. *J. Parenter. Enteral Nutr.* 11(1):93–96, 1987.
23. Landon, M.B., Gabbe, S. G., and Mullen, J. L. Total parenteral nutrition during pregnancy. *Clin. Perinatol.* 13(1):57–72, 1986.
24. Lee, R. V., et al. Total parenteral nutrition during pregnancy. *Obstet. Gynecol.* 68(4):563–571, 1986.
25. Levine, M. G., and Esser, D. Total parenteral nutrition for the treatment of severe hyperemesis gravidarum: maternal nutritional effects and fetal outcome. *Obstet. Gynecol.* 72(1):102–107, 1988.
26. Nugent, F. W., et al. Total parenteral nutrition in pregnancy: conception to delivery. *J. Parenter. Enteral Nutr.* 11(4):424–427, 1987.
27. Rayburn, W., et al. Parenteral nutrition in obstetrics and gynecology. *Obstet. Gynecol. Surv.* 41(4):200–214, 1986.
28. Rivera-Alsina, M. E., Saldana, L. R., and Stringer, C. A. Fetal growth sustained by parenteral nutrition in pregnancy. *Obstet. Gynecol.* 64(1):138–141, 1984.
29. Stellato, T. A., Danziger, L. H., and Burkons, D. Fetal salvage with maternal total parenteral nutrition: the pregnant mother as her own control. *J. Parenter. Enteral Nutr.* 12(4):412–413, 1988.
30. Tresadern, J. C., et al. Maintenance of pregnancy in a home parenteral nutrition patient. *J. Parenter. Enteral Nutr.* 8(2):199–202, 1984.

LACTOSE INTOLERANCE

31. Gray, G. Intestinal Disaccharidase Deficiencies and Glucose-Galactose Malabsorption. In J. B. Stanbury et al. (eds.), *The Metabolic Basis of Inherited Disease*. New York: McGraw-Hill, 1983.
32. Haverberg, L., Kwon, P.H., and Scrimshaw, N. S. Comparative tolerance of adolescents of differing ethnic backgrounds to lactose-containing and lactose-free dairy drinks: I. Initial experience with a double-blind procedure. *Am. J. Clin. Nutr.* 33:17, 1980.
33. Kwon, P. H., Rorick, M. H., and Scrimshaw, N. S. Comparative tolerance of adolescents of differing ethnic backgrounds to lactose-containing and lactose-free dairy drinks: II. Improvements of a double-blind test. *Am. J. Clin. Nutr.* 33:22, 1980.
34. Villar J., Kestler E., Castillo P., et al. Improved lactose digestion during pregnancy: A case of physiologic adaptation? *Obstet. Gynecol.* 71:697, 1988.

Selected Readings

Atlay, R. D., and Weekes, A. R. The treatment of gastrointestinal disease in pregnancy. *Clin. Obstet. Gynecol.* 13(2):335–347, 1986.

Creasy, R. K., and Resnik, R. (eds.). *Maternal-Fetal Medicine: Principles and Practice* (2nd ed.). Philadelphia: Saunders, 1989.

De Swiet, M. (ed.). *Medical Disorders in Obstetric Practice* (2nd ed.). Oxford: Blackwell, 1989.

Rustgi, V. K. and Cooper, J. N. (eds.). *Gastrointestinal and Hepatic Complications in Pregnancy.* New York: Wiley, 1986.

ANTIEMETIC THERAPY

Heinonen, O. P., Sloan, D., and Shapiro, S. *Birth Defects and Drugs in Pregnancy.* Littleton, MA: Publishing Sciences Group, 1977.

Nelson, M. M., and Forfar, J. O. Associations between drugs administered during pregnancy and congenital abnormalities of the fetus. *Br. Med. J.* 1:523–527, 1971.

PEPTIC ULCER DISEASE

Peden, N. R., et al. Women and duodenal ulcer. *Br. Med. J.* 282:866, 1981.

CIMETIDINE

Colin-Jones, D. G., et al. Post-marketing surveillance of the safety of cimetidine: twelve-month morbidity report. *Q. J. Med.* 54(215):253–268, 1985.

Frank, M., et al. Comparison of the prophylactic use of magnesium trisilicate mixture B.P.C., sodium citrate mixture or cimetidine in obstetrics. *Br. J. Anaesth.* 56(4):355–362, 1984.

McAuley, D. M., et al. Cimetidine in labour: absence of adverse effect on the high-risk fetus. *Br. J. Obstet. Gynaecol.* 92(4):350–355, 1985.

Qvist, N. and Storm, K. Cimetidine pre-anesthetic. A prophylactic method against Mendelson's syndrome in cesarean section. *Acta Obstet. Gynecol. Scand.* 62(2):157–159, 1983.

Qvist, N., Storm, K., and Holmskov, A. Cimetidine as pre-anesthetic agent for cesarean section: perinatal effects on the infant, the placental transfer of cimetidine and its elimination in the infants. *J. Perinat. Med.* 13(4):179–183, 1985.

Takacs, G. Usefulness of acid and gastric juice secretion decreasing action of cimetidine in anaesthesia for the prevention of aspiration. *Ther. Hung.* 37(1):43–45, 1989.

Thorburn, J. and Moir, D. D. Antacid therapy for emergency caesarean section. *Anaesthesia* 42(4):352–355, 1987.

GASTROENTERITIS

Anders, B. J., et al. Double-blind placebo controlled trial of erythromycin for treatment of *Campylobacter enteritis*. Paper presented at the 21st Interscience Conference on Antimicrobial Agents and Chemotherapy, Chicago, Nov. 1981.

Blaser, M. J., et al. *Campylobacter enteritis* in the United States. *Ann. Intern. Med.* 98:3760, 1983.

Brumfitt, W., and Pursell, R. Trimethoprim/sulfamethoxazole in the treatment of bacteriuria in women. *J. Infect. Dis.* 128 (Suppl.):S657–S663, 1973.

Landers, D. V., Green J. R., and Sweet, R. L. Antibiotic use during pregnancy and the postpartum period. *Clin. Obstet. Gynecol.* 26:391, 1983.

Sande, M. A., and Mandell, G. L. Antimicrobial Agents: Tetracyclines, Chloramphenicol, Erythromycin, and Miscellaneous Other Agents. In A. G. Goodman et al. (eds.), *The Pharmacological Basis of Therapeutics* (7th ed.). New York: MacMillan, 1985.

ANTIHELMINTHIC THERAPY

Kreutner, A. K., et al. Giardiasis in pregnancy. *Am. J. Obstet. Gynecol.* 140:895–901, 1981.

INFLAMMATORY BOWEL DISEASE

Donaldson, R. M., Jr. Management of medical problems in pregnancy—inflammatory bowel disease. *N. Engl. J. Med.* 312(25):1616–1619, 1985.

Hanan, I. M., and Kirsner, J. B. Inflammatory bowel disease in the pregnant woman. *Clin. Perinatol.* 12(3):669–682, 1985.

Khosla, R., Willoughby, C. P., and Jewell, D. P. Crohn's disease and pregnancy. *Gut* 25(1):52–56, 1984.

Korelitz, B. I. Pregnancy, fertility, and inflammatory bowel disease. *Am. J. Gastroenterol.* 80(5):365–370, 1985.

Miller, J. P. Inflammatory bowel disease in pregnancy: a review. *J. R. Soc. Med.* 79(4):221–225, 1986.

Moeller, D. D. Crohn's disease beginning during pregnancy. *South. Med. J.* 81(8):1067, 1988.

Porter, R. J., and Stirrat, G. M. The effects of inflammatory bowel disease on pregnancy: a case-controlled retrospective analysis. *Br. J. Obstet. Gynaecol.* 93(11):1124–1131, 1986.

Sorokin, J. J., and Levine, S. M. Pregnancy and inflammatory bowel disease: a review of the literature. *Obstet. Gynecol.* 62(2):247–252, 1983.

9 Hepatobiliary Disease

Mark C. Williams

Liver Abnormalities

I. Physiology

A. General function. The liver performs a wide variety of metabolic processes including protein synthesis; the metabolism of carbohydrates, lipids, and amino acids; and biotransformation of a myriad of different compounds. It is intimately involved in glucose homeostasis, through the countering influences of gluconeogenesis and glycogenolysis. It is directly responsible for the synthesis of most classes of proteins (excepting immunoglobulins) and synthesizes fibrinogen; prothrombin; factors V, VII, XIII, IX, X, XI, XII, and XIII; and thrombolytic factors such as antithrombin III, protein C, and protein S.

Pregnancy, medications, and certain disease states specifically alter hepatic function. It is necessary to understand the characteristic alterations of hepatic function common to pregnancy in order to differentiate normal physiologic changes from abnormalities attributable to disease states.

B. Pregnancy-related changes. Pregnancy is known to cause a significant increase in maternal plasma volume. Plasma albumin concentration decreases as a direct result of this phenomenon. Changes in other laboratory measures of hepatic function include the following:

Albumin	Approximately 20% decrease
Alkaline phosphatase	2 times normal
Bilirubin	No change
Ceruloplasmin	Elevated
Cholesterol	Often 2 times normal
Gamma globulins	Slight decrease
Gamma glutamyl transpeptidase	No change or slight increase
Haptoglobins	No change
Serum transaminases	No change
Total protein	No change or slight decrease (dilutional)
Transferrin	Elevated
Triglycerides	Gradual rise to term
Clotting factors	
Fibrinogen I	20% elevation at term
Prothrombin II	Minimal change
Factor V	50% elevation
Factor VII	25% elevation
Factor VIII	2 times elevation
Factor IX	30% elevation
Factor X	No change or slight rise
Factor XI	30% decrease
Factor XII (Hageman)	2–3 times normal at term
Factor XIII	30% decrease at term
Plasminogen	30% elevation at term
Antithrombotic factors	
Antithrombin III	No change or slight rise
Proteins C and S	Slight decrease at term

II. Evaluation of hepatic dysfunction. Mild hepatic dysfunction may remain undetected for extended periods. Jaundice or elevated hepatic enzymes often are the first indication of metabolic dysfunction. Except for the physiologic increase in serum alkaline phosphatase, significant elevations of the hepatic enzymes (serum transaminases, bilirubin, and gamma glutamyl transpeptidase) do not occur in pregnancy and, if present, should be investigated.

A. Jaundice

1. Pathophysiology. Bilirubin is normally produced from the metabolism of hemoglobin from senescent erythrocytes and other hemoproteins. Any process that causes increased destruction of erythrocytes (e.g., hemolysis, disseminated intravascular coagulation) will cause increased bilirubin to be produced. Bilirubin is cleared from the circulation by conjugation (usually with glucuronic acid) and excretion as a component of bile. Circulating bilirubin is found in two forms: conjugated and unconjugated. These are usually quantitated as direct (conjugated) and indirect (unconjugated). Conjugated bilirubin is soluble in water. When present in elevated quantities, it will darken urine and impart a characteristic yellow-green color. Elevations of circulating bilirubin may occur either as a result of altered hepatic metabolism or due to increased production of bilirubin.

Jaundice is caused by elevated serum and tissue concentrations of bilirubin and is not clinically apparent until circulating levels are greater than approximately 2.5 mg/dl.

2. Etiology. Jaundice occurs in 1 in 1500 pregnancies. It results from either hepatic dysfunction or increased bilirubin production (Tables 9-1 and 9-2).

B. Abnormal hepatic function tests. Viral hepatitis, cholelithiasis, and drug-induced hepatitis should be considered as potential causes of hepatic dysfunction.

Table 9-1. Jaundice in pregnancy

Hepatic dysfunction	Increased bilirubin production
Metabolic defect in conjugation or excretion	Disseminated coagulopathy
Hepatic cirrhosis	Drug reaction (e.g., oxidizing medication in glucose 6-phosphate dehydrogenase deficiency)
Hepatitis: viral or bacterial	Hemolytic anemia
Pregnancy-related disease	Sickle cell crisis
Toxic drug exposure	

Table 9-2. Etiologies of hepatic dysfunction in pregnancy

Dysfunction	Frequency (%)
Viral hepatitis	42
Intrahepatic cholestasis of pregnancy	21
Cholelithiasis	6
Hyperemesis gravidarum	6
Preeclampsic disorders	5
Hemolysis	3
All other disorders	10
No diagnosis	7

Source: Adapted from Rustigi, V. K., *Gastrointestinal and Hepatic Complications in Pregnancy.* New York: Wiley, 1986. P. 169.

During the third trimester, pregnancy-specific causes of hepatic dysfunction such as intrahepatic cholestasis of pregnancy (ICP), pregnancy-induced hypertension, and acute fatty liver of pregnancy (AFLP) may present with acute hepatic dysfunction. The presence of these pregnancy-related diseases should be excluded before proceeding to evaluate other disease etiologies. Prompt diagnosis and initiation of appropriate therapy will greatly minimize the potential complications of ICP, pregnancy-induced hypertension, and AFLP. See Table 9-3 for a listing of acute and chronic causes of hepatitis.

Hepatic dysfunction in pregnancy can be divided into two broad categories of diseases: (1) disease states specific to pregnancy, and (2) diseases coexistent with pregnancy. **It is important to first evaluate patients for pregnancy-specific diseases.** Although relatively uncommon, these diseases carry a high associated maternal mortality if left undiagnosed and untreated. After they have been excluded from the differential diagnosis, other more common etiologies should be evaluated.

III. Pregnancy-related hepatic disease states

A. Preeclampsia. Preeclampsia occurs in 7–10% of pregnancies. Its hallmarks are the triad of new-onset hypertension, proteinuria, and edema. More severe manifestations of preeclampsia include thrombocytopenia, diminished renal function, and liver function abnormalities. One particularly severe variant of severe preeclampsia is the **HELLP syndrome** (hemolysis, elevated liver enzymes, low platelets). Preeclampsia is discussed in Chap. 5 (see sec. **III.D.1** and **III.E.3**).

B. Acute fatty liver of pregnancy

1. Natural history. AFLP is a relatively rare obstetric disease that usually pre-

Table 9-3. Differential diagnosis for hepatitis in pregnancy

Acute hepatitis

Viral infection	Pregnancy-related disease
Hepatitis A	Severe preeclampsia or HELLP syndrome
Hepatitis B	Intrahepatic cholestasis of pregnancy
Hepatitis C (non-A, non-B)	Acute fatty liver of pregnancy
Hepatitis D (delta virus)	Nonviral infections
Cytomegalovirus	Liver abscess
Epstein-Barr	Leptospirosis
Yellow fever	Malaria
Coexistent disease	Q fever
Hepatic vein thrombosis	Salmonella
Inflammatory bowel disease	Syphilis
Medication induced	Toxoplasma
Primary biliary cirrhosis	
Wilson's disease	

Chronic hepatitis

Chronic infections	Medications and drugs
Hepatitis B	Acetaminophen
Hepatitis C (non-A, non-B)	Aspirin
Hepatitis D (delta virus)	Ethanol
Medical illnesses	Isoniazid
$Alpha_1$-antitrypsin deficiency	Methyldopa
Autoimmune	Nitrofurantoin
Idiopathic	Sulfonamides
Inflammatory bowel disease	
Primary biliary cirrhosis	
Wilson's disease	

sents at 34–36 weeks of pregnancy. It occurs in approximately 1 in 10,000 pregnancies. Previous estimates of maternal and fetal mortalities were as high as 80 and 75%, respectively. More recently, however, investigators have estimated maternal and fetal mortalities as approximately 18 and 23%, respectively. These differences may reflect a previous underdiagnosis of milder cases, of perhaps improved medical management of the many metabolic abnormalities associated with AFLP.

Findings frequently associated with AFLP include jaundice (> 90%); upper abdominal pain (40–60%); the preeclamptic symptom complex of hypertension, edema, and proteinuria (50%); nausea; and vomiting. Other common findings include ascites (40%), fever (45%), headache (10%), and pruritus. A high incidence of pancreatitis has been reported in postmortem examinations of AFLP patients. AFLP is seen in association with preeclampsia in 30–60% of cases, is noted more frequently in twin gestations (9–25%), and has a 3 : 1 predominance of male fetuses.

AFLP causes significant disarrangement of normal hepatic functions. These alterations cause significant maternal morbidity. Common findings include the following:

a. Leukocytosis: the white blood cells are usually in the range of 20,000–30,000/mm^3
b. Elevated liver transaminases are usually elevated 3–10 times normal, possibly higher if severe
c. Alkaline phosphatase is elevated 5–10 times normal
d. Bilirubin is frequently greater than 10 mg/dl
e. Hyperammonemia
f. Hypoglycemia is often undiagnosed
g. Hypoaminoacidemia
h. Prolonged prothrombin time is sometimes greater than 25 seconds
i. Thrombocytopenia is often less than 100,000/mm^3

2. **Etiology.** The precise etiology of AFLP remains uncertain. Predisposing conditions include viral infection, exposure to toxins, and preeclampsia. Abnormalities of ornithine transcarbamylase and carbamyl synthetase have been described in AFLP. Riley and colleagues [4] have recently suggested that AFLP and preeclampsia may be different manifestations of a common disease entity. Pathologic findings in this disorder include widespread microhemorrhages and fatty infiltration in the brain, bone marrow, gastrointestinal tract, kidneys, and liver. Liver biopsies in AFLP characteristically show panlobular microvesicular steatosis with periportal sparing, intrahepatic cholestasis, and often acute cholangitis. Reye's syndrome, carnitine deficiency, Jamaican vomiting sickness, and therapy with certain medications (sodium valproate, salicylates, and intravenous tetracycline) have similar pathologic findings.

3. **Diagnosis.** The diagnosis of AFLP is one of exclusion. Nausea, vomiting, and jaundice may be the presenting symptoms. These complaints necessitate immediate evaluation of any pregnant women. The differential diagnoses for AFLP include viral hepatitis, severe preeclampsia or the HELLP syndrome, extrahepatic obstruction of the biliary tract, and ICP.

   Initial evaluation should include testing for hepatitis A and B, cytomegalovirus (CMV), and Epstein-Barr virus (EBV). Serum transaminases, alkaline phosphatase, bilirubin, creatinine, and uric acid evaluations are helpful in characterizing the metabolic abnormalities in a given patient. If significant hepatic dysfunction is noted, coagulation studies such as prothrombin time and bleeding time should be obtained. The most definitive test for AFLP is the liver biopsy. Although this test can be very helpful in discriminating between fulminant viral hepatitis and AFLP, it is usually reserved for only the most severe cases. Recent studies indicate that ultrasound of the liver may be helpful in the diagnosis of AFLP [1], although a normal study does not exclude the possibility of AFLP. Computed tomography may offer some advantages over sonography. A low attenuation number on a noninfused computed tomography scan is indicative of fat deposition within the liver, a finding that favors the diagnosis of AFLP [2,3]. Magnetic resonance imaging and proton spectroscopy also appear to offer advantages in allowing more accurate diagnosis of AFLP.

4. **Management.** Maternal metabolic abnormalities can be significant. Proper management of the patient with AFLP centers on stabilization of the mother, assessment of the fetal status, and expeditious delivery of the fetus.

   a. Patients with significant hepatic dysfunction are likely to have abnormal coagulation parameters because of decreased hepatic synthesis of fibrinogen and vitamin K–dependent coagulation factors (II, VII, IX, X). They are at increased risk for hypoglycemia, hypoaminoacidemia, infection, gastrointestinal bleeding, hepatic encephalopathy, and renal failure. A **multidisciplinary team approach** to medical management for patients with this multisystem disease is recommended.

   b. Once the diagnosis of AFLP has been established, **delivery should be accomplished.** If the cervical exam is favorable for induction and no contraindications to labor induction or vaginal delivery are present, an attempt at labor induction is warranted. If the cervical examination is unfavorable or the maternal or fetal status is unable to tolerate labor, a cesarean section should be performed.

   c. **Optimal anesthesia** for labor or cesarean delivery is controversial. The risks of hepatotoxicity with general anesthesia and bleeding complications with regional anesthesia must be considered. These patients may be safely managed with regional anesthesia (epidural or spinal) if they have adequate coagulation parameters and an adequate platelet count. A bleeding time is also quite useful, as it allows evaluation of the clotting system as a whole.

   d. Patients who develop **bleeding abnormalities** should receive fresh-frozen plasma and vitamin K supplementation. It should be emphasized that hypoglycemia in AFLP can be significant, and maternal serum glucose should be followed carefully if any alteration in mentation is present.

C. Intrahepatic cholestasis of pregnancy

1. **Natural history.** Intrahepatic cholestasis of pregnancy is an uncommon condition thought to affect approximately 1 in 500 pregnancies. The exact incidence of this condition is difficult to determine, due to its wide spectrum of clinical presentations, which range from mild, generalized, third-trimester pruritus to overt jaundice accompanied by significant pruritus and maternal cholestasis. Because published series of ICP have not used uniform systems of patient classification, it is difficult to make comparisons among the studied populations. Nevertheless, the incidence of ICP is thought to be increased in Scandinavian and Mediterranean populations. An autosomal dominant inheritance pattern has been observed [9], with affected patients having a positive family history in 40–45% of cases. A recurrence rate of 45% has been reported in subsequent pregnancies. Affected pregnancies in many studies have shown an increased incidence of preterm labor and a possibly elevated incidence of unexplained fetal demise. Maternal malabsorption of fab-soluble vitamins may occur [12]. Postpartum hemorrhage is seen in 10–20% of cases, and this is possibly due to malabsorption of vitamin K or altered hepatic biosynthesis of vitamin K–dependent coagulation factors. Intrahepatic biliary stasis also appears to promote the occurrence of cholelithiasis [10]. Patients with ICP who are subsequently placed on oral contraceptive pills have a high chance of developing recurrent symptoms, and for this reason, oral contraceptives should be avoided or used with extreme care. Finally, resolution of symptoms has been reported with high-dose therapy with *S*-adenosyl-*L*-methionine [6].

2. **Mechanism.** Although the precise metabolic abnormality responsible for ICP has not been determined, **altered maternal intrahepatic metabolism of estrogens** seems the most likely cause. Patients with ICP have higher serum levels of estrogen sulfates and show reduced biliary and urinary excretion of various estrogen metabolites. An association between twin gestations (with their higher attendant estrogen levels) and ICP has recently been reported [7].
   The symptom of **generalized pruritus** is felt to be due to the deposition of bile

salts in the subcutaneous tissues. The association between bile salt deposition and subsequent pruritus has been noted among other nonpregnancy-related conditions with elevated serum bile acids [11].

Older literature frequently documented an increased rate of premature labor, neonatal mortality (probably directly attributable to prematurity), and unexplained intrauterine fetal demise [5]. The proposed mechanism for these changes was deposition of bile salts in the placenta with resultant alteration of placental function. Whether this in fact occurs is open to question, as more recent studies have not documented an increased rate of intrauterine fetal demise.

3. Diagnosis

a. Clinical findings

(1) Usually occurs between 36 and 40 weeks' gestation, almost never before 30 weeks' gestation

(2) Generalized pruritus

(3) Mild to moderate jaundice (variable rate of occurrence)

b. Laboratory findings

(1) Elevated conjugated bilirubin (2–5 times normal)

(2) Elevated alkaline phosphatase (7–10 times normal)

(3) Mild elevations of serum glutamic-oxaloacetic transaminase and serum glutamic-pyruvic transaminase

(4) Prolonged prothrombin time (usually corrects with vitamin K therapy)

(5) Elevated (10–100 times normal) serum cholic acid, chenodeoxycholic acid, and bile acids

4. Differential diagnosis

a. Infectious hepatitis (hepatitis A and B, EBV, CMV, and others)

b. Extrahepatic obstruction (cholelithiasis, cholangiocarcinoma, others)

c. Primary biliary cirrhosis

d. AFLP

e. Drug reactions (hemolytic)

f. Metabolic abnormalities (Dubin-Johnson syndrome, others)

5. Management

a. Symptomatic treatment. Current antepartum management recommendations usually center on palliation of pruritus with antihistaminic agents such as the following:

(1) Diphenhydramine (Benadryl), 25–50 mg PO q6–8h

(2) Promethazine (Phenergan), 12.5–25 mg PO q6–8h

(3) Phenobarbital, 25–50 mg PO q6–8h

b. Therapeutic treatment. Severe refractory pruritis in a patient too premature for elective delivery is an indication for medication to attempt to lower circulating bile acids.

(1) Cholestyramine (Questran), a nonabsorbable basic anion-exchange resin that binds bile salts into a complex that is then eliminated by fecal excretion, has proved effective in lowering bile acid levels. Cholestyramine should not be used during the first 20–24 weeks of pregnancy. Teratogenicity has not been noted, but there has not as yet been wide experience with this therapy. Cholestyramine therapy may interfere with normal fat absorption and promote steatorrhea, resulting in decreased absorption of such fat-soluble vitamins as A, D, and K. It has also been shown to interfere with the oral absorption of some medications and can cause hyperchloremic acidosis. The initial dose of cholestyramine is 3 gm/6 hours, with a daily maximum allowed dose of 20 gm. Vitamin K (10 mg SC q5–7d) should be administered and prothrombin times monitored.

(2) *S*-adenosyl-*L*-methionine. A final treatment option involves the use of high-dose *S*-adenosyl-*L*-methionine (SALM), which has been used to normalize serum bile acids [6]. Cholestyramine and SALM should be begun only after consultation with a maternal-fetal medicine specialist.

6. Perinatal risks. Affected pregnancies may be at increased risk for both preterm labor and unexplained intrauterine fetal demise. Because more recent studies have questioned these findings, the most reasonable recommendations at this time are the following:

a. Carefully discuss the signs of preterm labor with the patient, and possibly initiate home uterine contraction monitoring at 26–28 weeks' gestation.

b. Begin antepartum fetal surveillance at 30–32 weeks' gestation. Weekly contraction stress tests or twice-weekly nonstress testing have most commonly been used.

c. Fetal ultrasound evaluation to verify normal fetal growth and development should be performed at the time of diagnosis and every three to four weeks thereafter.

7. Delivery. The potential risk to the fetus in an ICP-affected pregnancy is not well known, and the need for elective delivery prior to spontaneous labor is controversial. Some authorities advocate induction of labor at 37–38 weeks' gestation after verification of fetal lung maturity by amniocentesis. Other authors feel that the risks to the fetus are not of sufficient magnitude to justify such intervention. They feel infants can be followed with careful surveillance and delivered at term. It is reasonable to induce labor by 41 weeks' gestation if it has not occurred spontaneously by that time.

IV. Concurrent hepatic diseases

A. Viral hepatitis. Viral hepatitis is the most common cause of jaundice in pregnancy. The **differential diagnosis** for viral hepatitis in pregnancy includes a wide range of viral, bacterial, and medical syndromes (Table 9-3).

1. Hepatitis A virus. Hepatitis A virus (HAV) is an RNA enterovirus that causes infection primarily involving the liver. It is usually acquired by eating contaminated food or contact with infected feces, often by contamination of water supplies with sewage (Table 9-4).

The incubation period is from 14–40 days from exposure, with maximum viral shedding noted in feces at an interval of two to three weeks from exposure.

a. Diagnosis. The infection usually presents as a flulike syndrome, with malaise, anorexia, headache, fatigue, fever, and arthralgia as predominant symptoms. Patients may not present until they have developed clay stools, jaundice, and dark (bilirubinuric) urine. The diagnosis is verified by demonstrating the presence of specific antibodies to the HAV. Anti-HAV immunoglobulin M (IgM) antibodies are usually present within 30 days of exposure and persist for 8 weeks or more. The IgG anti-HAV usually appears at 10–12 weeks from exposure and persists for many years (Fig. 9-1).

Table 9-4. Common hepatic viral pathogens in pregnancy

Agent	Type	Route	Incubation
Hepatitis A	RNA enterovirus	Fecal/oral/food	14–40 d
Hepatitis B	DNA	Parenteral/ intimate contact	30–180 d
Hepatitis C (non-A, non-B)	Unknown, 3 or more?	Parenteral/enteric	Various patterns
Hepatitis D (delta virus)	RNA, virion is incomplete	Parenteral	Variable
Cytomegalovirus	DNA herpesvirus	Parenteral/body fluids	20–60 d
Epstein-Barr, mononucleosis	DNA herpesvirus	Saliva	30–60 d
Herpes simplex	DNA herpesvirus	Mucosal contact	1–26 d
Varicella zoster	DNA herpesvirus	Respiratory	10–20 d

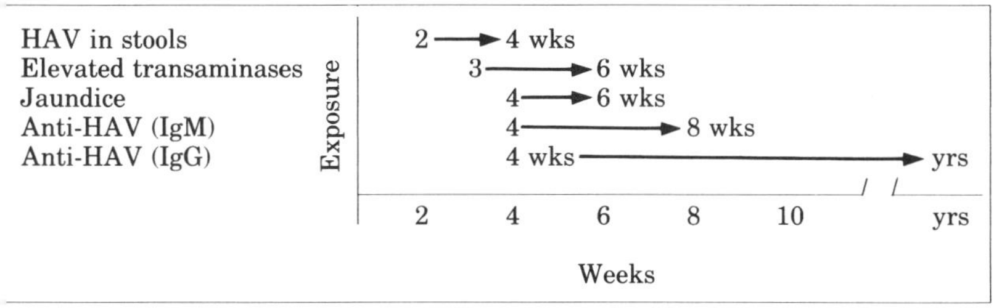

Fig. 9-1. Course of HAV infection in weeks after exposure.

b. Management. Recent reviews of HAV infection in pregnancy indicate that it has little or no effect on pregnancy [19, 27]. Nevertheless, it is recommended that hepatitis immunoglobulin be given for significant exposure if no evidence of previous exposure to HAV can be documented by the presence of an IgG anti-HAV.

Prophylaxis is effective in up to 80% of cases if given within two weeks of exposure. Hepatitis immunoglobulin with a high anti-HAV titer should be given at a dose of 0.02 mg/kg of maternal weight. Although the virus has not been shown to cross the placenta, the neonate is at some risk of acquiring it from the mother. For this reason, at-risk infants should receive prophylactic hepatitis immunoglobulin at a dose of 0.02 mg/kg after delivery.

It is recommended that pregnant women planning **travel** to areas where HAV is endemic receive passive immunization with hepatitis immunoglobulin. An active attenuated virus is now available, but its safety in pregnancy has not been evaluated.

2. Hepatitis B virus. Hepatitis B is a DNA virus. Infection by hepatitis B virus (HBV) is a significant cause of jaundice in pregnancy worldwide, especially in China and Southeast Asia, where it is endemic. It is transmitted almost exclusively via contaminated needles, blood products, or direct mucosal contact with contaminated body fluids. In certain populations, vertical transmission from mother to child is a significant problem. Chronic infection with HBV is associated with the development of hepatocellular carcinoma later in life.

a. Diagnosis

(1) The incubation period for HBV ranges from 30–110 days and may increase to as much as 180 days in chronic disease states. Serologic evidence of infection is usually present within six to seven weeks, but after highly infectious exposure, serologic evidence of infection may be present as soon as two weeks after exposure.

(2) Patients commonly present with **malaise, fever, and jaundice,** and **occasionally arthritis, urticarial rashes, and glomerulonephritis.** Ninety percent of patients experience complete recovery; 10% go on to suffer chronic hepatic disease, and approximately 1% suffers fulminant disease and liver failure.

(3) Serologic evidence of acute infection is used to confirm the diagnosis. HBV infection characteristically results in antibody response to the viral surface components (HBsAg), to the DNA core (HBcAg), and to other enzymatic components of the viral core called "e" antigens (HBeAg). Assays are available for these antigens and their respective antibodies, HBsAb, HBcAb, and HBeAb. Recently, IgM testing for these compounds has become available, further improving the differentiation of acute and chronic disease. Direct assay for virus-specific DNA segments is also available in some institutions. Patients who have been vaccinated against HBV infection should develop positive titers for HBsAb but should not show evidence of antibody response to the HBV core antigens (i.e., anti-HBcAb, anti-HBeAb).

The specific antigens and antibodies associated with HBV infection present at a given time vary over the course of the illness. Fig. 9-2 displays approximate time intervals for various serologic tests in HBV infection.

(4) All pregnant women in groups at risk for HBV infection should be screened. In the United States, such risk groups would include health care workers with exposure to blood or blood products, patients with a history of having lived or traveled in Southeast Asia, and patients with either a history of blood transfusions or IV substance abuse. The need for universal HBV screening of all pregnancies remains controversial. Its ultimate value will depend on considerations of disease prevalence and a societal cost-benefit analysis regarding perinatal infections prevented. Regardless, screening consists of testing maternal serum for the presence of HBsAg. Patients testing positive are then assessed for infective risk by evaluating for HBeAg and HBeAb.

b. Fetal risks. Transplacental passage of HBV does not usually occur, but indirect evidence of it has been reported [26]. The primary risk for perinatal infection is present during the birth process and the neonatal period. This risk is related to the quantity of HBV-DNA present in the maternal serum [18, 21, 24]. Maternal HBeAg and HBeAb status are closely correlated with subsequent vertical transmission to children in the first 18 months of life [14]. These correlations and the percentage of subsequent HBV infections are listed in Table 9-5.

The exact risk of vertical transmission varies among racial groups. It is as high as 95% in Asian populations, and on the order of 20% in some African populations. Cesarean section is not currently recommended to prevent vertical transmission of HBV. Nevertheless, Lee [25] analyzed the vertical transmission rates among 447 infants born to mothers at high risk of transmitting HBV to their infants (positive for HBeAg and HBsAg) and found that cesarean section may decrease the risk of perinatal transmission. HBV infection was found in 25% of 385 vaginally delivered infants and in 10% of 62 infants born by cesarean section.

c. Immunoprophylaxis. Patients at high risk of contracting HBV infection, such as certain health care workers, are recommended to be immunized against HBV prior to becoming pregnant. Vaccines for this purpose, such as Heptavax, are now produced in bacterial culture using recombinant DNA technology and carry no risk of transmitting other viral infections. The usual dosage schedule for vaccination in adults is 20 μg deep IM (deltoid or anterior thigh, not buttock) at 0, 1, and 6 months outside of pregnancy.

(1) Maternal. If HBV exposure occurs during pregnancy and no evidence of immunity to HBV can be demonstrated (i.e., neither HBsAb nor HBsAg

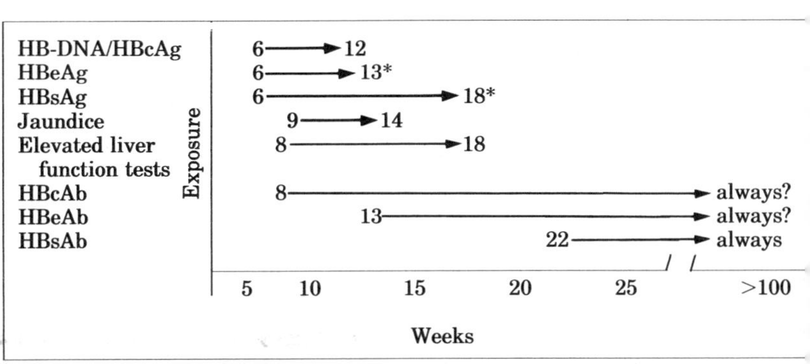

Fig. 9-2. Course of HBV infection in weeks after exposure. In cases of chronic disease, both HBeAg and HBsAg may remain positive for long periods and appear directly related to a patient's infectivity (see asterisks).

Table 9-5. Risk of HBV mother-child vertical transmission

Maternal HBeAg/Ab serology (known maternal HBV infection)	Risk category	Infection (%)
Positive HBeAg, negative HBeAb	High	57
Negative HBeAg, negative HBeAb	Intermediate	20
Negative HBeAg, positive HBeAb	Low	11

Source: From Beasley, R. P., and Hwang, L. Y. Postnatal infectivity of hepatitis B surface antigen-carrier mothers. *J. Infect. Dis.* 147(2):185–190, 1983.

is present), the patient should be passively immunized with hepatitis B immunoglobulin. Hepatitis B immunoglobin ideally should be administered within 12 hours of exposure, although it may have clinical efficacy if given up to 48 hours after exposure. Vaccination with viral surface components (e.g., Heptavax) during pregnancy against hepatitis B is not currently recommended, but several such occurrences have been reported with no documented fetal morbidity. Should significant exposure to hepatitis B occur during pregnancy, consultation with a specialist in maternal-fetal medicine or infectious diseases regarding the risks and benefits of active vaccination is recommended.

(2) Infant. It is recommended that infants born to HBsAg-positive mothers receive combined therapy with hepatitis B immunoglobulin and vaccination against HBV. Although an optimal neonatal immunization scheme has not been defined, early experience indicates that a 0-, 1-, 6-month schedule may be clinically efficacious [17]. Infants who have begun combined immunotherapy should be allowed to breast-feed. Proper hand-washing techniques, use of protective gloves, and careful handling of potentially infectious waste should be encouraged among those caring for both mother and child.

3. Non-A, non-B hepatitis (hepatitis C). The precise etiology of non-A, non-B hepatitis (NANBH), sometimes called **hepatitis C,** is unclear. Dienstag and Alter [16] and Shorey [29] have offered the opinion that at least three different agents may be involved—two that are blood borne and a third that is spread enterically (similar to hepatitis A). Enteric NANBH appears to be the cause of epidemics of NANBH in many underdeveloped countries worldwide [28]. Epidemiologic evaluation of post-transfusion infections indicates that at least two agents may be associated with blood-borne NANBH. One pattern resembles that of hepatitis B; another (associated with clotting factor administration) has a much shorter, 7–10 day, incubation period. It is likely that NANBH can also be transmitted venereally, as it is often seen in sporadic cases without an identifiable vector. NANBH is thought responsible for 90–95% of transfusion-associated hepatitis and 15–30% of sporadic cases of hepatitis. Blood-borne NANBH infections are initially less fulminant but progress to cirrhosis much more commonly than either hepatitis A or B. Some 40–60% of patients develop chronic hepatitis, and of these, 10–20% progress to cirrhosis [16].

Epidemic enteric NANBH does not usually progress to cirrhosis but has a high mortality rate among pregnant women [20, 28]. In a series of NANBH patients who developed fulminant hepatitis, Bal and colleagues [13] found that 32% were pregnant women, whereas pregnant women composed only 0.8% of patients with the milder nonfulminant variety of NANBH. Similar high attack rates were reported by Khuroo and colleagues [23] in an outbreak in the Kashmir valley, India, where 2.8% of men, 2.1% of nonpregnant women, and 17.3% of pregnant women became infected. Reported case fatality rates in pregnancy range from 20% [22] to 100% [15].

The prognosis for pregnancy complicated by chronic NANBH may be somewhat better than that for acute infection. Wejstal [30] has reported on 14 pregnancies among 11 patients with chronic NANBH, finding 12 term deliveries, 1 preterm birth, and 1 stillborn. Among the 13 surviving infants, 61% had transiently elevated liver enzymes and 15% developed chronic hepatitis.

a. **Diagnosis.** There are no specific tests for NANBH. Until they become available, the most effective means of reducing the spread of NANBH are to use nonspecific tests (such as liver function studies) to screen blood transfusion products, and the promotion of public sanitation measures in underdeveloped areas.

   The diagnosis of NANBH is made by exclusion, after other likely causes of hepatitis have been excluded.

4. **Hepatitis delta virus.** The hepatitis delta virus (HDV) is an incomplete RNA virus that is sometimes isolated from the contents of the hepatitis B viral core. An HDV infection is acquired at the time of infection with HBV. HDV is not capable of creating its own surface capsule but uses surplus HBV surface antigen to form its capsid, with which it can then penetrate host cell membranes.

   a. **Diagnosis.** Infection by HDV should be suspected if a patient convalescing from HBV infection develops suddenly worsening liver function. The diagnosis can be confirmed by serologic testing for IgM and IgG antibodies specific for the HDV, although these tests are not as yet widely available.

5. **Herpesviruses.** Two members of this family of viruses, CMV and EBV, can cause hepatic disease.

   a. **Cytomegalovirus,** a DNA herpesvirus, is of significance in obstetrics because if in utero infection occurs, significant fetal morbidity may result. CMV is endemic to most populations worldwide, and its prevalence rises with age. Among white, middle-class females, the incidence rises from 30% at age 20 to 60% at age 40. This rise in exposure to CMV coincides with the reproductive years for many women.

      Under normal circumstances, a patient who enters pregnancy with no serologic evidence of prior exposure to CMV has a 1% risk of acquiring CMV during pregnancy. It is reasonable to restrict the pregnant patient's exposure to known carriers of CMV and other identifiable sources of exposure to CMV in order to reduce the risk of primary infection, but routine work in nurseries and hospital laboratories is probably acceptable.

      (1) **Diagnosis.** The diagnosis of CMV should be considered when a flulike syndrome of malaise, intermittent high fevers, arthralgias, nausea, and vomiting presents. The differential diagnoses for these findings include other causes of viral hepatitis. Mononucleosis (Epstein-Barr infection) is almost indistinguishable from CMV infection by clinical examination.

      The diagnosis of CMV can be confirmed by a fourfold rise in paired antibody titer, obtained by enzyme-linked immunosorbent assay, fluorescent antibody, or indirect hemagglutination, over four to six weeks. A single positive titer for IgG directed against CMV does not indicate active disease. Complement fixation titers are no longer used because of a high rate of cross reactivity with other herpesviruses. Demonstration of either IgM against CMV or a positive viral culture from serum or urine is also sufficient to confirm the diagnosis. False-positive IgM determinations sometimes occur due to a cross reaction with circulating rheumatoid factor. Finally, DNA-DNA hybridization techniques now allow rapid detection of CMV in urine and serum specimens.

      (2) **Maternal risk.** CMV hepatitis during pregnancy is usually mild. It most often causes an illness quite similar to Epstein-Barr "mononucleosis" and rarely progresses to fulminant disease.

      (3) **Fetal risk.** CMV is the most frequent in utero fetal infection, with 0.5–2.5% of newborns showing evidence of infection at birth. Severely affected infants are found in approximately 1 in 15,000 births.

      Fetal risk is affected by prior maternal exposure to CMV. Fetal exposure to primary maternal CMV infection will result in transmission to the fetus in 30–40% of cases, with as many as 10% of infected fetuses being severely affected at birth. Infants born to mothers exposed to CMV before pregnancy have a 3–6% risk of becoming infected with CMV in utero and if infected will be severely affected in less than 1% of cases.

Fetal exposure to primary infection in the first two trimesters of pregnancy is associated with the highest incidence of severely affected infants. Congenital CMV infection is often not diagnosed at birth, but from 5–25% of infants with otherwise asymptomatic infections develop **significant developmental problems** over the next several years. These problems include hearing deficit, psychomotor difficulties, ocular deficit, and dental abnormalities. Infants thought to have been exposed to active disease in utero should have careful pediatric follow-up.

(4) **Management.** At present, no adequate prophylaxis for CMV exposure in pregnancy is available. The use of CMV hyperimmune globulin has proven effective in minimizing the CMV infectious morbidity associated with organ transplantation and bone marrow transplantation, but there is as yet no experience with this therapy in pregnancy.

After consideration of the risks of in utero CMV exposure before 20 weeks of gestation, termination of the pregnancy may be desired by some patients.

b. **Epstein-Barr virus** is a DNA herpesvirus responsible for causing mononucleosis.

(1) **Diagnosis.** EBV is characterized by a syndrome involving intermittent high fevers, malaise, headache, sore throat, and cervical and axillary lymphadenopathy. Splenomegaly occurs in 75%, hepatomegaly in 17%, and jaundice in 11%. It is essentially indistinguishable from acute CMV infection on a clinical basis.

Diagnosis can be readily confirmed by the presence of maternal IgM specific for the EBV. If IgM is not detected, evidence of a rising IgG titer or the presence of IgM against EBV nuclear antigen is also confirmatory.

(2) **Management.** Supportive care and maintenance of good nutrition are important aspects of care in these patients. Maternal EBV infection is not associated with any known fetal morbidity.

c. **Other herpesviruses.** Varicella zoster and herpes simplex infections are not usually associated with significant maternal hepatic involvement. They do have significant potential implications for the fetus should exposure or reactivation of these infections occur in pregnancy.

B. **Hepatic cirrhosis.** Hepatic cirrhosis is a state of chronic hepatic dysfunction resulting from a wide variety of infections, metabolic diseases, and toxic exposures. It is characterized by permanent changes in hepatic microarchitecture including fibrosis and areas of nodular regeneration. The spectrum of hepatic dysfunction ranges from minimal disease to congestive heart failure, ascites, portal hypertension, and gastrointestinal bleeding from gastric and esophageal varices. Hepatic cirrhosis often results in impaired fertility, possibly due to altered steroid metabolism. As a result, there has been only limited experience with the management of cirrhosis in pregnancy.

Recent reports indicate that pregnancy has little effect on hepatic function among most cirrhotics, although perhaps 20% of patients experience worsened disease. **Pregnancy-associated maternal morbidity** correlates well with the prepregnancy disease state. Maternal and fetal prognosis is best predicted by the extent of maternal metabolic disarrangement, as well as the presence or absence of esophageal varices.

Esophageal varices associated with **portal hypertension** account for much of the maternal morbidity. **Variceal bleeding** is more commonly observed in the third trimester, possibly relating to concomitant elevations in the circulating blood volume associated with pregnancy. Correction of portal hypertension by portal-systemic shunting prior to pregnancy seems to improve fetal outcome significantly and reduce maternal risk [31]. Recent advances in sclerotherapy of esophageal varices may offer the possibility of treatment of this potentially life-threatening condition if it is first noted during pregnancy.

1. **Primary biliary cirrhosis** (PBC) is an uncommon disorder that is often diagnosed after elevated alkaline phosphatase levels are noted in an otherwise

asymptomatic patient. Ninety percent of patients with PBC are female, most commonly between the ages of 35 and 60. Common symptomatology includes pruritus, jaundice, hepatosplenomegaly, bone pain, and hyperpigmentation of the skin. Late in the course of PBC, ascites and variceal bleeding may present. The long-term prognosis for patients with this disorder appears to be related to symptomatology. Asymptomatic patients have an essentially normal age-adjusted life expectancy; symptomatic patients have a life expectancy of 5–10 years.

There appears to be a strong association between PBC and various autoimmune diseases, such as autoimmune thyroiditis, renal tubular acidosis, the CREST syndrome (calcinosis, Raynaud's phenomenon, esophageal dysmotility, sclerodactyly, and telangiectasia), Sjögren's syndrome, and the sicca syndrome (dry eyes and mouth).

a. Diagnosis. If first noted during pregnancy or with oral contraceptive use, the symptomatology of PBC will often be ascribed to intrahepatic cholestasis of pregnancy (ICP). The differential diagnoses for PBC are identical to those for ICP.

When resolution of symptoms does not follow delivery or discontinuation of the medication, the diagnosis of PBC should be strongly considered. The distinction between PBC and ICP during pregnancy can be ascertained by using the following laboratory studies; findings in PBC include

(1) Alkaline phosphatase elevations of 2–6 times normal; occasionally up to 10 times normal
(2) Bilirubin normal or mildly elevated
(3) Serum bile acids often increased
(4) Serum cholesterol often increased
(5) Serum IgM elevated in 75% of patients
(6) Antimitochondrial antibody present in 95% of patients
(7) Hypoprothrombinemia
(8) Prolonged prothrombin time that usually corrects with vitamin K therapy
(9) Hypocalcemia related to malabsorption of vitamin D

b. Therapy. No corrective therapy is known for PBC, irrespective of pregnancy. Various medications have been tried in nonpregnant PBC patients, including azathioprine, corticosteroids, and D-penicillamine, without convincing benefit to the patient.

Management recommendations for pregnancy complicated by PBC are not widely agreed on, probably owing to the relative rarity of this pregnancy complication. PBC closely mirrors ICP, and management considerations are similar.

Early series of PBC in pregnancy documented a high fetal mortality but with no appreciable increase in maternal mortality. Modern obstetric management with increased use of antenatal fetal testing may reasonably be expected to improve fetal outcomes in PBC, just as it has in ICP.

2. Wilson's disease. Wilson's disease is an autosomal recessive disorder with a population incidence of 1 in 100,000 live births. The probable abnormalities of copper metabolism responsible for this disorder involve a decreased rate of incorporation of copper into the ceruloplasmin molecule, and an alteration of biliary copper excretion. The liver releases excess copper into the general circulation, which is then deposited into such tissues as the cornea, kidneys, lenticular nucleus of the brain, and muscles. The most frequent presentation for these patients is as a result of liver disease or neurologic abnormalities. Degenerative changes of the basal ganglia and hepatic cirrhosis may occur.

a. Diagnosis. Classic features of Wilson's disease include

(1) Kayser-Fleischer rings on slit-lamp examination of the cornea (not specific to Wilson's disease, however)
(2) Low plasma ceruloplasmin
(3) Elevated serum nonceruloplasmin copper
(4) Decreased total plasma copper
(5) Elevated urinary copper excretion

During pregnancy, the diagnosis of Wilson's disease may be made more difficult by the pregnancy-associated elevation of ceruloplasmin, which may mask otherwise low levels of this enzyme. Testing with radioisotopes of copper (^{64}Cu, ^{67}Cu) is contraindicated in pregnancy.

b. Management. Successful results have been reported using D-penicillamine [33] (35 patients) and trientine [32] (9 patients) chelation therapy for Wilson's disease. Although experience with chelation therapy in pregnancy has been good, the use of such medications cannot yet be routinely recommended, as potential fetal effects are documented and their etiology is as yet unclear. Patients on long-term therapy should be placed on a lower dose during pregnancy, or have therapy stopped altogether. Wilson's disease pregnancies should be followed with serial ultrasound evaluations to assess fetal growth. Antepartum testing should be initiated at 26–28 weeks of gestation. Oral zinc therapy has also been attempted in the past, but no experience is available for this therapy in pregnancy.

3. Hepatic vein thrombosis. Hepatic vein thrombosis (HVT), or Budd-Chiari syndrome, although generally a pediatric disease, has been noted to develop in adults. Associated factors include pregnancy, oral contraceptive use, abdominal trauma, and disease states associated with hypercoagulability, such as polycythemia rubra vera and paroxysmal nocturnal hemoglobinuria.

a. Diagnosis. The symptoms commonly associated with HVT include abdominal pain of either acute or gradual onset, and ascites. These symptoms are due to impeded outflow of blood from the liver and are common to all disease processes that share this alteration of outflow.

Laboratory findings include elevations of serum transaminases and bilirubin, although these are usually mild. Alkaline phosphatase may be elevated beyond normal pregnancy ranges. In pregnancy, demonstration of decreased hepatic venous blood flow with Doppler velocimetry is suggestive of the diagnosis. Liver biopsy showing centrilobular congestion in the absence of significant cardiac disease or hepatic outflow obstruction suggests the diagnosis of HVT. Occasionally it may be necessary to attempt hepatic venography, a procedure that allows precise diagnosis of this condition.

Patients with suspected HVT should also be evaluated for antithrombin III deficiency, the presence of a "lupus anticoagulant" type factor, polycythemia rubra vera, and paroxysmal nocturnal hemoglobinuria.

b. Management. Even in the nonpregnant state, HVT is associated with mortality rates as high as 50–90%. Nevertheless, various reports of successful pregnancy in HVT have been published. Additionally, successful pregnancies have been reported to one patient after having received an orthotopic liver transplant.

Management of maternal ascites associated with HVT is difficult, as diuretics are not frequently clinically efficacious, and their safety in pregnancy among patients with significant liver disease has not been well established.

4. Medication-induced hepatitis. A wide range of medications can potentially cause hepatitis. It is important to keep this in mind, as discontinuation of the medication will often lead to rapid resolution of the hepatic dysfunction. Table 9-6 lists potential hepatotoxic medications categorized by their characteristic hepatic lesion.

C. Hereditary hyperbilirubinemia. Certain inherited abnormalities of bilirubin metabolism may present as isolated elevations of either conjugated or unconjugated bilirubin. Genetic syndromes associated with isolated conjugated hyperbilirubinemia include Dubin-Johnson and Rotor's syndromes; unconjugated hyperbilirubinemia is seen in Crigler-Najjar (types 1 and 2) and Gilbert's syndrome. Crigler-Najjar (type 1) syndrome is usually fatal in early childhood, but the other conditions usually have a benign course. Many patients will be first diagnosed when serum chemistries drawn for other reasons reveal elevated bilirubin levels. Patients with the Dubin-Johnson syndrome will occasionally first manifest this condition in pregnancy, or after taking oral contraceptives for the first time. Fifty percent of patients with the Dubin-Johnson syndrome will develop jaundice in pregnancy.

The characteristic finding common to these syndromes is hyperbilirubinemia

Table 9-6. Medication-induced hepatitis: Characteristic alterations in liver microarchitecture

Mimic viral hepatitis	Fatty liver
Halothane	Alcoholic hepatitis
Isoniazid	Corticosteroids
Methyldopa	Tetracyclines
Phenytoin	Valproic acid
Sulfonamides	Other liver pathology
Cholestasis	Acetaminophen
Anabolic steroids	Aspirin
Androgens (17 alpha)	Carbon tetrachloride
Antithyroid medications	Oxacillin
Erythromycin estolate (and other macrolides)	
Estrogens (natural and synthetic)	
Phenothiazines	

without other significant biochemical abnormalities. Bilirubin levels in Crigler-Najjar type 2 syndrome are usually in the range of 8–18, although levels as high as 40 have been reported. Bilirubin levels of 2–5 mg/dl are usually found in patients having Dubin-Johnson, Rotor's, or Gilbert's syndromes.

A theoretic risk of kernicterus exists in infants exposed in utero to chronically elevated maternal bilirubin levels, but this concern has not proved to be of clinical concern when evaluated. Several reported cases of Dubin-Johnson syndrome have been associated with intrauterine fetal demise [34].

Gallbladder Disease

I. Cholecystitis is the second most frequent nonobstetric indication for surgery in pregnancy and usually results from obstruction by gallstones. Asymptomatic gallstones detectable by sonographic evaluation are reported to occur in 3.5–11.0% of patients during pregnancy. It has not been determined whether pregnancy is a risk factor for cholelithiasis. Cholecystectomy is required in approximately 1 in 1000 deliveries.

A. Diagnosis. Pregnancy does not alter the presentation or management of cholecystitis. Patients will usually complain of sudden-onset nausea, vomiting, and right upper quadrant pain with some radiation to the back. Dietary intolerance to fatty foods may not be present.

Laboratory findings characteristically include:

1. Hyperbilirubinemia (both conjugated and unconjugated)
2. Elevated serum transaminases
3. Bilirubinuria

The normal increase of alkaline phosphatase with pregnancy limits its usefulness in evaluating obstructions of the biliary tree.

The diagnosis of cholecystitis in pregnancy can most often be confirmed by **ultrasonographic evaluation** of the liver and gallbladder. Choleliths are generally quite echogenic, and if obstruction has occurred, some dilation of the biliary tree may also be present. If normal sonographic imaging fails to confirm the diagnosis and maternal symptomatology is severe, a radioisotope scan using radiolabeled technetium 99 may be considered [35]. Other methods of imaging the biliary tract that require fluoroscopy or other high radiation exposures are not recommended unless adequate fetal shielding can be provided.

B. Management. Proper management of cholecystitis in pregnancy requires the following:

1. Provide adequate narcotic analgesia (meperidine may cause less spasm of the sphincter of Oddi than morphine)

2. Maintain adequate hydration
3. Maintain total bowel rest for several days, then gradually advance diet
4. Use intermittent nasogastric suction to decrease stimulation of the gallbladder
5. Begin broad-spectrum antibiotic (i.e., ampicillin or cephalosporins) to decrease possibility of secondary infection

The decision to perform **cholecystectomy** should be individualized to the unique situation each patient presents. Patients with recurrent bouts of cholecystitis or patients with documented obstruction that does not resolve should be considered for percutaneous drainage or surgery. It is not advisable to delay indicated drainage or surgery until the postpartum interval, as such delay is associated with unacceptable maternal morbidity. Orally administered bile acids such as chenodeoxycholic acid have been used in **nonpregnant** patients to dissolve choleliths. **Such therapy is contraindicated in pregnancy, as similar compounds do cross the placenta and have been found teratogenic in primates.**

Pancreatic Disease

Our understanding of the effects of pregnancy on pancreatic function is incomplete. Glucagon and insulin, produced by the alpha and beta islet cells respectively, are increased. Insulin secretion is markedly elevated in late pregnancy. It is not clear if pregnancy alters serum amylase levels. They have been reported to either remain unchanged or to peak late in the second trimester. Electrophoresis reveals two categories of amylase isoenzymes: P and S isoamylases. P isoamylases tend to be produced by the pancreas and the S variety are produced at the various other sites. If elevated levels are encountered, electrophoresis may help identify the source of the elevation. Table 9-7 lists conditions predisposing to hyperamylasemia.

I. Pancreatitis. Pancreatitis complicating pregnancy occurs in 1 of 3000–10,000 pregnancies. A strong correlation exists between maternal biliary disease and pancreatitis. Episodes of pancreatitis may be somewhat more frequent in the third trimester. Various conditions that have been noted to predispose to pancreatitis are listed in Table 9-8.

A. Diagnosis. In pregnancy pancreatitis presents much as in the nonpregnant state. Nausea and vomiting are present in 70–90% of patients. Constant, extreme, sudden-onset epigastric pain radiating to the back is common. Hemorrhagic pancreatitis may lead to internal hemorrhage with blood dissecting through the retroperitoneal tissues and into the flanks (Grey Turner's sign) or the periumbilical area (Cullen's sign).

The differential diagnoses for pancreatitis include acute appendicitis, aortic aneurysm, bowel obstruction, cholecystitis, diabetic ketoacidosis, peptic ulcer disease, pyelonephritis, perinephric abscess, perforated viscus, and renal colic.

Common laboratory findings include:
1. Mild jaundice (bilirubin approximately 4 mg/dl in 15% of patients
2. Fever
3. Leukocytosis with white blood cell count of 15,000–30,000/mm^3

Table 9-7. Differential diagnoses for hyperamylasemia

Aortic aneurysm	Malignancies (esophagus, lung, ovary, pancreas)
Bowel disease (infarction, obstruction)	Mumps
Cerebral trauma	Pancreatic disease
Diabetic ketoacidosis	Peptic ulcer (penetrating)
Ectopic pregnancy (ruptured)	Peritonitis
Gallbladder disease	Pregnancy
Hepatitis (chronic)	Renal insufficiency
Macroamylasemia	Salivary gland disease

Table 9-8. Predisposing factors for pancreatitis

Infection
- Viral
  - Coxsackievirus, echovirus, enterovirus, mumps
- Bacterial
  - Actinomycosis, mycoplasma, *Salmonella typhi*
- Parasites
  - *Ascaris lumbricoides, Clonarchis sinensis*

Mechanical factors
- Pancreatic outflow obstruction
  - Tumor, stenosis, lithiasis
- Previous endoscopic retrograde cholangiopancreatography
- Penetrating duodenal ulcer

Medication/toxic exposure
- Diuretics
  - Ethacrynic acid, furosemide, thiazides
- Immunosuppressives
  - Azathioprine, corticosteroids, L-asparaginase
- Other medications
  - Ethanol, oral contraceptives, tetracyclines, isoniazid

Medical illness
- Biliary tract disease
- Collagen vascular disease
  - Lupus erythematosus, polyarteritis
- Hereditary
  - Cystic fibrosis, familial pancreatitis
- Pregnancy-related
  - Preeclampsia
- Other diseases
  - Hyperlipidemia, hyperparathyroidism, scarlet fever

4. Elevated serum amylase, often greater than 200 units/dl

Elevated serum amylase levels are used for diagnosing pancreatitis [36, 37]. Recent studies have shown that serum lipase elevations parallel those of serum amylase in pancreatitis. Unfortunately, normal values for lipase in pregnancy have not yet been established.

If pancreatitis is suspected, the patient should undergo radiologic evaluation for signs of free air within the peritoneum. Additionally, ultrasound evaluation of the pancreas may reveal calcifications, swelling, or possibly a developing pseudocyst. If pancreatitis is likely, the patient should be carefully followed for signs of worsening disease. Complications such as hypocalcemia, hypovolemia, hypomagnesemia, and hyperglycemia are fairly common. Patients are also at risk of developing renal failure, disseminated intravascular coagulopathy, adult respiratory distress syndrome, hemorrhage, and pseudocyst formation.

B. Management. In pregnancy pancreatitis is treated in much the same manner as among nonpregnant patients. Symptoms usually resolve with conservative management over three to seven days.

Management in pregnancy requires provision of adequate analgesia, careful attention to hydration status, and serial evaluation of certain biochemical parameters. Intravenous rehydration is essential, as most pancreatitis patients are quite dehydrated. Blood chemistries should be followed for evidence of hyperglycemia, hypocalcemia, and hypomagnesemia. Complete bowel rest is recommended until serum amylase (and lipase) levels have begun to normalize and there is evidence of normal bowel function (such as normal bowel sounds, or the passage of flatus or formed stool). Low intermittent nasogastric suction may provide symptomatic relief and facilitate recovery. Parenteral hyperalimentation has been successfully used in severe cases for prolonged nutritional support.

Low-grade fever (temperature $< 100.5°F$) is commonly associated with pancreatitis; however, persistent fevers should be evaluated and appropriate therapy instituted. Secondary infections involving necrotic tissues are common. Prophylactic antibiotics have not proved beneficial in several recent randomized trials involving nonpregnant patients.

Pancreatic pseudocysts and abscesses may form. These usually require either percutaneous or open surgical drainage. If such complications are noted to develop, they should be aggressively managed.

References

ACUTE FATTY LIVER OF PREGNANCY

1. Campillo, B., et al. Ultrasonography in acute fatty liver of pregnancy. *Ann. Intern. Med.* 105:383–384, 1986.
2. Coche, G., et al. Acute fatty liver of pregnancy: Apropos of 4 cases: Contribution of x-ray computed tomography. *J. Radiol.* 68:193, 1987.
3. McKee, C. M., et al. Acute fatty liver and diagnosis by computed tomography. *Br. Med. J.* 292:291–292, 1986.
4. Riley, C. A., et al. Acute fatty liver of pregnancy: A reassessment based on observations in nine patients. *Ann. Intern. Med.* 106:703, 1987.

INTRAHEPATIC CHOLESTASIS OF PREGNANCY

5. Fisk, N. M., Bye, W. B., and Storey, G. N. Maternal features of obstetric cholestasis: 20 years experience at King George V Hospital. *Aust. N.Z. J. Obstet. Gynaecol.* 28(3):172–176, 1988.
6. Frezza, M., et al. Reversal of intrahepatic cholestasis of pregnancy in women after high dose *S*-adenosyl-*L*-methionine administration. *Hepatology* 4(2):274–278, 1984.
7. Gonzalez, M. C., et al. Intrahepatic cholestasis of pregnancy in twin pregnancies. *J. Hepatol.* 9(1):84–90, 1989.
9. Holzbach, R. T., Sivak, D. A., and Braun, W. E. Familial recurrent intrahepatic cholestasis of pregnancy: a genetic study providing evidence for transmission of a sex-limited, dominant trait. *Gastroenterology* 85(1):175–179, 1983.
10. Kirkinen, P., et al. Gallbladder function and maternal bile acids in intrahepatic cholestasis of pregnancy. *Eur. J. Obstet. Gynecol. Reprod. Biol.* 18(1–2):29–34, 1984.
11. Lunzer, M., et al. Serum bile acid concentrations during pregnancy and their relationship to obstetric cholestasis. *Gastroenterology* 91(4):825–829, 1986.
12. Reyes, H., et al. Steatorrhea in patients with intrahepatic cholestasis of pregnancy. *Gastroenterology* 93(3):584–590, 1987.

VIRAL HEPATITIS

13. Bal, V., et al. Virological markers and antibody responses in fulminant viral hepatitis. *J. Med. Virol.* 23(1):75–82, 1987.
14. Beasley, R. P., and Hwang, L. Y. Postnatal infectivity of hepatitis B surface antigen-carrier mothers. *J. Infect. Dis.* 147(2):185–190, 1983.
15. Belabbes, E. H., et al. Epidemic non-A, non-B viral hepatitis in Algeria: strong evidence for its spreading by water. *J. Med. Virol.* 16(3):257–263, 1985.
16. Dienstag, J. L., and Alter, H. J. Non-A, non-B hepatitis: evolving epidemiologic and clinical perspective. *Semin. Liver Dis.* 6(1):67–81, 1986.
17. Esteban, J. I., et al. Immunoprophylaxis of perinatal transmission of the hepatitis B virus: efficacy of hepatitis B immune globulin and hepatitis B vaccine in a low-prevalence area. *J. Med. Virol.* 18(4):381–391, 1986.
18. Greenfield, C., et al. Perinatal transmission of hepatitis B virus in Kenya: its relation to the presence of serum HBV-DNA and anti-HBe in the mother. *J. Med. Virol.* 19:135–142, 1986.
19. Hieber, J. P., et al. Hepatitis and pregnancy. *J. Pediatr.* 91:545–549, 1977.
20. Hla Myint, et al. A clinical and epidemiological study of an epidemic of non-A non-B hepatitis in Rangoon. *Am. J. Trop. Med. Hyg.* 34(6):1183–1189, 1985.
21. Ip, H. M., et al. Prevention of hepatitis B virus carrier state in infants according to maternal serum levels of HBV DNA. *Lancet* 1(8635):406–410, 1989.

22. Kane, M. A., et al. Epidemic non-A, non-B hepatitis in Nepal. Recovery of a possible etiologic agent and transmission studies in marmosets. *J.A.M.A.* 252(22):3140–3145, 1984.
23. Khuroo, M. S., et al. Incidence and severity of viral hepatitis in pregnancy. *Am. J. Med.* 10:252, 1981.
24. Lee, S. D., et al. Prevention of maternal-infant hepatitis B virus transmission by immunization: the role of serum hepatitis B virus DNA. *Hepatology* 6(3):369–373, 1986.
25. Lee, S. D., et al. Role of caesarean section in prevention of mother-infant transmission of hepatitis B virus. *Lancet* 2(8615):833–834, 1988.
26. Ohto, H., et al. Intrauterine transmission of hepatitis B virus is closely related to placental leakage. *J. Med. Virol.* 21(1):1–6, 1987.
27. Palmvic, D. Acute viral hepatitis in pregnancy. Results of a prospective study of 99 pregnant women. *Lijec. Vjesn.* 108:296–300, 1986.
28. Ramalingaswami, V., and Purcell, R. H. Waterborne non-A, non-B hepatitis. *Lancet* 1(8585):571–573, 1988.
29. Shorey, J. The current status of non-A, non-B viral hepatitis. *Am. J. Med. Sci.* 289(6):251–261, 1985.
30. Wejstal R., and Norkrans, G. Chronic non-A, non-B hepatitis in pregnancy: outcome and possible transmission to the offspring. *Scand. J. Infect. Dis.* 21(5):485–490, 1989.

CIRRHOSIS/PORTAL HYPERTENSION

31. Schreyer, P., et al. Cirrhosis, pregnancy, and delivery: A review. *Obstet. Gynecol. Surv.* 37:304–312, 1982.

WILSON'S DISEASE

32. Walshe, J. M. Pregnancy in Wilson's disease. *Q. J. Med.* 46:73, 1977.
33. Walshe, J. M. The management of pregnancy in Wilson's disease treated with trientine. *Q. J. Med.* 58:81–87, 1986.

HEREDITARY HYPERBILIRUBINEMIA

34. Zoglio, J. D. D., and Cardillo, E. The Dubin-Johnson syndrome and pregnancy. *Obstet. Gynecol.* 42:560–563, 1973.

GALLBLADDER DISEASE

35. Hiatt, J. R., et al. Biliary disease in pregnancy: strategy for surgical management. *Am. J. Surg.* 151:263–265, 1986.

PANCREATITIS

36. Lankisch, P. G., et al. Specificity of increased amylase to creatinine clearance ratio in acute pancreatitis. *Digestion* 16:160, 1977.
37. Levitt, M. D., and Johnson, S. G. Is the Cam/Ccr ratio of value for the diagnosis of pancreatitis? *Gastroenterology* 75:118, 1978.

Selected Readings

Creasy, R. K., and Resnik, R. (eds.). *Maternal-Fetal Medicine: Principles and Practice* (2nd ed.). Philadelphia: Saunders, 1989.

DeSwiet, M. (ed). *Medical Disorders in Obstetric Practice* (2nd ed.). Oxford: Blackwell, 1989.

Rustgi, V. K. and Cooper, J. N. (eds.). *Gastrointestinal and Hepatic Complications in Pregnancy*. New York: Wiley, 1986.

LIVER ABNORMALITIES

Douvas, S. G., et al. Liver disease in pregnancy. *Obstet. Gynecol. Surv.* 38(9):531–536, 1983.

Lunzer, M. R. Jaundice in pregnancy. *Baillieres Clin. Gastroenterol.* 3(2):467–483, 1989.

Rolfes, D. B., and Ishak, K. G. Liver disease in pregnancy. *Histopathology* 10(6):555–570, 1986.

Rustgi, V. K. Liver disease in pregnancy. *Med. Clin. North Am.* 73(4):1041–1046, 1989.

Varma, R. R. Course and prognosis of pregnancy in women with liver disease. *Semin. Liver Dis.* 7(1):59–66, 1987.

ACUTE FATTY LIVER OF PREGNANCY

Bernau, J., et al. Non-acute fatty liver of pregnancy. *Gut* 24:340–344, 1983.

Bova, J. G., and Schenker, S. Acute fatty liver of pregnancy. *N. Engl. J. Med.,* 313:1608, 1985.

Burroughs, A. K., et al. Idiopathic acute fatty liver of pregnancy in 12 patients. *Q. J. Med.* 304:481–497, 1982.

Davies, M. H., et al. Acute liver disease with encephalopathy and renal failure in late pregnancy and early puerperium: A study of fourteen patients. *Br. J. Obstet. Gynaecol.* 87:1005–1014, 1980.

Hague, W. M., et al. Acute fatty liver of pregnancy. *J. R. Soc. Med.* 76:652–661, 1983.

Kaplan, M. M. Acute fatty liver of pregnancy. *N. Engl. J. Med.* 313:367–370, 1985.

Pockros, P. J., et al. Idiopathic fatty liver of pregnancy: findings in ten cases. *Medicine* (Baltimore) 63:1–11, 1984.

Varner, M., and Rinderknecht, N. K. Acute fatty metamorphosis of pregnancy. A maternal mortality and literature review. *J. Reprod. Med.* 24:177–180, 1980.

INTRAHEPATIC CHOLESTASIS OF PREGNANCY

Berg, B., et al. Cholestasis of pregnancy. Clinical and laboratory studies. *Acta Obstet. Gynecol. Scand.* 65(2):107–113, 1986.

Chowdhury, J. R., and Chowdhury, N. R. Conjugation and excretion of bilirubin. *Semin. Liver Dis.* 3(1):11–23, 1983.

Cotton, D. B. Infantile hepatic cholestasis with maternal Dubin-Johnson syndrome. *South. Med. J.* 77(9):1213–1214, 1984.

Dacus, J. V., and Muram, D. Pruritus in pregnancy. *South. Med. J.* 80(5):614–617, 1987.

Douvas, S. G., et al. Liver disease in pregnancy. *Obstet. Gynecol. Surv.* 38(9):531–536, 1983.

Fisk, N. M., and Storey, G. N. Fetal outcome in obstetric cholestasis. *Br. J. Obstet. Gynaecol.* 95(11):1137–1143, 1988.

Frezza, M., et al. Alteration in sulfobromphthalein hepatic storage capacity (S) in non-pregnant women previously affected with intrahepatic cholestasis of pregnancy (ICP). *Acta Obstet. Gynecol. Scand.* 65(6):577–580, 1986.

Haave, N. C., and Innis, S. M. Induction of 3-hydroxy-3-methylglutaryl coenzyme A reductase activity in foetal rats by maternal cholestyramine feeding. *J. Dev. Physiol.* 10(3):247–255, 1988.

Heikkinen, J. Effect of a standard test meal on serum bile acid levels in healthy nonpregnant and pregnant women and in patients with intrahepatic cholestasis of pregnancy. *Ann. Clin. Res.* 15(5–6):183–188, 1983.

Heikkinen, J. Serum bile acids in the early diagnosis of intrahepatic cholestasis of pregnancy. *Obstet. Gynecol.* 61(5):581–587, 1983.

Holland, R. L. Recurrent intrahepatic cholestasis of pregnancy. *S. D. J. Med.* 40(4):9–12, 1987.

Innis, S. M. Effect of cholestyramine administration during pregnancy in the rat. *Am. J. Obstet. Gynecol.* 146(1):13–16, 1983.

Innis, S. M. Effect of diet during pregnancy and lactation on the activity of HMG-CoA reductase in the developing rat. *J. Nutr.* 118(10):1177–1183, 1988.

Israel, E. J., Guzman, M. L., and Campos, G. A. Maximal response to oxytocin of the isolated myometrium from pregnant patients with intrahepatic cholestasis. *Acta Obstet. Gynecol. Scand.* 65(6):581–582, 1986.

Jiang, Z. H., et al. Intrahepatic cholestasis of pregnancy and its complications. Analysis of 100 cases in Chongqing area. *Chin. Med. J.* [Engl.] 99(12):957–960, 1986.

Kane, J. P., and Havel, R. J. Treatment of hypercholesterolemia. *Ann. Rev. Med.* 37:427–435, 1986.

Kauppila, A., et al. Low serum selenium concentration and glutathione peroxidase activity in intrahepatic cholestasis of pregnancy. *Br. Med. J.* [Clin Res] 294(6565):150–152, 1987.

Kreek, M. J. Female sex steroids and cholestasis. *Semin. Liver Dis.* 7(1):8–23, 1987.

Krejs, G. J. Jaundice during pregnancy. *Semin. Liver Dis.* 3(1):73–82, 1983.

Kuoppala, T., et al. Vitamin D and mineral metabolism in intrahepatic cholestasis of pregnancy. *Eur. J. Obstet. Gynecol. Reprod. Biol.* 23(1–2):45–51, 1986.

Laatikainen, T., and Tulenheimo, A. Maternal serum bile acid levels and fetal distress in cholestasis of pregnancy. *Int. J. Gynaecol. Obstet.* 22(2):91–94, 1984.

Landon, M. B., et al. Primary sclerosing cholangitis and pregnancy. *Obstet. Gynecol.* 69(3 Pt. 2):457–460, 1987.

Levitz, M., Kadner, S., and Young, B. K. Intermediary metabolism of estriol in pregnancy. *J. Steroid Biochem.* 20(4B):971–974, 1984.

Lunzer, M. R. Jaundice in pregnancy. *Baillieres Clin. Gastroenterol.* 3(2):467–483, 1989.

Noguera, X., Puig, L., and de Moragas, J. M. Prurigo gravidarum. *Cutis* 39(5):437–440, 1987.

Penzias, A. S., and Treisman, O. Vitamin K-dependent clotting factor deficiency in pregnancy. *Obstet. Gynecol.* 72(3 Pt. 2):452–454, 1988.

Qiu, Z. D., et al. Intrahepatic cholestasis of pregnancy. Clinical analysis and follow-up study of 22 cases. *Chin. Med. J.* [Engl.] 96(12):902–906, 1983.

Riely, C. A. Case studies in jaundice of pregnancy. *Semin. Liver Dis.* 8(2):191–199, 1988.

Rolfes, D. B., and Ishak, K. G. Liver disease in pregnancy. *Histopathology* 10(6):555–570, 1986.

Simon, J. A. Biliary tract disease and related surgical disorders during pregnancy. *Clin. Obstet. Gynecol.* 26(4):810–821, 1983.

Vore, M. Estrogen cholestasis. Membranes, metabolites, or receptors? *Gastroenterology* 93(3):643–649, 1987.

Wilson, J. A. Intrahepatic cholestasis of pregnancy with marked elevation of transaminases in a black American. *Dig. Dis. Sci.* 32(6):665–668, 1987.

Yip, D. M., and Baker, A. L. Liver diseases in pregnancy. *Clin. Perinatol.* 12(3):683–694, 1985.

VIRAL HEPATITIS

Beasley, R. P., et al. Prevention of perinatally transmitted hepatitis B virus infections with hepatitis B immune globulin and hepatitis B vaccine. *Lancet* 2(8359):1099–1102, 1983.

Boxall, E. H., and Tarlow, M. J. Hepatitis B vaccine in the prevention of perinatally transmitted hepatitis B infections: initial report of a study in the West Midlands of England. *J. Med. Virol.* 18:255–260, 1986.

Caredda, F., et al. Clinical features of sporadic non-A, non-B hepatitis possibly associated with faecal-oral spread (letter). *Lancet* 2(8452):444–445, 1985.

Heijtinkra, R. A., et al. Hepatitis B virus DNA in serum of pregnant women with HBsAg and HBeAg or antibodies to Hbe (letter). *J. Infect. Dis.* 150:462, 1984.

Levin, S., et al. Interferon treatment in acute progressive and fulminant hepatitis. *Isr. J. Med. Sci.* 25(7):364–372, 1989.

Lo, K. J., et al. Long-term immunogenicity and efficacy of hepatitis B vaccine in infants born to HBeAg-positive HBsAg-carrier mothers. *Hepatology* 8(6):1647–1650, 1988.

Mohite, B. J., et al. Mechanisms of liver cell damage in acute hepatitis B. *J. Med. Virol.* 22(3):199–210, 1987.

Morbidity and Mortality Weekly Report (M.M.W.R.). Enterically transmitted non-A, non-B hepatitis—Mexico. *M.M.W.R.* 36(36):597–602, 1987.

Morbidity and Mortality Weekly Report leads from M.M.W.R.: Recommendations against viral hepatitis. *J.A.M.A.* 254:197–198, 1985.

Morbidity and Mortality Weekly Report (M.M.W.R.). Recommendations for protection against viral hepatitis. *M.M.W.R.* 34:3313–3324, 1985.

Nouasria, B., et al. Fulminant viral hepatitis and pregnancy in Algeria and France. *Ann. Trop. Med. Parasitol.* 80(6):623–629, 1986.

Pongpipat, D., Suvatte, V., and Assateerawatts, A. Efficacy of hepatitis-B immunoglobulin and hepatitis-B vaccine in prevention of the HBsAg carrier state in newborn infants of mothers who are chronic carriers of HBsAg and HBeAg. *Asian Pac. J. Allergy Immunol.* 4(1):33–36, 1986.

Pongipat, D., Suvatte, V., and Assateerawatts, A. Vaccination against hepatitis B virus infection in neonates. *Helv. Paediatr. Acta* 39(3):231–236, 1984.

Shen, H. D., et al. Hepatitis B virus infection of cord blood leukocytes. *J. Med. Virol.* 22(3):211–216, 1987.

Snydman, D. R. Hepatitis in pregnancy. *N. Engl. J. Med.* 313(22):1398–1401, 1985.

HERPESVIRUSES

Balfour, C. L., and Balfour, H. H. Cytomegalovirus is not an occupational risk for nurses in renal transplantation and neonatal units. *J.A.M.A.* 256:1909, 1986.

Best, J. M. Congenital cytomegalovirus infection. *Br. Med. J.* 294:1440–1441, 1987.

Chandler, S. H., Alexander, E. R., and Holmes, H. R. Epidemiology of cytomegalovirus infection in a heterogenous population of pregnant women. *J. Infect. Dis.* 152:249, 1985.

Hanshaw, J. B. Congenital cytomegalovirus infection: A 15 year prospective study. *J. Infect. Dis.* 123:555, 1971.

Stagno, S., and Whitley, R. J. Herpesvirus infections of pregnancy. Part 1: Cytomegalovirus and Epstein-Barr virus infection. *N. Engl. J. Med.* 313:1270, 1985.

Stern, J., and Tucker, S. M. Prospective study of cytomegalovirus infection in pregnancy. *Br. Med. J.* 2:268, 1973.

CIRRHOSIS/PORTAL HYPERTENSION

Benhamou, J. P., and LeBrec, D. Non-cirrhotic intrahepatic portal hypertension in adults. *Clin. Gastroenterol.* 14:21–31, 1985.

Brown, S. E., et al. Pregnancy and esophageal varices. *Am. J. Surg.* 4:421–425, 1982.

Cheng, Y. S. Pregnancy in liver cirrhosis and/or portal hypertension. *Am. J. Obstet. Gynecol.* 128:812–822, 1977.

Huchzermeyer, H. Pregnancy in patients with liver cirrhosis and chronic hepatitis. *Acta Hepatosplenol.* (Stuttg) 18:294, 1971.

Varma, R. R., et al. Pregnancy in cirrhotic and non-cirrhotic portal hypertension. *Obstet. Gynecol.* 50:217–222, 1976.

Vujic, I., et al. Embolic management of rare hemorrhagic gynecologic and obstetric conditions. *Cardiovasc. Intervent. Radiol.* 9:69–74, 1986.

WILSON'S DISEASE

Danks, D. M. Hereditary Disorders of Copper Metabolism in Wilson's Disease and Menke's Disease. In J. B. Stanbury et al. (eds.), *The Metabolic Basis of Inherited Disease* (5th ed.). New York: McGraw-Hill, 1982. Pp. 1251–1266.

Lyle, W. H. Penicillamine in pregnancy. *Lancet* 1:606, 1978.

Morimoto, I., et al. Pregnancy and penicillamine treatment in a patient with Wilson's disease. *Jap. J. Med.* 25:59–62, 1986.

Scheinberg, I. H., and Sternlieb, I. Pregnancy in penicillamine treated patients with Wilson's disease. *N. Engl. J. Med.* 293:1300, 1975.

HEPATIC VEIN THROMBOSIS

Asherson, R. A., et al. Budd-Chiari syndrome, visceral arterial occlusions, recurrent fetal loss and the "lupus anticoagulant": in systemic lupus erythematosus. *J. Rheumatol.* 16(2):219–224, 1989.

Khuroo, M. S., and Datta, D. V. Budd-Chiari syndrome following pregnancy. Report of 16 cases with roentgenologic, hemodynamic, and histologic studies of the hepatic outflow tract. *Am. J. Med.* 68:113–121, 1980.

Krol-Van Straaten, J., and De Maat, C. E. Successful pregnancies in cirrhosis of the liver before and after portacaval anastomosis. *Neth. J. Med.* 27(1):14–15, 1984.

Krumbiegel, P., et al. Nuclear medicine liver function tests for pregnant women and children: 1. Breath tests with 14C-methacetin and 13C-methacetin. *Eur. J. Nucl. Med.* 10(3–4):129–133, 1985.

Lee, M. G., et al. Pregnancy in chronic active hepatitis with cirrhosis. *J. Trop. Med. Hyg.* 90(5):245–248, 1987.

Lewis, J. H., and Weingold, A. B. The use of gastrointestinal drugs during pregnancy and lactation. *Am. J. Gastroenterol.* 80:912–923, 1985.

Schalm, S. W., and van Buuren, H. R. Prevention of recurrent variceal bleeding: non-surgical procedures. *Clin. Gastroenterol.* 14(1):209–232, 1985.

Vons, C., et al. Successful pregnancy after Budd-Chiari syndrome (letter). *Lancet* ii:975, 1984.

Yip, D., and Baker, A. L. Liver diseases in pregnancy. *Clin. Perinatol.* 12(3):683–694, 1985.

HEREDITARY HYPERBILIRUBINEMIA

Arias, I. M. Inheritable and congenital hyperbilirubinemia. *N. Engl. J. Med.* 285:1416–1421, 1971.

Cohen, L., et al. Pregnancy, oral contraceptives, and chronic familial jaundice with predominantly conjugated hyperbilirubinemia (Dubin-Johnson syndrome). *Gastroenterology* 62:1182–1190, 1972.

Seligsohn, U., and Shani, M. The Dubin-Johnson syndrome and pregnancy. *Acta Hepatogastroenterol.* 27:167–169, 1977.

GALLBLADDER DISEASE

Chesson, R. R., and Gallup, D. G. Ultrasonographic diagnosis of asymptomatic cholelithiasis in pregnancy. *J. Reprod. Med.* 30:920–922, 1985.

Hill, L. M., et al. Cholecystectomy in pregnancy. *Obstet. Gynecol.* 9:291–293, 1975.

Palmer, A. K., and Heywood, R. Pathological changes in the rhesus fetus associated with oral administration of chenodeoxycholic acid. *Toxicology* 2:239–246, 1974.

Stauffer, R. A., et al. Gallbladder disease in pregnancy. *Am. J. Obstet. Gynecol.* 144:661–664, 1982.

Woodhouse, D. R., and Haylen, B. Gallbladder disease complicating pregnancy. *Aust. N. Z. J. Obstet. Gynecol.* 25:233–237, 1985.

PANCREATITIS

Bartelink, A. K., et al. Maternal survival after acute haemorrhagic pancreatitis complicating late pregnancy. *Eur. J. Obstet. Gynecol. Reprod. Biol.* 29(1):41–50, 1988.

Block, P., and Kelly, T. R. Management of gallstone pancreatitis during pregnancy and the postpartum period. *Surg. Gynecol. Obstet.* 168(5):426–428, 1989.

Corlett, R. C., and Mishell, D. R. Pancreatitis in pregnancy. *Am. J. Obstet. Gynecol.* 113:281–290, 1972.

De Chalain, T. M., Michell, W. L., and Berger, G. M. Hyperlipidemia, pregnancy and pancreatitis. *Surg. Gynecol. Obstet.* 167(6):469–473, 1988.

DeVore, G. R., et al. The amylase/creatinine ratio in normal pregnancies and pregnancies complicated by pancreatitis, hyperemesis gravidarum, and toxemia. *Am. J. Obstet. Gynecol.* 136:747–754, 1980.

Fitzgerald, O. Pancreatitis following pregnancy. *Br. Med. J.* 1:349, 1955.

Gineston, J. L., et al. Prolonged total parenteral nutrition in a pregnant woman with acute pancreatitis. *J. Clin. Gastroenterol.* 6(3):249–252, 1984.

Jouppila, P., et al. Acute pancreatitis in pregnancy. *Surg. Gyn. Obstet.* 139:879–882, 1974.

Kaiser, R., et al. Serum amylase changes in pregnancy. *Am. J. Obstet. Gynecol.* 122:283–286, 1975.

Kitzmiller, J. L., et al. Pancreatic alpha cell response to alanine during and after normal and diabetic pregnancies. *Obstet. Gynecol.* 56:440–445, 1980.

Klein, K. B. Pancreatitis in Pregnancy. In V. K. Rustgi and J. N. Cooper (eds.), *Gastrointestinal and Hepatic Complications in Pregnancy.* New York: Wiley, 1986. Pp. 138–166.

Langmade, C. F., and Edmondson, H. A. Acute pancreatitis during pregnancy and the post-partum period: report of 9 cases. *Surg. Gyn. Obstet.* 92:43–52, 1984.

Levine, R. I., Glauser, F. L., and Berk, J. E. Enhancement of the amylase-creatinine clearance ratio in disorders other than acute pancreatitis. *N. Engl. J. Med.* 292:329, 1975.

Rajala, B., et al. Acute pancreatitis and primary hyperparathyroidism in pregnancy: treatment of hypercalcemia with magnesium sulfate. *Obstet. Gynecol.* 70(3 Pt. 2):460–462, 1987.

Rivera-Alsina, M. E., Saldana, L. R., and Stringer, C. A. Fetal growth sustained by parenteral nutrition in pregnancy. *Obstet. Gynecol.* 64(1):138–141, 1984.

Stowell, J. C., Bottsford, J. E., Jr., and Rubel, H. R. Pancreatitis with pseudocyst and cholelithiasis in third trimester of pregnancy: management with total parenteral nutrition. *South. Med. J.* 77(4):502–504, 1984.

Wilinson, E. J. Acute pancreatitis in pregnancy: a review of 98 cases and a report of 8 new cases. *Obstet. Gynecol. Surv.* 28:281–303, 1973.

Williamson, S. L., and Williamson, M. R. Cholecystosonography in pregnancy. *J. Ultrasound Med.* 3:329–331, 1984.

Yamauchi, H., et al. Hyperlipidemia and pregnancy associated pancreatitis with reference to plasma exchange as a therapeutic intervention. *Tohoku J. Exp. Med.* 148(2):197–205, 1986.

10 Endocrine Disorders

Arthur T. Evans and
Mahmoud M. Benbarka

I. Diabetes mellitus. Diabetes mellitus is a metabolic disorder characterized by hyperglycemia resulting from either a relative deficiency of pancreatic insulin production, limited insulin release in response to carbohydrate challenge, or impaired effect of insulin at the cellular level. An exaggerated tendency exists toward hyperglycemia, increased fat and protein catabolism, and ultimately the risk of ketosis progressing to ketoacidosis. In the United States, 6.6% of all individuals ages 20–74 and 0.5% of pregnant women have diagnosed or undiagnosed overt diabetes [5]. Its etiology is multifactorial, with a contributory genetic component in adult-onset diabetes and a probable infectious viral component in childhood or juvenile-onset diabetes.

A. Physiology. Carbohydrate metabolism is significantly altered during pregnancy. There is a shift to hyperinsulinemia, lower fasting or premeal glucose values, progressive insulin resistance, and exaggerated ketone response to caloric restriction [6]. The two central, counteracting components of this metabolic change are the fetal-placental unit and the placental hormones. In order to ensure availability of adequate glucose to the fetus, **placental hormones** (primarily human placental lactogen, estrogen, and progesterone) act as hyperglycemic agents, interfering with insulin efficacy. Normal pregnancy fasting glucose values are 60–80 dl, and the upper limits of normal for one-hour postprandial values are 120–140 dl [2]. It is important to adjust the goals of diabetes management during pregnancy to these values rather than to those of the nonpregnant state.

1. Both the fetus and the placenta depend on **maternal glucose** as their primary energy source. Glucose is continually transported across the placenta from mother to fetus by facilitated diffusion, whereas insulin does not cross the placenta in either direction [23]. Fetal glucose levels are approximately 10–20 dl lower than maternal levels [3]. By 10–12 weeks' gestation, the fetal pancreas is able to produce and secrete insulin and glucagon [19]. Maternal hyperglycemia leads to fetal hyperglycemia and subsequent stimulation of the fetal pancreatic beta-cells to produce excess amounts of insulin. Fetal hyperglycemia and hyperinsulinemia appear to be directly related to, and perhaps causative for, most of the fetal and neonatal complications of infants of diabetic mothers. Thus the satisfactory outcome of diabetic pregnancies appears to be closely related to the degree of maternal and fetal euglycemia achieved before conception and throughout the pregnancy.

2. **The impact of pregnancy** on insulin requirements and blood glucose levels is biphasic. The first half of pregnancy is characterized by insulin sensitivity. This results in a 50% reduction from prepregnancy insulin requirements and is clinically expressed as an improvement in glucose control or insulin sensitivity [21]. The latter half of pregnancy is typified by a relative insulin resistance with an exaggerated diabetogenic effect of the placental hormones and a consequent rise in the insulin requirement to 50% above prepregnancy levels. This is clinically expressed as a continually increasing insulin dose requirement during late pregnancy.

   The biphasic effect of pregnancy on glucose metabolism explains why gestationally induced diabetes is usually not clinically apparent or detectable until 24–30 weeks' gestation. Only then is the degree of insulin resistance sufficient to interfere with normal carbohydrate metabolism in a way that can be detected by current biochemical testing.

B. Pathology. Pregnancy and diabetes present risks to each other, but seldom is pregnancy contraindicated solely because a woman has diabetes.

1. **Maternal.** With current diabetes management capabilities, avoidance of pregnancy is generally recommended for only two groups of women: those with coronary artery insufficiency (due to a maternal mortality rate of 50%) or other severe vascular disease from their diabetes; and those with extremely brittle diabetes due to the risk of unpredictable and severe insulin reactions, which can be life-threatening. Many of these women are able to be managed satisfactorily now with insulin pump therapy.

   A long-standing concern has been that pregnancy accelerates the progression of diabetes and its complications, such as retinopathy, nephropathy, and neuropathy. Current information suggests that this risk is directly related to the duration of diabetes. its severity, and the degree of metabolic control. With aggressive management of diabetes, it now appears that these risks, although increased, are acceptable and possibly not any greater than would occur over the same 9–12-month period [7, 8, 12, 16].

   Diabetic pregnancies are more at risk for maternal obstetric complications. Accelerated chronic hypertension, pregnancy-induced hypertension, and urinary tract infections are the most frequently encountered complications.

2. **Fetal.** The fetus is particularly at risk with a diabetic pregnancy. The degree of maternal glycemic control is the key factor in determining **fetal risks,** which include abortion, congenital anomalies, polyhydramnios, intrauterine fetal death, and growth abnormalities.

   Poor maternal glucose control during early pregnancy is associated with increased spontaneous abortion and congenital anomalies [11]. Tight control of maternal glucose levels and achievement of normal glycosylated hemoglobin values may virtually eliminate the risk of spontaneous abortion.

   Congenital anomalies continue to be the single greatest problem in diabetic pregnancies. They are the major cause of perinatal mortality for the infant of the diabetic mother. No anomaly is pathognomonic for diabetes; however, the organ systems most commonly involved are the neural tube (central nervous system), heart, skeletal, and gastrointestinal and urinary tracts [10]. The etiology of these anomalies appears to be hyperglycemia-induced hypoxic injury to the yolk sac during the initial four to six weeks of gestation [18]. It remains to be demonstrated whether tight preconception and early pregnancy glucose control with normalization of glycosylated hemoglobin values will eliminate or substantially reduce this risk.

   In the third trimester, diabetes places the fetus at risk for intrauterine death and abnormalities of growth. The **intrauterine death** risk is directly related to hyperglycemia and probable fetal hypoxia and acidosis. Historically, this risk was so significant that diabetic pregnancies were delivered prior to term to protect the fetus. Antepartum fetal surveillance by heart rate testing or ultrasound is now used in the third trimester of diabetic pregnancies to predict fetal well-being and to allow continuation to term. In combination with improved maternal glucose control capabilities, the risks of intrauterine fetal death have been reduced significantly although not eliminated.

   Abnormalities of fetal growth may be either macrosomia (excessive size) or growth retardation. Fetal **macrosomia** that occurs with diabetes is secondary to hyperglycemia although the exact mechanism is unclear. Subcutaneous fat and the size of the liver increase, whereas the head and brain remain normal size. The disproportion of the fetal head and the body can result in dystocia at birth with the body trapped in the birth canal. Fetal injury or even death can occur. **Growth retardation** is less frequent, occurring in conjunction with placental insufficiency resulting from maternal diabetic vascular disease.

   Controversy remains concerning the effects of diabetes on **fetal lung maturation.** It appears that when maternal glucose control is adequate, the fetal lung matures at the usual pace. Instances of delayed fetal pulmonary maturity with diabetes are typically observed when maternal hyperglycemia has been the rule rather than the exception.

C. Classification. The pregnant diabetic may be categorized by either the **White classification** [22], which is used only during pregnancy, or the **National Diabetes Data Group** (NDDG) nomenclature [13], which is applicable regardless of pregnancy status.

1. White classification

A_1. Gestational diabetes not requiring insulin
A_2. Gestational diabetes requiring insulin
B. Onset > 20 years old or duration < 10 years
C. Onset at 10–20 years old or duration 10–20 years
D. Onset < 10 years old or duration > 20 years
F. Nephropathy
R. Proliferative retinopathy or vitreous hemorrhage
H. Atherosclerotic heart disease clinically evident
T. Renal transplant

2. National Diabetes Data Group classification

Type 1. Insulin dependent (when not pregnant)
Type 2. Noninsulin dependent (when not pregnant). Note that these patients may experience increased insulin resistance during pregnancy and require insulin.
Type 3. Gestational diabetes
Type 4. Impaired glucose tolerance

D. Diagnosis

1. Overt diabetes. It is common for women with preexisting but undetected diabetes to be initially diagnosed during pregnancy. Symptoms include polydipsia, polyuria, weight loss, blurred vision, and lethargy. Glycosuria is common but not diagnostic or necessary for the diagnosis. Any woman suspected of having overt diabetes when she begins prenatal care should be tested to establish the diagnosis. A fasting blood glucose of greater than 110 dl prior to 20 weeks' gestation is virtually diagnostic for diabetes. Confirmation is made by a 50-gm glucola test demonstrating a one-hour postglucola value of greater than 200 dl. Performance of a 100-gm three-hour oral glucose tolerance test is only indicated when the 50-gm glucola value is greater than 140 mg/dl and less than 200 dl. The glycosylated hemoglobin will also be elevated in overtly diabetic patients but is not by itself diagnostic.

2. Gestational diabetes

a. Screening. All pregnant women should be screened for diabetes [4, 17]. Between 1 and 5% of all pregnancies will have gestationally induced diabetes. Historical risk factors include a previous pregnancy with diabetes, family history of diabetes, previous macrosomic infant, previous unexplained stillbirth, polyhydramnios, obesity, and advanced maternal age. Unfortunately, historical risk factors can only identify 50% of all gestational diabetics, and glycosuria does not reflect blood glucose levels accurately enough to be used for screening [15].

Universal glucola testing is the only approach that will detect virtually all gestational diabetes. The Second Workshop Conference on Gestational Diabetes, sponsored by the American Diabetes Association in 1984, recommended screening all pregnant women at 24–28 weeks' gestation who had not been previously identified as having glucose intolerance [20]. Those with risk factors other than pregnancy alone should be screened with the first prenatal visit to exclude overt or more severe, early-onset pregnancy carbohydrate intolerance. If normal, they should be rescreened again at 24–28 weeks' gestation. The standard (and most convenient method) of screening is with 50 gm of glucola followed by a single glucose determination one hour after the glucola. Patients may be ambulatory and nonfasting. Glucose determinations are performed on venous blood since the standardized values do not apply to capillary blood samples such as those from finger sticks. The upper limit of normal for 50-gm glucola screening is usually selected as either 135 or 140 dl. The latter value is used at the University of California, Davis (UCD). Values above this are considered abnormal and require further evaluation with a three-hour 100-gm oral glucose tolerance test (OGTT). The probability of any single screening value resulting in an abnormal OGTT (and the diagnosis of gestational diabetes) is as follows [1]:

Plasma glucose	Positive OGTT (%)
135–144	15
145–154	17
155–164	29
165–174	20
175–184	50
>185	95

Values greater than 200 dl are themselves diagnostic of gestational diabetes and do not require further confirmation of abnormality except evaluation for elevation of the fasting glucose.

b. Diagnosis. The 100-gm glucose, three-hour OGTT is the standard diagnostic test for diabetes during pregnancy. Elevation of two of the three hourly postglucose load values is required for the definition of diabetes. The fasting value need not be elevated for the diagnosis but when present indicates the need for insulin treatment. The most frequently used criteria for the OGTT are the following [1, 13, 14]:

Fasting	1 hour	2 hour	3 hour
> 105	> 190	> 165	> 145 NDDG (plasma)
> 95	> 180	> 155	> 140 Carpenter (plasma)
> 90	> 165	> 145	> 125 O'Sullivan (whole blood)

No universal agreement exists as to which set of cutoff values is most appropriate. The NDDG values are used at the University of California, Davis. Patients with significant risk factors such as previous pregnancies with gestational diabetes or macrosomic infants, who screen or test negative initially, should have screening evaluations repeatedly monthly until 36 weeks' gestation. Pregnant women with only a single abnormal screening value may still be at risk for perinatal complications, particularly fetal macrosomia. They are, therefore, often given dietary counseling and followed with weekly pre- and postprandial glucose values [9].

E. Antepartum management

1. Activity. Physical activity is a major determinant of the glucose level and insulin requirement. Significant changes in daily levels of physical activity can adversely effect glucose control. Therefore, a regular, repeatable level of daily activity and exercise should be maintained. If dramatic fluctuations occur, then appropriate alterations should be made in diet or insulin, or both. Patients with unusual work schedules should be encouraged to change to a more normal schedule, or their insulin program should be customized to their schedule. During hospitalization, daily activity levels should be maintained if at all possible.

2. Diet. Total caloric intake is calculated from 30–35 calories/kg/day. This results in 1800–2400 calories/day distributed as four to six meals/day including snacks. Calories are distributed as carbohydrates 200 gm/day and protein 90 gm/day. Salt intake is not restricted and diuretics are not used except for specific medical therapy.

3. Gestational diabetes

a. Class A_1. Dietary control is the primary management. Efficacy of treatment is initially monitored with daily fasting and one-hour postprandial glucose values performed after each meal by home glucose monitoring. If a normal, predictable pattern is achieved, monitoring can be decreased to every two to seven days with fasting and one-hour postprandial glucose values. When monitoring by reflectance colorimeter is not available, glucose strips are collected by the patient with the date and time recorded. These are read by meter at the next office visit. Patients who, despite diet management, develop persistently elevated values or those with borderline elevations in fasting values or unusually high postprandial values (> 140 dl) require insulin treatment.

b. Class A_2. These patients require insulin treatment for persistent fasting or preprandial values greater than 100 dl or one-hour postprandials greater than 140 dl. The goal is to achieve normalization of glucose values. Management is the same as for women with overt or prepregnancy diabetes.

c. Postpartum evaluation. Pre- and postprandial values are monitored after delivery to determine that carbohydrate intolerance does not persist. Once values are known to be normal, no further treatment is necessary. At six to eight weeks post partum, **a two-hour, 75-gm glucola GTT** is performed to fully exclude persistent carbohydrate intolerance [20]. The normal values are

fasting	< 140 dl
1 hour	< 200 dl
2 hours	< 140 dl

Patients with abnormal results should be referred for diabetes management and receive prepregnancy diabetic counseling.

4. Insulin-dependent diabetes

a. Maternal tests

(1) Initial evaluation includes routine prenatal blood tests plus electrolytes, creatinine, blood urea nitrogen, liver functions, uric acid, glycosylated hemoglobin, electrocardiogram, ophthalmology exam, urinalysis, urine culture, and 24-hour urine collection for total protein and creatinine clearance.

(2) Subsequent tests are maternal serum alphafetoprotein (MSAFP) at 15–20 weeks, serial glycosylated hemoglobin values, and repeat ophthalmology exam in the third trimester.

(3) Common complications

(a) Recognition of chronic hypertension
(b) Pregnancy-induced hypertension
(c) Discovery of nephropathy
(d) Aberrations in fetal growth
  (i) Macrosomia (class A–D)
  (ii) Intrauterine growth retardation (class D–T)
(e) Polyhydramnios
(f) Fetal distress

b. Fetal evaluation. The two important areas of fetal evaluation are growth/development and documentation of fetal well-being during the third trimester.

(1) Growth and development. Ultrasound measurements of fetal size are obtained as early as possible to confirm the gestational age and estimated date. It is repeated:

(a) 15–20 weeks' gestation age to evaluate fetal anatomy in conjunction with MSAFP screening
(b) 28–32 weeks' gestational age to evaluate serial growth, early evidence of macrosomia, growth retardation, abnormal anatomy or development, amniotic fluid volume (AFV)
(c) Prior to delivery to evaluate for fetal macrosomia

More frequent ultrasounds are required for the usual obstetric indications.

(2) Fetal well-being. The purpose is to test for uteroplacental insufficiency and fetal compromise. The available techniques are antepartum fetal heart rate testing (AFHRT) and biophysical scoring (BPS). Testing by either technique starts at 32–34 weeks' gestational age and continues until delivery. Exceptions to this are uncomplicated class A diabetes prior to 40 weeks; vascular complication diabetes (class F–T) where testing starts at 28–30 weeks; diabetes with superimposed complications (pregnancy-induced hypertension, intrauterine growth retardation, diabetic ketoacidosis [DKA], chronic hypertension, and brittle or poor glucose control) where testing starts as soon as 26 weeks or thereafter when the complication occurs.

(a) The primary testing technique is AFHRT. Each type of test—contraction stress test (CST) and nonstress test (NST)—is interpreted and managed in the standard fashion. Fetal testing is performed more frequently than in other high-risk pregnancies due to the inherent instability of maternal diabetic control. The following testing schemes are acceptable:

(i) The CST and NST alternating every three to four days (a Mon/Thurs or Tues/Fri schedule is used at UCD)

(ii) The CST and BPS alternating every three to four days as in previous example

(iii) The NST alone every two to three days

(b). The BPS is a secondary, supporting, or backup technique. It may be interchanged with the NST, used to evaluate AFV, or used to evaluate situations that are equivocal by AFHRT. In the unusual situation where it is used alone as the primary testing technique, it is repeated every one to three days depending on the stability of the clinical situation.

F. Insulin management. Attaining predictable control of maternal (and fetal) glucose levels depends on the interaction of three variables: insulin, diet, and physical activity. Changes in any of these variables will alter the level of glucose control. The daily insulin dose and schedule are important because they represent the most measurable and hence controllable variables in the equation.

1. **Goals.** Euglycemia of both pre- and postprandial glucose levels is desired. This means **all** fasting and premeal glucoses between 50 and 80 dl; one-hour postprandial glucoses less than 140 dl and preferably less than 120 dl with excellent control. Glucose levels down into the 40-dl range are usually well tolerated and safe in **well-controlled** diabetic pregnancies. Occasional mild insulin reactions are not harmful but should be avoided during the hours of sleep. This level of control may not be achievable in particularly brittle diabetics or during the first trimester. It is important to avoid the combination of hyperglycemia and acidosis for fetal well-being. **The overall goal of the program is to teach the diabetic patient to continuously manage her own diabetes throughout the day, in response to the glucose levels she measures.**
2. **Glucose monitoring.** Home glucose monitoring with a reflectance meter is the accepted standard of care. Fasting and preprandial glucose values are measured 4 times a day (30–45 minutes before each meal and the hs snack) every day during the pregnancy until delivery. The advantage of preprandial glucose monitoring is that it allows for immediate adjustment of the planned insulin program by adding additional regular insulin to compensate for any hyperglycemia already present prior to meals. One-hour postprandial values are measured as needed to ensure that the correlations between the preprandial glucose troughs and postprandial peaks remain predictable.

   Collection of paired pre- and postprandial values is often necessary when starting insulin therapy or during times of poor glucose control. This allows for evaluation of both insulin and dietary contributions to diabetic control. All values are recorded in a daily log along with the insulin dose and information on other variable factors (e.g., diet, exercise, illness). Ketones are monitored anywhere from daily to weekly with the first morning-voided urine to assess adequacy of caloric intake. **Urine glucose levels are not monitored.**
3. **Insulin adjustment.** A daily planned insulin dose is established to meet the guidelines of control already established. The dose is generally a combination of intermediate (NPH or lente) and short-acting (regular) insulins given in a

split-dosage schedule. Individualization of scheduling is needed to produce the desired results. The standard regimen during pregnancy is NPH and regular insulin given bid prebreakfast and presupper. The patient who experiences nocturnal hypoglycemia may be improved by changing the time of the presupper NPH dose to 30 minutes prior to the bedtime snack.

4. **Supplemental regular insulin scale.** Each time the fasting or preprandial glucose is measured, the patient refers to the supplemental regular insulin scale to determine if additional regular insulin is needed. This is done whether or not she is to receive a planned insulin dose at the time. **Prior to the hs snack or between 10 P.M.–6 A.M. only one-half the indicated supplemental regular insulin dose is used.** Alterations of the dose scale may be necessary for individual insulin sensitivity, particularly with extremely brittle diabetes.

Preprandial capillary glucose (mg/dl)	Additional units of regular insulin
< 100	0
100–140	2
140–160	3
160–180	4
180–200	5
200–250	6
250–300	8
> 300	10

When a pattern for additional regular insulin supplementation is identified over two to three days, that amount of insulin can then be added to the planned daily dose (e.g., 1 unit additional regular insulin at lunch is converted to 1 unit additional regular insulin at A.M. dose; 1 unit additional regular insulin prior to supper is converted to 1 unit additional NPH with the A.M. dose). This allows for a continuous, measurable increase in the insulin dose throughout pregnancy on an individual basis. Each patient may change the supplemental regular insulin scale as they gain experience with it.

5. **Special considerations**
   a. **Illness.** Whenever a diabetic patient is nauseated or unable to eat due to illness, the scheduled insulin dose is discontinued until the diet can be resumed. The patient remains NPO or on clear liquids only. Glucose levels are measured at the usual times or more frequently if necessary. Regular insulin is used in response to the glucose values as indicated by the supplemental regular insulin scale.
   b. **Somogyi effect** is a hypoglycemic episode in the early morning (12–6 A.M. with rebound hyperglycemia resulting in an elevated prebreakfast glucose value. This is verified with measurement of 2–4 A.M. glucoses if necessary and treated by either reduction in the evening NPH dose, an increase in hs snack calories, or a change in timing of the P.M. NPH dose.
   c. **Dawn phenomenon** is isolated early morning (4–7 A.M.) hyperglycemia not preceded by a Somogyi episode or preexisting hyperglycemia. This is due to exaggerated growth hormone or corticosteroid effect in conjunction with the morning waking process, resulting in prebreakfast hyperglycemia. Treatment involves cautious use of early A.M. (3–6 A.M.) regular insulin, properly timed to blunt the rapid rise in glucose prior to breakfast. Late evening NPH may also be helpful in these circumstances.
   d. **Humulin insulin,** available in all forms, is a purified, genetically engineered model of human insulin that has far less insulin antibody stimulation. All patients should be changed to it, but due to its greater potency, the dose may need to be reduced by one-third from beef/pork insulin doses.
   e. **Insulin pump.** Patients who cannot be adequately controlled by standard insulin regimens should be referred to a perinatal center for consideration of insulin pump therapy.
   f. **Injection site.** The site of insulin injection can affect absorption and bio-

availability. For example, exercise will accelerate absorption from extremity injection sites.

g. **Insulin schedules.** Individualized, multiple-dosage schedules, including all regular insulin programs, are sometimes necessary to produce euglycemia.

h. **Preterm labor.** Magnesium sulfate is the preferred tocolytic agent with diabetes. The use of beta-sympathomimetics should be approached with extreme caution due to the attendant risk of hyperglycemia. Steroids present a similar risk and the use of the two concurrently can cause refractory hyperglycemia.

G. **Hypoglycemia management**

1. **Symptoms** of hypoglycemia are hunger, headache, sweating, weakness, tremulousness, nausea, numbness, blurred or tunnel vision, confusion, stupor, loss of consciousness, coma, and seizure. In general, episodes of hypoglycemia fall into one of three categories:
   a. Symptomatic but alert and oriented
   b. Symptomatic with disturbed mental function (drowsy, lethargic, disoriented)
   c. Comatose, obtunded, or otherwise seriously disoriented
2. Guidelines for treating hypoglycemic episodes are as follows:
   a. Immediately measure the glucose level by finger stick and glucose meter.
   b. If vomiting, minimally responsive, confused, or unconscious, give **glucagon** (one vial IM or IV) immediately. Glucagon is preferred over intravenous D-10 or D-50. It is more physiologic and has less propensity for subsequent hyperglycemia.
   c. Treatment is initiated unless the glucose value is greater than 50 dl, in which case no glucose is given and the glucose value is repeated in 10–15 minutes.
   d. Glucose is given orally with 4 oz (one-half glass) of grape juice, apple juice, or orange juice (in that order of preference). Glucola may be substituted for juices if preferred by the patient. Foods such as milk, crackers, cheese, or fruit, which have less readily available glucose, should not be used due to their slower absorption and less rapid effect on the blood glucose. These foods will produce a more delayed and prolonged rise in the blood glucose and tend to overshoot the physiologic glucose range.
   e. The glucose value should be repeated within 10–20 minutes based on the symptoms and response to oral glucose.
   f. Repeat small amounts of juice can be given as necessary. It should be remembered that the purpose of treatment is to give just enough glucose to make the patient euglycemic (50–100 dl) and not hyperglycemic (> 100 dl).
   g. An appropriate person should remain with the patient until she becomes fully conscious, stable, and euglycemic. This should be a family member if she is at home or a medical person if she is in the hospital.
   h. Large amounts of IV glucose should not be given except in the most unusual circumstances where the patient has such a large amount of insulin on board that the glucose level continues to drop after the initial treatment.
3. **Glucagon** is a hormone with the opposite effect of insulin; it raises the blood glucose level by rapidly releasing glycogen stored in the liver. It is used to counteract severe hypoglycemic reactions due to insulin when the patient is unable to take calories orally. All diabetics on insulin should have glucagon at home with family members instructed in its use.

H. **Intrapartum management.** The overall goal is to obtain a mature fetus at term (37–40 weeks) with delivery timed to avoid the risks of fetal macrosomia, malpresentation, and fetal distress.

1. **Timing of delivery**
   a. Gestational class A_1 diabetics are allowed to progress to their estimated date and then delivered unless extenuating circumstances for continuation of the pregnancy (unfavorable cervix without fetal macrosomia or distress) are present. Fetal surveillance must then be started.
   b. Well-controlled class A_2, B, C, and D diabetics are allowed to progress to 38–40 weeks before delivery. The goal is to attain at least 39 weeks' gestation

whenever possible. Selection of the exact gestational age for delivery depends on the degree of diabetic control, cervical favorableness, and fetal status (well-being and size).

c. In the absence of poor glucose control, vascular involvement (hypertension, renal, retinal, or cardiac disease) or pregnancy complications (pregnancy-induced hypertension, intrauterine growth retardation), delivery should be accomplished by 39 and 0/7 weeks.

d. Delivery prior to 37 weeks should be reserved for specific maternal or fetal indications.

e. Under no circumstances should insulin-requiring pregnancies continue beyond 40 and 0/7 weeks.

f. Confirmation of fetal pulmonary maturity by amniocentesis is obtained unless the pregnancy is at or beyond 39 weeks' gestation by the American College of Obstetricians and Gynecologists (ACOG) criteria. If the studies are not indicative of maturity and the pregnancy is stable with good glucose control, delivery should be delayed for another week and fetal lung status reevaluated. In well-controlled diabetic pregnancies, standard nondiabetic fetal lung maturity indexes are considered valid. Use of steroids to advance fetal lung maturity prior to 34 weeks' gestation is controversial due to the risk of subsequent maternal (and fetal) hyperglycemia and should be approached with caution. Use beyond 34 weeks' gestation is contraindicated.

2. Route of delivery

a. Vaginal delivery is the preferred route if the fetus is vertex and not macrosomic by ultrasound evaluation immediately prior to the date of delivery. Induction of labor is acceptable. If the cervix is unfavorable for induction, prostaglandin E_2 gel may be used. After the second or third day of failed induction, the patient should be delivered by cesarean section unless there are appropriate circumstances to continue pregnancy (unfavorable cervix, < 40 weeks' gestation, reassuring fetal heart rate monitoring, and excellent glucose control).

b. Cesarean section is indicated for noncephalic presentation, fetal macrosomia, or the usual obstetric indications. Cesarean section should also be performed for nonreassuring fetal heart rate monitoring due to the potential for decreased fetal reserve in the presence of maternal diabetes.

c. Diabetics with a previous cesarean section are offered repeat cesarean section. Vaginal birth after cesarean (VBAC) may be considered if the pregnancy is uncomplicated, the diabetes well controlled, and VBAC delivery criteria are met.

d. External breech version with tocolysis may be considered with stable diabetes. Beta-sympathomimetics are relatively contraindicated due to the risk of hyperglycemia.

3. Insulin management for induction of labor or cesarean section

a. Day prior to delivery. Follow routine diet and insulin schedule on the day prior to delivery. Ultralente insulin should be discontinued the day prior to delivery due to its prolonged action.

b. Day of induction

(1) NPO after midnight.

(2) Discontinue usual insulin regimen.

(3) Finger stick glucose at 0600 and **each hour** during induction.

(4) If glucose values exceed 100–110 dl, continuous insulin infusion (CII) is started and maintained as by protocol.

(5) Urine ketones are checked every one to two hours. If positive at moderate amounts or greater, then IV glucose infusion is started along with CII and the capillary glucose is maintained at less than 100 dl.

(6) Routine intravenous fluids are administered as normal saline or other **nonglucose** solutions. **No insulin is added to the routine intravenous fluids.**

(7) Labor is induced by standard pitocin induction protocol.

(8) If induction fails and a repeat attempt is to be made the next day, discontinue the induction by late afternoon in order to allow resumption of the normal schedule of supper and hs calories and subcutaneous insulin. The exception to this is the patient on CII, which is continued and adjusted appropriately for the evening caloric intake and subsequent glucose values.

(9) For a second day of induction, the protocol is repeated.

c. Day of cesarean section

(1) NPO after midnight.

(2) Discontinue usual insulin regimen.

(3) Finger stick glucose at 0600 and hourly until delivery.

(4) If glucose values exceed 100–110 dl, CII is started per protocol and adjusted each hour until the fetus is delivered.

(5) Cesarean section should be scheduled for early in the morning.

I. Postpartum management

1. The goal for glucose management during the immediate three to five days after delivery is to prevent severe hyperglycemia (> 200 dl) and ketoacidosis.

2. Immediately after delivery, CII is discontinued, and IV fluids may be administered as either a nonglucose or 5% dextrose solution. After vaginal delivery, glucose infusion is generally not required. The postoperative patient will generally tolerate a 5% dextrose solution at 125–150 ml/hour while NPO without insulin due to the rapid onset of postpartum insulin sensitivity.

3. Glucose control may be followed by measurement of either glycosuria or fasting/preprandial finger stick glucoses.

a. Glycosuria. When a 2+ (0.25 mg) or greater value is obtained, a finger stick glucose is performed. If more than 200 dl, insulin is given as follows:

Blood glucose	Regular insulin
< 200 dl	None
200–300 dl	5 units
> 300 dl	10 units

4. Once the need for repeated doses of regular insulin is established, a routine schedule of insulin is resumed at approximately 50% of the prepregnancy dose or 25–33% of the end-pregnancy doses of regular and intermediate insulins. Supplemental doses of regular insulin are used preprandially for glucose values more than 200 dl and then converted to the subsequent day's longer-acting insulin dose.

5. Initial glucose control is relatively loose with fasting and preprandial glucoses less than 200 dl. Return to more rigorous control is individualized and takes place over the subsequent two to six weeks. This is achieved at home with self-glucose monitoring and insulin adjustment. Fasting and preprandial glucoses are gradually lowered to less than 140 dl.

J. Special insulin management situations

1. Continuous insulin infusion for DKA

a. Administer 10 units of regular insulin as an IV bolus loading dose. The dose may be increased up to 20 units with severe DKA and glucoses more than 600–700.

b. Then immediately begin CII at 10 units/hour. Additional bolus doses of regular insulin are given after the first hour if the glucose values remain more than 400–500.

c. Begin peripheral glucose infusion (5%D/½ normal saline at 125 ml/hour) when blood glucose decreases to 250–300 dl. At this point the rate of CII should be decreased, usually to 2–4 units/hour.

d. The CII rate is then adjusted to fluctuations in glucose levels and continued until **24 hours after ketosis has cleared.** It is often tempting to stop CII prior to this time; however, this usually results in return of ketosis.

e. During the 24-hour maintenance period, the CII rate is decreased to the maintenance range of 05.–2.0 units/hour. Following this a daily dose of regular- and intermediate-acting insulin (NPH or lente) is calculated and supplemented by sliding scale regular insulin based on blood glucose values.

f. Preparation of CII solution: 200 units of regular insulin added to 1000 ml normal saline. Resulting solution is 2 units regular insulin/10 ml normal saline.

g. Laboratory monitoring

(1) Hourly with CII for DKA: serum ketones, urine ketones, and serum potassium.

(2) At longer intervals: serum electrolytes, arterial blood gases, blood urea nitrogen, creatinine, blood acetone, complete blood count, serum osmolality.

2. CII for antepartum and intrapartum situations

a. Calculate the antepartum ratio of total daily caloric intake to total daily insulin (2000-calorie diet and 40 units insulin [1 unit insulin/50 calories]).

b. Estimate the caloric intake for the time span of the infusion. (NPO on 5%D/½ normal saline at 125 ml/hour × 24 hours = 3 liters = 150 gm glucose.)

c. Calculate the insulin dose required to cover the estimated caloric intake and then determine the rate of insulin infusion/hour.

d. Infusion rates are generally 0.25–3.0 units/hour. Rates calculated at more than 5 units/hour should be rechecked.

e. A separate peripheral 5%D solution is used with CII for hydration, caloric, and potassium supplementation. The suggested solution is 5%D/½ normal saline at 125 ml/hour.

f. Preparation of solution. 100 units regular insulin is added to 1000 ml normal saline. The resulting solution is 1 unit regular insulin/10 ml normal saline.

g. The plasma glucose is monitored hourly initially and the rate of CII is adjusted upward or downward gradually by estimation considering the initial rate calculation and the observed response. **A careful record must be kept of adjustments.**

h. If a patient is placed on an oral diet while on CII, the hourly rate must be adjusted with the meal to cover the calorie bolus. Calculate the number of calories to be ingested, and using the patient's known insulin-calorie ratio, calculate the units of additional regular insulin needed to cover the meal calories. Then divide this insulin bolus over three hours and add it to the basal insulin infusion rate starting with the meal. After three hours the CII rate is reduced to a maintenance level based on glucose values. (300 calories at a ratio of 1 unit/10 calories = 30 units regular insulin. Divided over three hours = 10 units/hour. If basal rate is 1 unit/hour, this gives a rate of 11 units/hour × 3 hours with the meal.)

3. Postpartum continuous infusion insulin

a. Normally CII is stopped at delivery due to the dramatic reduction that occurs in insulin requirement with delivery of the placenta.

b. If CII is required, the antepartum rate is no longer applicable and a new rate of infusion must be established.

c. Start at 0.5–1.0 unit/hour.

d. Adjust rate every two hours.

e. Goal is to simply maintain glucose less than 200 dl.

II. Thyroid Disease. During pregnancy minor changes in thyroid functions occur. The serum level of thyroxine-binding globulin is increased, due to increased hepatic production stimulated by the high level of estrogen found in pregnancy. This increase in thyroxine-binding globulin level results in an elevation in the serum concentration of thyroxine (T4) and triiodothyronine (T3), with a reciprocal reduction in T3 resin uptake (T3RU). The serum concentrations of free T4 (FT4) and free T3 (FT3) are essentially unchanged. The serum level of thyroid-stimulating hormone (TSH) is normal during pregnancy. Human chorionic gonadotropin produced by the placenta has a weak thyroid-stimulating activity [31].

Enlargement of the maternal thyroid gland during pregnancy and an increase in radioactive iodine uptake have been reported [43]. These changes are felt to be secondary to an increase in renal iodide excretion and are more evident in iodine-deficient populations [29]. Fetal thyroid can concentrate iodine and produce thyroid hormones by the tenth to twelfth weeks of gestation. The fetal serum T4 level increases from 2–3 μg/dl by the end of the first trimester to 10 μg/dl in the third trimester. The fetal serum T3 level is low. Fetal serum TSH is detectable as early as 10 weeks [32]. After birth, the neonatal serum TSH level sharply rises with a peak in two to four hours with a return to normal levels within two days. This TSH rise is stimulated by extrauterine cooling and is followed by a rise in serum T4 and T3 concentrations [30].

The placenta is relatively impermeable to thyroid hormones (T4 and T3). Only minimal transfer of thyroid hormones across the placenta occurs at physiologic serum concentrations; however, at higher serum concentrations, some transfer may occur (T3 > T4). Antithyroid drugs (propylthiouracil [PTU] and methimazole), as well as iodine, cross the placenta without difficulty. Thyroid-stimulating immunoglobulins (TSIs) can cross the placental barrier and produce fetal or neonatal hyperthyroidism. Thyrotropin-releasing hormone crosses the placenta, but TSH does not [45].

A. **Hyperthyroidism.** The incidence of hyperthyroidism in pregnancy is about 0.1–0.2% [25, 44]. The most common cause is Graves' disease. Other causes include toxic nodular goiter (multinodular or single nodule), hydatidiform mole, choriocarcinoma, ovarian teratoma, and iatrogenic thyrotoxicosis.

1. **Graves' disease** is by far the most common cause of hyperthyroidism in pregnancy.

   a. **Etiology.** The cause of Graves' disease is not known. Familial predisposition is strong. About 15% of patients with Graves' disease have a relative with the same disorder, and about 50% of relatives of patients with Graves' disease have positive circulating thyroid autoantibodies. The female-male ratio is about 5 : 1. There is an increased frequency of HLA-B8 and DR3 in Graves' disease patients. Over 90% of patients with Graves' disease have detectable serum TSI.

   b. **Clinical features.** Clinical diagnosis of mild to moderate hyperthyroidism may be difficult in pregnant women because symptoms of hyperdynamic circulation occur normally in pregnancy.

   Helpful clinical clues include weight loss despite a good appetite and persistent tachycardia. The presence of exophthalmos and pretibial myxedema indicates Graves' disease. Other helpful clinical findings include tremor, weakness, and onycholysis. The thyroid gland is usually enlarged and has a bruit.

   c. **Laboratory findings.** The total T4 level, T3RU, and free thyroxine index (FTI) are elevated. The FT4 level is elevated (a better parameter than total T4). The T3 radioimmunoassay (RIA) is also elevated. The T3RIA level should be checked if the T4 is normal and hyperthyroidism is strongly suspected (to rule out T3 toxicosis).

   The TSH is significantly suppressed (when a sensitive TSH assay is used). The presence of a suppressed TSH level obviates the need for a thyrotropin-releasing hormone stimulation test. The serum TSI is positive.

   d. **Maternal and fetal considerations**

      (1) Untreated hyperthyroidism during pregnancy has a very poor prognosis to the fetus. The major risks are abortion, premature delivery, and neonatal thyrotoxicosis [38, 46].

      (2) Neonatal hyperthyroidism results from transfer of maternal TSI across the placenta. The TSI stimulates the fetal thyroid to produce thyroid hormones causing fetal (intrauterine) or neonatal hyper-

thyroidism. Neonatal hyperthyroidism depends on maternal TSI and not on maternal thyroid status. Therefore, infants of euthyroid women with previous history of Graves' disease are also at risk. Measurement of the maternal TSI level is useful to predict the likelihood of neonatal hyperthyroidism [38, 39, 46].

(3) Antithyroid drugs readily cross the placenta and inhibit fetal thyroid hormone secretion [34]. This will lead to fetal hypothyroidism and goiter. These effects cannot be reversed by administering thyroid hormone to the mother, since thyroid hormones do not cross the placenta [40]. The presence of a large fetal goiter may cause hyperextension of the fetal neck and head. The resultant abnormal presentation may require delivery by cesarean section [46].

(4) Neonatal hyperthyroidism is usually transient, lasting only one to three months, since the half-life of TSI in the neonate is approximately two weeks.

(5) Both PTU and methimazole are transferred into breast milk; however, PTU is present in only one-tenth the concentration of methimazole. In low doses, PTU is unlikely to affect the breast-fed baby's thyroid function [33].

(6) The long-term consequences of mild intrauterine hypothyroidism are not clear. Burrow and colleagues [26] reported no differences in median IQ in children who had been exposed to antithyroid drugs in utero when compared with their unexposed siblings. Similar results were obtained in another study when infants were compared with age-matched controls [35].

(7) After delivery, the neonate should be examined for evidence of goiter. Neonatal thyroid function tests should be obtained.

e. Treatment. The therapeutic choices of Graves' disease in pregnancy include the antithyroid medications (PTU and methimazole) or surgery. Radioactive iodine ablation is contraindicated during pregnancy.

f. Medical management. The therapeutic goal is to achieve a euthyroid or slightly hyperthyroid mother and prevent fetal hypothyroidism. Both PTU and methimazole are transported across the placenta; however, only about one-fourth the concentration of PTU crosses as compared to methimazole [34].

Both PTU and methimazole inhibit the synthesis of thyroid hormones primarily by the inhibition of iodide organification. Specifically, they inhibit the incorporation of oxidized iodide into tyrosine residues. Additional actions of antithyroid drugs include inhibition of the coupling reaction between iodothyronines (monoiodotyrosine and diiodotyrosine) to form iodothyronines (T3 and T4). The PTU inhibits the peripheral conversion of T4 to T3 [27]. In pregnant hyperthyroid women, PTU is the preferred drug because of its lower potency and limited placental transfer. Another reason for PTU as the drug of choice is the reported association of congenital scalp defects (aplasia cutis) [36] in infants exposed to methimazole in utero. Suppression of the fetal thyroid by PTU is generally dose dependent: the lower the dose, the lower the risk. Therefore, the goal is always to reduce the PTU dose as low as possible.

(1) Obtain baseline thyroid function tests (T4 and T3RU, or preferably FT4, T3RIA, TSH, and TSI).

(2) Start treatment with PTU at an initial dose of 100–150 mg q8h. More severe hyperthyroid patients may require a higher initial dose.

(3) PTU doses should be as small as possible to maintain T4 levels in the high-normal range for pregnant women.

(4) Monitor patients clinically and biochemically by measurement of FT4 level every two weeks. When T4 levels stabilize in the high-normal range for pregnant women, the dose of PTU can be gradually decreased to a maintenance dose of 50–150 mg/day.

(5) The time required to achieve euthyroidism after starting antithyroid drug treatment is usually two to four months.

(6) If hyperthyroidism recurs when the PTU dose is reduced, increase the dose to produce adequate suppression.

g. **Side effects.** The important side effects of antithyroid drugs include rash, urticaria, arthralgia, and occasionally frank arthritis. Transient leukopenia (white blood cell count $< 4000/mm^3$) occurs in up to 10–12% of patients. Since untreated Graves' disease by itself may cause mild leukopenia, a baseline leukocyte count should be obtained prior to initiation of antithyroid therapy.

The most serious complication of antithyroid drugs is agranulocytosis. Agranulocytosis is characterized by fever, evidence of bacterial infection (e.g., sore throat), and decreased granulocyte count ($< 250/mm^3$). Both methimazole and PTU can cause agranulocytosis. The onset is usually sudden and routine monitoring of white cell count is not helpful. If agranulocytosis develops, antithyroid drugs should be discontinued. The patients should be advised to report fever, sore throat, or any other symptoms of infection [27].

h. **Surgical treatment.** Subtotal thyroidectomy has a limited role in the management of Graves' disease in pregnancy. Surgery is reserved for those patients who are unable to take antithyroid medications or have large goiters causing significant tracheal obstruction. To reduce the vascularity of the gland, patients are treated with antithyroid drugs and a saturated solution of potassium iodide prior to surgery.

B. **Hypothyroidism.** Pregnancy in hypothyroid women is uncommon. Untreated hypothyroidism is associated with decreased fertility. If pregnancy occurs, abortions, stillbirths, and congenital malformations are more prevalent. Treatment with thyroxine prior to pregnancy usually corrects these abnormalities [37].

1. **Etiology.** The most common cause of hypothyroidism is autoimmune thyroiditis (Hashimoto's). Other causes include ablation of the thyroid gland (^{131}I or surgery), iodine deficiency, treatment with antithyroid drugs (PTU and methimazole), and less commonly hypothalamic-pituitary disease.

2. **Clinical presentation.** Hypothyroid patients usually complain of easy fatigability, cold intolerance, excessive weight gain, dryness of the skin, and constipation.

The physical examination usually reveals a dry, scaly skin; hoarse voice; and puffy face; and, in primary hypothyroidism, a goiter is usually present. The tendon reflexes are slow with a prolonged relaxation phase.

3. **Laboratory findings.** Low serum total T4, low T3 resin uptake, low FT4, and an elevated serum TSH levels are diagnostic of primary hypothyroidism. Serum T3RIA is usually low but may be in the normal range. Positive antimicrosomal and antithyroglobulin antibodies suggest Hashimoto's thyroiditis.

In pituitary hypothyroidism, FT4 and FTI are low but serum TSH levels are not elevated. If pituitary hypothyroidism is suspected, full evaluation of the pituitary gland functions is required.

4. **Management.** Treatment of hypothyroidism is straightforward. L-thyroxine is the treatment of choice. Start with a dose of 75–100 μg/day. Monitor TSH and FT4 levels in four weeks. Adjust the dose to maintain the TSH in the normal range.

For patients with underlying heart disease, start with a smaller dose (25–50 μg/day), and gradually increase the dose by 25 μg every 1–2 weeks until the optimal dose is achieved.

5. **Maternal and fetal considerations**

a. Since thyroxine does not cross the placenta, L-thyroxine taken by hypothyroid pregnant women has no effect on the fetal hypothalamic-pituitary-thyroid axis.

b. Untreated hypothyroid pregnant women have an increased incidence of stillbirths and spontaneous abortions [38].

c. A study [37] of 11 pregnancies in 9 hypothyroid women reported 9 normal births, 1 stillborn infant, and 1 infant with Down's syndrome and ostium primum defect (mother's age was 41 years).

C. Silent (painless) thyroiditis. Silent thyroiditis is an acute inflammatory disorder of the thyroid gland. The incidence of silent thyroiditis is not well known. In some reports in the literature, it accounted for 14–15% of all cases of hyperthyroidism [28, 41]. An incidence of 5.4% and 8.9% was found in the postpartum period in Japanese and American women, respectively [24, 42].

1. Clinical features. Patients with silent thyroiditis usually present with symptoms of thyrotoxicosis (hyperthyroid phase). This phase lasts one to four months. Subsequently, a hypothyroid phase that lasts one to two-and-one-half months usually develops. After the hypothyroid phase, patients usually recover, and thyroid function tests return to the normal range [47]. The thyroid gland is enlarged in 50–60% of the patients.

2. Laboratory. In the hyperthyroid phase, serum levels of total T4, T3 resin uptake, FT4 index, and FT4 are elevated. Serum TSH levels are suppressed. Radioactive iodine uptake is very low. Antimicrosomal and antithyroglobulin antibody titers may be positive. Conversely, when patients present with hypothyroidism, the total T4, T3RU, and FT4 are low, and the TSH levels are elevated [47].

3. Management. Treatment depends on the phase of presentation. In the hyperthyroid phase, Inderal usually provides symptomatic relief. Methimazole and PTU are not effective in this situation. When hypothyroidism develops, thyroxine replacement may be required for four to eight weeks.

III. Parathyroid disease. Parathyroid hormone (PTH) is secreted as an 84 amino acid polypeptide. It acts directly on bone and kidney and, indirectly (through its effect on synthesis of 1,25[OH]2-D) on the intestine to raise serum calcium. The PTH increases bone resorption, decreases renal calcium clearance, and increases calcium absorption from the gastrointestinal tract. Serum concentration of ionized calcium is the major regulator of PTH secretion.

Circulating PTH consists of the intact 84 amino acid polypeptide and multiple hormone fragments (C-terminal and the biologically active N-terminal fragments).

A. Hyperparathyroidism. Primary hyperparathyroidism in pregnancy is rare. About 80 cases have been described in the medical literature [56]. The most common cause of primary hyperparathyroidism is a single parathyroid adenoma (about 80% of cases). Multiple-gland involvement (parathyroid hyperplasia) is seen in 20% of the cases. Parathyroid carcinoma accounts for less than 2% of the cases.

1. Clinical presentation. Most patients with hyperparathyroidism are asymptomatic or have nonspecific symptoms such as weakness and easy fatigability. When symptoms are present, they include emotional lability, depression, loss of memory for recent events, anorexia, nausea, vomiting, constipation, polyuria, polydypsia, and nocturia. Evidence of renal calculi may be present. Somnolence and coma may develop in the presence of severe hypercalcemia.

2. Laboratory findings. The diagnosis of primary hyperparathyroidism is confirmed by finding an elevated PTH level in the presence of an elevated serum calcium level. (Note the total serum calcium levels fall during normal pregnancy; thus, it can mask mild hyperparathyroidism in pregnancy.)

3. Management. Untreated primary hyperparathyroidism is associated with high complication rates (up to 80% in some series) [51]. The most common complications are neonatal tetany and neonatal hypocalcemia, spontaneous abortion, stillbirth, and premature delivery [50, 52]. The treatment of choice for primary hyperparathyroidism during pregnancy is parathy roidectomy [51]. The optimal time for surgery is during the second trimes ter when all the fetal systems have developed and before the third trimeste when there is a greater likelihood of premature labor. Three cases o parathyroidectomy performed in the third trimester are reported in th literature; two had excellent outcome, the other resulted in a stillbor fetus [49, 56].

If parathyroidectomy is contraindicated, oral phosphate therapy is ap propriate. It has proved safe and effective in a few case reports. The dos is usually 1.5–3.0 gm/day of inorganic phosphate to maintain materna serum phosphate levels in the high-normal range [53].

4. **Maternal and fetal considerations**
   - **a.** Maternal PTH levels normally increase in late pregnancy at the tim of maximum calcification of the fetal skeleton [48].
   - **b.** Calcium crosses the placenta by the process of active transport, whic allows the fetal serum calcium to exceed that of the mother.
   - **c.** During pregnancy, calcium absorption in the mother increases fron 150 mg/day to about 400 mg/day at 20 weeks of pregnancy.
   - **d.** The PTH does not cross the placenta [55].
   - **e.** The newborn has low circulating PTH levels with suppressed respons of hypocalcemia, but calcitonin levels are relatively high.
   - **f.** In the full-term infant, serum calcium shows a modest decrease, whic reaches a nadir at 24–48 hours.
   - **g.** In the fetus, vitamin D and its metabolites are mostly derived from th maternal circulation. The fetal kidney is capable of 1,25(OH)2-D syn thesis [54].

B. Hypoparathyroidism. Hypoparathyroidism in pregnancy is uncommon. Th major causes of PTH-deficient hypoparathyroidism are postsurgical, idi opathic, and functional hypoparathyroidism (secondary to hypomagnese mia). Pseudohypoparathyroidism is a rare familial disorder characterize by target tissue resistance to PTH. The idiopathic form of hypoparathy roidism may be associated with other endocrine deficiency syndromes.

1. **Clinical presentation.** Patients usually present with symptoms and sign of increased neuromuscular excitability. Tetany may be the presentin symptom. This usually starts with paresthesia and is followed by spasn of the muscles of the extremities and face. Two provocative signs, whe positive, can detect latent tetany: Chvostek's sign (tapping the facial nerv just anterior to the ear lobe) and Trousseau's sign (carpal spasm when sphygmomanometer cuff is inflated above systolic blood pressure for tw minutes). Pseudohypoparathyroidism is usually associated with short fourt metacarpal bones.
2. **Laboratory.** Serum calcium levels (total and ionized) are low and th serum phosphorus is elevated. Reduced serum PTH levels in the presenc of hypocalcemia confirm the diagnosis of primary hypoparathyroidism.
3. **Management.** With appropriate treatment, the prognosis is good as lon as the patient remains normocalcemic. Treatment consists of calcium an vitamin D. Elemental calcium, 2 gm/day, is the usual dose required ir pregnancy. Several vitamin D preparations are available. Ergocalcifero (vitamin D_2) in a daily dose of 25,000–50,000 units; dihydrotachystero (Hytakerol), 0.2–1.0 mg/day; calcifediol (Calderol), 20–200 μg/day; or cal citriol (Rocaltrol), 0.25–5.0 μg/day can be used.
4. **Maternal and fetal considerations**
   - **a.** If hypoparathyroidism remains untreated, high maternal and fetal mor tality ensue.
   - **b.** Neonatal hyperparathyroidism may develop as a response to materna hypocalcemia.
   - **c.** Vitamin D is secreted in breast milk. Therefore, breast-feeding ma cause hypervitaminosis D in the infant.

IV. Adrenal disease. During pregnancy plasma corticosteroid-binding globulin and total cortisol levels increase. A small but progressive rise in plasma adrenocorticotropic hormone (ACTH) levels is associated with a two- to threefold increase in total and unbound plasma cortisol. The increased plasma-free cortisol levels during pregnancy poorly suppress ACTH [48].

A. Cushing's syndrome. Cushing's syndrome is rare. The coexistence of Cushing's syndrome and pregnancy is very uncommon, occurring in about two per million population. The causes of Cushing's syndrome include pituitary adenoma, adrenal adenoma, ectopic ACTH production, and adrenal carcinoma.

1. Clinical presentation. Patients usually present with characteristic moon facies, buffalo hump, and central obesity. Other physical findings include purple abdominal striae, hirsutism, hypertension, and proximal muscle weakness. Psychological disturbances have been described in 40% of Cushing's syndrome patients.

2. Laboratory findings. In Cushing's syndrome, a continuous, spontaneous, and autonomous production of adrenal steroids takes place.

a. An overnight dexamethasone suppression test is used as an initial screen. Dexamethasone, 1 mg, is taken orally at 11 P.M. and the serum cortisol is checked at 8 A.M. the next morning. A serum cortisol level less than 5 μg/dl rules out Cushing's syndrome, a serum cortisol level above 10 μg/dl is highly suspicious, and a serum cortisol between 5–10 μg/dl is "borderline."

b. A 24-hour urinary free cortisol is an equally effective screening test for Cushing's syndrome. (Note that urinary free cortisol is elevated in normal pregnancy.)

Patients with an abnormal overnight dexamethasone suppression test or elevated urinary free cortisol levels require endocrinology consultation for further investigation using the standard low-dose and high-dose dexamethasone suppression tests.

After biochemical diagnosis of Cushing's syndrome is established, one can proceed with imaging studies (computed tomography scan) to localize the lesion [57].

3. Management. Treatment depends on the underlying diagnosis and the stage of pregnancy. In the first trimester, termination of pregnancy and surgical removal are recommended for adrenal carcinoma. Pituitary adenomas should be removed surgically. In the third trimester, or after delivery of the infant, definitive therapy can be given. Metyrapone has been used to delay delivery. In the second trimester, most pregnancies will end with a miscarriage; however, for those pregnancies that continue, the choice is between medical (metyrapone) or surgical therapy [58, 63].

4. Maternal and fetal considerations

a. The prognosis for pregnancy associated with Cushing's syndrome is poor. About 50–60% of the pregnancies end in abortion, premature labor, or stillbirth.

b. The ACTH does not cross the placenta; however, glucocorticoids cross without difficulty [71]. Elevated maternal glucocorticoid levels can suppress the fetal hypothalamic-pituitary axis, resulting in adrenal insufficiency in the newborn.

B. Adrenal insufficiency. Primary adrenal insufficiency is a rare disorder. Its prevalence is about 40 cases/million. It is more common in females, with a female-male ratio of 2.5 : 1.0.

1. Etiology. The most common cause of primary adrenal insufficiency in the United States is autoimmune adrenalitis, which accounts for 80% of the cases. Tuberculosis accounts for about 20%. Other rare causes include adrenal hemorrhage and infarction, fungal infection, metastatic tumors, and amyloidosis.

2. Clinical presentation. Patients with adrenal insufficiency present with nonspecific symptoms. They usually complain of fatigue, weakness, anorexia, nausea, vomiting, and postural dizziness. Physical findings includ skin hyperpigmentation and postural hypotension.

3. **Laboratory findings.** In Addison's disease, both glucocorticoids and min eralocorticoids are deficient. Deficiency of glucocorticoids produces hy poglycemia and hyponatremia, and mineralocorticoid deficiency produce hyponatremia and hyperkalemia.

   Definitive diagnosis of Addison's disease is achieved by the ACTH stim ulation test.

   a. Obtain a baseline plasma cortisol level.
   b. Administer 250 μg of synthetic ACTH (Cortrosyn) IV or IM.
   c. Obtain blood samples for plasma cortisol at 30 and 60 minutes. A norma response is an increase in plasma cortisol of 7 μg/dl and a peak leve of greater than 18 μg/dl.

4. **Management.** Patients with Addison's disease require treatment wit both glucocorticoids and mineralocorticoids. Daily replacement doses c glucocorticoids can be achieved by giving hydrocortisone PO 20 mg in th morning and 5–10 mg in the afternoon. Alternatively, prednisone, 5 m PO in the morning and 2–5 mg in the afternoon, can be used. Mineral ocorticoids are given as fludrocortisone (Florinef) 0.05–0.1 mg/day PC Patients should be advised to increase their glucocorticoid dose (two- t threefold) for minor illnesses [65].

C. **Acute adrenal crisis.** Acute adrenal crisis is a state of acute deficiency c adrenocortical hormones. The clinical presentation consists of anorexia, nau sea, vomiting, and abdominal pain. Because of severe intravascular volum depletion, hypotension and shock usually develop.

1. **Management.** Adrenal crisis is a medical emergency, and immediat treatment is mandatory. Therapy consists of intravenous steroids (hy drocortisone, 100 mg IV q6h for the first 24 hours) and intravenous fluid to restore intravascular volume. If improvement occurs and the patien is stable, the steroid dose can be gradually decreased [65].

2. **Maternal and fetal considerations**

   a. Untreated adrenal insufficiency during pregnancy has an increase rate of fetal death (40–50%) and a high incidence of postpartum adrena crisis.
   b. Early in pregnancy, nausea and vomiting in patients with undiagnose adrenal insufficiency may be mistaken for symptoms of pregnancy.
   c. During labor, increased doses of parenteral hydrocortisone are recom mended (100 mg q6h throughout labor). After delivery, the dose can b gradually reduced to a maintenance dose [64].
   d. No contraindication exists to breast-feeding.

D. **Congenital adrenal hyperplasia (adrenogenital syndrome).** Congenital ad renal hyperplasia (CAH), as its name implies, is a hereditary disorder char acterized by enlargement of the adrenal glands. Several possible enzymati defects in the biosynthesis of cortisol lead to reduced circulating cortisc levels and an increase in ACTH levels in the serum. Excessive ACTH stim ulation of the adrenal glands is responsible for the adrenal hyperplasia an the increase in androgen secretion. 21-Hydroxylase deficiency is the mos common (95%) of the enzymatic abnormalities. A much less common forr of CAH is associated with a defect in 11-hydroxylation [59]. Untreated pa tients with CAH rarely become pregnant. On the other hand, a fertility rat of 64% was reported in a group of 20 patients with CAH first treated betwee the ages of 6 and 20 years [70].

1. **Clinical features.** The syndrome is most commonly recognized at the tim of birth of a female infant by noting the presence of ambiguous genitali The male infant, on the other hand, is unlikely to be diagnosed at birt unless an associated salt-losing tendency exists. The syndrome should b suspected in any infant or child who has frequent, refractory episodes c dehydration and whose genitalia are ambiguous. Patients who reac

adulthood undiagnosed usually present with menstrual disturbances, infertility, and hirsutism [67].

2. **Laboratory findings.** The diagnosis of CAH can be confirmed by finding depressed levels of plasma cortisol, elevated basal circulating levels of 17-hydroxyprogesterone, and an exaggerated response of 17-hydroxyprogesterone to intravenous injection of ACTH.
3. **Management.** Chronic treatment requires glucocorticoids to suppress ACTH secretion. Mineralocorticoids may be required for those patients who have the salt-losing form of the disorder. During episodes of stress (labor and delivery), the glucocorticoid dose should be increased, and these patients should be managed similarly to those patients with Addison's disease [66, 69].

E. **Primary aldosteronism.** Primary hyperaldosteronism (Conn's syndrome) is the association of hypertension, hypokalemia, and increased production of mineralocorticoids by the adrenal glands. With the primary increase in aldosterone levels, the circulating renin levels are greatly suppressed. Primary hyperaldosteronism is very uncommon during pregnancy, and the maternal-fetal effects are not well known. Maternal aldosterone crosses the placental barrier [68].

1. **Clinical presentation.** Patients usually come to medical attention when hypokalemia and hypertension are noted during a routine physical examination.
2. **Laboratory findings.** Hypokalemia and increased urinary excretion of potassium are usually noted. The diagnosis of primary hyperaldosteronism is confirmed by the absence of renin stimulation in response to volume depletion and the lack of aldosterone suppression in response to volume expansion (saline infusion test). Endocrine consultation should be obtained when primary hyperaldosteronism is suspected [74].
3. **Management.** Treatment of primary hyperaldosteronism depends on the etiologic diagnosis (adenoma 60% versus hyperplasia 40%) or rarely carcinoma. Medical management with antihypertensives and potassium-sparing diuretics may be adequate in benign lesions. Malignant lesions require surgery. Hypertension and hypokalemia of adrenal adenoma may respond to surgical removal of the tumor [60, 75].

F. **Pheochromocytoma.** Pheochromocytomas are tumors of the chromaffin tissues. They produce increasing amounts of epinephrine, norepinephrine, or both. Undiagnosed pheochromocytoma may be fatal in pregnant women during delivery or in patients undergoing surgical procedures for other disorders.

In adults, 85% of pheochromocytomas arise in the adrenal glands. Extra adrenal sites include the kidney, the organ of Zuckerkandl, and along the sympathetic chain. Pheochromocytoma may be part of multiple endocrine neoplasia. Less than 10% of pheochromocytomas are malignant [62].

1. **Clinical presentation.** Some patients are asymptomatic; others may present with episodic symptoms. Common findings during an episode include headaches, sweating, palpitations and forceful heartbeats, anxiety, and chest pain. Between episodes patients may complain of exhaustion and fatigue. More than 50% of the patients have paroxysmal hypertension. These paroxysms characteristically occur from several times a month to several times a day and last from one minute to several hours, but usually less than one hour. Because of increased metabolic rate, weight loss may be noted.
2. **Laboratory findings.** The diagnosis of pheochromocytoma requires the demonstration of excess catecholamine secretion. Measurement of 24-hour urine catecholamines and their metabolites, vanillylmandelic acid and total metanephrines, is widely used. Urinary creatinine should be measured with the 24-hour urine to assess the adequacy of the urine collection. Significantly elevated catecholamines, vanillylmandelic acid, and meta-

nephrines support the diagnosis of pheochromocytoma. If the results are normal, but there is a strong clinical suspicion of the disease, a urine collection can be obtained during a symptomatic attack to increase the diagnostic yield. Several drugs and foods interfere with catecholamines determination and should be avoided during the urine collection.

If diagnosis cannot be confirmed on the basis of urinary measurements a clonidine suppression test can be used. Plasma catecholamine levels are obtained before and three hours after oral ingestion of 0.3 mg of clonidine In patients with pheochromocytoma, plasma catecholamines fail to suppress in response to clonidine. A computed tomography scan of the adrenal glands is very helpful in tumor localization; however, it exposes the fetus to considerable irradiation. Radioisotope scanning is contraindicated during pregnancy. Ultrasound scanning may be the imaging study of choice in pregnancy.

3. **Management.** Untreated pheochromocytoma carries increased maternal and fetal mortality. Treatment in pregnancy includes adequate alpha adrenergic blockade to control hypertension. The most commonly used is phenoxybenzamine, 10–80 mg/day in divided doses, adjusting the dose according to blood pressure responses.

   Additional antihypertensive medications may be required. Beta-blockers should not be used. In early pregnancy, surgical removal of the tumor may be considered [61].
4. **Maternal and fetal considerations**
   a. Plasma catecholamines do not change in pregnancy; however, there is an increase during labor.
   b. Untreated pheochromocytoma in pregnancy has a poor prognosis. One study of 89 patients reported maternal mortality of 48% and fetal mortality of 54%. The same study revealed that maternal prognosis improved significantly if the diagnosis was made in the antenatal period and appropriate therapy was initiated; however, fetal mortality did not change [72].
   c. Epinephrine and norepinephrine traverse the placenta [73].

V. **Pituitary disease.** In pregnant women, the pituitary gland enlarges in size by about one-third. High plasma-estrogen concentrations during pregnancy stimulate hyperplasia of the lactotrophs in the anterior pituitary accounting for the pituitary gland enlargement. During normal pregnancy, serum prolactin concentrations rise to levels of 100–200 ng/ml.

The placenta is impermeable to hormones of the anterior pituitary gland including growth hormone, thyrotropin (TSH), gonadotropins, and ACTH [77]. Evidence also indicates that no placental transfer of the posterior pituitary hormones vasopressin and oxytocin occurs [81].

A. **Prolactinomas.** Prolactinomas are the most common secretory tumors of the pituitary gland. In women, about 50% of the tumors are microadenomas (< 10 mm), whereas the remainder are macroadenomas (> 10 mm). Most prolactinomas are confined to the pituitary fossa, but upward, lateral, or downward extension may occur.

1. **Clinical presentations.** Women with prolactinomas usually present with amenorrhea, galactorrhea, and infertility.
2. **Laboratory findings.** Although hyperprolactinemia may be seen in other pathologic conditions, prolactinomas are clinically the most important. Prolactinomas may account for up to 70% of all pituitary tumors. Elevated serum prolactin levels greater than 100 ng/ml are highly suggestive of prolactinoma Patients with prolactinomas usually have subnormal prolactin response to thyrotropin-releasing hormone. Normals usually have a twofold increase in prolactin levels in response to thyrotropin-releasing hormone stimulation Computed tomography scanning or magnetic resonance imaging of the sella helps to localize the tumor.
3. **Management.** Therapeutic options for prolactinomas are transsphenoidal surgery or bromocriptine.

a. **Transsphenoidal surgery.** In experienced hands, successful transsphenoidal microsurgery is achieved in 60–85% of microadenomas (< 10 mm). Success is defined as normal prolactin, normal menses, and cessation of galactorrhea. Transsphenoidal surgery is less successful in macroadenomas (> 10 mm). Recurrence rates vary considerably in the literature [80].

b. **Bromocriptine.** Bromocriptine is a dopamin-receptor agonist. It has proved to be effective in lowering serum prolactin levels, as well as reducing the size of prolactin-producing adenomas. Start with a small dose: 1.25–2.5 mg/day. The dose can be gradually increased to a maximum dose of 7.5–10.0 mg/day. Side effects of bromocriptine include nausea, vomiting, dizziness, and postural hypotension. In patients with microadenomas, bromocriptine is successful in normalizing circulating prolactin levels in over 90% of cases [82, 83].

4. **Pregnancy and prolactinomas.** Bromocriptine treatment of patients with pituitary microadenomas restores ovulation and fertility. There has been great concern if patients with prolactinomas became pregnant after bromocriptine therapy the adenoma will increase in size under the influence of placental estrogens and cause problems (e.g., visual field defects). Although a few case reports support this notion, reported experience with several hundred pregnancies suggests that clinically significant expansion of a prolactinoma during pregnancy is uncommon. Moreover, if a complication (increase in the size of an adenoma) occurs, it is rapidly reversible with the resumption of bromocriptine therapy, which may be required throughout pregnancy. In pregnant women with prolactinomas, monitoring of prolactin levels and visual field exams are recommended. Very high prolactin levels (> 500 ng/ml) in pregnant suggest tumor expansion [79].

B. **Diabetes insipidus.** Diabetes insipidus (DI) is a disorder characterized by the production of large amounts of very dilute urine. The disorder is due to deficiency of vasopressin (central DI) or failure of the kidneys to respond to circulating vasopressin (nephrogenic DI).

1. **Etiology.** Central DI may result from surgeries in the hypothalamic-pituitary region. Damage to the pituitary gland results in transient DI. Other causes of central DI include idiopathic, familial, and metastatic tumors to the hypothalamus. Nephrogenic DI is a rare congenital disorder.
2. **Clinical features.** Patients usually present with polyuria, polydipsia, and nocturia.
3. **Laboratory findings.** Early morning urine and serum osmolality determinations may be used as an initial screen. A urine osmolality greater than 800 mOsm/kg excludes the diagnosis of DI. The next step is to evaluate the effect of water deprivation on urine osmolality (water deprivation test). This should be performed in an inpatient setting under supervised conditions.
4. **Management.** Central DI is treated with vasopressin. At present, the drug of choice is desmopressin (DDAVP), a synthetic analog of vasopressin. It is administered intranasally in doses of 0.05–0.1 ml q12h.
   Nephrogenic DI is treated with diuretics and salt restriction. The aim is to keep the patient in a state of mild sodium depletion, which reduces the solute load on the kidney. This will enhance proximal tubular reabsorption.
5. **Maternal and fetal considerations**
   a. Vasopressin does not cross the placental barrier [81].
   b. Hime and Richardson [76] reviewed the course of DI in pregnancy in 67 patients. Most of the patients had deterioration in their disease, and the dose of DDAVP had to be increased. Few patients showed improvement in their disease.
   c. Data regarding lactation in the presence of DI are very limited.

C. **Sheehan's syndrome.** Sheehan's syndrome is a form of pituitary hypofunction that develops after obstetric bleeding or shock. The anterior pituitary gland enlarges during normal pregnancy and, lacking a direct arterial blood supply, is vulnerable to infarction during shock from excessive uterine bleeding during labor. The degree of loss of pituitary function is variable.

1. **Clinical presentation.** The first manifestation of this syndrome is lack of postpartum milk production, presumably secondary to low circulating prolactin levels. Other signs of anterior pituitary hormone deficiency may manifest later (e.g., failure of menses to resume, hypothyroidism, and adrenal insufficiency).
2. **Laboratory findings.** Patients may have laboratory evidence of hypothyroidism, adrenal insufficiency, and decreased gonadotropin hormone (TSH and leutinizing hormone) levels. Since the lesion is in the pituitary gland, TSH levels will not be elevated [78].
3. **Management.** Replacement therapy with thyroxine, glucocorticoids, and sex steroids is usually required. Mineralocorticoids are not required.

References

DIABETES

1. Carpenter, M. W., and Coustan, D. R. Criteria for screening tests for gestational diabetes. *Obstet. Gynecol.* 144:768, 1982.
2. Coustan, D. R., et al. Tight metabolic control of overt diabetes in pregnancy. *Am. J. Med.* 68:845–852, 1980.
3. Coustan, D. R., and Felig, P. Diabetes Mellitus. In G. N. Burrows and T. F. Ferris (eds.), *Medical Complications During Pregnancy* (3rd ed.). Philadelphia: Saunders, 1988.
4. Gestational diabetes mellitus: Position statement. *Diabetes Care* 1(Suppl. 13):5, 1990.
5. Harris, M. I. et al. Prevalence of diabetes and impaired glucose tolerance and plasma glucose levels in U.S. population aged 20–74 years. *Diabetes* 36:523, 1987.
6. Hollingsworth, D. R., and Moore, T. R. Diabetes and Pregnancy. In R. K. Creasy and R. Resnik (eds.), *Maternal-Fetal Medicine: Principles and Practice* (2nd ed.). Philadelphia: Saunders, 1989. Pp. 925–988.
7. Horvat, M., et al. Diabetic retinopathy in pregnancy: A 12 year prospective survey. *Br. J. Ophthalmol.* 64:398, 1980.
8. Kitzmiller, J. L. Diabetic nephropathy and perinatal outcome. *Am. J. Obstet. Gynecol.* 141:741, 1981.
9. Leiken, E. L., et al. Abnormal glucose screening tests in pregnancy: A risk factor for fetal macrosomia. *Obstet. Gynecol.* 69:570, 1987.
10. Mills, J. L., Baker, L., and Goldman, A. S. Malformations in infants of diabetic mothers occur before the seventh gestational week. *Diabetes* 28:292, 1979.
11. Mills, J. L., et al. Incidence of spontaneous abortion among normal and insulin dependent diabetic women whose pregnancies were identified within 21 days of conception. *N. Engl. J. Med.* 319:1617, 1988.
12. Moloney, J. B. M., and Drury, M. I. The effect of pregnancy on the natural course of diabetic pregnancies. *N. Engl. J. Med.* 93:745, 1982.
13. National Diabetes Data Group. Classification and diagnosis of diabetes mellitus and other categories of glucose intolerance. *Diabetes* 28:1039–1057, 1979.
14. O'Sullivan, J. B., and Mahan, C. M. Criteria for the oral glucose tolerance test in pregnancy. *Diabetes* 13:278, 1964.
15. O'Sullivan, J. B., et al. Screening for high-risk gestational diabetes patients. *Am. J. Obstet. Gynecol.* 116:895, 1973.
16. Phelps, R. L., Sakol, P., and Metzger, B. E. Changes in diabetic retinopathy during pregnancy. Corrections with regulation of hyperglycemia. *Arch. Ophthalmol.* 104:1806, 1986.
17. Position statement on gestational diabetes mellitus: Formulated by the American Diabetes Association. *Am. J. Obstet. Gynecol.* 156:488, 1987.
18. Reece, E. A., and Hobbins, J. C. Diabetic embryopathy: Pathogenesis, prenatal diagnosis and prevention. *Obstet. Gynecol. Surv.* 41:325, 1986.
19. Schaeffer, L. D., Wilder, M. L., and Williams, R. H. Secretion and content of insulin and glucagon in human fetal pancreatic slices in vitro. *Proc. Soc. Exp. Biol. Med.* 143:314, 1973.

20. Second International Workshop-Conference on Gestational Diabetes Mellitus. *Diabetes* 34:123, 1985.
21. Tyson, J. E., and Felig, P. Medical aspects of diabetes in pregnancy and the diabetogenic effects of oral contraceptives. *Med. Clin. North Am.* 55:947, 1971.
22. White, P. Classification of obstetric diabetes. *Am. J. Obstet. Gynecol.* 130:227, 1978.
23. Wolf, H., et al. Evidence for impermeability of the human placenta for insulin. *Horm. Metab. Res.* 1:274, 1969.

THYROID

24. Amino, N., et al. High relevance of transient postpartum thyrotoxicosis and hyperthyroidism. *N. Engl. J. Med.* 306:849, 1982.
25. Burrow, G. N. Maternal-fetal considerations in hyperthyroidism. *Clin. Endocrinol. Metab.* 7:115, 1978.
26. Burrow, G. N., Klatskin, E. H., and Genel, M. Intellectual development in children whose mothers received propylthiouracil during pregnancy. *Yale J. Biol. Med.* 51:151, 1978.
27. Cooper, D. S. Antithyroid drugs. *N. Engl. J. Med.* 311:1353, 1984.
28. Dorfman, S. G., et al. Painless thyroiditis and transient hyperthyroidism without goiter. *Ann. Intern. Med.* 86:24, 1977.
29. Dowling, J. T., et al. Effects of pregnancy on iodine metabolism in the primate. *J. Clin. Endcrinol. Metab.* 21:779, 1961.
30. Fisher, D. A., and Klein, A. H. Thyroid development and disorders of thyroid function in the newborn. *N. Engl. J. Med.* 304:702, 1981.
31. Harada, A., et al. Comparison of thyroid stimulators and thyroid hormone concentrations in the sera of pregnant women. *J. Clin. Endocrinol. Metab.* 48:793, 1979.
32. Innerfield, R., and Hollander, C. S. Thyroid complications of pregnancy. *Med. Clin. North Am.* 61:81, 1977.
33. Kampmann, J. P., et al. Propylthiouracil in human milk: revision of a dogma. *Lancet* 1:736, 1980.
34. Marchant, B., et al. The placental transfer of propylthiouracil, methimazole, and carbimazole. *J. Clin. Endocrinol. Metab.* 45:1187, 1977.
35. McCarroll, A. M., et al. Long-term assessment of children exposed in utero to carbimazole. *Arch. Dis. Child.* 51:532, 1976.
36. Milham, S., Jr., and Elledge, W. Maternal methimazole and congenital defects in children. *Teratology* 5:125, 1972.
37. Montoro, M., et al. Successful outcome of pregnancy in women with hypothyroidism. *Ann. Intern. Med.* 94:31, 1981.
38. Montoro, M., and Mestman, J. H. Graves' disease and pregnancy. *N. Engl. J. Med.* 305:48, 1981.
39. Munro, D. S., et al. The role of thyroid stimulating immunoglobulin of Graves' disease in neonatal thyrotoxicosis. *Br. J. Obstet. Gynaecol.* 85:837, 1978.
40. Myant, N. B. Passage of thyroxine and triiodothyronine from mother to fetus in pregnant women. *Clin. Sci.* 17:75, 1958.
41. Nikolai, T. F., et al. Lymphocytic thyroiditis with spontaneously resolving hyperthyroidism (silent thyroiditis). *Arch. Intern. Med.* 140:478, 1980.
42. Nikolai, T. F., Turney, S., and Roberts, R. The prevalence and clinical course of postpartum thyroiditis. Program of the 64th Annual Meeting of the Endocrine Society, San Francisco, June 16–18, 1982.
43. Pochin, E. E. The iodine uptake of the human thyroid throughout the menstrual cycle and in pregnancy. *Clin. Sci.* 11:441, 1952.
44. Ramsay, I. Thyroid disease in pregnancy. *Hosp. Update* 6:685, 1980.
45. Roti, E., Gnudi, A., and Braverman, L. E. The placental transport function. *Endocr. Rev.* 4:131, 1983.
46. Serup, J. Pregnancy and birth associated with thyrotoxicosis. *Dan. Med. Bull.* 26:74, 1979.
47. Woolf, P. D. Transient painless thyroiditis with hyperthyroidism: A variant of lymphocytic thyroiditis? *Endocr. Rev.* 4:411, 1980.

PARATHYROID

48. Burrow, G. N. Pituitary, Adrenal, and Parathyroid Disorders. In G. N. Burrow and T. F. Ferris (eds.), *Medical Complications During Pregnancy*. Philadelphia: Saunders, 1982.
49. Clark, D., Seeds, J. W., and Cefalo, R. C. Hyperthyroid crisis and pregnancy. *Am. J. Obstet. Gynecol.* 140:840, 1981.
50. Delmonico, F., et al. Hyperthyroidism during pregnancy. *Am. J. Surg.* 131:328, 1976.
51. Deutsch, A. A., et al. The diagnosis and management of hyperparathyroidism during pregnancy. *Am. J. Obstet. Gynecol.* 140:840, 1981.
52. Johnston, R. E., II, Kreindler, T., and Johnstone, R. E. Hyperparathyroidism during pregnancy. *Obstet. Gynecol.* 40:580, 1972.
53. Montoro, M. N., Collea, J. V., and Mestman, J. Management of hyperparathyroidism in pregnancy with oral phosphate therapy. *Obstet. Gynecol.* 55:4, 1980.
54. Moore, E. S., et al. Role of fetal 1,25 (OH)2 D production in intrauterine phosphorus and calcium homeostasis. *Pediatr. Res.* 19:566, 1985.
55. Northrop, G., Misenhimer, H. R., and Becker, F. O. Failure of parathormone to cross the non-human primate placenta. *Am. J. Obstet. Gynecol.* 129:449, 1977.
56. Patterson, R. Hyperparathyroidism in pregnancy. *Obstet. Gynecol.* 70:457, 1987.

ADRENALS

57. Aron, D. C., et al. Cushing's syndrome: Problems in diagnosis. *Medicine* (Baltimore) 60:25, 1981.
58. Aron, D. C., et al. Cushing's syndrome: Problems in management. *Endocr. Rev.* 3:229, 1982.
59. Bongiovanni, A. M., Elberlein, W. R., and Cara, J. Studies on the metabolism of adrenal steroids in the adrenogenital syndrome. *J. Clin. Endocrinol. Metab.* 14:409, 1954.
60. Bravo, E. L., et al. The changing clinical spectrum of primary aldosteronism. *Am. J. Med.* 74:641, 1983.
61. Bravo, E., and Gifford, R. W. Pheochromocytoma: Diagnosis, localization, and management. *N. Engl. J. Med.* 311:298, 1984.
62. Brown, M. J. Catecholamine measurements in clinical medicine. *Postgrad. Med.* 59:479, 1983.
63. Gormley, M., et al. Cushing's syndrome in pregnancy—treatment with metyrapone. *Clin. Endocrinol.* 16:283, 1982.
64. Hendon, J. R., and Melick, R. A. Pregnancy in Addison's disease. *Obstet. Gynecol. Surv.* 10:498, 1955.
65. Irvine, W. J. J., Toft, A. D., and Feek, C. M. Addison's Disease. In V. H. T. James (ed.), *The Adrenal Gland*. New York: Raven, 1979.
66. Jones, H. W. A long look at the adrenogenital syndrome. *Johns Hopkins Med. J.* 145:143, 1979.
67. Jones, H. W., and Verkauf, B. S. Congenital adrenal hyperplasia: Age at menarche and related events at puberty. *Am. J. Obstet. Gynecol.* 196:292, 1971.
68. Lauritzen, C., and Klopper, A. Estrogens and Androgens. In F. Fuchs and A. Klopper (eds.), *Endocrinology of Pregnancy* (3rd ed.). Philadelphia: Harper & Row, 1983. P. 73.
69. Lee, P. A., et al. (eds.). *Congenital Adrenal Hyperplasia*. Baltimore: University Park, 1977.
70. Klingensmith, G. J., et al. Glucocorticoid treatment of girls with congenital adrenal hyperplasia: Effects on height, sexual maturation, and fertility. *J. Pediatr.* 90:996, 1977.
71. Miyakawa, I., Ikeda, I., and Maeyama, M. Transport of ACTH across human placenta. *J. Clin. Endocrinol. Metab.* 39:440, 1974.
72. Schenker, J. G., and Chowers, I. Pheochromocytoma and pregnancy. *Obstet. Gynecol. Surv.* 26:739, 1971.

73. Sodha, R. J., Proegler, M., and Schneider, H. Transfer and metabolism of norepinephrine studied from maternal-to-fetal and fetal-to-maternal sides in vitro profused human placental lobe. *Am. J. Obstet. Gynecol.* 148:474, 1984.
74. Weinberger, M. Primary aldosteronism: Diagnosis and differentiation of subtypes. *Ann. Intern. Med.* 100:300, 1984.
75. Weinberger, M. H., et al. Primary aldosteronism: Diagnosis, localization, and treatment. *Ann. Intern. Med.* 90:386, 1979.

PITUITARY

76. Hime, M. C., and Richardson, J. Diabetes insipidus and pregnancy. *Obstet. Gynecol. Surv.* 33:375, 1978.
77. Laron, A., et al. Lack of placental transfer of human growth hormone. *Acta Endocrinol.* (Copenh.) 53:687, 1966.
78. Miller, M., et al. Recognition of partial defects in antidiuretic hormone secretion. *Ann. Intern. Med.* 73:721, 1970.
79. Molitch, M. E. Pregnancy and the hyperprolactinemic woman. *N. Engl. J. Med.* 312:364, 1985.
80. Schlecte, J. A., et al. Long-term follow up of women with surgically treated prolactin-secreting tumors. *J. Clin. Endocrinol. Metab.* 62:1296, 1986.
81. Stegner, H., et al. Permeability of the sheep placenta to 124-arginine vasopressin. *Dev. Pharmacol. Ther.* 7:140, 1984.
82. Vance, M. L., et al. Bromocriptine. *Ann. Intern. Med.* 100:78, 1984.
83. Warfield, A., et al. Bromocriptine treatment of prolactin secreting pituitary adenomas may restore pituitary function. *Ann. Intern. Med.* 101:783, 1984.

Selected Readings

Fuhrmann, K., et al. Prevention of congenital malformations in infants of insulin dependent diabetic mothers. *Diabetes Care* 6:219, 1983.

James, D. K., et al. Maternal diabetes and neonatal respiratory distress: I. Maturation of fetal surfactant. *Br. J. Obstet. Gynaecol.* 91:316, 1984.

Komis, J. L., Snyder, P. F., and Schwarz, R. H. Hyperthyroidism in pregnancy. *Obstet. Gynecol. Surv.* 30:527, 1975.

Miller, E., et al. Elevated maternal hemoglobin A.C. in early pregnancy and major congenital anomalies in infants of diabetic mothers. *N. Engl. J. Med.* 304:1331, 1981.

Mujtaba, Q., and Burrow, G. N. Treatment of hyperthyroidism in pregnancy with propylthiouracil and methimazole. *Obstet. Gynecol.* 46:282, 1975.

Van Der Spuy, Z. M., and Jacobs, H. S. Management of endocrine disorders in pregnancy. Part I—Thyroid and parathyroid disease. *Postgrad. Med.* 60:245, 1984.

Van Der Spuy, Z. M., and Jacobs, H. S. Management of endocrine disorders in pregnancy. Part II—Pituitary, ovarian, and adrenal disease. *Postgrad. Med.* 60:312, 1984.

11 Infectious Disease Complications

Stuart H. Cohen and
Elliot Goldstein

I. Use of antibiotics in pregnancy. Except for the additional consideration of fetal toxicity, the selection of antibiotics for treatment in pregnant women is the same as for nonpregnant women. Antimicrobial efficacy and toxicity are almost always unaltered in pregnancy. The two distinctive considerations in pregnancy are the potential toxicity for the fetus or mother of some commonly used antibiotics (e.g., sulfonamides, tetracyclines) and the occasional need for higher drug dosages owing to the expanded blood volume, increased renal blood flow, and increased glomerular filtration rate, which reduce drug levels below the therapeutic range [14, 34, 38]. Appropriate microbial smears and cultures should be obtained before therapy is instituted to identify pathogens and to determine their antimicrobial susceptibility patterns. If the smear is not helpful diagnostically, treatment is instituted on the basis of an educated guess concerning the likely pathogens for a particular infection (e.g., urinary tract infections are most often caused by *Escherichia coli*). Interpretation of culture results from the female genital tract requires knowledge of the normal flora. This flora, which is unchanged by pregnancy, consists of aerobic and anaerobic bacteria and small numbers of fungi, usually *Candida* sp.

A. Normal vaginal flora of pregnancy

1. **Commonly isolated flora** include *Staphylococcus epidermidis**, *Enterococcus faecalis**, *Lactobacillus* sp., *Corynebacterium* sp., *Bacteroides fragilis**, *Fusobacterium* sp., *Veillonella* sp., *Peptococcus* sp., and *Peptostreptococcus* sp.
2. **Occasionally isolated flora** include *Staphylococcus aureus**, *Streptococcus* sp.*, *Clostridium perfringens**, *Candida* sp., *E. coli**, *Proteus* sp.*, *Klebsiella* sp.*, *Actinomyces* sp., and *Mobiluncus* sp.
3. **Potential pathogens** are *Pseudomonas* sp., *Streptococcus pneumoniae, Listeria monocytogenes, Neisseria gonorrhoeae, Chlamydia trachomatis,* and *Haemophilus aphrophilus*.

B. Effect of selected antibiotics and antiviral agents on mother and fetus (Table 11-1)

1. **Penicillins.** Penicillins are safe in pregnancy. There is no increase in maternal toxicity and no known fetal toxicity [14, 38].
2. **Cephalosporins.** Cephalosporins are safe and do not cause increased fetal toxicity. Information about the newer cephalosporins (ceftazidime, cefotaxime, cefoperazone, ceftriaxone, cefuroxime) is limited, but these agents appear to have unaltered toxicity in pregnancy and to be nontoxic to the fetus [14, 38].
3. **Tetracyclines.** Parenteral tetracycline can cause fulminant maternal hepatitis and pancreatitis when administered during the third trimester of pregnancy. Oral tetracycline causes staining and deformity of deciduous teeth as well as inhibition of bone growth in the fetus [14, 38].
4. **Sulfonamides.** Maternal toxicity does not increase with sulfonamides. Fetal toxicity occurs in the perinatal period, when the inability of the neonatal liver to conjugate sulfonamides results in hyperbilirubinemia and kernicterus caused by blockage of the binding sites necessary to conjugate bilirubin. When used prior to the perinatal period, the maternal liver removes sulfonamide from the fetal bloodstream [14, 38].

*Significant pathogen.

Table 11-1. Antibiotics and antiviral agents and pregnancy[a]

Antimicrobial agent	Problem in pregnancy	Passes placenta	Harmful to fetus	Harmful to neonate
Acyclovir		Yes		No
Amantadine	Possible			
Amikacin	No[b]	Yes	Possible[c]	Possible[c]
Amoxicillin/clavulanate	No[b]	Yes	No[b]	
Amphotericin B	No[b]	Yes		
Ampicillin	No[b]	Yes	No[b]	No
Ampicillin/sulbactam	No[b]	Yes	No[b]	
Aztreonam	No[b]	Yes	No[b]	
Cefaclor	No[b]	Yes	No[b]	
Cefadroxil	No[b]	Yes	No[b]	
Cefamandole	No[b]	Yes	No[b]	No[b]
Cefazolin	No[b]	Yes	No[b]	
Cefonicid	No[b]	Yes	No[b]	
Cefoperazone	No[b]	Yes	No[b]	
Ceforanide	No[b]	Yes	No[b]	No[b]
Cefotaxime	No[b]	Yes	No[b]	No
Cefotetan	No[b]	Yes	No[b]	
Cefoxitin	No[b]	Yes	No[b]	Possible[d]
Ceftazidime	No[b]	Yes	No[b]	No
Ceftizoxime	No[b]	Yes	No[b]	Possible[d]
Ceftriaxone	No[b]	Yes	No[b]	No[e]
Cefuroxime	No[b]	Yes	No[b]	
Cephalexin	No[b]	Yes	No[b]	
Cephradine	No[b]	Yes	No[b]	
Chloramphenicol	No[b]	Yes	No[b]	Yes
Ciprofloxacin	Yes	Yes	Possible	Yes
Clindamycin		Yes		No[b]
Cloxacillin	No	Yes	No[b]	No
Dapsone	Possible	Yes	Possible	Possible
Dicloxacillin	No	Yes	No[b]	
Doxycycline	Yes	Yes	Yes	Yes
Erythromycin		Yes	No[b]	
Ethambutol	No[b]	Yes	No[b]	
Fluconazole		Yes	Possible	Possible
Flucytosine		Yes	Possible[f]	
Ganciclovir		Yes	Possible	Possible[g]
Gentamicin	No[b]	Yes	Possible[c]	Possible[c]
Imipenem/cilistatin	No[b]			
Isoniazid	No	Yes	One report unconfirmed	No[b]
Kanamycin	No[b]	Yes	Possible[c]	Possible[c]
Ketoconazole		Yes	Possible[h]	Possible[h]
Methenamine mandelate				
Methicillin	No	Yes	No[b]	No
Metronidazole	Yes[b,i]	Yes	Yes[i]	
Mezlocillin	No	Yes	No[b]	No

Table 11-1. (continued)

Antimicrobial agent	Problem in pregnancy	Passes placenta	Harmful to fetus	Harmful to neonate
Minocycline	Yes	Yes	Yes	Yes
Nafcillin	No	Yes	No[b]	No
Nalidixic acid	Yes[j]	Yes	Yes[j]	Yes[k]
Netilmicin	No	Yes	Possible[c]	Possible[c]
Nitrofurantoin		Yes		Yes
Norfloxacin	Yes	Yes	Yes	Yes
Oxacillin	No[b]	Yes	No[b]	
Penicillin G	No	Yes	No[b]	
Penicillin V potassium	No			
Pentamidine				
Piperacillin	No[b]	Yes	No[b]	
Pyrazinamide				
Pyrimethamine	Yes	Yes	Yes[l]	
Rifampin	No[b]	Yes	Possible[b]	
Spectinomycin				
Streptomycin	No	Yes	Rare[b]	
Sulfonamides	No[m]	Yes	No[b,m]	Yes
Tetracycline	Yes	Yes	Yes	Yes
Ticarcillin/clavulanate	No[b]	Yes	No[b]	
Tobramycin	No[b]	Yes	Possible[c]	Possible[c]
Trimethoprim and sulfamethoxazole	Yes	Yes	Yes[m,n]	Yes
Vancomycin			Possible[c]	Possible[c]
Zidovudine	Possible			

Notes: Breast milk levels of greater than 50% of maternal serum levels are seen with acyclovir, ampicillin, carbenicillin, chloramphenicol, erythromycin, isoniazid, metronidazole, tetracycline, and sulfonamides. Breast milk levels of less than 25% of maternal levels are seen with aztreonam, cefazolin, cefotaxime, cefoxitin, clindamycin, nalidixic acid, nitrofurantoin, methicillin, oxacillin, penicillin G, penicillin V potassium, and pyrimethamine.

[a]Blank spaces indicate information not well known.

[b]Not known to be harmful, but no adequate and well-controlled studies have been performed for pregnant women; therefore, should be used during pregnancy only if clearly needed.

[c]Ototoxicity and nephrotoxicity are potential consequences of use.

[d]Safety in infants from birth to 3 months has not yet been established. In older children, the drug's use has been associated with high incidence of increased eosinophils and elevated serum aspartate aminotransferase.

[e]Ceftriaxone should not be given to hyperbilirubinemic neonates, especially prematures.

[f]Teratogenic effects have been seen in rats that metabolize flucytosine to fluorouracil.

[g]Ganciclovir should be used with extreme caution in neonates due to the probability of carcinogenicity.

[h]Has been shown to be teratogenic to rats in high doses (10 times maximum human doses). Has also been shown to be embryotoxic in rats during the first trimester in the same dosage. Dystocia was noted in rats receiving ketoconazole in the third trimester. It probably is excreted in breast milk; therefore, mothers who are on ketoconazole should not breast-feed their children.

[i]A potential carcinogen.

[j]Safety established for second and third trimesters only.

[k]Increased central nervous system side effects in neonates.

[l]Significant teratogenic effect in the first and probably the second trimesters. Safe in the third trimester if clinically warranted. Used for treatment of toxoplasmosis.

[m]If given in large doses shortly before delivery, hyperbilirubinemia and kernicterus may occur in the neonate.

[n]Not recommended; trimethoprim is a folate antagonist.

Source: Adapted from L. D. Sabath, Use of Antibiotics in Obstetrics. In D. Charles and M. Finland (eds.), *Obstetrics and Perinatal Infections*. Philadelphia: Lea & Febiger, 1973. P. 564.

5. **Chloramphenicol.** No increase in maternal toxicity occurs with chloramphenicol. Inability of the neonatal liver to conjugate chloramphenicol results in the "gray-baby syndrome," which is characterized by gray facies, generalized flaccidity, hypothermia, and cardiovascular collapse [14, 38].
6. **Aminoglycosides.** The risk of ototoxicity and nephrotoxicity secondary to use of gentamicin, kanamycin, netilmicin, streptomycin, amikacin, or tobramycin is the same in the pregnant and nonpregnant woman. Fetal toxicity to the eighth cranial nerve has occurred after prolonged use of streptomycin in treating tuberculosis. Streptomycin should not be used unless isoniazid, ethambutol, or rifampin is contraindicated. These drugs may also cause nephrotoxicity in the fetus; therefore, their use should be limited as much as possible [25, 38, 40].
7. **Erythromycin.** No increase in maternal toxicity and no known fetal toxicity occur with erythromycin. The estolate form of this drug causes transient, self-limited elevations of serum transaminases, particularly in the latter half of pregnancy, so treatment with this agent is considered inadvisable [30, 38].
8. **Clindamycin.** Maternal or fetal toxicity is not known to increase with clindamycin. Because the drug enters fetal bone in high concentrations after parenteral administration, bone growth should be followed in infants exposed prenatally to clindamycin [14, 38].
9. **Trimethoprim-sulfamethoxazole.** Maternal toxicity does not increase with trimethoprim and sulfamethoxazole, but folic acid antagonists may increase anemia. Although unproved clinically, trimethoprim has the potential for teratogenicity, and therefore this drug should not be used unless absolutely indicated [38, 39].
10. **Isoniazid.** Maternal or fetal toxicity does not increase. Isoniazid is recommended for treatment of active tuberculosis. Chemoprophylaxis is not recommended during pregnancy [25, 40].
11. **Rifampin and ethambutol.** No increase in maternal toxicity and no known toxic effect on the fetus occur with rifampin or ethambutol, but experience is insufficient to certify their safety. Because fetal limb deformities of uncertain relationship to rifampin have occurred, ethambutol appears safer than rifampin [25, 40].
12. **Pyrimethamine.** Although no increase in maternal toxicity is known, pyrimethamine should not be used in the first or second trimester because it is potentially teratogenic. If absolutely warranted, pyrimethamine can be used in the third trimester [12, 28].
13. **Pentamidine.** Safety of pentamidine during pregnancy has not been established. Therefore, it should be used with caution [32].
14. **Acyclovir.** No established indications exist for the use of acyclovir during pregnancy. Animal studies and anecdotal use in humans suggest it is safe. Therefore, it should be used with caution to treat only life-threatening maternal infections [8, 14].
15. **Zidovudine.** Zidovudine (AZT) is the only therapy proved to prolong life in persons infected with the human immunodeficiency virus (HIV). Bone marrow suppression is caused by AZT, and its carcinogenicity and teratogenicity have not been studied. Presently, AZT is not recommended for use during pregnancy [32].

C. Causes of antibiotic failure

1. **Human factors**
   - **a.** Incorrect diagnosis
   - **b.** Treatment initiated too late
   - **c.** Antibiotic not given or taken improperly owing to prescription error or lack of compliance
2. **Drug factors**
   - **a.** Inadequate dose or inappropriate dose interval. (Pregnant women may require higher dosages than nonpregnant women because of altered pharmacokinetics.)
   - **b.** Inadequate course of therapy

c. Wrong route of administration
d. Failure of drug to reach site of infection
e. Incompatibility of antibiotics and other drugs present in the intravenous infusion
f. Drug fever

3. **Pathogen factors**
a. Microbial resistance
b. Bacteria in dormant state
c. Superinfection

4. **Host factors**
a. New, unrelated infection elsewhere in body
b. Rapid degradation of the antibiotic (e.g., acetylation of isoniazid)
c. Failure to institute appropriate supportive measures (e.g., surgical drainage, debridement, or dilatation and curettage)
d. Normal variation in clinical course
e. Impaired host defenses resulting from underlying illness or immunosuppressive therapy

II. Cell-mediated and humoral immunity in pregnancy

A. Investigations of the immunocompetency of pregnant women indicate selective depressions of cell-mediated and humoral immunity of uncertain clinical significance [44].

B. Pregnant women, particularly in their third trimester of pregnancy, have greater susceptibility to some infections.

1. **Viral illnesses.** The severity of illness is increased with infection caused by poliovirus, hepatitis A and B, influenza, and smallpox. Primary herpes progenitalis and disseminated herpes simplex are more apt to occur in pregnant women, and reactivation rates for cytomegalovirus (CMV) and Epstein-Barr virus are increased.
2. **Bacterial illnesses.** Pregnancy confers heightened susceptibility to infection with *L. monocytogenes, Salmonella typhi, S. pneumoniae,* and *N. gonorrhoeae,* as well as an increased risk of miliary tuberculosis.
3. **Fungal illnesses.** The risk of dissemination following a primary infection with *Coccidioides immitis* is increased in pregnant women.
4. **Protozoan illnesses.** The severity of infection with *Entamoeba histolytica, Giardia lamblia,* and *Toxoplasma gondii* is increased during pregnancy, as are the incidence and rate of complications of malaria.

III. Viral diseases

A. **Influenza** is an acute, communicable infection that occurs primarily in winter months [4, 26, 27]. Because of its high infectivity and frequency of genetic mutation, novel strains of orthomyxovirus influenza, the etiologic agent, often cause major epidemics.

1. **Diagnosis**
a. Generalized symptoms of headache, fever, myalgia, malaise, cough, and substernal chest pain appear abruptly within one to two days after infection.
b. Physical examination may reveal basilar rales.
c. The chest roentgenogram may show bilateral interstitial infiltrates.
d. Gram's stains of sputum show insignificant numbers of bacteria and mononuclear cells.
e. Identification of the virus within exfoliated epithelial cells after reaction with fluorescent conjugates of an influenza antiserum is the only rapid method of definitive diagnosis.
f. The virus can be cultured from nasopharyngeal washings, nasal swabs, and throat swabs.
g. Serum antibody is detectable two to three weeks after infection by hemagglutination-inhibition, neutralization, or complement-fixation antibody testing. Paired specimens are necessary for the diagnosis.

2. **Prognosis.** Influenza generally is a self-limited disease, but serious morbidity and mortality do occur.
a. **Mother.** Pregnant women are a high-risk group during influenzal epidem-

ics. Increased mortality is caused by viral pneumonia itself and by superimposed staphylococcal and gram-negative enteric pneumonias. Rates of spontaneous abortion are as high as 25–50%.

b. Influenza virus can be transplacentally transmitted to the fetus. Many studies of large numbers of patients have failed to link influenza and congenital malformations. However, serious maternal illness with hypoxia can cause premature labor and abortion.

3. Management

a. Amantadine hydrochloride, an orally administrable antiviral agent, reduces the incidence and severity of influenza A infections when given before and in the initial period of clinical symptomatology. The drug has not been investigated extensively in pregnancy, and its effect on the fetus, if any, is unknown. Amantadine at higher than therapeutic doses is embryotoxic and teratogenic in rats. As such, this drug should be used only if the potential benefit justifies the risk to the embryo or fetus [14]. In addition, amantadine is found in breast milk [14].

b. Pregnant women who are seriously ill should be hospitalized.

c. Prophylactic treatment with nafcillin and gentamicin is indicated to prevent or minimize superinfection in severely ill patients.

d. Immunization with type-specific vaccines is indicated before or in the first trimester of pregnancy if cardiopulmonary disease or diabetes is present. Influenza vaccine is an inactivated virus considered nonhazardous to the fetus (Table 11-2).

B. Measles (rubeola) is a highly contagious, exanthematous, common childhood disease with peak incidence in the spring [10, 27]. Widespread vaccination had reduced the number of cases in the United States from 200,000–400,000/year to fewer than 1500 cases reported in 1983. Due to vaccine failures, the number of cases of measles is increasing with more than 14,000 cases reported in 1989 [10].

1. Diagnosis

a. Small, irregular, bright red spots (Koplik's spots) that are diagnostic of measles appear on buccal and sometimes other mucosal membranes at the end of the 10- to 14-day incubation period.

b. Catarrhal symptoms of coryza, cough, keratoconjunctivitis, and fever are prominent early in the illness.

c. The maculopapular rash begins on the face and spreads downward to the extremities.

d. The rash, which often becomes confluent, fades in the same sequence.

e. Patients who are partially immune have milder catarrh, fewer Koplik's spots, and a more discrete and fainter rash.

f. Measles virus can be identified by immunofluorescent testing in smears from nasal secretions, sputum, and oropharyngeal surfaces and by culture of these specimens.

g. Fourfold or greater increases in hemagglutination-inhibition, neutralizing, or complement-fixing antibodies can be demonstrated in convalescent serum drawn two to three weeks after infection.

2. Prognosis

a. Mother. Morbidity from the respiratory symptoms and rash and mortality from the infrequent complications of encephalitis and myocarditis are the same for pregnant and nonpregnant women. Spontaneous abortions and premature deliveries are common.

b. Fetus. Measles virus penetrates the placenta, and neonates are born with or develop typical exanthematous lesions. Most reports, but not all, indicate no increase in congenital malformations in infants born to infected mothers [27].

3. Management

a. Supportive measures of bed rest, fluids, antipyretics, expectorants, and steam inhalation reduce morbidity.

b. Immune serum gamma globulin (0.5 ml/kg) given within six days after exposure minimizes or prevents measles symptomatology.

Table 11-2. Immunization for viral infections during pregnancy

	Influenza	Measles	Rubella	Mumps	Poliomyelitis	Hepatitis B
Risk of disease to pregnant women	Increase in morbidity and mortality, particularly during epidemics	Significant morbidity; low mortality; not altered by pregnancy	Low morbidity and mortality, not altered by pregnancy	Low morbidity and mortality, not altered by pregnancy	Increased incidence and severity in pregnancy	Possible increase in severity in pregnant women from nutritionally deprived backgrounds
Risk of disease to fetus or neonate	Increased rate of abortion; no increase in malformations	Significant increase in abortion rate; no malformations reported	High rate of abortion and congenital rubella syndrome in first trimester	Slightly increased fetal mortality in serious infections; no confirmed congenital abnormalities	Anoxic fetal damage reported; 25% mortality in neonatal disease; paralysis but no increase in congenital abnormalities	Hepatitis B is transmitted transplacentally, sometimes causing neonatal hepatitis; no increase in congenital defects or abortions
Vaccine	Inactivated type A and type B virus vaccines	Live attenuated virus vaccine	Live attenuated virus vaccine	Live attenuated virus vaccine	Live attenuated virus vaccine (Sabin) or killed virus vaccine (Salk)	Recombinant subunit vaccine (HBsAg)

Risk of vaccine to fetus	None confirmed	None confirmed	None confirmed; teratogenicity is suspected	None confirmed	None confirmed	Unknown
Indications for vaccination during pregnancy	Recommended for patients with serious underlying disease	Contraindicated	Contraindicated	Contraindicated	Not recommended for adults except in epidemics or close contact with a suspected case	Recommended for pregnant women at high risk
Comments	Amantadine may be of value in influenza A infections, but because of possible teratogenicity, its use should be avoided	0.25 ml/kg immune serum globulin to exposed susceptible women within 6 d of exposure	Serologic testing of women in childbearing age should determine need for vaccination	Passive immunization with mumps is not indicated	Salk vaccine indicated for nonimmunized women traveling in endemic areas (see text for details)	Immune serum globulin has failed to prevent hepatitis B in neonates; hepatitis B immune globulin and vaccine should be given to neonates (see text for details)

Source: Adapted from E. A. Leontic, Respiratory disease in pregnancy. *Med. Clin. North Am.* 61:111, 1977.

c. Secondary bacterial complications, particularly pneumonia, are treated with appropriate antibiotics (Table 11-3).

4. **Prevention**

a. Pregnant women who are exposed to measles and who are susceptible (i.e., do not have antibody) should receive gamma globulin [10]. Infants born to women with active measles should receive gamma globulin (0.25 ml/kg).

b. Women who have not had measles or documented measles immunity should receive two doses of the live virus vaccine, one month apart, at least 30 days prior to becoming pregnant [10]. Vaccine is contraindicated during pregnancy (see Table 11-2).

c. Women who were born after 1956 and were vaccinated prior to 1980 should be revaccinated with two doses of the live virus vaccine before becoming pregnant, owing to waning immunity [10].

C. **Rubella** (German measles) is a highly contagious, exanthematous disease of childhood and early adulthood. Despite the availability of effective vaccines, up to 20% of women in the childbearing age do not possess rubella antibody [9, 35].

1. **Diagnosis**

a. Fever, cough, conjunctivitis, headache, arthralgias, and myalgias occur after a 14- to 21-day incubation period and a 1- to 5-day prodromal period.

b. Postauricular, occipital, and cervical lymphadenopathy are prominent early findings. Arthritis is a frequent occurrence in adult women.

c. The maculopapular rash begins on the face, spreads downward, and subsequently fades in the same top-to-bottom order.

d. The illness lasts from a few days to two weeks.

e. Rubella virus can be isolated from pharyngeal secretions, blood, urine, and stools.

f. Increases in hemagglutination-inhibition, neutralizing, and complement-fixing antibodies are demonstrable two to four weeks after infection. Most laboratories presently use enzyme-linked immunosorbent assay (ELISA) or latex agglutination testing of paired sera to detect recent infection.

2. **Prognosis**

a. **Mother.** Morbidity from the rash, respiratory illness, arthritis, and infrequent encephalitis is the same for pregnant and nonpregnant women. Fatality is rare. Spontaneous abortion and stillbirth are 2–4 times more frequent in pregnancies complicated by rubella.

b. **Fetus.** Direct infection of the fetus occurs. If the disease is acquired during the first trimester of pregnancy, the risk of fetal malformation or death ranges from 10–34%. Acquisition of infection later in pregnancy results in fewer and usually less deleterious fetal abnormalities. Manifestations of congenital rubella include cataracts, blindness, cardiac anomalies (patent ductus arteriosus, ventricular septal defect, pulmonary valve stenosis), deafness, mental retardation, cerebral palsy, violaceous birthmarks, hepatosplenomegaly, thrombocytopenic purpura, hemolytic anemia, lymphadenopathy, encephalitis, and cleft palate.

3. **Management**

a. Supportive measures of bed rest, fluids, and aspirin for treatment of headache and arthritis usually suffice for this mild, self-limited illness.

b. Therapeutic abortion should be considered except in instances in which infection is known to occur in the third trimester of pregnancy. In 1989 only three cases of congenital rubella were reported to the Centers for Disease Control in Atlanta.

c. Methods to diagnose congenital rubella prenatally are improving but have not come into general use.

4. **Prevention.** Prepubertal and nonpregnant postpubertal women without documented antirubella antibodies should be immunized with live attenuated rubella vaccine. Women who are vaccinated should not become pregnant for three months after vaccination. Neither accidental immunization of a pregnant woman nor exposure to virus shed by recently immunized children has resulted in fetal infection (see Table 11-2).

Table 11-3. Recommended antibiotic treatment of selected sites of infection in pregnancy and the postpartum state

Infection	Usual causative organisms	Antibiotic regimen	Alternative regimen
Bacteriuria	*Escherichia coli*	Cephalexin, 500 mg PO qid for 7–10 d	Sulfisoxazole, 1 gm PO qid[a] for 7–10 d; or ampicillin 500 mg PO qid for 7–10 d
	Enterococcus faecalis	Ampicillin, 500 mg PO qid for 7–10 d	Based on bacterial susceptibility
	Proteus mirabilis	Ampicillin, 500 mg PO qid for 7–10 d	Cephalexin, 0.5–1.0 gm PO qid for 7–10 d
	Non–*Proteus mirabilis* sp.	Carbenicillin, 1–2 tablets PO qid for 7–10 d	Based on bacterial susceptibility
	Klebsiella sp.	Cephalexin, 500 mg PO qid	Sulfisoxazole, 1 gm PO qid[a] for 7–10 d
Endometritis and postpartum sepsis	Group A or B beta-hemolytic streptococcus	Penicillin G, 1×10^6 units IV q4–6h	Cefazolin, 50 mg/kg/d q8h
	Staphylococcus aureus	Nafcillin, 150–200 mg/kg/d IV q4h	Cefazolin, 1 gm IV q8h; or clindamycin, 25–35 mg/kg/d q8h
	E. coli	Gentamicin, 5 mg/kg/d IV q8h	Cefazolin, 50 mg/kg/d IV q8h; or ceftizoxime 1 gm IV q8h
	Bacteroides fragilis	Clindamycin, 25–35 mg/kg/d q8h	Ampicillin/sulbactam 1.5–3.0 gm IV q6h or metronidazole, 15 mg/kg loading dose followed by 7.5 mg/kg q8h[b]
Postinstrumentation (e.g., after dilatation and curettage or after instillation of abortifacients)	Mixed flora consisting of *B. fragilis*, group D streptococci, microaerophilic streptococci, gram-negative bacilli, *Clostridium perfringens*	Ampicillin, 150–200 mg/kg/d IV q4h; gentamicin, 5 mg/kg/d IV q8h; and clindamycin, 25–35 mg/kg/d IV q8h	Cefotetan 2 gm IV q12h (based on bacterial susceptibility)

Table 11-3. (continued)

Infection	Usual causative organisms	Antibiotic regimen	Alternative regimen
Pelvic abscess	Mixed aerobic and anaerobic flora consisting of *E. fecalis* group B beta-hemolytic streptococci, *E. coli,* peptostreptococcus, *B. fragilis*	Ampicillin, 150–200 mg/kg/d IV q4h; gentamicin, 5 mg/kg/d IV q8h; and clindamycin, 25–35 mg/kg/d IV q8h	Cefotetan, 2 gm IV q12h (based on bacterial susceptibility)
Pyelophlebitis	*Bacteroides* sp. or mixed flora of group D streptococci and gram-negative rods	Ampicillin, 150–200 mg/kg/d IV q4h; clindamycin, 25–35 mg/kg/d IV q8h; and gentamicin, 5 mg/kg/d IV q8h	Cefotetan, 2 gm IV q12h
Pneumonia	*Streptococcus pneumoniae*	Penicillin G, 1×10^6 units IV q6h; or penicillin G procaine, 600,000 units IM q12h	Erythromycin, 0.5 gm IV or PO q6h
	Mycoplasma pneumoniae	Erythromycin, 0.5 gm PO q6h	
	Haemophilus influenzae	Cefuroxime, 750 mg IV q8h	Ampicillin, 150–200 mg/kg/d IV q4h
	S. aureus	Nafcillin, 150–200 mg/kg/d IV q4h	Cefazolin, 50 mg/kg/d IV q8h; or clindamycin, 25–35 mg/kg/d PO or IV q8h
	Gram-negative enteric bacilli: *E. coli, K. pneumoniae, Enterobacter* sp., etc.,	Gentamicin or tobramycin, 5 mg/kg/d IV q8h	Ceftizoxime, 50 mg/kg/d IV q8h (based on bacterial susceptibility)
	Pseudomonas aeruginosa	Tobramycin, 5 mg/kg/d IV q8h; and piperacillin, 200–300 mg/kg/d IV q6h	Based on bacterial susceptibility
Cellulitis	*S. aureus*	Nafcillin, 150–200 mg/kg/d IV q4h	Cefazolin, 50 mg/kg/d IV q8h
	β-Hemolytic streptococci	Aqueous penicillin G, 1×10^6 units IV q4h	Cefazolin, 50 mg/kg/d IV q8h

Gonorrheal infection	*Neisseria gonorrhoeae* including penicillinase-producing *N. gonorrhoeae*		
Acute urethritis		Ceftriaxone, 250 mg IM	Amoxicillin, 3 gm PO, and probenecid, 1 gm (areas without resistant gonococci); or spectinomycin 2 gm IM (except for pharyngitis)
Arthritis, gonococcemia		Ceftriaxone, 1 gm IV or IM qd for 7–10 d	Erythromycin, 500 mg IV q6h for 7 d, or aqueous penicillin G, 10–12 $\times$ 10^6 units IV in q4h doses for 3 d, followed by ampicillin 500 mg PO qid for 5–7 d (if penicillin-susceptible)
Syphilis	*Treponema pallidum*		
Primary or secondary		Benzathine penicillin G, 2.4 $\times$ 10^6 units IM; or aqueous procaine penicillin G, 0.6–1.2 $\times$ 10^6 units IM qd for 10 d	Erythromycin, 500 mg q6h for 15 d
Tertiary		Benzathine penicillin G, 2.4 $\times$ 10^6 units/wk IM for 3 wk; or aqueous procaine penicillin G, 0.6–1.2 $\times$ 10^6 units IM qd for 15–20 d; or aqueous penicillin G, 2 $\times$ 10^6 units IV q4h for 10 d for neurosyphilis	Erythromycin, 500 mg q6h for 15–30 d[c]
Tuberculosis	*Mycobacterium tuberculosis*		
Pulmonary, minimal		Isoniazid, 300–600 mg PO qd, ethambutol, 15 mg/kg/d, and rifampin, 600 mg PO qd initially, and if susceptible isoniazid and ethambutol for 9 mo–1 yr	Isoniazid plus ethambutol, 15 mg/kg qd, and streptomycin, 1 gm qd for 2 mo
Cavitary disease, advanced		Isoniazid, 300–600 mg PO qd; rifampin, 600 mg PO qd; and ethambutol, 15 mg/kg/d for 9 mo–1 yr	

Table 11-3. (continued)

Infection	Usual causative organisms	Antibiotic regimen	Alternative regimen
Extrapulmonary, including genital		Isoniazid, 300–600 mg PO qd; rifampin, 600 mg PO qd; and ethambutol, 15 mg/kg/d for 9 mo–1 yr	
Vaginitis	*Trichomonas vaginalis*	Clotrimazole, two 100-mg vaginal tablets hs for 7 d	Metronidazole[b] should be avoided
	Candida sp.	Clotrimazole, 1 dose intravaginally hs for 7 d	Miconazole, 1 dose intravaginally hs for 7 d
	Herpes simplex virus	Acyclovir (see sec. **IV.A**)	
Toxoplasmosis	*Toxoplasma gondii*	Pyrimethamine, 100 mg PO for 1 d, then 25 mg PO qd for 1 mo, and sulfadiazine, 4 gm PO qd for 1 mo	Spiramycin 2–4 gm qd for 1 mo. Trimethoprim-sulfamethoxazole should be avoided owing to potential teratogenicity. Pyrimethamine teratogenic in first and probably second trimesters
Gas gangrene	*C. perfringens*	Aqueous penicillin G, 3×10^6 units IV q4h	Chloramphenicol, 50 mg/kg/d IV q6h[d]. Hysterectomy often necessary
Systemic mycoses	*Coccidioides immitis, Cryptococcus neoformans, Candida* sp., *Histoplasma capsulatum, Aspergillus* sp.	Amphotericin B beginning with 0.10–0.25 mg/kg body weight IV qd and gradually advancing daily to 0.75–1.0 mg/kg/qd	Ketoconazole, 200–600 mg PO qd, or fluconazole, 100–400 mg qd[e]

[a]Sulfonamides should not be used in the latter weeks of pregnancy owing to an increased incidence of kernicterus of the neonate.
[b]Metronidazole should be avoided in pregnancy as it may be mutagenic or carcinogenic.
[c]Not of proved efficacy.
[d]Chloramphenicol causes so-called gray-baby syndrome if given near term.
[e]Safety in pregnancy is not proved. These drugs should be used only with appropriate consultation.

D. Mumps is a common contagious disease of children and young adults [21, 27].

1. **Diagnosis**
   a. Fever, myalgia, malaise, and headache of variable severity occur after a two- to three-week incubation period.
   b. Parotitis is the most prominent feature, and this finding establishes the diagnosis.
   c. Mastitis and oophoritis can occur in postpubertal women.
   d. The demonstration of immunoglobulin M (IgM) antibody by immunofluorescent techniques or a fourfold or greater increase in serum complement-fixing antibody confirms the diagnosis.
2. **Prognosis**
   a. **Mother.** The morbidity from parotitis and the complications of mastitis, oophoritis, and encephalitis are the same for pregnant and nonpregnant women. Abortions are more frequent in women who are infected during the first trimester of pregnancy.
   b. **Fetus.** Congenital malformations do not appear to be increased in infants born to infected mothers. The postulated association between gestational mumps and endocardial fibroelastosis remains controversial.
3. **Management**
   a. Administer symptomatic treatment with fluids and aspirin to relieve the discomfort of fever and parotitis.
   b. Passive immunization with hyperimmune mumps immunoglobulin is no longer recommended as the drug is not of value.
4. **Prevention.** Vaccination with live attenuated mumps virus is suggested for nonpregnant postpubertal women who have not had mumps parotitis (see Table 11-2).

E. Poliomyelitis, currently a rare illness in pregnancy, was, in the prevaccine era, more common and more severe in pregnant than in nonpregnant women of similar age [13]. This increase in incidence was attributed to hormonal changes in pregnancy and to greater exposure to young children.

1. **Diagnosis**
   a. Fever, headache, coryza, nausea, vomiting, and sore throat precede the characteristic paralytic phase, which is marked by hyperesthesia, muscle pain, and flaccid paralysis.
   b. Poliovirus can be isolated from feces, serum, and cerebrospinal fluid.
   c. Increases in neutralizing and complement-fixing antibodies are demonstrable in serum obtained at two and four weeks after infection.
2. **Prognosis**
   a. **Mother.** In the prevaccine era, morbidity and mortality were higher than in the nonpregnant state. The incidence of abortion is increased.
   b. **Fetus.** Paralysis and growth retardation occur in infants infected during gestation. Neonatal poliomyelitis has a mortality of approximately 25%. There is no increase in the incidence of congenital abnormalities.
3. **Management**
   a. Isolation procedures are required for infected mothers and neonates to prevent spread of the infection through excretory products.
   b. Supportive care to prevent deformities and, if necessary, to maintain adequate maternal ventilation is indicated during the acute illness.
4. **Prevention.** If immediate protection against poliomyelitis is needed due to travel to an endemic area, a single dose of oral vaccine is given unless time permits the schedule required for the inactivated vaccine (see Table 11-2). The inactivated vaccine is recommended for booster injections, as the live attenuated oral vaccine has on rare occasions caused poliomyelitis in adults.

F. Coxsackieviruses serotypes A and B cause a wide spectrum of brief, self-limited illnesses involving one or more organ system [13].

1. **Diagnosis**
   a. Herpangina, lymphonodular pharyngitis, and rhinopharyngitis indistinguishable from rhinovirus-induced common colds occur in pregnant women

infected with coxsackievirus A. Aseptic meningitis is caused by both stereotypes. Pleurodynia is caused by infections with coxsackievirus B.

b. Coxsackievirus can be isolated from pharyngeal secretions and feces, but for practical purposes culture is rarely performed.

c. Because of the large numbers of serotypes, serologic proof of infection—demonstration of fourfold or greater increases in neutralizing or complement-fixing antibody—is impractical except in epidemics.

2. **Prognosis**

a. **Mother.** The coxsackievirus–induced illnesses are self-limited and are not associated with significant maternal mortality or increases in incidence of abortion.

b. **Fetus.** Coxsackievirus A infections are of no consequence to the fetus. Coxsackievirus B infections cause serious illness (myocarditis and encephalitis) and fetal mortality in the perinatal period. The most common defect associated with coxsackievirus B infection is tetralogy of Fallot, but definitive evidence linking this or other congenital abnormality to coxsackievirus B infections is lacking.

3. **Management.** Symptomatic treatment is indicated for the mother, and supportive treatment is indicated for the fetus with myocarditis or encephalitis. Neonates that survive infection usually do not have residual defects.

4. **Prevention.** No vaccine is available.

G. **Varicella** (chickenpox), a common contagious disease of childhood, can occur during pregnancy [21].

1. **Diagnosis**

a. Prodromal symptoms of fever and malaise are soon followed by the characteristic vesiculopapular rash. Approximately one-third of infected adults develop clinical and roentgenographic findings of pneumonia.

b. The diagnosis is established by clinical criteria. It is confirmed by histologic identification of intranuclear inclusion bodies or by immunofluorescent identification of varicella zoster antigen in vesicles or cells from desquamated tracheobronchial mucosa. The virus can also be cultured from vesicular fluids. Increases in antibodies appear in serum two to four weeks after infection.

2. **Prognosis**

a. **Mother.** Varicella pneumonia by itself or complicated by bacterial superinfection is an ominous occurrence and is associated with mortalities as high as 41%. No evidence exists that chickenpox in the absence of pneumonia is more serious in pregnant women. The incidence of abortion and premature delivery does not appear to be increased.

b. **Fetus.** The virus crosses the placenta. Infections acquired in the last 10 days of pregnancy result in variably severe fetal infections, with neonatal mortality as high as 34%. Fetal mortality increases with the proximity of the maternal infection to term. If contracted early in pregnancy, varicella infection may result in congenital defects such as paralysis, limb atrophy, cutaneous scars, rudimentary digits, convulsive disorders, and cortical atrophy. The risk of the congenital varicella syndrome is estimated at 4.9% if infection occurs in the first trimester.

3. **Management**

a. Calamine lotion helps to alleviate pruritus. Bacitracin ointment is useful in treating vesicular lesions that are secondarily infected with bacteria.

b. Treatment of varicella pneumonia is similar to that of influenza pneumonia.

c. In life-threatening cases of pneumonia, acyclovir, 30 mg/kg/day, is given despite a lack of established indications in pregnancy [8, 19, 21].

4. **Prevention.** Varicella zoster immune globulin (VZIG) may be of value in susceptible gravidas exposed to varicella. The drug should be given to infants of mothers who contract varicella from five days before to two days after birth. A vaccine made from an attenuated strain has been useful in children with leukemia, but its value in pregnancy is unknown. Women of childbearing

age who are susceptible to varicella could be an important population to immunize when the vaccine is introduced in the United States.

H. Cytomegalovirus (CMV) is a herpesvirus that, on the basis of antibody testing, infects 50–60% of women of childbearing age [18]. The virus is present in the urine of approximately 5% of pregnant women. Increased cervical excretion of CMV is seen in the third trimester. Virus shedding is much more common in women under the age of 30. Interestingly the majority of congenital CMV infections occur in infants of women less than 30 years of age [18].

1. Diagnosis

a. Adult infections usually are asymptomatic. Symptomatic infections resemble infectious mononucleosis and present with low-grade fever, malaise, lymphadenopathy, and hepatosplenomegaly.

b. Laboratory studies show leukocytosis with atypical lymphocytes, abnormalities in hepatocellular function, and a negative heterophile antibody test for mononucleosis.

c. CMV can be cultured from blood, saliva, urine, and cervical mucus. Since many patients excrete CMV, the demonstration of increases in antibody titers by a number of methods in convalescent serum is the most accurate means of documenting a newly acquired infection.

2. Prognosis

a. Mother. Cytomegalovirus infection is self-limited without increase in morbidity or mortality in pregnancy. The infection also is not known to increase the incidence of abortion and premature delivery.

b. Fetus. Infection of the fetus occurs either in utero by the passage of the virus through the placenta or at birth when the fetus traverses an infected birth canal. It has been estimated that the prevalence of intrauterine CMV infections is between 0.2 and 2.5% of births. Abnormalities of variable severity affect approximately 10% of infected infants and include microcephaly, diminished mentation, chorioretinitis, hearing loss, intracranial calcifications, and hepatosplenomegaly. Intrauterine infection also results in stillbirth. Additionally, 5–20% of asymptomatic infants congenitally infected will develop late manifestations that include neuromuscular disturbances, auditory damage, and visual impairment [18].

3. Management. Administer symptomatic treatment with aspirin and fluids to relieve discomfort. Ganciclovir, a new antiviral agent, is efficacious in the treatment of CMV retinitis and gastrointestinal disease. Its value in pregnancy is unknown [18]. CMV immune globulin may protect against disease in renal transplant recipients. Its efficacy in preventing primary CMV infections in pregnant women is unknown [41].

4. Prevention. No vaccine is currently available. A live attenuated vaccine is in clinical trials. Prenatal diagnosis by culturing amniotic fluid is of limited value.

I. Variola infections (smallpox), once a dreaded disease, has not occurred since 1977, and vaccination is no longer necessary.

J. Viral hepatitis (hepatitis A, B, or non-A, non-B [C]) is one of the most serious diseases in the United States and is the most common cause of jaundice during pregnancy [43, 46]. Hepatitis A has an incubation period of 25–40 days. Infection is transmitted by the fecal-oral route. Maternal transmission to the fetus does not occur. Hepatitis B has a 50- to 180-day incubation period and is transmitted by contaminated blood, saliva, breast milk, and semen. Pregnant women who are infected transmit the virus transplacentally to the fetus and at birth. Neonatal hepatitis seldom occurs if the mother is a chronic carrier or acquires hepatitis early in pregnancy; the risk is high when infection occurs late in pregnancy. Non-A, non-B hepatitis, which occurs in the same settings as hepatitis B, has an incubation period of approximately six weeks. Recently, a small single-stranded RNA virus now known as hepatitis C virus has been shown to be the cause of the majority of parenterally transmitted non-A, non-B hepatitis [1]. Indirect evidence suggests maternal-to-infant transmission does occur. The availability of tests to detect antibodies to hepatitis C will allow studies to determine patterns of transmission.

1. **Diagnosis**
   a. Except for fever being more common in hepatitis A and prodromal arthralgias occurring in 20% of patients with hepatitis B, the clinical presentations of both viruses are similar, being marked by anorexia, nausea, and malaise.
   b. Jaundice with hepatic tenderness and enlargement occurs in the first weeks following the onset of symptoms. Pruritus may also be present.
   c. In hepatitis A, the onset of jaundice is associated with rapid improvement in symptoms. Hepatitis B infection causes more prolonged symptomatology and jaundice.
   d. Aspartate aminotransferase (AST), alanine aminotransferase (ALT), and lactate dehydrogenase (LDH) are markedly elevated, signifying hepatocellular damage. The serum bilirubin also is increased significantly, whereas the serum alkaline phosphatase is minimally elevated.
   e. Hepatitis A infection is diagnosed by demonstrating hepatitis A IgM antibody or by culturing the virus from stool. Hepatitis B infection is diagnosed by demonstrating hepatitis B surface antigen (HBsAg) in serum and increases in hepatitis B core antibody (HBcAb) and hepatitis B surface antibody (HBsAb). Hepatitis Be antigen (HBeAg) is present in HBsAg-positive sera, and its persistence is associated with chronic hepatitis and increased infectiousness.
2. **Prognosis**
   a. **Mother.** An increased severity of illness has been reported in pregnant women from nutritionally deprived backgrounds. Whether this association applies in developed countries is uncertain. Viral hepatitis is associated with premature labor.
   b. **Fetus.** Fetal survival depends on the time of infection. Hepatitis B virus is transferred from mother to infant in 75% of cases when infection occurs in the last trimester of pregnancy and in only 10% of cases when infection occurs earlier. Consequently, neonatal hepatitis is more common in infants when mothers are infected in the last trimester. Congenital defects are not increased in infants born to infected mothers.
3. **Management**
   a. Bed rest and diet should accord with the patient's desires and tolerance.
   b. Although recommended in the past by some physicians, corticosteroids are no longer considered beneficial.
   c. Hepatitis B immune globulin is recommended for neonates born to HBsAg-positive women, particularly in infections occurring in the second half of pregnancy. Vaccine should be given concomitantly with additional doses at one and six months.
4. **Prevention**
   a. Human immune serum globulin, 0.02 ml/kg to a total of 2.0 ml, is given to prevent hepatitis A.
   b. Human immune serum globulin, 0.04 ml/kg to a total of 4.0 ml, is given to prevent hepatitis B. Alternatively, hepatitis B immune globulin, 0.05–0.07 ml/kg, can be given twice, once within 7 days of exposure and again 25–30 days after the first injection.
   c. Hepatitis B vaccine is available for individuals at high risk of infection, and pregnancy is not considered a contraindication.

K. **Rabies** is an almost invariably fatal infection that is transmitted by exposure to salivary secretions containing the neurotropic virus [4]. Most human cases result from bites or licks of an infected animal, usually a dog. On occasion, respiratory infection occurs when persons enter caves inhabited by rabid bats. Because **prevention is paramount** in this disease, which has an incubation period of 10 days–1 year, the critical decisions relate to prophylaxis. The following are guidelines for determining prophylaxis:

1. Dogs and cats that are considered healthy should be observed for signs of rabies: If disease does not develop in 10 days, prophylaxis is unnecessary. If the animal dies, the brain should be examined for the presence of virus. Rabies is proved by identifying viral antigen, by virus isolation, or by finding Negri bodies. If rabies is found, the patient is treated with a single dose of rabies immune globulin, 20 IU/kg, and a course of human diploid cell vaccine, five 1-ml doses IM, to be given on days 0, 3, 7, 14, and 28. Serum for rabies antibody testing should be collected two to three weeks after the last dose. If no antibody response occurs, a booster dose should be given.
2. If the animal escapes or is suspected of being rabid or if the bite is from a wild animal (e.g., skunks, raccoons, or foxes), treatment with rabies immune globulin and human diploid cell vaccine is instituted.

L. Acquired immunodeficiency syndrome (AIDS) is a disease caused by the human retrovirus HIV [15]. Homosexual men, intravenous drug users, hemophiliacs, and sexual partners of AIDS patients are the highest risk groups for infection with HIV. AIDS is defined by infections and malignancies that demonstrate a profound immunodeficiency. It is estimated that approximately 7% of patients with AIDS are women of reproductive age [33] and that 80% of the 1000 pediatric cases of AIDS were acquired perinatally [33]. Since the majority of HIV-infected patients are asymptomatic, patients with risk factors should be tested for HIV antibody with their consent.

1. Diagnosis

a. AIDS is diagnosed in persons with no known cause for immunosuppression who develop opportunistic infections or malignancies owing to defects in cell-mediated immunity.

b. There is a reversal in the ratio of T helper (CD4) and T suppresser cells (CD8) owing to a decrease in the number of T helper cells, producing a ratio of less than one.

c. Antibodies to HIV are detected using ELISA, immunofluorescence, and immunoblotting (Western blot). The ELISA test is used for screening, and the two others, particularly the Western blot, are used to confirm specificity. Although infrequent, false-positive and false-negative results occur with all tests. At present no practical means exist to detect the infrequent occurrence of a false-negative antibody test. The ability to detect HIV nucleic acid with the newly developed polymerase chain reaction (PCR) test may detect false-negative tests and should soon be more readily available. A positive antibody test is diagnostic for HIV infection and does not indicate AIDS.

2. Prognosis

a. **Mother.** Although the data are limited, the prognosis of HIV infection appears similar in pregnant and nonpregnant women.

b. **Fetus.** Mother-to-infant transmission occurs with a rate of 20–60% [33]. The existence of congenital abnormalities related to HIV infection is uncertain. Some evidence suggests that persons with AIDS are more infectious than those with asymptomatic HIV infection [24]. HIV can be transmitted to the neonate in breast milk.

3. Management

a. The treatment of choice for HIV infection is AZT. It is not presently recommended for use during pregnancy owing to the lack of knowledge regarding teratogenicity.

b. Treatment of opportunistic infections is the same as in nonpregnant patients. Despite the teratogenic potential of trimethoprim-sulfamethoxazole, this drug should be used in infections caused by *Pneumocystis carinii*.

c. Universal precautions are indicated for blood and body fluids.

4. Prevention. No vaccine is available for HIV infection.

M. Parvovirus B19. Human parvovirus B19, a small DNA virus, is responsible for erythema infectiosum (fifth disease), aplastic crisis in patients with chronic hemolytic anemia, and arthropathy [2, 11]. It is presumed to be transmitted via respiratory secretions. The incubation period is usually 4–14 days but may be as long as 20 days. Secondary attack rates are as high as 50–60%.

1. Diagnosis

a. The typical "slapped cheek" rash of erythema infectiosum is seen in childhood.

b. The IgM antibodies detected by ELISA are present in acute infection. IgG antibodies are usually present by day seven and persist for years.

2. Prognosis

a. Mother. The morbidity of B19 infections appears to be unchanged in pregnant women.

b. Fetus. Parvovirus infections in pregnancy are associated with fetal death manifested as hydrops fetalis. The risk of fetal death is 5–20% and most commonly occurs from the tenth through the twentieth weeks of pregnancy. To date, no evidence exists that clearly relates B19 infection with congenital anomalies.

3. Management

a. Exposure to infected persons should be avoided.

b. If exposure occurs, antibody tests should be used to document either infection or immunity.

c. Diagnostic ultrasound has been recommended in women with acute B19 infections although the utility of this test has not been proved.

4. Prevention

a. No vaccine is available.

b. Studies to determine efficacy of serum immune globulin for prevention have not been conducted. Therefore, use of immune globulin is not recommended.

N. Papillomavirus. Human papillomavirus, a small DNA virus, is associated with condyloma acuminata, cervical intraepithelial neoplasia, and invasive carcinomas [17].

1. Diagnosis

a. Flat warts or condyloma may be seen on external genitalia and cervix.

b. Colposcopy and acetowhitening are used to improve the clinical diagnosis by demonstrating shiny white patches with poorly defined borders and an irregular surface.

2. Prognosis

a. Mother. Clinically or cytologically visible infections with human papillomavirus are thought to be increased in pregnant women. Viral replication is enhanced during pregnancy as demonstrated by an increased number of viral copies determined by DNA hybridization.

b. Fetus. Genital human papillomavirus infections in the mother can be transmitted to the fetus and cause juvenile laryngeal papillomata.

3. Management

a. Podophyllin, topical 5-fluorouracil (5FU), and topical bleomycin should not be used in pregnancy as they may be absorbed and lead to serious fetal complications.

b. Electrocautery, cryocautery, or laser therapy offer alternatives to topical trichloroacetic acid.

4. Prevention. The risk of upper respiratory papillomata in the neonate is relatively low. Therefore, cesarean sections are not recommended.

IV. Genital infections

A. Herpes simplex. Herpetic infections usually are caused by type 2 virus, but type 1 is responsible for 15% of genital herpes infections [19]. Both viruses are transmitted by person-to-person contact and occur in approximately 1% of pregnant women.

1. Prognosis

a. Herpetic vesicles 1–22 mm in diameter develop on the genitalia and skin surfaces. These pruritic lesions rupture in two to three days, forming painful, shallow ulcers.

b. Accompanying signs and symptoms include low-grade fever, malaise, and regional adenopathy. Jaundice and encephalitis are infrequent complications.

c. The illness lasts from 7–10 days; recurrences are common.

d. Pregnant women infected for the first time shed virus for 8–100 days; patients with recurrences shed virus for 6–40 days.

e. The appearance and distribution of the lesions permit a presumptive clinical diagnosis. Substantiation of a viral etiology is obtained by identifying intranuclear inclusion bodies in Tzanck- or Papanicolaou-stained preparations. Definitive proof of herpes infection requires identification of virus in infected specimens by direct immunofluorescent testing or by culturing virus in tissue cultures. Serologic tests exist but are of limited clinical use.

2. **Prognosis**

a. **Mother.** The morbidity from these self-limited infections and the rarity of death, usually from encephalitis, are unaffected by pregnancy. Herpetic infection is associated with an increased incidence of abortion and premature delivery.

b. **Fetus.** Fifty percent of newborns delivered to mothers with primary herpes and five percent to those with recurrent disease develop local (skin or central nervous system) or disseminated herpetic infections. Disseminated infections are associated with high mortality and serious neurologic sequelae in survivors. Infections in newborns with intrauterine herpes simplex infections are characterized by a rash at birth, congenital malformations, and a less fulminant course. The congenital malformations include microcephaly, encephalitis, chorioretinitis, and cerebral atrophy.

3. **Management.** Acyclovir decreases the duration of a primary genital herpes infection. Acyclovir also decreases the duration of recurrent attacks. Recurrences are suppressed when 200 mg of the drug is given prophylactically, 2–5 times/day. Acyclovir has not been tested in pregnancy, and the manufacturers do not recommend its use.

4. **Prevention**

a. Patients should be examined for genital lesions in the third trimester. Cultures for cervicovaginal shedding in patients with chronic recurrent herpes are of limited use late in the third trimester. Patients with active lesions should be delivered by cesarean section before rupture of membranes or within 6–12 hours of membrane rupture [3, 19]. Amniocentesis for viral culture is no longer recommended before the decision for cesarean section is made.

b. Following delivery, the mother and the infant are separated until the maternal infection is inactive.

c. Newborn infants from infected mothers are isolated and examined for 12–14 days for the development of herpetic infection.

B. **Syphilis.** *Treponema pallidum,* the etiologic agent of syphilis, is transmitted through sexual contact. In recent years, the incidence of primary and secondary syphilis in the United States has increased to approximately 40,000 cases/year, with peak incidences in young adults [45]. Infections are transmitted readily from mother to fetus.

1. **Diagnosis**

a. The chance of primary syphilis is usually found on vaginal and cervical membranes. Chancres also occur extragenitally, most often in oral and anal regions. The lesions begin as nontender papules and subsequently ulcerate. Healing occurs within three to six weeks. Clinical features of primary syphilis are infrequently seen in pregnancy.

b. Manifestations of secondary syphilis appear 2–12 weeks after the primary chancre and include skin rashes of various types (e.g., macular, papular, pustular, bullous), which often occur on the palms and soles; condylomas in perigenital areas; alopecia; generalized adenopathy; and low-grade fever. Condylomas are the most commonly observed lesions of secondary syphilis in pregnancy.

c. **Testing.** Using dark-field microscopy, the diagnosis is established by identifying *T. pallidum* in specimens from suspicious lesions. In the absence of a positive dark-field examination, a presumptive diagnosis is made by detecting antibody to reagin (a cardiolipin-lecithin antigen) with the Venereal Disease Research Laboratory (VDRL) or rapid plasma reagin card (RPRC) test. Because false-positive results occur with these tests, positive results are confirmed with the fluorescent treponemal antibody absorption test (FTA-ABS) or the microhemagglutination assay (MHATP) for antibodies to *T. pallidum*. The diagnostic accuracy of the FTA-ABS or MHATP test is nearly 100% in cases of secondary syphilis, and the rate of false-positive results is less than 1%.

d. The manifestations of congenital syphilis may occur at birth, but more often they appear in the first weeks of life. The most common clinical findings are skin eruptions of the type and distribution observed in adults, osteitis of nasal bones resulting in characteristic saddle nose deformities, periostitis and osteochondritis of long bones, hepatosplenomegaly, frontal bossing, notched incisors, mulberry molars, eighth nerve deafness, and neurosyphilis.

2. Prognosis

a. Mother. The morbidity of primary and secondary syphilis is the same in pregnant and nonpregnant women.

b. Fetus. If the mother is untreated, 25% of fetuses will die in utero, 25–30% will die shortly after birth, and 40% of survivors will develop syphilis after the third week of life.

3. Management

a. Treat pregnant patients with primary, secondary, or tertiary syphilis with one to three weekly injections of 2.4 million units IM of benzathine penicillin G (Table 11-3).

b. Patients allergic to penicillin should receive 500 mg of erythromycin PO q6h for 14 days. Because of fetal toxicity, tetracycline is an unacceptable alternative drug for patients with penicillin allergy (Table 11-3).

c. If the serologic titer as measured by serial quantitative VDRL tests does not decrease, a second course of therapy is indicated. Patients with a history of previous treatment of syphilis should be retreated if doubts exist regarding the adequacy of therapy.

d. Adequate treatment of the syphilitic mother before the sixteenth week of gestation prevents congenital syphilis; after the sixteenth week, treatment cures the infection but may not prevent the stigmata of congenital syphilis.

4. Prevention. Pregnant women should be tested serologically for syphilis at their first prenatal examination.

C. Gonorrhea. Currently, gonococcal infections are epidemic in the United States, with yearly incidence of nearly 800,000 [23]. Infections are transmitted primarily through sexual contact. Asymptomatic carriers, male as well as female, are the primary source of infection.

1. Diagnosis

a. Gonorrhea is an asymptomatic infection in 80% of women. Pain and tenderness in the pelvic region, cervical discharge, dysuria, and fever are the most common findings in patients with symptomatic infection. Pustular skin lesions, migratory arthralgias, and tenosynovitis culminating in a monoarticular septic arthritis indicate disseminated infection.

b. The diagnosis is established by demonstrating gram-negative diplococci within polymorphonuclear leukocytes from vaginal and cervical exudates. The microscopic impression is confirmed by culturing the exudates on Thayer-Martin media. Newer laboratory techniques employing immunofluorescent antibody or ELISA are being used for rapid diagnosis, but their value is uncertain.

c. Gonococci can be cultured from pharyngeal and rectal swabs, blood, septic joints, and skin pustules.

2. Prognosis

a. Mother. Women who become infected during the last 20 weeks of gestation or in the puerperium have an increased incidence of gonococcal arthritis.

Women who harbor gonococci in the genital tract may have a flare-up of their latent disease during labor or immediately post partum. There may be an increased risk of gonococcemia in such women. Abortion may occur because of premature rupture of the membranes secondary to gonococcal infection. Chronic pelvic inflammatory disease is an important cause of ectopic pregnancy.

b. **Fetus.** Neonatal gonorrhea is acquired in utero or during delivery when the fetus traverses an infected birth canal. Infection in utero results in chorioamnionitis and subsequent neonatal sepsis. Infections acquired during delivery cause conjunctivitis (ophthalmia neonatorum), otitis externa, and vulvovaginitis.

3. **Management**

   a. Treat pregnant patients with urogenital, rectal, or oropharyngeal infections with ceftriaxone, 250 mg IM, followed by erythromycin, 500 mg qid for 7–10 days, in order to eradicate coexisting *C. trachomatis* infection (Table 11-3).

   b. Patients with disseminated infections are treated with 1 gm of ceftriaxone IV or IM once daily for 7–10 days. If patients are improving and the organism is found to be penicillin susceptible, the patients can be switched to amoxicillin after 3 days at a dose of 500 mg PO q6h for a total of 7–10 days of therapy (Table 11-3).

   c. Patients allergic to beta-lactams are treated with spectinomycin, but it must be emphasized that this drug is ineffective in syphilis (Table 11-1) and is potentially ototoxic to the fetus.

   d. Ophthalmia neonatorum is prophylaxed with topical erythromycin. If the prevalence of penicillinase-producing *N. gonorrhoeae* is high, 1% aqueous silver nitrate solution is used.

   e. To validate cures, pregnant patients should be recultured five to seven days after termination of the treatment.

4. **Prevention**

   a. Pregnant women should have cervical cultures for *N. gonorrhoeae* at the first prenatal visit. A second culture is obtained late in the third trimester in high-risk women.

   b. Sexual contacts should be identified and treated.

   c. A vaccine made from gonococcal pili is being investigated.

D. **Streptococcal infections.** Groups A and B beta-hemolytic streptococci are the major causes of perinatal infection [6, 7, 22]. In the past, group A streptococci *(Streptococcus pyogenes)* were responsible for most puerperal fevers. Recently, the less virulent group B streptococci *(S. agalactiae),* which is a normal constituent of the genital tract in 5–25% of pregnant women, has become the most common cause of perinatal infection. Transmission of group B streptococci from parturient women to the neonate results in infections of varying severity, particularly in the premature infant.

1. **Diagnosis**

   a. Streptococcal infection is suspected in patients with prematurely ruptured membranes, septic abortions, endometritis, chorioamnionitis, or pelvic peritonitis.

   b. The diagnosis is established by culturing group A or B streptococci from genital exudates or blood.

2. **Prognosis**

   a. **Mother.** Puerperal infections that are caused by group A streptococci and are untreated have a grave prognosis. With penicillin treatment, the outcome is much more favorable: Death is infrequent. Group B streptococcal infections usually cause less serious, self-limited perinatal infections. Life-threatening puerperal infections occur on occasion, particularly in women with prolonged rupture of membranes. Stillbirths and septic abortions are infrequent complications.

   b. **Fetus.** Early-onset infection of the fetus with group B streptococci occurs during the late intrauterine or intrapartum period [6, 7]. Twenty-five percent of infants born to mothers harboring the bacteria become colonized.

Neonatal sepsis, including meningitis, is a major complication. Pneumonia is the principal cause of morbidity and mortality in premature infants.

3. **Management**
   a. Puerperal fever is treated with high doses of parenteral penicillin or ampicillin (Table 11-3).
   b. Infected newborns also are treated with high doses of penicillin or ampicillin.
4. **Prevention.** Group A streptococcal infection is acquired by person-to-person contact. Use of aseptic techniques during delivery has significantly reduced the incidence of this once common disease. A recent study has demonstrated that neonatal colonization and bacteremia with group B streptococci could be decreased by use of intrapartum ampicillin. Difficulties in implementing this approach include accuracy of a single culture for group B streptococci and maternal risk for life-threatening adverse reactions to ampicillin [22].

E. **Chlamydial infections.** *C. trachomatis,* an obligatory intracellular parasite, is recognized as the most common sexually transmitted disease in the United States and the cause of nongonococcal urethritis, lymphogranuloma venereum, epididymitis, pelvic inflammatory disease, and conjunctivitis in adults, and of inclusion conjunctivitis, pneumonia, otitis media, and vaginitis in infants who are born through infected birth canals [37]. The small, 0.2- to 0.7-μm bacterial microorganisms can be isolated from the genital tract of approximately 25% of sexually active nonpregnant women, approximately 5% of pregnant women, and less than 5% of women without a history of sexual contact.

1. **Diagnosis**
   a. Most genital infections with *C. trachomatis* are asymptomatic. Some result in cervicitis, discharge, and discomfort.
   b. Gram's stains of the exudate show polymorphonuclear leukocytes and an absence of gram-negative intracellular bacteria.
   c. Definitive diagnosis requires the identification, by means of the Giemsa stain, of typical intracytoplasmic inclusion bodies; demonstration of elementary bodies within genital cells, with fluorescent monoclonal antibodies; isolation of *C. trachomatis* in tissue cultures using irradiated McCoy cells treated with cycloheximide; or the demonstration of increases in serum antibody to chlamydia by immunofluorescent testing. Of these tests, the fluorescent method using monoclonal antibodies is the most useful.
2. **Prognosis**
   a. **Mother.** Morbidity and mortality are the same for pregnant and nonpregnant women. The effect, if any, of chlamydial infection on the incidence of abortion and premature labor is uncertain.
   b. **Fetus.** Newborn infants may develop inclusion conjunctivitis, nasopharyngitis, pneumonia, or vaginitis after passage through an infected birth canal. Transplacental infection also occurs. Inclusion conjunctivitis occurs in 20–50% of exposed newborn infants. The incidence of pneumonia is much lower (10–20%). Most infections are mild and self-limited.
3. **Management**
   a. Because chlamydial infections are readily transmitted to sexual partners and to offspring, treatment is indicated in pregnant women with proved infection. The importance of chemoprophylaxis in patients with asymptomatic chlamydial infection is unknown.
   b. Treatment is also indicated for women whose sexual partners develop nongonococcal or postgonococcal urethritis.
   c. Pregnant women should be treated with erythromycin, 250 mg PO qid for 14–21 days or 500 PO qid for 7 days. Tetracycline, another effective drug, should be avoided in pregnancy.
4. **Prevention.** All sexual contacts, regardless of symptomatology, require treatment.

V. **Miscellaneous infections of importance in pregnancy**

A. **Toxoplasmosis.** Toxoplasmosis is a common worldwide infection [20, 28, 36]. The causative microorganism, *Toxoplasma gondii,* is a protozoan with infectious cystic forms that are found in cat feces (oocyst) and herbivorous and carnivorous animal tissue (tissue cyst). Infection results from the ingestion of cyst-containing animal tissues or foods contaminated with cat feces and by transplacental transmission when women are infected during pregnancy.

1. **Diagnosis**
   - a. Asymptomatic lymphadenopathy is the most common manifestation.
   - b. More severe infections resemble infectious mononucleosis with fever, myalgias, sore throat, lymphadenopathy, macular rashes, migratory polyarthritis, and hepatosplenomegaly.
   - c. Meningoencephalitis, the most dreaded complication, usually occurs in immunocompromised patients. Chorioretinitis is rare in acquired toxoplasmosis. Toxoplasmosis also simulates viral pneumonia.
   - d. The diagnosis is established by identification of the protozoa in tissue sections, smears, or body fluids, or by demonstrating eightfold or greater increases in antibody titer using either the Sabin-Feldman dye test or immunofluorescent testing for IgM or IgG antibody. In cases limited to a single test, only elevated IgM antibody titers permit the diagnosis of acutely acquired toxoplasmosis [20]. *T. gondii* can be isolated from infected tissue by inoculation into tissue culture or intraperitoneally in mice.
2. **Prognosis**
   - a. **Mother.** Maternal morbidity and mortality are unaffected by pregnancy. Infection increases the incidence of abortion and premature labor to 10–15% in women infected in the first and second trimesters of pregnancy. Complications are rare in women infected before conception; only one case of congenital toxoplasmosis has occurred when the mother acquired the infection prior to conception [36].
   - b. **Fetus.** The incidence of congenital infection varies with the trimester in which maternal infection occurs. The lowest incidence is in the first trimester, and the highest is in the third trimester. Congenital infection may lead to stillbirth, premature birth, or full-term pregnancy. Although the incidence of fetal infection is high (approximately 65%) in the third trimester, almost 90% of newborns are without clinical signs of disease. Infection acquired during the first trimester results in congenital infection in only 25%. But serious disease is most common. Immediate manifestations are low birth weight, microcephaly, intracranial calcifications, hydrocephalus, chorioretinitis, hepatosplenomegaly, jaundice, and thrombocytopenia. Delayed manifestations include mental retardation, seizure activity, and chorioretinitis. Treatment of the mother can reduce the incidence of congenital infection by 60% [36].
3. **Management**
   - a. No treatment is necessary for asymptomatic seropositive patients.
   - b. For active progressive disease, pyrimethamine, alone or in combination with sulfadiazine, is recommended (Table 11-3). Pyrimethamine should be avoided in the first and probably the second trimester of pregnancy, as it is teratogenic. Sulfadiazine and erythromycin have been used in the first and second trimesters; alternatively, sulfadiazine and pyrimethamine can be used, followed by therapeutic abortion. Spiramycin, an experimental drug that can be obtained from the Food and Drug Administration (FDA), appears to be less toxic than pyrimethamine and safer during the first trimester of pregnancy and is recommended therapy at a dose of 3 gm/day.
   - c. Although the risk of congenital toxoplasmosis occurring in the first trimester is low, the probability of severe disease in the fetus is so high that therapeutic abortion should be considered.
4. **Prevention.** Hygienic measures to prevent transmission of *T. gondii* through infected feces or animal products are the only available methods for reducing the incidence of illness. Pregnant women should avoid exposure to cat feces, wash their hands after contact with meat and soil, and cook their meat adequately. Serologic testing should be considered based on a recent French study [16] that demonstrated improved outcomes in treated, prenatally diagnosed cases of toxoplasmosis in women who wished to continue their preg-

nancies. In order to make testing more cost-effective, a three-test regimen has been recommended. Antibody testing is obtained on the diagnosis of pregnancy. If this is positive, IgM testing is done on the same serum sample. If positive, the decision regarding therapy or therapeutic abortion could be considered. If the IgG test is negative, the woman is retested at 10–12 weeks and at 20–22 weeks to determine whether infection was acquired in the interim [16, 38].

B. Malaria, one of the most common infections of humans, causes significant morbidity and mortality in medically indigent areas of the world [5, 29]. Acute life-threatening illnesses are invariably caused by *Plasmodium falciparum,* whereas relapsing chronic infections are caused by *P. vivax* or, in selected endemic areas, *P. ovale* or *P. malariae.*

1. Diagnosis

a. Episodic paroxysms of high spiking fever, headache, and myalgia distinguish malaria from virtually every other illness. Splenic enlargement is present in chronic infections.

b. A history of residence in or passage through an endemic area usually is obtained.

c. In the United States, the possibility of illicit intravenous drug use should be considered, since malaria is transmitted by contaminated blood.

d. Microscopic identification of the parasite in blood smears confirms the diagnosis.

e. Chronic infections are diagnosed by demonstrating high levels of indirect fluorescent antibody in serum.

2. Prognosis

a. Mother. Malarial attacks, especially those caused by *P. falciparum,* are particularly severe in pregnant patients. Abortions, prematurity, and stillbirths are increased in women who undergo malarial attacks during the first trimester of pregnancy.

b. Fetus. On occasion in nonimmune mothers, malarial parasites cross the placenta, initiating fetal infection. Congenital malaria results in intrauterine growth retardation. Infection neonates have fever, jaundice, hepatosplenomegaly, seizures, and, occasionally, pulmonary edema 48–72 hours after delivery.

3. Management. Treat pregnant women with malaria caused by *P. vivax, P. ovale,* and nonchloroquine-resistant *P. falciparum* with 1.0 gm of chloroquine phosphate PO for 1 dose, followed by 0.5 gm at 6, 24, and 48 hours. Nonpregnant patients with infections caused by *P. vivax* and *P. ovale* should receive 26.3 mg of primaquine phosphate PO for 14 days. However, because fetal red blood cells are relatively deficient in glucose 6-phosphate dehydrogenase and glutathione, the fetus is at risk for intravascular hemolysis. Therefore, primaquine is not recommended in pregnancy [14]. Relapses are treated with chloroquine, and primaquine is used after delivery. Falciparum malaria resistant to chloroquine is treated with 650 mg of quinine sulfate PO tid for 10 days, combined with pyrimethamine, 50 mg/day PO for 3 days, followed by 500 mg of sulfadiazine PO qid for 5 days. It should be emphasized that pyrimethamine is a highly teratogenic drug. Some experts recommend Fansidar (pyrimethamine and sulfadoxine) in combination with folinic acid to treat chloroquine-resistant *P. falciparum,* as quinine is an abortifacient in early pregnancy and can lead to premature labor in later pregnancy. Fansidar-resistant malaria is treated with quinine and tetracycline despite the risks of teratogenicity. Mefloquine is now available in the United States, but data to support its use in pregnancy are lacking.

4. Prevention. Chloroquine can cause retinal and cochleovestibular damage but is generally considered sufficiently safe in pregnancy to be recommended if travel to an endemic area is required. Chloroquine phosphate, 500 mg PO, is given 1 week prior to leaving and once weekly while the patient must remain in endemic areas. The drug should be continued for 6 weeks after the patient has left the endemic area. Fansidar is no longer recommended as prophylaxis in areas with chloroquine-resistant *P. falciparum* due to severe drug reactions. It is recommended that Fansidar should be carried by travelers to these areas and taken therapeutically at the first sign of illness. Pregnant women should be informed of the risk of teratogenicity before they take Fansidar [14]. Mefloquine should not be used in pregnancy. Proguanil, a drug that is not licensed by the FDA, is used in many countries in addition to chloroquine to prevent chloroquine-resistant *P. falciparum.* No adverse effects on the pregnancy or fetus have been established [5]. Because safe, effective therapy is unavailable for chloroquine-resistant *P. falciparum,* nonimmune pregnant women should be discouraged from traveling to endemic areas unless absolutely necessary.

C. Lyme disease is caused by *Borrelia burgdorferi,* a tick-borne spirochete [42]. The organism is transmitted by the bite of Ixodes ticks, generally during the spring and summer.

1. Diagnosis

a. Early infection is characterized by a distinctive rash (erythema migrans) that has advancing serpiginous borders with central clearing.

b. Later disease can involve the heart, neurologic system, musculoskeletal system (arthritis), and eyes.

c. The diagnosis is made clinically by noting a history of tick bite followed by a rash consistent with erythema migrans in association with a positive antibody test with the ELISA being the preferred test. Serologic test results must be interpreted with caution as false-positive and false-negative results occur with all assays.

2. Prognosis

a. Mother. Infection is similar in pregnant women and nonpregnant women.

b. Fetus. Transplacental transmission of *B. burgdorferi* has been reported and was associated with congenital cardiac malformations and encephalitis. Serosurveys suggest that although *B. burgdorferi* can cause an adverse fetal outcome, it is uncommon [42].

3. Management

a. Early infection is treated with amoxicillin, 500 mg PO qid for 10–30 days. Doxycycline is contraindicated in pregnancy.

b. Arthritis is treated with amoxicillin, 500 mg PO qid plus probenecid 500 mg qid for 30 days. Ceftriaxone 2 gm IV qd for 14 days or penicillin 3×10^6 U IV q4h for 14 days is an alternative.

c. Severe cardiac or neurologic disease is treated with ceftriaxone 2 gm IV qd for 14 days or penicillin 3×10^6 U IV q4h for 14 days.

4. Prevention. No vaccine is available. Avoidance of tick bites is the only method of prevention.

VI. Parasitic infections that can cause infertility secondary to maternal debilitation include amebiasis, giardiasis, visceral leishmaniasis, malaria, trypanosomiasis, ascariasis, trichuriasis, schistosomiasis, fascioliasis, fasciolopsiasis, paragonimiasis, and clonorchiasis. Amebiasis, ascariasis, enterobiasis, filariasis, schistosomiasis, and hydatid disease reduce fertility by directly damaging female reproductive organs. Malaria, *P. carinii,* toxoplasmosis, trypanosomiasis, and, possibly, visceral leishmaniasis cause congenital infections [5].

VII. Mycotic infections. Except for vaginal infections secondary to *Candida* sp., mycotic infections in healthy pregnant women are uncommon [31]. Disseminated candidiasis, cryptococcosis, aspergillosis, and histoplasmosis occur as opportunistic infections in immunocompromised patients. Pregnancy predisposes to dissemination of an otherwise acute, self-limited respiratory infection caused by *C. immitis* [31].

A. Diagnosis

1. *Candida* sp. commonly cause oral thrush and vaginitis. The spectrum of candidiasis also includes skin infections, colonization and infection of the gastrointestinal tract, septicemia, and invasion of internal organs (e.g., endophthalmitis, endocarditis). Disseminated disease occurs in pregnancies complicated by immunosuppression.

2. *C. immitis* and *Histoplasma capsulatum* generally cause self-limited respiratory illnesses. Both fungi disseminate to extrapulmonary sites in a small proportion of cases. *C. immitis* has a predilection for causing meningitis and osteomyelitis, and *H. capsulatum* tends to invade the reticuloendothelial system, causing hepatic, splenic, and lymph node infection.

3. *Cryptococcus neoformans,* like *C. immitis* and *H. capsulatum,* disseminates to extrapulmonary sites in a small percentage of patients. In these cases the fungus can infect all organs, with a predilection for the brain. Most cases of dissemination occur in immunocompromised patients.
4. *Aspergillus* sp. are frequently cultured saprophytes that cause primarily pulmonary and, less often, disseminated infections, usually involving the brain or kidneys, in immunocompromised patients.
5. Cryptococcosis, histoplasmosis, and coccidioidomycosis are diagnosed by culturing the fungus or by identifying it in tissue specimens. Since *Candida* sp. and *Aspergillus* sp. are human commensals, proof of infection requires culture from an abscess or blood or the identification of tissue invasion.
6. Complement-fixing tests permit accurate diagnosis of coccidioidal infections and are useful in diagnosing histoplasmosis when rising titers of complement-fixing antibody are demonstrated. Cryptococcosis also is diagnosed with some degree of assurance by demonstrating cryptococcal antigen in cerebrospinal fluid and serum. The value of serologic tests in diagnosing candidal infection is uncertain with the present assays. Serologic tests for diagnosing invasive aspergillosis have been developed but are not yet commercially available.

B. Prognosis

1. **Mother.** Except for an increased incidence of vaginitis, morbidity and mortality from candidiasis are unaffected by pregnancy. Neither the incidence nor the severity of cryptococcal or histoplasmal infections is known to be affected by pregnancy. In contrast, coccidioidomycosis can be very severe in pregnancy, and disseminated infections usually are fatal if untreated.
2. **Fetus.** Thrush is common in infants who pass through a birth canal infected with *Candida* sp. Fetal loss may be as high as 50% in instances in which *C. immitis* invades the placenta. Infants born to mothers with cryptococcosis are without illness, indicating absence of placental transfer of the fungus. Data on the effects, if any, of maternal histoplasmosis on the fetus are scarce.

C. Management

1. Amphotericin B is the drug of choice for most systemic mycoses. Data concerning the use of amphotericin B in the first trimester of pregnancy are scarce. Patients with coccidioidomycosis and cryptococcosis have been treated successfully in their second and third trimesters without harm being done to the fetus (Table 11-3).
2. Flucytosine has been used in the treatment of disseminated candidiasis and cryptococcosis. The teratogenic potential of the drug is unknown (Table 11-1).
3. Ketoconazole, an antifungal agent, is useful in the treatment of coccidioidomycosis, candidiasis, and histoplasmosis. The drug is given for prolonged periods of 1 or more years at dosages of approximately 400–600 mg/day. Because its toxicity and potential for teratogenicity are unknown, it should not be used in pregnancy without obtaining appropriate consultation.
4. Fluconazole is a new antifungal agent that is useful in treating cryptococcal meningitis and other fungal infections. The potential for teratogenicity in humans is unknown; therefore, it should not be used in pregnancy without obtaining appropriate consultation.

VIII. Immunization during pregnancy. Pregnancy is considered a contraindication for immunization with live virus vaccines in nonepidemic settings. A nonpregnant woman of childbearing age receiving a live virus vaccine should avoid pregnancy during the subsequent three months. Use of inactivated virus vaccines is considered nonhazardous to the fetus. The specifics of immunization are given in Table 11-2.

References

1. Alter, H. J., et al. Detection of antibody to hepatitis C virus in prospectively followed transfusion recipients with acute and chronic non-A, non-B hepatitis. *N. Engl. J. Med.* 321:1494, 1989.
2. Anderson, L. J., and Hurwitz, E. S. Human parvovirus B19 and pregnancy. *Clin. Perinatol.* 15:273, 1988.
3. Arvin, A. M. Antiviral treatment of herpes simplex infection in neonates and pregnant women. *J. Am. Acad. Dermatol.* 18:200, 1988.
4. Arvin, A. M., and Yeager, A. S. Other Viral Infections of the Fetus and Newborn. In J. S. Remington and J. O. Klein (eds.), *Infectious Diseases of the Fetus and Newborn Infant* (3rd ed.). Philadelphia: Saunders, 1990. Pp. 516–527.
5. Arvin, A. M., Ruskin, J., and Yeager, A. S. Protozoan and Helminthic Infections. In J. S. Remington and J. O. Klein (eds.), *Infectious Diseases of the Fetus and Newborn Infant* (3rd ed.). Philadelphia: Saunders, 1990. Pp. 528–573.
6. Baker, C. J. Group B streptococcal infection in newborns: Prevention at last. *N. Eng. J. Med.* 314:1702, 1986.
7. Baker, C. J., and Edwards, M. S. Group B Streptococcal Infections. In J. S. Remington and J. O. Klein (eds.), *Infectious Diseases of the Fetus and Newborn Infant* (3rd ed.). Philadelphia: Saunders, 1990. Pp. 742–833.
8. Brown, Z. A., and Baker, D. A. Acyclovir therapy during pregnancy. *Obstet. Gynecol.* 73:526, 1989.
9. Centers for Disease Control. Elimination of rubella and congenital rubella syndrome—United States. *M.M.W.R.* 34:65, 1985.
10. Centers for Disease Control. Measles prevention: Recommendations of the Immunization Practices Advisory Committee (ACIP). *M.M.W.R.* 38(S9):1, 1989.
11. Centers for Disease Control. Risks associated with human parvovirus B19 infection. *M.M.W.R.* 38:81, 1989.
12. Charles, D. *Infections in Obstetrics and Gynecology.* Philadelphia: Saunders, 1980. Pp. 362–427.
13. Cherry, D. Enteroviruses. In J. S. Remington and J. O. Klein (eds.), *Infectious Diseases of the Fetus and Newborn Infant* (3rd ed.). Philadelphia: Saunders, 1990. Pp. 325–366.
14. Chow, A. W., and Jewesson, P. J. Pharmacokinetics and safety of antimicrobial agents during pregnancy. *Rev. Infect. Dis.* 7:287, 1985.
15. Curran, J. W., et al. The epidemiology of AIDS: Current status and future prospects. *Science* 229:1353, 1985.
16. Daffos, F., et al. Prenatal management of 746 pregnancies at risk for congenital toxoplasmosis. *N. Engl. J. Med.* 318:271, 1988.
17. Ferenczy, A. HPV-associated lesions in pregnancy and their clinical implications. *Clin. Obstet. Gynecol.* 32:191, 1989.
18. Forbes, B. A. Acquisition of cytomegalovirus infection. *Clin. Microbiol. Rev.* 2:204, 1989.
19. Freij, B. J., and Sever, J. L. Herpesvirus infections in pregnancy: Risks to embryo, fetus, and neonate. *Clin. Perinatol.* 15:203, 1988.
20. Fung, J. C., et al. Serologic diagnosis of toxoplasmosis with emphasis on the detection of toxoplasma-specific immunoglobulin M antibodies. *Am. J. Clin. Pathol.* 83:196, 1985.
21. Gershon, A. A. Chickenpox, Measles, and Mumps. In J. S. Remington and J. O. Klein (eds.), *Infectious Diseases of the Fetus and Newborn Infant* (3rd ed.). Philadelphia: Saunders, 1990. Pp. 395–445.
22. Gotoff, S. P., and Boyer, K. M. Prevention of group B streptococcal early onset sepsis: 1989. *Pediatr. Infect. Dis. J.* 8:268, 1989.
23. Hansfield, H. H. *Neisseria gonorrhoeae.* In G. L. Mandell, R. G. Douglas, and J. E. Bennett (eds.), *Principles and Practices in Infectious Diseases* (3rd ed.). New York: Churchill-Livingstone, 1990. Pp. 1613–1631.
24. Ho, D. D., et al. Quantitation of human immunodeficiency virus type 1 in the blood of infected persons. *N. Engl. J. Med.* 321:1621, 1989.

25. Jacobs, R. F., and Abernathy, R. S. Management of tuberculosis in pregnancy and the newborn. *Clin. Perinatol.* 2:305, 1988.
26. Klein, J. O., and Remington, J. S. Current Concepts of Infections of the Fetus and Newborn Infants. In J. S. Remington and J. O. Klein (eds.), *Infectious Diseases of the Fetus and Newborn Infant* (3rd ed.). Philadelphia: Saunders, 1990. Pp. 1–16.
27. Korones, S. B. Uncommon virus infections of the mother, fetus and newborn: Influenza, mumps and measles. *Clin. Perinatol.* 2:259, 1988.
28. Lee, R. V. Parasites and pregnancy: The problems of malaria and toxoplasmosis. *Clin. Perinatol.* 2:351, 1988.
29. Main, E. K., Main, D. M., and Krogstad, D. J. Treatment of chloroquine-resistant malaria during pregnancy. *J.A.M.A.* 249:3207, 1983.
30. McCormack, W. M., et al. Hepatotoxicity of erythromycin estolate during pregnancy. *Antimicrob. Agents Chemother.* 12:630, 1977.
31. Miller, M. J. Fungal Infections. In J. S. Remington and J. O. Klein (eds.), *Infectious Diseases of the Fetus and Newborn Infant* (3rd ed.). Philadelphia: Saunders, 1990. Pp. 475–515.
32. Minkoff, H. L., and Feinkind, L. Management of pregnancies of HIV infected women. *Clin. Obstet. Gynecol.* 32:467, 1989.
33. Nanda, D., and Minkoff, H. L. HIV in pregnancy—Transmission and immune effects. *Clin. Obstet. Gynecol.* 32:456, 1989.
34. Philipson, A. The use of antibiotics in pregnancy. *J. Antimicrob. Chemother.* 12:101, 1983.
35. Preblud, S. R., and Alford, C. A. Rubella. In J. S. Remington and J. O. Klein (eds.), *Infectious Diseases of the Fetus and Newborn Infant* (3rd ed.). Philadelphia: Saunders, 1990. Pp. 196–240.
36. Remington, J. S., and Desmonts, G. Toxoplasmosis. In J. S. Remington and J. O. Klein (eds.), *Infectious Diseases of the Fetus and Newborn Infant* (3rd ed.). Philadelphia: Saunders, 1990. Pp. 89–195.
37. Ross, S. M. Sexually transmitted diseases and pregnancy. *Clin. Obstet. Gynecol.* 9:565, 1982.
38. Schwarz, R. H. Considerations of antibiotic therapy during pregnancy. *Obstet. Gynecol.* (Suppl. 5):955, 1981.
39. Smithells, R. W. Co-trimoxazole in pregnancy. *Lancet* 2:1142, 1983.
40. Snider, D. E., et al. Treatment of tuberculosis during pregnancy. *Am. Rev. Respir. Dis.* 122:65, 1980.
41. Stagno, S. Cytomegalovirus. In J. S. Remington and J. O. Klein (eds.), *Infectious Diseases of the Fetus and Newborn Infant* (3rd ed.). Philadelphia: Saunders, 1990. Pp. 241–281.
42. Steere, A. C. Lyme disease. *N. Engl. J. Med.* 321:586, 1989.
43. Steven, C. E., et al. Perinatal hepatitis B virus transmission in the United States. *J.A.M.A.* 253:1740, 1985.
44. Weinberg, E. D. Pregnancy-associated depression of cell-mediated immunity. *Rev. Infect. Dis.* 6:814, 1984.
45. Wendel, G. D. Gestational and congenital syphilis. *Clin. Perinatol.* 15:287, 1988.
46. Zeldis, J. B., and Crumpacker, C. S. Hepatitis. In J. S. Remington and J. O. Klein (eds.), *Infectious Diseases of the Fetus and Newborn Infant* (3rd ed.). Philadelphia: Saunders, 1990. Pp. 574–600.

12 Neurologic Complications

Stephen D. Collins

Pregnancy per se does not produce neurologic disease; however, a number of preexisting conditions may be adversely affected by the physiologic changes of pregnancy. Other conditions may not be altered by pregnancy but become difficult to diagnose or treat due to pregnancy. The most important single clinical dictum in treating women with neurologic problems in pregnancy is that **the neurologist and obstetrician need to remain in close, frequent communication.** Clinic visits will generally be scheduled at a much higher frequency than is the norm in neurologic practice, and the length of the visit is much longer than is the norm in obstetric practice. As in other high-risk obstetric settings, a defined treatment plan needs to be established early in the course of pregnancy and understood by all parties involved.

I. Epilepsy. Epilepsy is defined as the recurrent discharge of groups of brain cells causing the stereotyped disturbances of mentation or movement, or both, known as **seizures.** The high prevalence of the epilepsies in the general population (up to 1%) is mirrored by a similarly high prevalence in pregnancy (0.3–0.6%) [9, 33]. Although seizures and their therapies may increase the risk for adverse pregnancy outcomes, the precise risks are unknown at this time. Most authors state a 2–3% increase or an approximate doubling of overall risk for fetal malformation [42]. Thus, it should be stressed to the epileptic woman that the great majority (over 90%) of children born to epileptics are healthy.

Classification of epilepsies may be made on various grounds, with the most useful for therapy being that which describes the clinical symptomatology of individual seizures. The following is a synopsis of the International Classification of Epileptic Seizures as adopted by the International League Against Epilepsy in 1981.

A. Partial seizures (begin locally)

1. Simple (without alteration of consciousness)

a. Motor

b. Sensory

c. Autonomic

2. Complex (with alteration of consciousness)

a. Progressing from simple partial

b. Immediate impairment of consciousness

B. Generalized seizures (diffuse onset)

1. Absence

2. Myoclonic

3. Clonic, tonic, and **tonic-clonic**

4. Atonic

Seizures may occur for a number of reasons, and a pregnant woman who presents with her first seizure (1) does not yet have a diagnosis of epilepsy, (2) needs an extensive workup for the cause of her seizure, and (3) may or may not need to begin anticonvulsant treatment. Many conditions may resemble epilepsy including syncopy, vasovagal episodes, breath-holding spells, migraine, benign paroxysmal vertigo, transient ischemic attacks, narcolepsy, nonconvulsive epilepsy (pseudoseizures), hysteria, malingering, and intoxications. Evaluation of an initial seizure in pregnancy needs to consider these nonepileptic possibilities, and an outline of this workup will be presented later. Prediction of individual epileptic seizure patterns in pregnancy is extremely difficult. A widely cited retrospective study by Knight and Rhind [30] of 84 women with "idiopathic epilepsy" showed no change in seizure frequency in 50%, an increase in 45%, and a decrease in 5% of these women. Risk factors for increases were a history of frequent seizures (> one/month) and possibly the presence of catamenial seizures. A prospective study by Schmidt and colleagues [38] of 136 pregnancies in 122 women with sundry types of epilepsy showed no change in seizure frequency in 50%, an increase in 37%, and no change in 13%. Numerous factors may lead to increased seizures in any one patient, including noncompliance (due to fear of teratogenicity of anticonvulsants), anxiety, loss of sleep, alterations in steroid hormones, increases in clearance, decreases in bioavailability, and alterations in protein binding.

C. Status epilepticus. In the setting of noncompliance or "physiologic" subtherapeutic anticonvulsant levels, or both, a serious and mortal threat to mother and child is status epilepticus. Status epilepticus is simply defined as recurrent seizures without return of consciousness between seizures. Tonic-clonic generalized status is the most common type and produces hyperthermia and renal and cerebral damage with a resultant mortality of 3–20% [22]. Even in paralyzed, respirated animals, prolonged seizure activity may result in severe cerebral damage and death. Status epilepticus must be immediately recognized and treated if significant morbidity or mortality is to be avoided. **The goals of treatment** are (1) to maintain adequate respiration and blood pressure at all times, (2) to identify precipitating factors and correct the same, (3) to prevent complications of ongoing seizure activity, and (4) to rapidly provide an anticonvulsant with long serum half-life.

While rapid, deliberate, and step-wise treatment is requisite, **the elimination of seizures in seconds should not be the goal.** Too rapid administration of anticonvulsants resulting in a respiratory arrest is to be avoided as avidly as a protracted "treat and watch" approach. Benzodiazepines are particularly prone to cause rapid respiratory depression.

1. A general paradigm for treatment of status epilepticus follows:

a. History. Have separate members of the team obtain a careful history from whomever is available (family, friends, witnesses) paying particular attention to possible precipitating factors, including the following:

(1) Head trauma
(2) Systemic infection, or central nervous system (CNS) infection
(3) Tumor
(4) Systemic disease, e.g., diabetes requiring insulin use
(5) Prior history of epilepsy, prior episodes of status epilepticus or anticonvulsant noncompliance history, or a combination
(6) Illicit drug use
(7) Sleep deprivation
(8) Symptoms or signs of CNS hemorrhage

b. Vital functions

(1) Place patient in prone position, head turned, and slightly down to prevent aspiration.
(2) Pad the environment, especially the area near the patient's head.
(3) Take rectal temperature, pulse, and blood pressure. Place patient on cardiac monitor.
(4) If patient is hyperthermic (> 40°F), begin intubation immediately, since the most significant predictor of bad outcome is hyperthermia, and general anesthesia will eliminate seizures and attendant muscle activity. Continue to monitor blood pressure and heart rate closely, especially during and after anticonvulsant infusion.
(5) Place an oral airway, if possible, i.e., without forcing teeth apart.
(6) Obtain blood for
(a) complete blood count
(b) serum electrolytes, including calcium and magnesium
(c) serum glucose
(d) arterial blood gas
(e) serum toxicology screen
(f) anticonvulsant levels

(7) Obtain urine for toxicology screen

c. **Correction of medical problems and initiation of anticonvulsants**

(1) Dextrose 50 gm IV push (after giving thiamine 100 mg IV push).

(2) Clear line of glucose with normal saline solution.

(3) **Phenytoin** load, 15–20 mg/kg or approximately 1000–1500 mg, given at a maximum rate of 50 mg/minute by a physician as an injection close to the IV site, **not** into an infusion solution hanging at bedside. Blood pressure and respiration must be monitored closely during all anticonvulsant infusions, particularly if benzodiazepines have been previously administered. If a clear history of high-grade arrhythmia is present, phenobarbital may be the initial dose of choice. Do not give "half" doses on the theory that the patient may already have "some" anticonvulsant in her system; ataxia from high serum levels is preferable to continuing seizures. Intramuscular phenytoin is never indicated for treatment of status epilepticus due to slow and erratic uptake. A loading dose of 15 mg/kg will take 20 minutes to administer.

(4) If seizures continue following a load to 20 mg/kg then proceed to **phenobarbital** load as necessary to 13 mg/kg or approximately 1 gm, at a maximum rate of 100 mg/minute. Again blood pressure and respiratory rate need to be followed continuously, due to the combined depressant effects of phenytoin and barbiturates. If seizures still persist, endotracheal intubation and induction with general anesthesia should proceed at once, since generalized convulsions beyond one hour show significant morbidity and mortality [19]. The use of intravenous diazepam or lorazepam, while common, carries significant risk of respiratory depression and hypotension while exerting a significant anticonvulsant effect for a very brief period. Brown and Penry [13] found 26 cases of respiratory or cardiac depression, or both, in 401 cases of status epilepticus treated with diazepam. If intravenous benzodiazepines are to be used, experienced anesthesiologists should be at hand and ready to provide emergency intubation. In no case should benzodiazepines be given in the place of longer-acting anticonvulsants.

(5) Paraldehyde, once a mainstay of treatment, is an effective drug in the treatment of status epilepticus, but is not currently available in the United States. Dosage is 5 ml per buttock as a deep, IM injection, using glass syringes only.

(6) Initial laboratory studies should be available during the course of anticonvulsant infusion, and correction of acid-base disorders, hypocalcemia, and so forth should be aggressively pursued. Hyperthermia should be addressed through induction of general anesthesia and not solely through the use of ice packs.

D. **Effects on pregnancy.** Maternal and paternal epilepsy in the absence of anticonvulsant drug treatment poses a real, although poorly delineated, **risk of fetal malformation.** To date, the only anticonvulsants with definite teratogenic potential are trimethadione [20] and valproic acid, the latter associated with a high incidence of neural tube deficits [10], especially when used in polytherapy. It should be noted that some patients, especially those with frequent atonic seizures, may need to remain on valproic acid throughout their pregnancy. Ideally, these patients (and all epileptics) would be placed on monotherapy and their doses kept to the minimum possible to prevent seizures. Experimental and retrospective clinical data indicate high serum dosage and polytherapy to be risk factors for fetal malformation. **High-resolution ultrasound and serum/amniotic fluid testing for neural tube deficits should occur early** enough in pregnancy to allow termination of pregnancy if so desired. Alterations of anticonvulsants should not occur solely to "decrease teratogenic effects" since maternal seizure type, frequency of seizures, and prior response to anticonvulsants need to dictate therapy. No anticonvulsant at present is without fetal risk.

1. **General principles of antiepileptic drug therapy in the pregnant woman** are difficult to state due to the large variety of epilepsies and anticonvulsants. Generally accepted principles follow:

- **a.** Plasma concentrations of anticonvulsants should be maintained at the lowest possible level previously established to be effective in seizure control in that patient.
- **b.** Monotherapy should be attempted, and if seizures are very rare or can be safely endured without treatment (for example, simple partial seizures), a few women may be able to become pregnant free of drugs.
- **c.** Since organ system development is largely completed by six to eight weeks of fetal growth, and all anticonvulsants pose possible fetal risks, the sudden discontinuation or rapid tapering off and substitution of anticonvulsants may place the patient at greater risk for morbidities from breakthrough seizures than the benefits gained from substituting "safer" anticonvulsants.
- **d.** Epileptic women need to be seen and examined at least monthly during pregnancy, due to alterations of anticonvulsants secondary to the physiologic changes of pregnancy. All examinations should include a check of the patient's seizure calendar and compliance record, and examination for the occurrence of possible toxicities (lethargy, double vision, ataxia); the exam should note nystagmus, upper and lower limb ataxia, and gait and station.
- **e.** Expect dose increases secondary to increases in volume of distribution, increases in hepatic and renal clearance, and decreases in bioavailability. Emphasize to the patient and family that dose increases do not necessarily imply serum, brain, or **fetal** increases in free drug levels.

E. Additional effects of epilepsy on pregnancy. Various retrospective studies using different populations, and analyzed by different techniques, have alternately suggested or refuted other maternal and fetal risks. These risks include vaginal hemorrhage, delay in labor, toxemia, spontaneous abortion, stillbirth, or complicated delivery, either due to epilepsy itself or anticonvulsants [26, 40]. Neonates may demonstrate sedation to the point of respiratory compromise (especially with barbiturates or magnesium sulfate used as "eclampsia prophylaxis"). Neonatal hemorrhage secondary to vitamin K–dependent clotting factor deficiency has been documented [11], and therefore the current recommendation is to treat all women at 36 weeks or time of delivery, or both, with phytonadione (vitamin K). The neonate should be treated intravenously at birth, and cord bloods should be obtained for clotting studies with appropriate use of fresh-frozen plasma, if vitamin K–dependent clotting factors are deficient.

Maternal folic acid deficiency may increase fetal malformation rate, placental abruption, and spontaneous abortion. A small prospective study [6] showed no worsening of seizures on folic acid supplementation and an absence of congenital malformations in women treated with folic acid. A separate study by different authors [17] corroborated the findings, and so folic acid supplementation during pregnancy is recommended.

F. Effect of anticonvulsants on infant care. Breast-feeding is not impaired by epilepsy or anticonvulsant medications. Since breast milk is an ultrafiltrate of serum, milk concentrations of anticonvulsants mirror serum free drug levels. Kaneko and colleagues [27] measured milk to serum concentrations and found valproic acid as 5%, phenytoin as 18%, phenobarbital as 36%, carbamazepine as 40%, and primidone as 70%. Although phenobarbital and primidone have been shown to have associated infant feeding difficulties and decreased weight gain, the abrupt withdrawal of anticonvulsants in infants who experienced these drug in utero has been associated with neonatal convulsions. Anticonvulsant effects on brain development secondary to breast milk transfer are unknown. The American Academy of Pediatrics considers most anticonvulsants to be compatible with breast-feeding [14]. Case-by-case decisions should be made with mother and family regarding the risk/benefit of breast-feeding.

G. Evaluation of new-onset seizures. The onset of seizures in pregnancy may represent significant underlying pathology and, therefore, particularly in the case of focal epilepsies, needs an extensive and careful evaluation. This evaluation begins with the following:

1. A careful history from patient and family delineating seizures needs to be obtained.

a. Special care should be taken in describing presence or absence of premonitory signs or symptoms. Following an open-ended questioning, a list of common auras should be detailed, since the patient may consciously or unconsciously ignore/suppress some symptoms. Examples include rising feelings in the stomach, micropsia, macropsia, alterations in smell or hearing, vertiginous sensations, and "headrushes."
b. The patient's own prenatal and early natal history should be examined, looking for hypoxic, infectious, or traumatic episodes.
c. Prior seizure history, possibly only noted as blank stares, and information about school or behavioral problems should be sought.
d. Family history of seizures, strokes, hemorrhages, migraine, tuberous sclerosis, neurofibromatosis, and cardiac disease need to be ascertained.
e. Illicit and prescription drug ingestion history needs to be taken.
f. Trauma history should be elicited.
g. Headaches of a new, particularly progressive, or postural type must be looked for.
h. It should be determined if the seizure began focally, as focal seizure with or without generalization demands immediate structural evaluation.

2. A neurologic exam should attempt to uncover a focal or lateralizing postictal deficit.
3. The laboratory exam needs to screen for metabolic, infectious, and toxic abnormalities. Lumbar puncture is requisite if intracranial hemorrhage or infection is suspected and should occur immediately following a high-resolution computed tomography (CT) scan without contrast. Even high-resolution CT scans may not discern all subarachnoid bleeds, and so a "negative" CT does not rule out intracranial hemorrhage. If CNS bacterial infection is suspected, an immediate loading dose of appropriate antibiotics should be followed by CT scan, then the lumbar puncture, if not contraindicated.

H. Eclampsia. While magnesium sulfate has been in use for a number of years as a presumed prophylactic for seizures in preeclampsia, its efficacy is questionable, at best. Numerous trials are now in progress comparing phenytoin and magnesium sulfate for efficacy and safety to mother and child. Early results favor the use of the phenytoin but will need to be extended to large numbers of patients before definitive protocols can be delineated.

II. Headache. Headache is one of the most common presenting complaints to general practitioners. For obstetricians, two concerns repeatedly form the basis for neurologic consult: The first relates to the possibility of serious underlying pathology, and the second relates to safe and adequate treatment of "benign" head pain.

A. "Pathologic" headache. That it is difficult to determine the "malignancy" of a headache is understandable, because (1) the majority of migraines (60–75%) occur in women, (2) the presenting age of migraine overlaps the peak fertility period of women, and (3) some serious conditions associated with or exacerbated by pregnancy initially present as head pain. Additionally, obstetricians are not accustomed to diagnosing serious neurologic diseases, and last, differential symptoms and signs between "benign" and serious causes of headache may be subtle, at best.

1. A partial list of conditions with serious underlying pathology and with predilection for pregnancy that produce headache includes
   a. Sinus thrombosis (venous occlusive disease)
   b. Arterial thrombosis
   c. Severe preeclampsia
2. Conditions that may be worsened or precipitated by pregnancy include
   a. Pseudotumor cerebri
   b. Subarachnoid hemorrhage, secondary to rupture of arteriovenous malformations (AVMs), aneurysms, and fistulae
   c. CNS tumors, e.g., meningiomas, neurofibromas, pituitary adenomas, and choriocarcinomas
3. Last, conditions that are not related to pregnancy but that need to be recognized include the following:

- **a.** CNS infections (with acquired immunodeficiency syndrome [AIDS] an increasing specter)
- **b.** Drug abuse, especially cocaine and alcohol
- **c.** "Cry for help," the abused, depressed, or socially distressed woman seeking help via an oblique complaint

4. Diagnosis. The majority of women presenting with headache will not have serious underlying pathology, so how does one differentiate these patients from those needing rapid, complete neurologic evaluation? Patients with a long-standing history of head pain of a particular character are most likely to have "benign" headache. The patient who presents with headache of a new type, especially if progressive; constant; and associated with exertion, change of position, bowel movements, awakening the patient from sleep, or neurologic deficit, should have immediate evaluation. The overworked saw of medical school, "The worst headache of my life," is far less elucidating than "The first time I've had this headache in my life."

Since most patients with headache do not have abnormal neurologic exams, **the key to successful differential diagnosis lies in accurate history taking.** The location of pain will usually be offered spontaneously by the patient, as well as its severity. Unfortunately, neither of these historical details is as helpful as the character of pain, e.g., sharp, dull, constant, throbbing, ramping. Obtaining details about time of onset and duration of pain (as thoroughly documented in Raskin [36]) significantly aids in the differential diagnosis of migraine, cluster, "tension," hemorrhage, or tumor types of head pain. Patients may state that the pain is "always" there, in which case, the examiner must focus on onset and duration of severe periods of pain. Likewise, the chronology of onset may need to be determined by relating it to known events, such as high school graduation, marriage, or a new job. Inquiring if this type of pain necessitated time off from school or work in the past can reveal prior chronicity in many patients who are at first unable to set dates for initiation of pain. The examiner should first attempt to elicit precipitating factors in an open-ended manner, then by listing such common migraine triggers as chocolate, heavy cheeses, or wine.

5. Pertinent points to search for on physical exam are the following:

- **a.** Neck stiffness or straight-leg-raising pain, or both
- **b.** Retinal hemorrhages, at the optic nerve head, as in subarachnoid hemorrhage, or in the fundus, as associated with hypertension or preeclampsia
- **c.** Asymmetry of strength, particularly of cranial nerves III, IV, VI, and VII. The presence or absence of pronator drift needs to be ascertained
- **d.** Maintenance of motor speed, e.g., fast finger movements such as finger tapping
- **e.** Sensory loss, which the patient will often complain of prior to the examination
- **f.** Gait

Given a high-risk patient, immediate neurologic consultation with appropriate radiologic examination is mandatory.

B. Treatment of "benign" headache. Since no medicine is totally "safe" for the treatment of headache in pregnancy, obstetricians or neurologists treating pregnant women with frequent headache may end up with headaches themselves. Many patients need to be constantly reassured that even severe, classic migraine in itself bears no risk to the fetus. Severe, unremitting headache with nausea, vomiting, and potential dehydration does, however, pose significant risk to the fetus and forms the basis for the more aggressive treatment of head pain during pregnancy.

C. Effects of pregnancy on headache. Somerville [39] reported on 38 women who complained of migraine headaches in pregnancy. Seven (18%) said their migraines started in pregnancy, usually in the first trimester. Of the 31 women with preexisting migraine, 24 (78%) reported some improvement in pain during pregnancy, usually in the second and third trimesters. It can be gleaned from this small study that women will not **of necessity** experience worsened migraine during pregnancy, although in 14 of 38 (37%) migraines began, continued unabated, or worsened during pregnancy.

1. **General principles for treatment of headache in pregnancy** are easy to state (but hard to live with).
   a. Attempt to identify and eliminate precipitating factors associated with headache, e.g., lack of sleep and exercise, and imbibition of chocolate, cheese, and wine.
   b. Attempt nonmedical therapies such as relaxation techniques, behavioral modification, and hypnosis.
   c. Recommend avoiding fasts and maintaining a regular schedule of eating and sleeping.
   d. If medical therapy must be used, attempt control of minor pain with **acetaminophen** alone. More severe pain should be treated with **meperidine.** This agent has been in use for many years, and in 1100 exposures anytime in pregnancy, a zero relationship to major or minor fetal malformations was found [23]. Although obstetric anesthesia with meperidine has resulted in fetal respiratory depression, doses used in normal oral treatment have not been associated with significant fetal blood levels or respiratory distress.
   e. **Aspirin and other prostaglandin inhibitors should be avoided** due to the high incidence of maternal and fetal hemorrhage past 32 weeks' gestation and the risk of premature closure of ductus associated with nonsteroidal anti-inflammatory drug (NSAID) use.
   f. Raskin [36] recommends a **cocoa butter–based suppository of meperidine** as helpful when migraines associated with nausea or vomiting, or both, preclude oral delivery. Physical dependence can occur with any opiate or opiate congener, but doses less than 400 mg/day have not been associated with dependence [24].
   g. **Ergot preparations are to be avoided** since ergonovine has been implicated in fallopian tube motility changes (potentially interfering with pregnancy attempts) [15] and produces chromosomal alterations in human lymphocytes, indicating possible teratogenic potential [28]. Ergotamine tartrate taken orally probably does not have an oxytocic action as the parenterally applied form has been shown to have [18], but animal toxicity studies, albeit with large doses, indicate significant potential teratogenicity.
   h. **Propranolol** might be considered in a woman with meperidine-insensitive, intractable headache. Unfortunately, oxytocic effects, intrauterine growth retardation, hypoglycemia, bradycardia, and respiratory depression have been observed [12] even in low-dose treatment. Women with severe nausea or vomiting secondary to migraine, who fail to improve with meperidine might be candidates for beta-blockade. Extensive discussion of risk and benefits with the patient would need to occur and be documented.

D. **Effects of headache on pregnancy.** As noted before, headache per se does not bear significant risk to fetal outcome unless dehydration from continued nausea and vomiting supervenes. No evidence exists for earlier suppositions that headache predilects for preeclampsia or eclampsia.

III. **Cerebrovascular disease.** Neurologic dysfunction may be due to seizures, infections, tumors, vascular compromise, or drugs. Sudden onset of dysfunction with residual deficit lasting greater than 24 hours due to cerebrovascular disease is termed **stroke.** If the defect lasts less than 24 hours, the term **transient ischemic attack** (TIA) is used. Stroke is usually categorized as ischemic (embolic and thrombotic subcategories) or hemorrhagic (intraparenchymal and subarachnoid).

A. **Ischemic stroke.** Nonhemorrhagic or ischemic stroke is uncommon in nonpregnant young women. Pregnancy increases the risk approximately to 3–4 times normal by the late second and third trimester [16], and that risk remains high during the puerperium. Most ischemic strokes are caused by arterial, as opposed to cerebral, venous occlusions [4, 5, 16].

1. **Arterial occlusive disease.** As in most strokes, the carotid distribution is the favored site of arterial occlusion with middle cerebral artery occlusions being

the most common. Oral contraceptive use predisposes to vertebrobasilar occlusions [7]. Determining the etiology of a stroke may be difficult; the three major categories are thrombotic, embolic, and vasculitic.

a. **Thrombotic occlusions** are felt to be the most common. They may be preceded by transient ischemic attacks or may be progressive in nature with step-wise, serial loss of function. Women with preexisting conditions such as diabetes or hypertension are at increased risk due to the presence of atheromatous plaques, but thrombus formation without previous arterial disease is certainly possible. Associated risks for thrombus formation include hematologic conditions (sickle cell disease, thrombotic thrombocytopenic puerpera, systemic lupus erythematosus, anemia), preeclampsia, and infection (septicemia, meningovascular syphilis, tuberculosis).

b. **Embolic occlusion** classically presents with maximum deficit at onset with gradual clearing thereafter. An exception to this rule may be when secondary local edema formation in the infarction territory produces secondary loss of function in the hours or first day following the onset of symptoms. The potential sources of emboli are numerous and include cardiac problems (cardiomyopathy, valvular disease, dysrhythmias, patent cardiac defects); vascular complications (carotid or paradoxical from pelvic vein with patent cardiac defects); infections (subacute bacterial endocarditis with septic or bland emboli); drugs (intracarotid injection of illicit drugs mixed with talc, chalk, and so forth); and, more rarely, fat (after crisis in sickle and S/C disease); air (due to vaginal delivery or cesarean section, abortion, or vaginal insufflation); and amniotic fluid.

c. **Vasculitic occlusion.** Infections such as meningovascular syphilis and tuberculosis may present as small-vessel strokes. Collagen vascular disease and systemic erythematosus may cause arteritis leading to stroke. Illicit street drugs such as brown heroin and amphetamines have been shown in angiography to cause arterial spasms, and cocaine is presumed to cause stroke through similar mechanisms. Migraine can cause stroke, presumably through arterial spasm.

d. **Diagnosis**

(1) Etiology may be favored by historical evidence; however, clinical judgment is inadequate to distinguish ischemic from hemorrhagic stroke, and **laboratory studies** need to be initiated early, since treatment will be radically different given differing etiologies of stroke. Laboratory studies should include

(1) Cell blood count including platelet count
(2) Red blood cell morphology
(3) Erythrocyte sedimentation rate
(4) Serum electrolytes
(5) Serum lipid levels
(6) Prothrombin and partial thromboplastin
(7) Electrocardiogram

(2) **A CT scan** needs to be performed initially and rapidly since it best delineates ischemic from hemorrhagic infarction. **It does not** rule out subarachnoid hemorrhage and cannot supplant lumbar puncture in the evaluation of possible bleeds.

(3) **Lumbar puncture.** A CT exam should precede lumbar puncture unless it is unavailable, in which case patients with signs of herniation should not be tapped. These patients require neurosurgical evaluation. Cerebrospinal fluid (CSF) obtained within hours of a subarachnoid hemorrhage may not demonstrate red blood cells or xanthochromia. A "traumatic" tap generally shows decreasing numbers of red cells on successive tubes; however, xanthochromia will be absent since freshly lysed red blood cells will not release reduced hemoglobin. Hence, the physician should personally centrifuge a tube of CSF and examine for the presence of yellow supernatant.

(4) **Angiography.** Atheromatous lesions, as well as vasculitic and spastic

arteries, carotid dissections, and other structural causes of ischemic stroke, can be determined by angiography of the major vessels. Extensive shielding of the abdomen will substantially reduce radiation exposure to the fetus. Contrast loads are low and felt to be safe for the fetus.

(5) **Echocardiography.** Cardiac embolic sources need to be sought, as well as paradoxical emboli ruled out with use of bubble testing for patent foramina.

(6) **Magnetic resonance imaging.** After CT examination to rule out recent hemorrhage (for which magnetic resonance imaging [MRI] still is less sensitive), MRI may be especially helpful in elucidating etiologies such as cavernous angiomas and venous occlusion. MRI "angiography," an evolving technique, should supplant invasive angiography in the next few years.

e. Treatment

(1) Blood pressure should not be lowered unless diastolic pressures remain greater than 120 mm or signs of fetal distress are found on monitoring. If hypotensive agents are delivered, they should be able to be rapidly discontinued, e.g., nitropaste on chest or intravenous agents.

(2) Intravenous solutions with excess free water should be kept to a minimum, since these may increase cerebral edema and extend infarct size.

(3) Antiembolism stockings and careful skin care must be used to prevent secondary complications of pulmonary embolus and decubitus ulcers.

(4) Anticonvulsants should be begun if seizures occur.

(5) Surgically accessible disease, e.g., carotid disease or cardiac valvular disease, should proceed as in the nonpregnant patient. Inaccessible disease, nonsurgical disease, or postoperative patients may have thrombi or surgical sites, or both, which will serve as embolic sources, and may need to be anticoagulated. Due to fetal wastage and teratogenicity [41], warfarin should not be used. Heparin given in the intravenous or subcutaneous route is the anticoagulant of choice.

(6) Vaginal delivery is preferred if stroke has occurred early in pregnancy. A woman with a completed stroke and resolution of causation (e.g., valvoplasty), may deliver vaginally without further intervention. A completed stroke with presumed or known thrombus still in situ may dictate operative assistance of vaginal delivery with regional anesthesia at onset of labor to prevent the increased intracranial pressure associated with bearing down. If a stroke occurs near labor, cesarean section may be necessary.

2. **Venous occlusive disease.** Septic thrombophlebitis was a common problem in preantibiotic times. In women in their first trimester of pregnancy, venous thrombosis is generally associated with abortion or hematologic abnormality such as sickle cell disease or polycythemia. The majority of cases occur in the puerperium, 80% in the second and third weeks post partum. Neither maternal age nor parity is a predisposing factor, and the preceding labor and delivery are usually normal. Clinical presentation is usually manifested by headache of a progressive, severe, and analgesic-resistant nature. Transient neurologic deficits may or may not be noticed, but commonly seizures will bring the patient to medical attention. These seizures are often focal, and the presence of a focal seizure should **not** predispose the evaluating physician against a midline process, i.e., sagittal vein thrombosis.

a. Diagnosis. As in arterial occlusive disease, the clinical picture of headache followed by seizure in a postpartum woman implies, but does not prove, a venous occlusion. Structural anomalies, illicit drug use, or complicated migraine may also occur in this time period. Laboratory studies as in occlusive arterial disease need to be obtained. Postcontrast CT imaging may disclose the so-called delta sign (a filling deficit at the confluence of sinuses), but the sensitivity and specificity of this sign are both low. MRI is very sensitive for venous occlusive disease as is digital subtraction angiography.

Occasionally the diagnosis of postpartum eclampsia is considered, but the absence of other indicators of preeclampsia and the often significant delay in time from delivery both would help differentiate venous disease from eclampsia.

b. Treatment. Although some authors quote a 30% mortality in this entity, the reporting bias for series with autopsied material may exaggerate its presumed high mortality rate. The clinical grade of neurologic deficit does correlate with prognosis, and obtundation, coma, rapid progression, and subarachnoid blood are poor signs.

No proved effective treatment exists for venous thrombosis. Anticoagulation has been used, but intracranial (two of three patients [21]) and uterine bleeding have been documented [29]. Some centers have begun thrombectomy via catheters under radiologic guidance, but extensive experience in this technique is still lacking. General measures as in arterial occlusive disease should be effected. Vaginal delivery with regional anesthesia and operatively assisted at the second stage of labor is recommended if thrombus occurs early in pregnancy. If thrombus occurs very near or in labor, cesarean section may be necessary.

B. Hemorrhagic stroke. Ischemic stroke, from whatever cause, may have secondary bleeding, particularly in the instance of large ischemic insults. **Small-vessel hemorrhage** can be seen in patients with diabetes, hypertension, and eclampsia. These can be limited to small petechial lesions on CT or MRI or may coalesce to form truly massive bleeds that totally occupy the deep brain structures that are predilected to small-vessel disease.

Subarachnoid hemorrhage may be due to ruptured aneurysm or vascular malformation (arteriovenous malformations, cavernous angiomas, venous angiomas). Some authors [37] have suggested an increased tendency for arteriovenous malformations to rupture in pregnancy, but others [25, 35] have not supported these observations.

The presentation of subarachnoid hemorrhage generally includes sudden and severe headache of a different quality than previously experienced headache—progressive, unremitting, and unresponsive to analgesic (see sec. **II.A** for differentiation of subarachnoid hemorrhage headache from migraines). Nausea, vomiting, stiff neck, seizures, and focal neurologic deficits may be present. Rapid progression to obtundation and coma are poor prognostic signs and demand immediate neurosurgical evaluation. Focal neurologic deficits tend to occur with arteriovenous malformations slightly more frequently than with aneurysm, and third trimester bleeds are slightly more common with aneurysmal ruptures. Intralabor bleeds are uncommon with either anomaly. An increase in frequency in the first postpartum days is seen, presumably secondary to large shifts of intravascular volume that occur as a physiologic change following deliveries. The larger blood loss generally seen in delivering by cesarean section may, in fact, produce larger vascular volume shifts. Therefore cesarean section potentially could increase the risk of postdelivery vascular bleeds if loss of intravascular volume is a potential mechanism for postpartum hemorrhage.

1. Diagnosis

a. Diagnostic evaluation proceeds as in ischemic stroke, with **early CT and lumbar puncture** (LP). If the CSF exam is negative for blood, but was performed close in time to the onset of symptoms, repeat exam may be necessary 12–24 hours later. If focal deficits reappear, then repeat CT exam and LP are requisite.

b. Angiography needs to be performed in all vessels, as significant numbers of multiple aneurysms or coexisting arteriovenous malformations and aneurysms, or a combination of these, are found. Angiography may be "falsely" negative in the case of some angiomas, due to spasms of feeding vessels or low flow rate. Cavernous angiomas are classically cryptic on angiography and can usually be discerned on MRI.

2. Treatment

a. Blood pressure control, as opposed to ischemic stroke, is effected in order to keep blood pressure in normal ranges. Again, agents that can rapidly be discontinued are used since hypotension not only can extend previously damaged CNS insult, but fetal hypotension may cause significant morbidity and mortality.

b. **Antiedema agents** such as mannitol are only indicated if herniation ensues, and then for the period of time while the patient is being prepared for surgery. Steroids are generally not felt to be helpful in management of edema from hemorrhage.

c. **Anticonvulsants** should be administered early in the course of evaluation, since seizures can significantly worsen bleeding from either arteriovenous malformations or aneurysms. Intravenous phenobarbital or phenytoin is the agent of choice. Care needs to be exercised in administration of these drugs to prevent hypotension (see sec. **I.C.1.c** on appropriate delivery of anticonvulsants).

d. **Aneurysms** have a significant risk of rebleeding with high mortality and morbidity in the days and weeks following initial hemorrhage. **Surgery** should therefore be attempted as soon as possible, if indicated by radiologic findings and patient clinical grade. Hypotension should be avoided intraoperatively, but hypothermia has been used with good success and is well tolerated by the fetus [37]. Antivasospastic agents such as nimodipine are beginning to be used widely and show great promise in the prevention of postoperative spasm. No literature exists to date on its use in pregnancy.

e. **Arteriovenous malformations** have a much lower rate of rebleed in the weeks following initial hemorrhage, and embolization and surgery may be able to be delayed until after delivery.

f. **The woman with a surgically resected aneurysm may undergo normal labor and vaginal delivery.** Untreated aneurysms and AVMs do not fair better with cesarean section, since, as described before, bleeds in women with known vascular anomalies generally do not occur during labor, but rather may increase pre- and post partum. The latter may be due to loss of intravascular volume, a normal process that may be worsened by larger blood loss associated with cesarean section. Thus, a regional anesthesia placed early in labor with operative assistance of vaginal delivery at the second stage of labor is recommended for appropriate patients.

g. **No convincing case can be made for sterilization** of women with vascular anomalies, as has been suggested in older literature.

C. Other vascular anomalies

1. **Dural arteriovenous malformations.** Anomalous shunts between dural sinuses may present in pregnancy or in the puerperium. Anteroinferior dural shunts may present with eye signs such as ocular bruits, proptosis, conjunctival bleeds, or diplopia. Superior-posterior shunts may present with signs of subarachnoid hemorrhage, seizures, or focal neurologic deficit. Either entity may present as headache. Papilledema may be present in either category of AVM. Angiography is usually diagnostic and embolization with invasive neuroradiologic techniques may be adequate to treat these lesions.

2. **Spinal arteriovenous malformation.** Pregnancy can clearly be shown to worsen spinal AVMs, although the mechanism for this is unknown. Once having bled, spinal AVMs generally rebleed, and mortality on first or subsequent bleeds is high. Often, those who live progress to incontinence and paraplegia. As stated, presentation can be with death or with upper and lower motor neuron deficits in lower extremities and sensory loss to the spinal segment involved. The diagnostic exam of choice is MRI, especially since angiography may not reveal feeding vessels and involves large quantities of contrast dye, and the fetus can rarely be shielded adequately from radiation. Surgical treatment must not be delayed if progressive cord compression and even death are to be prevented. Dural or intradural and extramedullary lesions offer good promise of surgical ablation. Anterior and intraspinal lesions offer more poor surgical outcomes.

IV. Neuropathy

A. Mononeuropathies

1. **Bell's palsy.** Bell's palsy or **idiopathic facial palsy** has a clear association with

pregnancy, with an increase of incidence from 17 in 100,000 per year (all women) to 57 in 100,000 per year in pregnant women [2]. Nearly all (76%) occur in the third trimester or puerperium with no known predisposing factor. Presentation is usually as a sudden onset of unilateral facial weakness in a forehead-to-chin distribution. Taste may be involved and hyperacusis may be noted. On questioning, most patients will remember a postauricular pain in the day or so preceding weakness.

Prognosis in cases of partial paralysis is very good, with complete or near complete recovery the rule. When paralysis is complete, taste is affected, and hyperacusis present, the prognosis drops to 50%. Short-course treatment with prednisone at 40–50 mg/day in these severe cases may improve recovery to 80% [1]. No ill effects of this short-term treatment should occur to mother or fetus, providing the mother is not diabetic, in which case steroid treatment should not be used.

2. **Carpal tunnel syndrome.** While up to one-fifth of pregnant women complain of some sort of hand pain during pregnancy [32], the majority of these cases are not true carpal tunnel syndrome (CTS) but rather instances of transient, distal finger-tip tingling. True CTS involves painful tingling of the thumb and first fingers, often awakening the patient or first noted on awakening. Relief is found at first from elevation of the hand or vigorous shaking, but when symptoms continue into the day, the patient will generally seek medical help. The cause of CTS, median nerve compression, can be treated conservatively in almost all cases by discontinuation of extremes of flexion or extension of the wrist. This may require retraining or refitting job tools, e.g., computer keyboards, or discontinuation of certain hobbies. The use of night-time splints is generally quite successful. Regression following delivery of the child is nearly universal, so therapy may need to be performed for only a short time. If conservative therapy has proved unsuccessful after good-faith tries, then local injection of steroids may be attempted. This will only afford temporary relief, but it may be adequate until delivery and subsequent loss of interstitial edema. Surgery would rarely be indicated.
3. **Meralgia paresthetica.** Lateral femoral nerve compression is seen in pregnant women and in persons with significant pannus. One symptom is a stinging pain in the middle to upper lateral thigh, worsened by standing and relieved by flexion at the hip. Third-trimester presentation is most common, and delivery remits symptoms in nearly all cases within weeks.
4. **Femoral nerve.** Operations on true pelvis or lower abdomen, e.g., cesarean sections and hysterectomies, may predispose to femoral nerve compression. This is commonly reported in thin women when retractors are placed on or about the psoas muscle. Clinically, the patient notes weakness on first ambulation following surgery, unilaterally, and of the quadriceps and possibly the iliopsoas muscles. Knee jerks are absent or decreased. Sensory loss is variable, from negligible to numbness and paresthesias of anterior thigh. Prognosis is usually excellent but may take weeks to many months for full recovery to occur.
5. **Obturator nerve.** Much less common is damage to the obturator nerve, exiting near the pelvic brim and through the obturator canal. Predisposing factors for this compression include large fetal size with prolonged labor, pelvic hematoma, or pelvic mass, or a combination. Weakness is found on leg adduction without reflex abnormalities. Sensory deficits can be found in the upper, inner thigh. Prognosis, as in other compressive neuropathies, is generally excellent.

B. Polyneuropathy

1. **Guillain-Barré syndrome.** The Guillain-Barré syndrome (idiopathic polyneuritis) has no association with pregnancy. Plasmaphoretic therapy for patients with Guillain-Barré can decrease recovery time and so it may be of benefit in pregnant women with significant neurologic dysfunction. Care needs to be taken with plasmaphoresis in the maintenance of intravascular volume, especially since autonomic instability is the hallmark of severe Guillain-Barré.

C. Root and plexus lesions

1. Lumbar root lesions. Pregnancy does not predispose women to lumbar disk prolapse, but the lordosis imposed by the enlarging fetus may significantly worsen underlying lumbar disease. Acute prolapse is characterized by sharp, radiating pain from buttock to knee or foot and is worsened by standing, stretching the root (e.g., straight-leg raises) and increases in intracranial pressure, for example, those caused by Valsalva maneuvers. In the presence of progressive neurologic deficit, surgery may be necessary, otherwise strict bed rest and analgesia are the treatments of choice. Most acute prolapsed disks will respond to such conservative treatments.

2. Lumbosacral plexus lesions. Injury to the plexus may occur with compression of nerve from the fetal head or by the use of forceps. Predisposing factors are prolonged labor, large fetal size, short maternal stature, and mid-forcep rotations. Diagnosis is usually obvious since symptoms are noted on first ambulation following delivery, almost always unilateral and of characteristic clinical type. The woman displays a foot drop with weakness of flexion and eversion at the ankle. Sensory disturbances such as "pins and needles" numbness on the dorsum of the foot and lateral leg may also be found. Compression of the lateral peroneal nerve, generally following long surgical procedures with inadequate padding of the fibular head, will lack eversion weakness, lack sensory symptoms above the knee, and lack straight-leg-raising pain. Prognosis is generally good with either compression, but nerve conduction studies will help prognosticate proximal compressions. If normal distal peroneal conduction velocities are found one week after injury, then full recovery is the rule. Recovery may take months, however, and so a foot drop must be corrected with orthopedic appliances, since permanent heel cord shortening may ensue.

V. Muscle disease

A. Myasthenia gravis. The pregnant woman who has myasthenia gravis should be in the care of a neurologist who specializes in muscle disease. No particular effects of pregnancy on myasthenia can be stated, merely that significant improvement in symptoms or drastic worsening may occur [34]. The obstetrician should have injectable (IV/IM) anticholinesterase (e.g., neostigmine methyl sulfate, 0.5 mg IV, IM) available in case of myasthenic crisis and for use during labor when nausea may preclude oral administration. Labor proceeds as in the nonmyasthenic patient. Regional anesthesia is preferred to general anesthesia since the weaning of a myasthenic from intubation may prove difficult. Sedatives and narcotic analgesics should be used sparingly and with careful measurement of vital capacities. Arterial blood gases are not indicated in following respiratory function since deficits in oxygenation are not present until the patient is in extremis.

Neonatal myasthenia gravis develops in approximately 10% of babies born of myasthenic mothers [31]. No prenatal prognostic factors or testing have yet identified babies at increased risk for this problem. Thus, the pediatrician must be equipped with full resuscitation equipment at birth and the child must be observed in a monitored situation for several days following delivery. Weakness may appear up to four days following birth, although it will generally be noticeable in the first day of life.

VI. Movement disorders. In the preantibiotic era, **chorea gravidurum,** the sudden, brief involuntary movements of the face, limbs, and trunk with onset in pregnancy, was a common occurrence. This was due to the prevalence of acute rheumatic fever and Sydenham's chorea, i.e., basal ganglionic arteritis and petechial hemorrhage. A modern review [43] disclosed 1 case in 140,000 deliveries, and, therefore, other rare causes of abnormal movements, e.g., Wilson's disease, must be excluded if choreatic movements are seen in a pregnant woman.

More common today are the dyskinesias and dystonias associated with phenothiazine use. Prochlorperazine (Compazine) for use in nausea and vomiting may produce dystonic reactions and these may be truncated by intravenous or intramuscular use of diphenhydramine. Tardive dyskinesias associated with chronic phenothiazine use in psychiatric practice is a much more difficult entity and most likely will have been chronic prior to pregnancy. The obstetrician and psychiatrist will need to make case-to-case decisions on treatment for this entity.

VII. **Tumors.** No CNS tumors are strictly associated with pregnancy; however, some may be preferentially exacerbated by pregnancy. These include **meningiomas, acoustic neuromas, pituitary adenomas, and cerebellar hemangioblastomas.** Numerous theories have been proposed for these pregnancy-associated exacerbations, including sex steroid hormone induction of tumor or vasculature, and intrinsic intravascular volume expansion. However, proof exists for no one etiology. Symptomatic tumors of pregnancy do share a predilection for localization to areas where expansion will cause direct pressure effects on a nerve or the brain. Thus, parasellar meningiomas or pituitary adenomas produce visual field deficits, acoustic neuromas produce hearing loss, and cerebellar hemangioblastomas produce multitudinous brainstem signs and symptoms. Worsening of symptoms by third trimester and remission of symptoms following delivery with recrudescence in subsequent pregnancies have been noted by many authors [3, 8].

Choriocarcinoma is a primary germ cell tumor much less frequently seen in Western countries than in Africa and Asia. Metastatic choriocarcinoma can initially present with central nervous symptoms of headache or mild alteration of consciousness, and signs can include stiff neck, focal neurologic deficit, seizure, or gross obtundation. Choriocarcinoma can present after abortion or molar or normal pregnancy. Chest x rays need not be abnormal, but head CT scans should nearly always show hemorrhagic lesions. Treatment of solitary CNS metastases may include surgery (if in an appropriate location) as well as chemotherapy. Recent advances in treatment of primary germ cell tumors with good survival at five years should be reflected in treatment outcomes of these "high-risk" categories of choriocarcinoma.

Any tumor may present as a solitary infarction, CNS bleed, or mass lesion with the full panoply of associated signs and symptoms. Appropriate workup for these presentations has been described earlier (see secs. **I, II, and III**). It is important to remember to include tumor in the differential diagnosis of all of the "benign" conditions that will of necessity form the majority of presentations to obstetricians. **No solitary management course can be presented for the case of a woman with a CNS tumor in pregnancy.** It is possible to state that treatment should occur as in the nonpregnant woman. That is, tumors that have caused neurologic deficit, especially spinal cord compression or posterior fossa symptoms, need immediate diagnostic workup and treatment. Delay to postdelivery dates may be appropriate for some "benign" tumors such as meningiomas or pituitary adenomas since delay results in a decrease of vascularity of tumor beds. These patients would clearly require close follow-up during pregnancy to monitor for progression of symptomatology. Delivery of the woman with a CNS mass has been discussed in sec. **III.**

A. **Pseudotumor cerebri.** Also known as **"benign" intercranial hypertension,** the syndrome of pseudotumor cerebri is one of an elevation of intracranial pressure in the absence of intracranial mass or other clear etiology. These patients present with headache and may have visual complaints of blurring, obscuration, or diplopia, or a combination.

1. **Physical exam** may reveal significant papilledema, visual field deficits, and abducens palsy. Computed tomography or MRI by definition will not disclose a space-occupying lesion; the follow-up lumbar puncture will disclose elevation of pressure.
2. Pregnancy alone (as well as any other cause of increased intraabdominal and thus intrathoracic pressure) can elevate CSF pressures to approximately 250 ml of water. **Measurements of opening CSF pressure need to be performed in all cases,** with good patient relaxation and with legs extended to obviate false-positive pressure elevations.
3. No etiology is known for pseudotumor cerebri.
4. **Treatment.** Numerous treatment regimens have been tried over the years, with the most common being repeat lumbar puncture. The efficacy of any regimen is debatable. Pseudotumor generally presents in midtrimester; it may spontaneously regress in weeks or may only remit after delivery. Progression of

intracranial hypertension may occur in the face of repeat lumbar puncture, diuretic treatment, or glucocorticoid treatment. Diuretic therapy must be performed with caution in order to preserve intravascular volume and to prevent oligohydramnios. Chronic and progressive cases with worsening visual field loss may require optic nerve decompression.

5. No fetal disease accompanies the maternal intracranial hypertension.

References

1. Adour, K. K. The bell tolls for decompression? *N. Engl. J. Med.* 292:748, 1975.
2. Adour, K. K., and Wingerd, J. Idiopathic facial paralysis (Bell's palsy) factors effecting severity and outcome in 446 patients. *Neurology* 24:112, 1974.
3. Allen, J., et al. Acoustic neuroma in the last months of pregnancy. *Am. J. Obstet. Gynecol.* 119:516, 1974.
4. Amias, A. G. Cerebral vascular disease in pregnancy: I. Hemorrhage. *J. Obstet. Gynaecol. Br. Comm.* 77:100, 1970.
5. Amias, A. G. Cerebral vascular disease in pregnancy: II. Occlusion. *J. Obstet. Gynaecol. Br. Comm.* 77:312–325, 1970.
6. Biale, Y., and Lewenthal, H. Effect of folic acid supplementation on congenital malformations due to anticonvulsant drugs. *Eur. J. Obstet. Gynecol. Reprod. Biol.* 18:211, 1984.
7. Bickerstaff, E. R. *Neurological Complications of Oral Contraceptives.* Oxford: Clarendon, 1975.
8. Bickerstaff, E. R., et al. The relapsing course of certain meningiomas in relation to pregnancy and menstruation. *J. Neurol. Neurosurg. Psychiatry* 21:89, 1958.
9. Bjerkedal, T., and Bahna, S. L. The course and outcome of pregnancy in women with epilepsy. *Acta Obstet. Gynecol. Scand.* 52:245, 1973.
10. Bjerkedal, T., et al. Valproic acid and spina bifida. *Lancet* 2:1096, 1982.
11. Bleyer, W. A., and Skinner, A. L. Fatal neonatal hemorrhage after anticonvulsant treatment. *J.A.M.A.* 235:626, 1976.
12. Briggs, G. G., et al. (eds.). *Drugs in Pregnancy and Lactation* (2nd ed.). Baltimore: Williams & Wilkins, 1987.
13. Brown, T. R., and Penry, J. K. Benzodiazepines in the treatment of epilepsy: A review. *Epilepsia* 14:277, 1973.
14. Committee on Drugs, American Academy of Pediatrics. The transfer of drugs and other chemicals into human breast milk. *Pediatrics* 72:75, 1983.
15. Coutinho, E. M., et al. The response of the human fallopian tube to ergonovine and methyl ergonovine, *in vivo. Am. J. Obstet. Gynecol.* 126:48, 1976.
16. Cross, J. N., Castro, P. O., and Jennett, W. B. Cerebral strokes associated with pregnancy and the puerperium. *Br. Med. J.* 3:214–218, 1968.
17. Dansky, L., et al. Anticonvulsants, folate levels, and pregnancy outcome: A prospective study. *Ann. Neurol.* 21:176, 1987.
18. Davis, M. E., et al. The present status of oxytocics in obstetrics. *J.A.M.A.* 107:261, 1936.
19. Delgado-Escueta, A. V., et al. Medical intelligence: Current concepts in neurology: Management of status epilepticus. *N. Engl. J. Med.* 306(22):1337, 1982.
20. Feldman, G. L., et al. The fetal trimethadione syndrome. *Am. J. Dis. Child.* 131:1389, 1977.
21. Gettelfinger, D. M., and Kokmen, E. Superior sagittal sinus thrombosis. *Arch. Neurol.* 34:2–6, 1977.
22. Hauser, W. A. Epidemiology, Morbidity, and Mortality of Status Epilepticus. In A. V. Delgado-Escueta et al. (eds.), *Status Epilepticus: Mechanisms of Brain Damage and Treatment.* New York: Raven, 1982.
23. Heinonen, O., et al. *Birth Defects and Drugs in Pregnancy.* Littleton, MA: Publishers Scientific Group, 1973.
24. Himmelsbach, C. K. Further studies of the addiction liability of Demerol. *J. Pharmacol. Exp. Ther.* 79:5, 1943.
25. Hoades, J., Andrews, B., and Collins, S. D. Subarachnoid hemorrhage in pregnancy. Unpublished. 1989.

26. Janz, D., and Back-Mannagetta, G. Complications of Pregnancy in Women with Epilepsy: Retrospective Study. In D. Janz et al. (eds.), *Epilepsy, Pregnancy, and the Child.* New York: Raven, 1982.
27. Kaneko, S., et al. The Problems of Antiepileptic Medication in the Neonatal Period: Is Breast Feeding Advisable? In D. Janz et al. (eds.), *Epilepsy, Pregnancy, and the Child.* New York: Raven, 1982.
28. Kato, T., and Jarvik, L. F. LSD-25 and genetic damage. *Dis. Nerv. Syst.* 30:42, 1969.
29. Kendall, D. Thrombosis of intracranial veins. *Brain* 71:386, 1948.
30. Knight, A. H., and Rhind, E. G. Epilepsy in pregnancy: A study of 153 pregnancies in 59 patients. *Epilepsia* 16:99, 1975.
31. Namba, T., et al. Neonatal myasthenia gravis: Report of two cases and a review of the literature. *Pediatrics* 45:458, 1970.
32. Nicholis, G. G., et al. Carpal tunnel syndrome in pregnancy. *Hand* 3:80, 1971.
33. Niswander, K. R., and Gordon, M. *The Collaborative Perinatal Study of the National Institute of Neurological Diseases and Stroke: Women and Their Pregnancies.* DHEW publication no. NIH 73-379. Washington, D.C.: GPO, 1972.
34. Osserman, K. E. Myasthenia Gravis. In J. J. Rovinsky and A. F. Guttmacher (eds.), *Medical, Surgical, and Gynecologic Complications of Pregnancy* (2nd ed.). Baltimore: Williams & Wilkins, 1965.
35. Parkinson, D., and Bachers, G. Arteriovenous malformations: Summary of 100 consecutive supratentorial cases. *J. Neurosurg.* 53:285, 1980.
36. Raskin, N. H. *Headache.* Philadelphia: Saunders, 1988.
37. Robinson, I. L., et al. Arteriovenous malformations, aneurysms, and pregnancy. *J. Neurosurg.* 43:63, 1974.
38. Schmidt, D., et al. Change of seizure frequency in pregnant epileptic women. *J. Neurol. Neurosurg. Psychiatry* 45:751, 1983.
39. Somerville, B. W. A study of migraine in pregnancy. *Neurology* 22:824, 1977.
40. Watson, J. D., and Spellacy, W. N. Neonatal effects of maternal treatment with the anticonvulsant drug diphenylhydantoin. *Obstet. Gynecol.* 37:881, 1971.
41. Wiebers, D. O. Ischemic cerebrovascular complications in pregnancy. *Arch. Neurol.* 42:1106, 1985.
42. Yerby, M. Teratogenicity of Antiepileptic Drugs. In T. A. Pedley and B. S. Meldrum (eds.), *Advances in Epilepsy.* Edinburgh: Churchill-Livingstone, 1988.
43. Zegart, K. N., and Schwarz, R. H. Chorea gravidarum. *Obstet. Gynecol.* 32:24, 1968.

Selected Readings

Aminoff, M. J. Neurologic Disorders. In R. K. Creasy and R. Resnik (eds.), *Maternal Fetal Medicine.* Philadelphia: Saunders, 1988.

Donaldson, J. O. *Neurology of Pregnancy.* Philadelphia: Saunders, 1978.

Raskin, N. H. *Headache.* Philadelphia: Saunders, 1988.

13 Dermatologic Complications

Arthur C. Huntley
and Debra Ann Horney

Pregnancy is a temporary period of profound metabolic, endocrinologic, and immunologic changes. The pregnant woman is subject to both physiologic and pathologic alterations that can occur in the skin, hair, and nails. Pregnancy-related cutaneous changes can be classified in five broad categories: (1) physiologic changes secondary to the hormonal milieu; (2) cutaneous tumors influenced by pregnancy; (3) diseases specifically related to pregnancy; (4) genital infections of perinatal importance; and (5) other dermatologic diseases or diatheses that are influenced by pregnancy. Comments on dermatologic diagnosis and therapy precede the discussion of these five categories.

I. Dermatologic diagnosis

A. History and physical examination. The most important part of dermatologic diagnosis is often the history. Not all skin problems that arise during pregnancy are the result of that condition. One needs to review the medication history and ascertain whether the dermatologic condition has been aggravated by environmental exposure. How long has the eruption been present, and what seem to be the aggravating factors? Do other members of the family suffer from a dermatologic condition? On what part of the body did the reaction start, and what was the initial morphology?

In performing the physical examination, it is important to use adequate lighting and to inspect all of the skin, mucous membranes, and adnexal structures as deemed necessary. If the morphology of the eruption has changed, look for a primary rather than a secondary manifestation (examples of secondary manifestations include lichenification, excoriations, impetiginization).

B. Laboratory aids. In addition to standard laboratory procedures, the following may be useful:

1. Skin biopsy of an early, typical nontraumatized lesion
2. Potassium hydroxide preparation for fungal and yeast elements
3. Gram's stain for the presence of bacteria
4. Tzanck smear for acantholytic cells in pemphigus vulgaris or multinucleate epithelial giant cells in herpes simplex or herpes zoster
5. Culture of skin lesions for bacterial, fungal, or viral disease
6. Dark-field examination for *Treponema pallidum*
7. Examination for fluorescence of infected skin (*Pseudomonas* species = green, erythrasma = coral red)

II. Dermatologic therapy. Most inflammatory skin eruptions commonly associated with pregnancy will resolve after delivery. During gestation, significant relief may be afforded by topical and systemic therapy.

A. Topical therapy. Topical therapy has the advantage of delivering medication to the symptomatic area of skin with little or no systemic absorption. When sufficient, it is the method of choice. Topical measures include gently cleansing and debriding the skin; cooling the skin and reducing pruritus; modifying the rate of water loss from the skin; and delivering medications (e.g., antibacterial, antifungal, anti-inflammatory) to the skin.

1. Applications of water with or without solutes (showers, baths, soaks, and compresses) are useful for acute moist, weeping eruptions. Room-temperature tap water, aqueous Burow's solution 1:100, or aqueous potassium permanganate solution 1:10,000 are well tolerated.

2. Applications of an insoluble powder or shake lotion (zinc oxide, calamine lotion, talc) are useful in subacute eruptions as they are cooling, drying, and somewhat protective.
3. Applications of an oil, either liquid or semisolid (Aquaphor, Eucerin, Vaseline), are useful in dry, chronic eruptions. These help to reduce water loss from the skin.
4. Addition of anti-inflammatory agents to lotions, creams, or ointments. Commonly used in pregnancy are hydrocortisone 1% and triamcinolone acetonide 0.1%.

B. Systemic therapy. The systemic medications used for dermatoses that occur in pregnancy often include one or more of the following:
1. Antipruritic (antihistamines or acetaminophen [Tylenol])
2. Antibiotics
3. Anti-inflammatory agents

C. General therapeutic considerations
1. The medications chosen should be suitable for use during pregnancy.
2. Consider need versus risk, especially in early pregnancy.
3. Keep the therapy as uncomplicated as possible.
4. Avoid known sensitizers and irritants.
5. If there is failure to improve, consider
   a. Intolerance or allergy to medications
   b. Noncompliance
   c. Reappraisal of diagnosis
   d. Adjustment of therapy
   e. Consultation

III. Physiologic changes of pregnancy

A. Pigmentation changes

1. **Hyperpigmentation.** Localized hyperpigmentation is common in pregnancy, especially in darker-skinned individuals. Darkening of the nipples, areolae, linea alba, and external genitalia have the clinical manifestations most commonly appreciated. Other skin areas that may become hyperpigmented include those prone to friction such as the medial aspect of the thighs. In addition, nevi, freckles, and recent scars may darken during pregnancy. This pigment change is believed to be related to melanocyte stimulation by increased serum levels of estrogen and progesterone. Most of these pigment changes regress post partum.

2. **Melasma**

Melasma (chloasma, the so-called mask of pregnancy) is a symmetric, light- to dark-brown pigmentation involving the skin of the forehead, cheeks, and sometimes upper lip. It is said to occur in two-thirds to three-fourths of all pregnancies. Increased levels of serum estrogen and progesterone are thought to be responsible for this condition. The pigmentation usually fades after delivery. Sun exposure plays a major role in inducing this hyperpigmentation. Similar changes may occur in nonpregnant women, patients receiving oral contraceptives, and even in some men. It should be differentiated from postinflammatory hyperpigmentation, which follows various dermatoses.

The most important aspect of treatment for this condition involves decreasing the amount of ultraviolet light penetration into the skin. This may be accomplished by avoiding sun exposure or by the use of potent sun-blocking agents, or both. Topical creams containing bleaching agents such as hydroquinone may also be of assistance in removing some of this hyperpigmentation. This effect may be enhanced by the addition of topical tretinoin. If inflammation results from the application of these two agents, then the addition of a topical corticosteroid is also warranted. The combination of these ingredients (tretinoin 0.1%, hydroquinone 5%, dexamethasone 0.1%) has been as effective for this condition [9]. When resolution has been achieved, it is important for the patient to continue using a sun-blocking agent to prevent melanocyte stimulation and reacquisition of pigment.

B. Hair. The physiologic state of pregnancy apparently affects hair by prolonging the anagen (growing) phase. In some persons this results in hirsutism, i.e., increased hair on the face, legs, and back. This hirsutism regresses post partum. One additional effect of prolonging the anagen phase during pregnancy is that of postponing the telogen (resting) phase of hair. As a result, in many women following delivery, the major portion of the scalp hair is cycled into the telogen phase. Approximately three months post partum, this results in a major shedding of scalp hair, the so-called telogen effluvium. Hair lost in the telogen effluvium is replaced by normal anagen hair. Following several additional months (the hair grows at about ½ in./month), the patient regains scalp hair approaching prepartum density.

C. Vascular changes

1. **Palmar erythema.** Erythema appears on the palms in a diffuse or localized distribution. There are no symptoms, and resolution occurs after delivery.
2. **Spider telangiectasis** lesions appear as multiple red macules approximately 2–10 mm in diameter with small central pulsating papules. They appear on the face, trunk, and upper extremities. Pressure on the central arteriole will obliterate the lesion transiently. Resolution without treatment is expected shortly after delivery but failure to resolve has been reported in 20–50% of individuals.

D. Striae distensae. "Stretch marks" appear frequently and in varying degrees during pregnancy. Initially, they are slightly erythematous, linear, flat-to-barely raised areas appearing most commonly on the breasts, abdomen, and hips. After pregnancy, they fade to approach normal skin color. There is no known prevention or satisfactory cure. Striae are probably caused by increased corticosteroid serum levels rather than by increased abdominal girth as previously thought, although their localization is probably owing to physical factors.

IV. Cutaneous tumors. These lesions appear for the first time, increase in number, or enlarge in size during pregnancy.

A. Skin tags (acrochordons). These lesions are 1–3 mm in diameter, skin-colored, tan, or brown-black papules that appear on the neck, chest, axillae, and groin during pregnancy. Clothing and jewelry may irritate them and they may become swollen and tender. Treatment is not required for asymptomatic lesions. When the lesions are symptomatic or for purposes of cosmesis, most skin tags are easily removed by clipping the unanesthetized base with surgical scissors and applying a styptic solution (ferric sulfate or aluminum chloride) to the wound. Another method of removal involves simple destruction by freezing the lesions with liquid nitrogen. One note of caution: It may be difficult to differentiate the skin tags from pedunculated nevi. Rarely, a malignant melanoma may be pedunculated. Often, excision is favored over simple destruction due to the importance of submitting questionable lesions for a pathology examination.

B. Nevi. Moles may enlarge, darken, or first become apparent during pregnancy. Any mole that appears to change in a manner unlike the other moles present should be carefully evaluated, and consideration should be given to removal and histopathologic examination.

C. Pyogenic granuloma (granuloma gravidarum, pregnancy tumor). This lesion looks like a small, dome-shaped hemangioma, often with a peripheral collarette of scale. It appears most commonly on the gums in association with extensive gingivitis. Pyogenic granuloma is a misnomer, for this is not a pustular or infectious process. Histologically, the lesion consists of granulation tissue. The lesion usually resolves partially or completely postpartum.

V. Diseases specifically related to pregnancy

A. Pruritus gravidarum is a common problem in pregnancy and consists of intense, generalized pruritus and the absence of skin lesions. It tends to occur late in the pregnancy and resolves with parturition. The cause is said to be estrogen inhibition of glucuronyl transferase resulting in impaired bilirubin conjugation and excretion, cholestasis, and increased levels of circulating bile salts [6, 16].

1. **Clinical findings.** The physical examination is important in differentiating this common phenomenon from other pruritic conditions in pregnancy. This condition is characterized by pruritus in the absence of preceding skin lesions. Patients may scratch enough to produce excoriations, and these areas may become secondarily infected. Thus the exam may reveal linear erythema or even abrasions, some of which have a golden crust and a surrounding erythema. But physical examination does not reveal a primary lesion.
2. **Laboratory findings.** Laboratory examination often reveals elevation of serum alkaline phosphatase, serum glutamic oxaloacetic transaminase, or bilirubin. These patients are usually anicteric. Skin biopsy is unhelpful.
3. **Therapy.** If treatment is necessary, emollients and antihistamines are first-line therapy. Oatmeal baths or cooling lotions containing menthol 0.25% or camphor 0.25% (Sarna lotion) may also be of benefit. For patients with more severe pruritus (those not responding to first-line therapy), oral cholestyramine (4 gm bid–tid) or activated charcoal (10 gm tid mixed with water or juice) may be required.
4. **Course and prognosis.** No maternal or fetal complications have been reported in pruritus gravidarum. Patients affected by this condition during pregnancy may have a similar condition if given oral contraceptives after delivery. Cholestatis of pregnancy is a severe form of this disorder in which the patients are usually jaundiced. Also, this more severe form has been associated with premature labor, low-birth-weight infants, and postpartum hemorrhage [4].

B. **Pruritic urticarial papules and plaques of pregnancy.** Since its description in 1979 [8, 20], this condition has been generally recognized as a distinct clinical entity. It is characterized by urticarial papules and plaques first beginning on the trunk and later appearing on the proximal extremities of women in the third trimester of pregnancy. It is most common in primigravidas. This may be the most common skin eruption of pregnancy.

1. **Clinical findings.** It is generally a disease of the first pregnancy. The skin eruptions usually start in the third trimester with pruritic, erythematous papules and urticarial plaques that develop suddenly over the abdomen. In half the patients, the initial lesions appear in the abdominal striae distensae. The eruption gradually becomes more generalized with extension to the thorax and proximal extremities. Individual lesions consist of 1–2 mm erythematous juicy papules that blanch on pressure.
2. **Laboratory findings.** No abnormalities have been found in serology, chemistry, or blood count. Biopsy of typical lesions reveals a superficial perivascular lymphohistiocytic infiltrate with papillary edema and epidermal parakeratosis with focal spongiosis.
3. **Therapy.** Most patients can be managed with topical corticosteroids, but occasionally patients with severe symptoms require prednisone up to 40 mg/day.
4. **Course and prognosis.** Most lesions resolve rapidly within one week of delivery. Fetal wastage and morbidity have not been reported, and there is usually no recurrence in subsequent pregnancies.

C. **Herpes gestationis.** Herpes gestationis, also known as **pemphigoid gestationis,** is a rare recurrent polymorphous, usually vesiculobullous, dermatosis of pregnancy in the puerperium [17]. The presentation with vesicles or pustules on an erythematous base is herpetiform but not due to the viral infection. The incidence is 1 in every 3000–5000 pregnancies. The etiology is unknown, although many believe this disease is immunologically similar to bullous pemphigoid. The disease may recur with subsequent pregnancies, menstruation, or treatment with progesterone-containing medications, suggesting that hormonal modulation plays a role.

1. **Clinical findings.** Although the disease may begin at any time during gestation or early puerperium, in the majority of cases its onset is in the second or third trimester. Clinically often an early prodrome of malaise, chills, fever, nausea, and headache is present. Erythematous papules, vesicles, and bullae appear on the extremities, abdomen, buttocks, and mucous membranes. Occasionally target lesions similar to those that occur in erythema multiforme may also be seen [16]. Involvement of the oral mucosa occurs rarely.
2. **Laboratory findings.** Eosinophilia and elevated erythrocyte sedimentation are often present. Biopsy of a characteristic lesion reveals superficial and deep perivascular infiltrate of eosinophils, lymphocytes, and histiocytes. Depending on the stage of the lesion biopsied, there is either a marked dermal edema or a subepidermal split. Direct immunofluorescence of perilesional and normal-appearing skin reveals a linear deposition of C3 with or without immunoglobulin G (IgG) at the basement membrane zone [3]. A circulating herpes gestationis factor is often present in the serum. This factor has been shown to be an IgG capable of fixing complement by the classic pathway, and it may be responsible for herpes gestationis–like skin lesions in the newborn. Generally the disease activity is unrelated to the titer of herpes gestationis factor.
3. **Therapy.** In mild cases of herpes gestationis, symptomatic therapy with oral antihistamines and topical steroids may be sufficient. Pyridoxine hydrochloride has also been reported to be of value. However, most patients require oral prednisone, 20–80 mg/day in divided doses. With clearing, the dosage can be tapered and eventually administered on an alternate-day schedule and continued until after delivery.
4. **Course and prognosis.** Resolution usually occurs within three months after delivery. If the onset of lesions is late in pregnancy, resolution may take even longer. Maternal prognosis is generally excellent. The prognosis for the infant has been debated for many years. Holmes and Black [7] reported that the incidence of small-for-gestational-age infants is increased, but perinatal mortality is not increased. It is not known whether steroid therapy alters fetal prognosis. Occasionally, transient blisters are noted in the newborn. Herpes gestationis tends to recur during subsequent pregnancies, generally presenting with an earlier onset and more severe manifestations.

D. **Impetigo herpetiformis** is a rare condition characterized by sheets of pustules on an erythematous base. It is a rare condition of pregnancy and has its usual onset in the third trimester.

1. **Clinical findings.** The primary skin lesion is a small pustule appearing on an erythematous base. Large erythematous areas studded with pustules usually appear first in the inguinal folds and axillae. Progression may occur, with widespread involvement and occasional development of mucous membrane lesions. The pustules tend to coalesce and dry while new ones appear toward the periphery of the expanding erythematous areas. These patients are often extremely ill with malaise, chills, fever, diarrhea, vomiting, and sometimes tetany [16].
2. **Therapy.** Treatment consists of correction of the underlying metabolic disturbance, oral prednisone, 15–30 mg/day, and antibiotics in the event of secondary infection. Termination of pregnancy should be considered if the patient's condition worsens on appropriate therapy.
3. **Course and prognosis.** With the use of corticosteroids and antibiotics, maternal mortality is now low; however, stillbirth and placental insufficiency still occur even when the disease appears to be controlled with prednisone. The disease remits promptly post partum but may recur in subsequent pregnancies.

E. **Spangler's papular dermatitis of pregnancy** was initially described in 1962 by Spangler and colleagues [18] and has been seen only in a handful of patients [12]. The etiology is unknown. The initial reports of this condition raise some doubt on its existence, but it is included here because of the reported fetal mortality.

1. **Clinical findings.** This disorder is characterized by intensely pruritic generalized papules, 3–5 mm in diameter with central, elevated, slightly firmer papules usually covered by a hemorrhagic crust, 1–2 mm in diameter [12]. These papules are not grouped and may occur on any area of the trunk or extremities. In 7–10 days these lesions heal, usually leaving macules of postinflammatory hyperpigmentation.
2. **Laboratory findings.** Spangler reported the characteristic finding of increased urine levels of human chorionic gonadotrophin and decreased plasma levels of estrogen and cortisol [18]. Biopsy of the skin lesion from one patient demonstrated normal epidermis overlying superficial perivascular infiltrate of lymphocytes and eosinophils with occasional extravasated red blood cells.
3. **Therapy.** The recommended treatment has been prednisone 40–200 mg/day [12]. The eruption is curtailed within 24–48 hours. Concomitant treatment for the pruritus could include oral antihistamines and topical antipruritic measures.
4. **Course and prognosis.** The primary concern of this syndrome is the reported 27% fetal loss [18]. Treatment with corticosteroids is said to markedly improve the fetal outcome. This condition may recur with subsequent pregnancies.

VI. Genital infections of perinatal importance

A. Herpes simplex. Of major concern to both mother and fetus is the development of primary herpes simplex after the twenty-sixth week of pregnancy. Such an event is occasionally accompanied by encephalitis, myocarditis, and hepatitis. Mortality for disseminated infection for both mother and fetus approaches 50%.

Recurrent genital herpes simplex has been of concern because of the possibility of transmission at parturition to the newborn. This concern has led to the recommendation that weekly cultures be done on the vaginal pool beginning at 34 weeks' gestation, and that a positive culture is grounds for a cesarean section. More recently these guidelines have been questioned because the risk of transmission appears to be low (5%) for recurrent infection [11]. Proposed modification of the management guidelines has suggested that the management decisions be based solely on examination and culture at the time of admission to the labor and delivery unit. Cesarean section should be considered for patients who demonstrate clinical evidence of infection at the time of admission. Cultures should be available in three days, and if positive, the infant should be recalled for observation and possible treatment.

The major agent available for treatment of herpes simplex infection is acyclovir. However, the safety to the fetus has not been determined. Pending further studies, routine administration of acyclovir to prevent the occurrence of an outbreak of this infection prior to parturition is not recommended.

B. Chlamydia. *Chlamydia trachomatis* causes an asymptomatic infection of the cervix and can cause inclusion conjunctivitis or pneumonia in neonates who pass through an infected birth canal.

C. Condylomata acuminata (anogenital warts)

1. **Clinical findings.** The appearance of warts varies among other aspects, according to the surface that they occupy. Warts on the vulva often exist as dry papules with a horny surface, which on close inspection consist of multiple projections. These individual islands of hyperkeratosis are characteristic of warts. When the wart exists in an area that receives friction, such as in the groins or buttocks crease, the hyperkeratosis may not be as evident; one sees a papule surfaced by micropapules in a cobblestone appearance. Often lesions in folds have moist surfaces. Constant moisture may lead to maceration, secondary infection, and malodor. The lesions on

mucous membranes are similar to those that occur on occluded skin. Identifying small lesions on mucous membranes may prove to be a challenge, but moistening the surface with dilute acetic acid (vinegar) results in a whitish surface of these hyperkeratotic papules, which sets them apart from the normal mucosa.

2. **Laboratory findings.** Most lesions suspected of being warts are treated without laboratory confirmation. When a biopsy is performed, it reveals epidermal hyperplasia with hyperkeratosis and parakeratosis. The dermal papillae have widely dilated vessels. In young verrucae there are large vacuolated cells in the upper stratum malphighi and in the granular layer. Immunofluorescent antibodies can be used to confirm the presence of a wart virus in tissue or smears, but currently these agents are only available as investigational tools.
3. **Therapy.** Traditional treatment of warts is hampered by the lack of an effective antiviral antibiotic. Destructive measures such as electrodesiccation, cryotherapy, and laser therapy are the treatments of choice for smaller lesions. Larger lesions may need to be "debulked" prior to treatment of the base. Podophyllin, a topical agent often used in treating moist warts, is contraindicated in pregnancy because of reported maternal toxicity and fetal death. Resistant lesions may be injected with interferon, but this is also not recommended during pregnancy.

VII. Skin diseases aggravated by pregnancy

A. Infections. It is normal for cell-mediated immunity to be depressed during pregnancy. This results in aggravation of many infections that are ordinarily kept in check by this arm of the immune system (Table 13-1).

1. **Herpes simplex.** Refer to sec. **VI.**
2. **Varicella zoster.** Varicella during pregnancy can have disastrous consequences to both the mother and fetus. Varicella occurring in adulthood carries the risk of serious pneumonia or encephalitis. Varicella can also lead to premature labor. During the first trimester of pregnancy, maternal varicella can result in congenital varicella syndrome in the fetus. Zoster occurring during pregnancy apparently carries no special risk to the mother or baby.
3. **Leprosy.** Pregnancy and the subsequent first six months of lactation are said to result in an exacerbation of leprosy in about one-third of patients. The fetal effects are said to include low birth weights, small placentae, and a high incidence of infant mortality. Dapsone appears to be a safe drug for treatment [19].

B. Rheumatologic diseases

1. **Lupus erythematosus.** Pregnancy has been said to improve, to leave unaffected, and to worsen systemic lupus erythematosus. Thus the response in a given individual cannot be predicted. The effects of systemic lupus erythematosus on fetal outcome are generally proportional to the severity of maternal disease. Neonatal lupus syndrome with heart block, skin lesions, and liver or hematologic abnormalities is an occasional complication [19]. (See also Chap. 14, sec. **I.A.**)
2. **Systemic sclerosis.** There are few reports of systemic sclerosis and pregnancy. This may reflect the fact that systemic sclerosis tends to have its onset several years after childbearing. The information gleaned from those patients reported can be summarized as follows: Pregnancy has no adverse effect on the disease status of the patient with systemic sclerosis. In fact, some patients seem to have improvement, albeit temporary. Patients with systemic sclerosis carry an increased risk of hypertension and preeclampsia. The reports on fetal outcome are variable from relatively unaffected to 66% mortality [2].
3. **Polymyositis/dermatomyositis.** Polymyositis/dermatomyositis (PM/DM) appears to carry high risk for both fetus and mother during pregnancy. Pregnancy appears to be a precipitating factor in the onset and in the exacerbation of PM/DM. The disease may begin during pregnancy. Half

Table 13-1. Skin diseases of note in pregnancy

Infections	Fetal risk	Maternal risk
Herpes simplex	Primary infection after wk 26 has risk of fetal myocarditis, encephalitis, hepatitis	? increased mortality from disseminated infection
Varicella	Varicella syndrome, first trimester premature labor	Varicella in adult may be accompanied by pneumonia, encephalitis
Leprosy	Increased fetal mortality	Aggravation
Rheumatologic diseases		
Lupus erythematosus	Neonatal lupus syndrome	Variable
Systemic sclerosis	Unaffected other than maternal complications	Hypertension, preeclampsia
Polymyositis	50% fetal loss	Often onset or worsening of disease
Bullous diseases		
Pemphigus	12% fetal loss, neonatal pemphigus	Often onset or worsening of disease
Porphyria		Worsening in some
Inherited disorders		
Ehlers-Danlos syndrome type I, IV		25% fatal outcome
Pseudoxanthoma elasticum		Gastrointestinal bleed
Neurofibromatosus	Increased fetal mortality	Tumor growth; vascular rupture
Malignancies		
Melanoma		Tumors of onset in pregnancy have poor prognosis
Acquired immunodeficiency syndrome (AIDS)	Perinatal transmission	Increases complications

of those patients with inactive PM/DM will undergo an exacerbation during pregnancy. The frequency of spontaneous abortions and perinatal death increases to about 50% in patients with this condition [5].

C. Bullous diseases

1. **Pemphigus.** Pemphigus vulgaris may have its onset during pregnancy or with the administration of oral contraceptives. It may have a clinical presentation similar to herpes gestationis. The evaluation of a patient with bullous diseases should include a skin biopsy for histopathology and immunofluorescence. Pemphigus may also have adverse consequences on the fetus. This diagnosis carries an increased risk of stillbirth (about 12%) and live infants with neonatal pemphigus. Live births with neonatal pemphigus usually have clearing of the cutaneous findings within weeks and have a good prognosis [14].
2. **Porphyria cutanea tarda.** Pregnancy appears to cause a worsening of porphyria cutanea tarda in some patients. This might be as expected because estrogens are known precipitating factors for this condition. The fetal outcome appears to be unaffected.

D. Inherited disorders

1. **Ehlers-Danlos syndrome.** Of the many types of Ehlers-Danlos syndrome (EDS), those with type I (gravis) and type IV (ecchymotic) tend to have problems with pregnancy. Pregnant women with either type may develop postpartum bleeding, poor wound healing, wound dehiscence, uterine lacerations, bladder and uterine prolapse, and abdominal hernias [19]. Patients with type IV Ehler-Danlos syndrome (EDSIV) appear to have a high incidence of complications of pregnancy. In addition to the aforementioned complications, they may also develop rupture of the bowel, aorta, vena cava, or uterus; and vaginal lacerations. The overall risk of maternal death for each pregnancy in patients with EDSIV is 25% [15].
2. **Pseudoxanthoma elasticum.** Pseudoxanthoma elasticum is an inherited disorder of connective tissue that has its primary manifestations on the degeneration of elastic tissue in the skin, eye, gastrointestinal tract, and blood vessels. It is clinically recognized by the presence of cutaneous yellow papules, usually on the upper back and neck region, and by the presence of angioid streaks, hemorrhages, and retinal scarring on ocular examination. The chief complication during pregnancy is gastrointestinal bleeding and hematemesis. No fetal risk is proved.
3. **Neurofibromatosis.** Neurofibromatosis is an autosomal dominant inherited disease that is clinically characterized by the presence of café au lait macules, and tumors of peripheral nerves. Pregnancy appears to aggravate this condition. The skin tumors may appear to enlarge during pregnancy. Growth of these tumors during pregnancy may result in invasion of vascular walls and vascular rupture. Hypertension is also a common occurrence during the pregnancy of patients with neurofibromatosis. The fetal risks include a high incidence of spontaneous abortion and stillbirth [1].

E. Malignancies

1. **Melanoma.** Malignant melanoma is an increasingly common tumor among the fairer-skinned population in the Western world. The prognosis of this tumor seems to best relate to the extent of vertical growth as determined by tumor thickness, at the time of diagnosis. The most common form of this condition, superficial spreading malignant melanoma, is often excised before it develops extensive vertical growth, and thus has a more favorable prognosis. The reports of the effect of pregnancy on melanoma vary, but it appears that melanoma arising during pregnancy has a worse prognosis [13]. However, women with a previous melanoma not related to pregnancy apparently do not have increased risk of reactivation of the tumor due to pregnancy.
2. **Acquired immunodeficiency syndrome.** Acquired immunodeficiency syndrome (AIDS) may have poor consequences for the mother and the pregnancy and may have disastrous consequences for the fetus. Premature rupture of the membranes, chorioamnionitis, and postpartum sepsis or hemorrhage appear to be common. Children born to affected mothers tend to have lower birth weights. Perinatal transmission of AIDS to the fetus is a major risk that does not seem to be affected by performing cesarean rather than vaginal delivery [10].

   Cutaneous manifestations of AIDS are several. At or around the time of seroconversion, there is often fever and an evanescent maculopapular eruption on the trunk. This syndrome consists of erythematous macules and faint papules located on the trunk and occasionally on the palms, sometimes with an associated enanthema, adenopathy, and low-grade fever. Patients with AIDS are also subject to more persistent or extensive involvement with common cutaneous infections by such agents as *Candida,* herpes simplex (types I and II), and by wart viruses. These patients may also have skin infections produced by organisms usually not pathogenic, such as *Mycobacterium avium* and *Bartonella* sp. The most common later finding of AIDS is that of Kaposi's sarcoma, usually noted as erythematous-to-purple macules and nodules.

References

1. Ansari, A. H., and Nagamani, M. Pregnancy and neurofibromatosis (von Recklinghausen's disease). *Obstet. Gynecol.* 47:25–29s, 1976.
2. Ballou, S. P., Morley, J. J., and Kushner, I. Pregnancy and systemic sclerosis. *Arthritis Rheum.* 27:295–298, 1984.
3. Carruthers, J. A., et al. Immunopathologic studies in herpes gestationis. *Br. J. Dermatol.* 96:35, 1977.
4. Dacus, J. V., and Muram, D. Pruritus in pregnancy. *S. Med. J.* 80:614, 1987.
5. Gutierrez, G., Dagnino, R., and Mintz, G. Polymyositis/dermatomyositis and pregnancy. *Arthritis Rheum.* 27:291, 1984.
6. Hanno, R., Salecky, E. R., and Krull, E. A. Pruritic eruptions of pregnancy. *Dermatol. Clin.* 1:553, 1983.
7. Holmes R. C., and Black, M. M. The fetal prognosis in pemphigoid gestationis (herpes gestationis). *Br. J. Dermatol.* 110:67, 1984.
8. Lawley, T. J., et al. Pruritic urticarial papules and plaques of pregnancy. *J.A.M.A.* 241:1696, 1979.
9. Kligman, A. M., and Willis, I. A new formula for depigmenting human skin. *Arch. Dermatol.* 111:40, 1975.
10. Minkoff, H., et al. Pregnancies resulting in infants with acquired immunodeficiency syndrome or AIDS-related complex. *Obstet. Gynecol.* 69:285, 1987.
11. Prober, C. G., et al. Low risk of herpes simplex virus infections in neonates exposed to the virus at the time of vaginal delivery to mothers with recurrent genital herpes simplex virus infections. *N. Engl. J. Med.* 316:240, 1987.
12. Pruett, K. A., and Kim, R. Papular dermatitis of pregnancy. *Obstet. Gynecol.* 55:38s, 1980.
13. Reintgen, D. S., et al. Malignant melanoma and pregnancy. *Cancer* 55:1340, 1985.
14. Ross, M. G., et al. Pemphigus in pregnancy: A reevaluation of fetal risk. *Am. J. Obstet. Gynecol.* 155:30, 1986.
15. Rudd, N., et al. Pregnancy complications in type IV Ehlers-Danlos syndrome. *Lancet* 1:50, 1983.
16. Sasseville, D., Wilkinson, R. D., and Schnader, J. Y. Dermatoses of pregnancy. *Int. J. Dermatol.* 20:223, 1981.
17. Shornick, J. K. Herpes gestationis. *J. Am. Acad. Dermatol.* 17:539, 1987.
18. Spangler, A. S., et al. Papular dermatitis of pregnancy. A new clinical entity. *J.A.M.A.* 181:97, 1962.
19. Winton, G. B. Skin diseases aggravated by pregnancy. *J. Am. Acad. Dermatol.* 20:1, 1989.
20. Yancey, K. B., Hall, R. P., and Lawley, T. J. Pruritic urticarial papules and plaques of pregnancy. *J. Am. Acad. Dermatol.* 10:473, 1984.

14 Immunologic Complications

Lorraine A. Milio
and Gary A. Comstock

I. Collagen-vascular or rheumatic diseases. The collagen-vascular diseases, also referred to as **rheumatic, autoimmune,** or **connective tissue diseases,** are a group of acquired autoimmune disorders in which chronic inflammation of various connective tissues and joints is the common finding. Since these diseases occur predominantly in women and tend to have their onset during childbearing years, the obstetrician is likely to encounter these chronic diseases more often than their prevalence in the general population would indicate. Three points must be considered in treating pregnant women with collagen-vascular diseases: several major organ systems are often involved; severity of the disease may vary greatly from patient to patient; the course of the disease during pregnancy is often unpredictable. For these reasons, the treatment program must be highly individualized, and a multidisciplinary approach involving a rheumatologist or experienced internist and a perinatologist/obstetrician is recommended for the duration of the pregnancy.

A. Systemic lupus erythematosus

1. **Clinical presentation and laboratory findings.** Systemic lupus erythematosus (SLE) is a chronic multisystem inflammatory disease of as yet undetermined etiology. The disease is most frequent in women during the reproductive years, with clinical evidence occurring for the first time during pregnancy or the postpartum period in up to 14% of all cases [6]. Although the cause of SLE is unresolved, the underlying pathophysiology is hyperactivity of the B-lymphocyte population with subsequent production of autoantibodies [13]. Antinuclear antibodies can be detected in the serum of virtually all patients with SLE, with those directed against double-stranded or native DNA being highly specific for the disease. Antinuclear antibody titers have not been found to be elevated in normal pregnancy or preeclampsia. Antibodies to DNA histones, although not specific for SLE, are present in up to 75% of SLE sera and are the source of the lupus erythematosus phenomenon. A chronically false-positive VDRL (Venereal Disease Research Laboratory) test or rapid plasma reagin test is seen in 10–20% of patients.

   Clinical manifestations of SLE mostly result from circulating antigen-autoantibody complexes or the reaction of autoantibodies with fixed tissue antigens in vessel walls. Frequent manifestations include arthritis or arthralgias (90%), skin rash (70–80%), nephritis (46%), fever, neuropsychiatric disorders, pleurisy, and pericarditis. Hematologic abnormalities include anemia (57–78%), leukopenia (50%), and a positive direct Coombs' test. Table 14-1 summarizes the American Rheumatism Association criteria for SLE. For both the 1971 criteria and the 1982 revision, four or more criteria are required for diagnosis of SLE. In Table 14-2, the main laboratory abnormalities of SLE are presented.

2. **Effect on pregnancy.** Overall fertility rates in patients with SLE are normal. Amenorrhea may occur during exacerbations of the disease or as a result of steroid treatment. Conception does tend to occur more frequently in periods of remission or mild disease activity. There is a marked increase in fetal loss in patients with SLE with spontaneous abortion rates ranging between 10 and 40%. Women with SLE who conceive during a period of disease quiescence and who demonstrate no evidence of renal disease have the best fetal outcome. In patients with lupus nephritis, a maternal serum creatinine of 1.5 mg/dl is

Table 14-1. Diagnosis of systemic lupus erythematosus*

1971 Criteria	1982 Revision
Facial erythema, butterfly rash	Malar rash
Discoid lupus	Discoid lupus
Raynaud's phenomenon	Photosensitivity
Alopecia	Oral ulcers
Photosensitivity	Arthritis
Oral or nasopharyngeal ulceration	Antibody to DNA or Sm or LE cells or false-positive STS
Arthritis without deformity	Proteinuria > 0.5 gm/d or cellular casts
Lupus erythematosus cells	Pleuritis and pericarditis
Chronic false-positive serologic test for syphilis	Psychosis or seizures
Profuse proteinuria > 3.5 gm/24 h	Hemolytic anemia or leukopenia or thrombocytopenia
Cellular casts	
Pleuritis or pericarditis, or both	
Psychosis or convulsions, or both	
Hemolytic anemia or leukopenia or thrombombocytopenia	

*For each set of criteria, four or more are required for diagnosis of SLE.
Source: C. H. Syrop and M. V. Varner, Systemic lupus erythematosus. *Clin. Obstet. Gynecol.* 26(3), 1983.

Table 14-2. Main laboratory abnormalities in systemic lupus erythematosus

Abnormality	Patients (%)
Hematology	
Anemia (hemoglobin < 11 gm/dl)	73
Leukopenia (white blood cells < 4500/μl)	61
Thrombocytopenia (< 100,000/μl)	15
Positive direct Coombs' test	14
Circulating anticoagulants	Rare
Immunology	
Positive test for antinuclear antibodies	99
Positive lupus erythematosus cell tests	60–80
Hypocomplementemia	75
Increased globulin (> 1.5 gm/dl)	60–77
Positive tests for rheumatic factors	20
Biologic false-positive tests for syphilis	15

Source: T. R. Harrison, *Principles of Internal Medicine* (8th ed.). New York: McGraw-Hill, 1977. P. 428.

associated with a 50% fetal loss rate; decreased creatinine clearance and proteinuria are associated with an 80% loss rate [14]. Around 20–30% of patients with SLE have circulating anticardiolipin antibody (IgG), which has been associated with fetal loss and vascular thrombosis [11]. However, no increased incidence of congenital abnormalities associated with SLE, with steroids, or with immunosuppressive therapy has been reported.

Maternal complications are associated most closely with the presence of nephropathy. Premature births are seen in 10–36% of the cases. The incidence of preeclampsia and intrauterine growth retardation is increased, particularly in the presence of maternal hypertension or renal involvement. Unfortunately, it is difficult to clinically distinguish between the development of preeclampsia and a lupus flare with renal involvement. The presence of other systemic SLE manifestations (such as rash or arthralgias), a decrease in serum complement, and an elevated anti-DNA antibody level are more associated with a lupus flare. Preeclampsia, often severe, may occur as early as 24–26 weeks in the patient with underlying lupus.

3. **Effect of pregnancy**
   a. **Course of pregnancy.** Pregnancy does not predictably alter the course of SLE. Each pregnancy is a separate event during which the disease may remain stable, exacerbate, or go into remission. The prognosis in a later pregnancy cannot be anticipated from the course in an earlier one. A worsening of the disease during gestation, particularly in the first half of pregnancy, may occur. There also is evidence demonstrating that the risk of exacerbation increases as much as sevenfold in the first eight weeks post partum. The release of DNA by the involuting uterus is thought to account for this high rate of recrudescence. In patients with complete clinical remission of SLE of at least six months' duration before the onset of pregnancy, a correlation between clinical remission and improved maternal outcome has been seen. Remission persisted during pregnancy in two-thirds of such patients, and the rate of successful live birth was 92%. Patients with exacerbations of SLE during the six months prior to conception had a less favorable course during pregnancy and in the postpartum period, and successful pregnancy outcome was reduced by 25%. Therefore, it is advisable for a patient who desires a pregnancy to conceive during a period of remission.
   b. **Mortality.** Pregnancy, itself, does not significantly increase mortality in patients with SLE. Although an increased risk of exacerbation may be associated with pregnancy, no permanent sequelae are seen as long as severe cardiac or renal involvement is absent.
   c. **Renal function.** In general, lupus nephropathy, even in its severe forms, is often compatible with one or more successful pregnancies without recurrence of disease activity, provided that pregnancy occurs after a complete, sustained remission of at least three to six months [6]. In patients with mild renal insufficiency only, at the time of conception, pregnancy should not worsen subsequent renal function. However, with moderate or severe renal failure at the time of conception, the effect of pregnancy on long-term renal function is less clear.
   d. **Abortion.** Therapeutic abortion has not been found to ameliorate the underlying disease process, and symptoms of lupus fairly frequently flare up following this intervention.
4. **Maternal management**
   a. **Routine management during pregnancy.** Pregnant women with SLE must be closely followed throughout pregnancy, and any evidence of disease activity warrants a complete physical and laboratory evaluation. Low-dose prednisone and one pediatric aspirin (80 mg) is one maintenance regimen used in pregnant lupus patients without evidence of increased disease activity [8]. Prednisone is the drug of choice in treating acute SLE exacerbations and should be given in a dosage adequate to suppress disease activity; the usual dosage is 40–60 mg/day. After induction of remission, the daily dose can be tapered by 5–10 mg at weekly intervals. Immunosuppressive agents, such as cyclophosphamide and azathioprine, are used to treat SLE patients in the nonpregnant state. These agents are indicated in life-threatening disease uncontrolled by corticosteroids alone and for the benefit of their steroid-sparing effect in patients who develop intolerable side effects from corticosteroids. Cyclophosphamide should be avoided in pregnancy, especially in the first trimester, due to its teratogenic effects. Azathioprine, a purine analog, has been used routinely in pregnant women with renal transplants with good fetal outcomes. If an immunosuppressive agent is

required in pregnancy, azathioprine would be the prudent choice. The antimalarial drugs, such as chloroquine, are contraindicated in pregnancy because of their association with chromosomal and retinal damage.

b. **Fever.** Patients with SLE frequently have fever. Since steroids may mask symptoms of infection, it is mandatory, even in the asymptomatic patient, that infection be ruled out before an elevated temperature is attributed to the underlying disease. Aspirin may then be used for treatment of this symptom.

c. **Lupus nephritis.** In general, patients with lupus nephritis do poorly during pregnancy. In this group of patients intrapartum and postpartum maternal death may occur. During pregnancy, the nephritis may worsen with an increase in proteinuria, azotemia, and hypertension. The clinical picture of lupus nephritis may thus be identical to that of preeclampsia as discussed before. Also, superimposed preeclampsia occurs in 18–25% of patients with lupus nephritis. Management of the pregnant SLE patient with lupus nephritis or preeclampsia, or both, presents a clinical dilemma when the two disease processes cannot be differentiated. For the patient who has completed 32–34 weeks of pregnancy, delivery is probably the best option. A trial of high-dose corticosteroids for presumed lupus nephritis may be warranted when an earlier gestational age is involved. Unfortunately, neither drug therapy nor expectant management of severe or superimposed preeclampsia has been found to improve fetal outcome, and delivery of an infant with extreme prematurity may be nonpreventable.

   Patients with severe renal failure should be given the benefit of hemodialysis or peritoneal dialysis, which have both been successfully employed during pregnancy. Close attention must be paid to the patient's blood pressure, blood urea nitrogen, and fluid balance. An increase in the frequency and duration of dialysis during pregnancy is often indicated. Dialysis should maintain the blood urea nitrogen at approximately 30 mg/dl. All drug dosages should be altered appropriately for renal insufficiency.

d. **Fetal surveillance.** Accurate pregnancy dating is essential in SLE patients due to their propensity for both fetal growth retardation and early obstetric intervention. Serial ultrasound examinations (every 4 weeks) should be performed between 24 weeks and term to evaluate interval fetal growth. Antenatal surveillance using fetal monitoring should be employed in all lupus pregnancies to reduce the incidence of intrauterine demise. Semiweekly nonstress tests or weekly contraction stress tests starting at 30–32 weeks' gestation may be used in the uncomplicated pregnancy. However, in the pregnancy complicated by lupus exacerbations, nephritis, fetal growth retardation, or preeclampsia, biophysical profile evaluations may be started as early as 26 weeks. As in other high-risk pregnancies, electronic fetal monitoring should be employed throughout labor.

e. **Valvular heart disease secondary to systemic lupus erythematosus.** Patients with valvular heart disease secondary to SLE should have an echocardiogram performed during pregnancy to assess current cardiac function. Prophylactic antibiotics against endocarditis are given at the time of delivery.

f. **Management during labor.** Any patient with SLE who has been treated with steroids for two weeks or longer in the year prior to labor and delivery should be considered to have adrenal suppression and be treated with high-dose steroids during the intrapartum and immediate postpartum period. Recommendations for these patients are as follows:

   (1) **Normal labor and delivery.** Beginning with the onset of labor, cortisone acetate, 100 mg IM or IV q8h, should be given until delivery has occurred.

   (2) **Cesarean section and elective surgery.** For an emergency cesarean section, 100 mg cortisone acetate IM or IV should be given, followed by 100–200 mg of hydrocortisone sodium succinate IV during surgery. A similar regimen is used for elective surgery, with an additional 100 mg of cortisone acetate given IM 24 hours prior to the operation.

(3) Follow-up management. If, at any time, signs of adrenal insufficiency appear (i.e., unexplained abdominal pain, severe nausea and vomiting, or hypotension), an additional 100 mg of hydrocortisone succinate should be given IV. These additional doses of steroids should then be tapered over the next several days to the patient's maintenance level unless complications arise. It is recommended that the maintenance dosage not be tapered for at least eight weeks' post partum, since some evidence shows that continuation of the maintenance regimen may prevent the flare-ups that are seen during this period.

g. Mode of delivery. The method of delivery for the patient with SLE should be individualized and based on obstetric indications. Alone, SLE is not an indication for cesarean section. For the fetus with congenital heart block, no evidence shows that cesarean section is of benefit, although fetal monitoring during labor is problematic.

5. Effect of systemic lupus erythematosus on the newborn. A familial component exists in SLE. Genetic studies have demonstrated an increased frequency of HLA DR2 and DR3 in patients with SLE. Family members of SLE patients are more likely to have SLE or another rheumatic disease. Twin studies have revealed a high but incomplete concordance of lupus among monozygotic twins. Fraternal twins do not have a higher frequency of SLE than other first-order relatives. Presently, however, potential genetic transmission cannot be determined by prenatal diagnosis.

a. Mortality. Much of the neonatal mortality seen in infants of SLE mothers is due to extreme prematurity. Unfortunately, a number of preterm deliveries prior to 30 weeks' gestation are necessitated by maternal or fetal decompensation. Complete congenital heart block leads to death in as many as 25% of affected fetuses and accounts for much of the neonatal mortality following SLE pregnancies.

b. Other complications. Transplacental passage of antibodies of the IgG class may cause a transiently positive antinuclear antibody in the infant but is not associated with disease activity. Lupus erythematosus cells have also been found in newborns of patients with SLE. Placental passage of antibodies to blood components may be seen, causing a temporary leukopenia, thrombocytopenia, or hemolytic anemia in the newborn. Although these problems are self-limited, the thrombocytopenia or anemia may require treatment with corticosteroids.

Neonatal lupus is usually dermatologic or cardiac in nature and is a separate entity from familial lupus, which usually appears later in life [14]. Skin lesions are erythematous, scaly macules and plaques, involving the sun-exposed face and upper thorax, which resolve within the first year of life. Congenital heart block is a permanent sequela of maternal SLE. Atrioventricular conduction is impeded by underlying endocardial fibroelastosis and fibrosis of the atrioventricular conducting system. Today, most cases are discovered antenatally by auscultatory findings of fetal bradycardia. The heart block is associated with other congenital cardiac defects in 15–20% of affected infants, and fetal/neonatal M-mode echocardiography should be done at the time of diagnosis. Nearly all infants with congenital heart block are born to mothers who have anti-Ro (SSA) antibodies, a type of antinuclear antibody [13]. Fifty percent of these women will not have clinically apparent lupus. Although some infants with congenital heart block require pacemakers in infancy or later in life, the prognosis for children who survive the neonatal period is very good.

6. Prevention of pregnancy. All women of childbearing age with SLE should receive preconceptual counseling and effective contraception as needed. Since pregnancy termination carries increased risk for women with lupus, unplanned pregnancies should be avoided in these patients.

a. Oral contraception. The relationship between the use of oral contraceptives and the development of lupuslike symptoms is still unclear. However, since oral contraception containing even low-dose estrogen has been associated with thrombosis, hypertension, and disease exacerbation in women with established lupus, this form of contraception should be avoided. A pure progestogen with its antigonadotrophic and antiestrogenic effects has been suggested as an alternative [14].

b. Intrauterine devices. Dysmenorrhea, menorrhagia, and frequent infections necessitate removal of 50% of the intrauterine devices placed in women with lupus. The SLE patients on corticosteroid or immunosuppressive therapy are particularly at risk for endometrial infection.

c. Barrier contraception. Mechanical methods, including the diaphragm or condom with contraceptive foam/jelly, are often the safest choice for SLE patients. No contraindications to barrier contraception exist for this population.

d. Sterilization. Sterilization should be seriously considered by the women with SLE who has decided firmly against future pregnancies. Since unplanned pregnancies may place a patient with SLE at an unnecessary, increased risk of complications and the more effective methods of contraception are often contraindicated, family planning is an essential topic to be considered in all female lupus patients.

B. Rheumatoid arthritis

1. Clinical presentation. Rheumatoid arthritis (RA) is a chronic systemic inflammatory disease characterized by swelling, tenderness, and pain of symmetric synovial (hinged) joints, usually involving the upper extremities first. The American Rheumatism Association Diagnostic Criteria [1] are as follows:

a. Morning stiffness in and around joints lasting at least one hour before maximum improvement

b. Soft tissue swelling (arthritis) of three or more joint areas observed by a physician

c. Swelling (arthritis) of the proximal interphalangeal, metacarpophalangeal, or wrist joints

d. Symmetric swelling (arthritis)

e. Rheumatoid (subcutaneous) nodules

f. Presence of rheumatoid factor

g. Radiographic erosions or periarticular osteopenia, or both, in hand or wrist joints, or both

Criteria a through d must have been present for at least six weeks. An RA is defined by the presence of four or more criteria [4]. Female-male ratio is 3:1 with peak incidence at ages 35–40. The etiology of RA is unknown. It is suggested to be an inherited disease with a strong association to the histocompatibility complex antigen HLA DR4. Although RA is a progressive disease without cure, spontaneous remission is common. Vasculitis is a life-threatening complication of advanced RA and manifests with fever, leukocytosis, mononeuritis multiplex, scleritis, mesenteric infarction, and gangrene.

2. Laboratory findings. Rheumatoid factors are IgM and IgG antibodies against the Fc region of IgG and are measured by the latex fixation test. Titers increase with age in normal persons. Although nonspecific for RA, the rheumatoid factors are positive in 70–85% of patients with RA.

3. Effect on pregnancy. Negative effects of RA on pregnancy are rare. No increase occurs in rates of either spontaneous abortion or preterm labor. A mild anemia that frequently accompanies RA may be aggravated by the physiologic anemia of pregnancy. In a few cases, where the disease has caused marked deformity of the hips and lower extremities, vaginal delivery may be difficult or impossible. The rheumatoid factor does not cross the placenta, and there are no specific effects of the disease on the fetus [16].

4. Effect of pregnancy. Pregnancy generally has a beneficial effect on the symptoms of RA, with most patients experiencing a remission shortly after conception. The ameliorating effect of pregnancy may be the result of elevated maternal cortisone levels, although the slight generalized suppression of the immune response in pregnancy may also account for this effect. A few patients have an unchanged course, and, rarely, an exacerbation may occur. Occasionally, the onset of RA may occur during pregnancy. The improvement often seen during pregnancy is only temporary, and the disease usually flares up by the second month post partum.

The etiology of the improved clinical picture of RA in pregnancy is unclear. Although elevated maternal cortisol levels have been implicated, no correlation between disease remission and corticosteroid level has been demonstrated. Infusion of plasma from either pregnant or nonpregnant patients without RA results in sudden improvement in many patients with RA. This effect focuses attention on nonhormonal plasma constituents such as ceruloplasmin, alpha fetoprotein, and pregnancy-associated glycoprotein. These substances have an overriding effect on suppresser T cells and lead to a decreased antibody (rheumatoid factor) production.

5. **Maternal management.** The use of pharmacologic agents in treatment of RA during pregnancy is significantly restricted. Antimalarials, D-penicillamine, and the cytotoxic agents—methotrexate and cyclophosphamide—are teratogenic and, therefore, contraindicated during pregnancy. Although salicylates are the mainstay of therapy in the nonpregnant patient, their use in pregnancy is controversial. Aspirin modifies the arachidonic acid cascade and interferes with prostaglandin synthesis; the clinical result may be a prolonged bleeding time, maternal anemia, delayed parturition, or postpartum hemorrhage. Rare bleeding or bruising problems have been observed in the newborn. A therapeutic salicylate blood level of 20 mg/100 ml usually requires ingestion of 3.6–4.0 gm/day of acetylsalicylic acid. If used during pregnancy, aspirin should be discontinued at least one week prior to delivery. Other nonsteroidal anti-inflammatory drugs have similar biochemical effects and are not recommended during pregnancy. Corticosteroids in low doses are effective for syptomatic relief of RA and are relatively safe in pregnancy. The placenta converts the active steroid to its inactive 11-keto form, and at low steroid doses, neonatal adrenal suppression is rare. One recommended regimen is prednisone 5 mg in the morning and 2.5 mg in the evening. If a patient is receiving corticosteroids prior to delivery, a booster dose must be given intrapartum. Intraarticular, long-acting steroid injections are used in pregnancy and may provide several months of symptomatic relief for local joint inflammation. The intramuscular injection of gold salts to induce remission of RA has been used in pregnancy with relative safety since the gold salts cross the placenta poorly. However, unless necessary, treatment should be postponed until after delivery. If a cytotoxic drug is needed for treatment, azathioprine is the drug of choice, having been used routinely in pregnant women following kidney transplants without harmful fetal effects.

   Unless the hip is significantly involved in the disease process, patients with RA can anticipate a normal labor and delivery.
6. **Effect of rheumatoid arthritis on the newborn.** Perinatal morbidity or mortality does not increase due to maternal RA. Neonatal effects of various therapeutic regimens are discussed previously.
7. **Contraception and rheumatoid arthritis.** Oral contraceptive pills are safe in the patient with RA and may have a beneficial effect. In RA patients on chronic steroid therapy, intrauterine devices should be avoided due to the increased risk of infection.

C. **Scleroderma (systemic sclerosis).** Scleroderma is a chronic and progressive disease similar to other collagen-vascular disorders and of unclear etiology. The underlying pathology is excess collagen production, which may be seen in skin, muscles, joints, tendons, nerves, and certain internal organs such as the esophagus, intestinal tract, lungs, breast, and kidneys [5]. Involvement of small arterioles and capillaries produces end-organ vascular insufficiency. Clinically, scleroderma is often divided into two categories: **acrosclerosis or linear scleroderma,** in which the disease is limited to the skin and musculoskeletal system, and **progressive systemic sclerosis** (PSS), in which internal organs are involved. Because patients with only skin manifestations may nevertheless rapidly develop acute renal disease, severe hypertension, or pulmonary hypertension, this differentiation is of limited use.

1. **Clinical presentation and course.** The onset and severity of symptoms with scleroderma is highly variable [2]. Table 14-3 summarizes the clinical presentation.

   The course of scleroderma is also variable. Patients with only skin and esophageal involvement may have slow, progressive deterioration, while patients with cardiac, pulmonary, or renal involvement may have rapid deterioration and early death.

   Laboratory tests are nonspecific. Since scleroderma is an immune-mediated disease, hypergammaglobulinemia 12G antibodies are present in up to 50% of

Table 14-3. Clinical features of scleroderma

Organ	Clinical presentation
Skin	
Sclerosis may involve a limited or diffuse area	Tight abdominal wall with compression of viscera; sclerosis of lower legs resulting in painful limbs; flexion contractures of arms limiting mobility and venous access; anesthetic difficulties due to microstomia
Joints	
Polyarthralgias and polyarthritis	Stiff painful joints and functional disability
Tendons	
Contractures and friction subs	Limited mobility of upper extremities
Skeletal muscles	
Wasting and weakness of various muscle groups	Tiredness and weakness
Heart	
Pericarditis, arrhythmias, congestive cardiac failure	Cardiac failure
Lungs	
Dyspnea, cough, pulmonary fibrosis, pulmonary hypertension	Increasing dyspnea; sudden pulmonary hypertension
Kidneys	
Proteinuria, hypertension, renal failure, microangiopathic hemolytic anemia	Malignant hypertension and irreversible renal failure
Esophagus	
Dysphagia, reflux, formation of strictures, esophagitis	Increased reflux and esophagitis; worsening dysphagia
Small bowel	
Ileus, diarrhea; malabsorption	Possible malnutrition
Large bowel	
Constipation, diarrhea; partial obstruction, perforation, ulceration	Constipation, diarrhea, abdominal pain

Source: Adapted from C. M. Black and W. M. Stevens, Scleroderma. *Rheum. Dis. Clin. North Am.* 15(2), 1989.

patients. Rheumatoid factor is found in 25–30% and antinuclear antibodies in 30–40% of patients with clinical disease. The electrocardiogram identifies non-specific abnormalities in about 50% of patients. Radiological studies may be more helpful in progressive disease. The chest x ray in pulmonary scleroderma shows a diffuse reticular pattern with a honeycomb appearance in lower lung fields that may progress to dense interstitial fibrosis. Other radiologic findings include soft-tissue atrophy, calcinosis, absorption of terminal phalanges, a dilated atomic esophagus, colonic diverticulum, and duodenal/jejunum abnormalities.

2. **Effect on pregnancy.** Although scleroderma has a definite female preponderance, it is uncommonly associated with pregnancy due to its peak incidence age range of 35–55 years. Data on the disease's effects on fertility are inconclusive. An increased incidence of spontaneous abortion has been substantiated in two retrospective studies, and, indeed, a poor obstetric history may precede development of clinical disease. Intrauterine fetal demise is not more likely in women with scleroderma, but an increased risk of prematurity and intrauterine growth retardation is present.
3. **Effect of pregnancy.** Anecdotal reports have indicated an increase in maternal morbidity and mortality in women with scleroderma. In most cases, malignant hypertension or acute renal failure in the third trimester lead rapidly to maternal demise. A recent retrospective case-controlled study of 223 pregnant patients with scleroderma revealed no statistical increase in the rate of maternal morbidity or mortality. Overall, patients without renal disease or pulmonary hypertension tend to have successful pregnancy outcomes. When renal, pulmonary, or cardiac disease is present, termination of the pregnancy should be seriously considered. The sudden onset of malignant hypertension or renal failure in this subgroup is the major cause of maternal mortality in pregnancies complicated by scleroderma and a major cause of death in the disease itself.
4. **Maternal management**
   a. **Preconceptual counseling.** In view of the maternal and fetal risks described, the extent of organ involvement should be evaluated prior to pregnancy. However, the effect of pregnancy on the disease process remains unclear. Women with scleroderma need to be cautiously advised about future pregnancies.
   b. **Antenatal care.** Systemic manifestations of scleroderma need to be carefully monitored during pregnancy. Renal function and blood pressure should be assessed frequently. Evidence of preeclampsia is a particular concern, as renal scleroderma may present as third-trimester preeclampsia. Attention to esophageal and intestinal symptoms, nutritional status, skin care, and musculoskeletal complaints is important. Symptomatic treatment and nutritional support should be provided.
   c. **Fetal surveillance.** As with lupus, accurate pregnancy dating and serial ultrasound evaluations should be used to assess fetal growth. The use of antenatal FHR testing in the patients has not been studied.
   d. **Labor and delivery.** Patients with scleroderma may undergo normal labor and vaginal delivery; cesarean section should be reserved for obstetric indications. These patients are potential anesthetic problems, however, and a preanesthetic evaluation is essential. An epidural block is the preferred method of anesthesia, as it avoids the difficulties of intubation and the pulmonary complications of general anesthesia.

D. **Antiphospholipid antibodies in pregnancy.** The association between antiphospholipid antibodies and adverse pregnancy outcomes such as habitual abortion, intrauterine fetal demise, preeclampsia, and intrauterine growth retardation has received much recent attention. The offending antibodies are autoantibodies directed against membrane phospholipids; they include lupus anticoagulant, anticardiolipin antibody, and antiphosphatidylserine antibody. Although these autoantibodies were first identified in patients with known collagen-vascular disease, they are also present in the absence of clinical disease. Whether the incidence of these antibodies is significantly higher in women with adverse pregnancy outcomes versus women with normal pregnancies remains controversial [7, 10].

As the majority of habitual aborters have no clear etiology for their poor obstetric outcomes, the possibility of identifying antiphospholipid antibodies in these patients and developing treatment options is a cause for hope.

1. **Diagnosis** includes a prolonged activated partial thromboplastin time (APTT)—such as the Russell's viper venom time—to identify the lupuslike anticoagulant, and solid-phase radioimmunoassay (RIA) or enzyme-linked immunoassay (ELISA) tests to detect anticardiolipin and other antiphospholipid antibodies. The presence of antinuclear antibodies is of less clinical importance, although it is reported to occur in 40 to 70% of patients with antiphospholipid antibodies.
2. **Therapy.** Various treatment regimens have been developed, with improved pregnancy outcome reported in most cases. Therapy often includes prednisone 20–60 mg/day, with or without aspirin 75–80 mg/day. Another alternative is IV heparin. A multicenter clinical trial is currently under way to determine an optimum treatment plan. Because high-dose steroids, aspirin, and heparin are all associated with some maternal and fetal risk, drug therapy should be given only on protocol and with consultation. The use of antepartum fetal assessment to prevent fetal death in late pregnancy has been suggested in this patient population.

E. Idiopathic or immunologic thrombocytopenia purpura (ITP). ITP is an autoimmune disease caused by maternal antiplatelet antibodies. These IgG autoantibodies are produced by the mother and are capable of traversing the placenta to the fetus. Antiplatelet antibodies function to damage circulating platelets. They are then sequestered and destroyed in the reticuloendothelial system, resulting in thrombocytopenia.

1. **Diagnosis.** A decreased platelet count without depression of other blood factors is the initial indication of ITP. The disease is also associated with the presence of large platelets on the peripheral blood smear and increased megakaryocytes in the marrow. Confirmation is made by the detection of antiplatelet antibody in the maternal serum. Isolated thrombocytopenia without any other cause should be considered to be ITP.
2. **Maternal effects.** The primary maternal complication is hemorrhage from severe thrombocytopenia. This rarely occurs with platelet counts above 30,000/μl [9]. Maternal mortality is exceedingly rare. The need for blood transfusion during pregnancy is unusual in these women.
3. **Fetal and neonatal effects.** Fetal and neonatal effects are secondary to thrombocytopenia from transplacentally acquired maternal antiplatelet antibody. The perinatal mortality has been reported to be 6–17%; however, it appears to be significantly lower in recent studies [15].
   a. **Hemorrhagic complications** that have been reported include intracranial hemorrhage, periumbilical bleeding, gastrointestinal bleeding, hematuria, and generalized bleeding. The critical level for fetal and neonatal platelet counts is approximately 50,000/μl. With counts above this level, significant hemorrhage requiring intervention or therapy is rare. The primary fetal risk occurs during the labor and delivery process, with the greatest concern being intracranial hemorrhage.
   b. It is important to recognize that **there is no specific correlation or predictive relationship between the maternal and fetal platelet counts** [3]. There is no way to determine which ITP-pregnancy fetus is at risk for intrapartum hemorrhage from thrombocytopenia based on the maternal platelet count. There have been conflicting results on the predictive value of maternal antiplatelet antibody levels for fetal platelet counts. Therefore, the only reliable indicator at present is the actual platelet count determined from a **fetal scalp blood sample.** Values of less than 50,000/μl indicate risk for thrombocytopenic hemorrhage.
   c. **Neonatal thrombocytopenia** from ITP is self-limiting, since it is a passively acquired disease. Once the maternal IgG antibodies have been eliminated,

the thrombocytopenia disappears. Recovery usually occurs within six weeks of delivery. Platelet transfusions may be necessary in the acute neonatal situation.

4. **Management.** Pregnancies complicated by ITP must be carefully followed with serial maternal platelet counts. If the platelet count is greater than 100,000/μl, it may be repeated every three to four weeks without any further therapy.
   a. **Severe thrombocytopenia** is treated with corticosteroid therapy, 60 to 80 mg of prednisone daily. Splenectomy is only used for extreme situations with persistent, severe thrombocytopenia despite high-dose steroids; it is associated with a significant risk for preterm labor. Severe thrombocytopenia that is refractory to steroids may be treated with intravenous immunoglobulin G to attempt to suppress antiplatelet antibody activity. Maternal platelet transfusions are not helpful except in an acute hemorrhagic emergency and should be reserved solely for such cases. Destruction of exogenous platelets occurs rapidly, so the benefit is short-lived.
   b. Decisions on the **route of delivery** should be based on the fetal platelet count as determined from a fetal scalp blood sample taken at the time of labor. If the count is less than 50,000/μl, delivery is immediately carried out by cesarean section unless there is a maternal contraindication [12]. Vaginal delivery is permitted with fetal scalp platelet counts greater than 50,000/μl. Difficult operative vaginal delivery, lacerations, and large episiotomies should be avoided.
5. **Contraception.** Because pregnancy may intensify ITP, contraception is important. Women with ITP who desire future pregnancies may use a low-dose oral contraceptive agent. Those not planning additional pregnancies should consider having a permanent sterilization procedure either at the time of cesarean section or later, when the platelet count is normal.

References

1. Arnett, F. C., et al. The American Rheumatism Association 1987 revised criteria for the classification of rheumatoid arthritis. *Arthritis Rheum.* 31(3):315, 1988.
2. Black, C. M., and Stevens, W. M. Scleroderma. *Rheum. Dis. Clin. North Am.* 15(2):193, 1989.
3. Cines, D., et al. Immune thrombocytopenic purpura and pregnancy. *N. Engl. J. Med.* 306:826–831, 1982.
4. El-Roeiy, A., Myers, S. A., and Gleicher, N. The prevalence of autoantibodies and lupus anticoagulant in healthy pregnant women. *Obstet. Gynecol.* 75(3 Pt. 1):390, 1990.
5. Goplerud, C. P. Scleroderma. *Clin. Obstet. Gynecol.* 26(3):587, 1983.
6. Hayslett, J. P., and Lynn, R. I. Effect of pregnancy in patients with lupus nephropathy. *Kidney Int.* 18:207, 1980.
7. Hayslett, J. P., and Lynn, R. I. Effect of pregnancy in patients with SLE. *Am. J. Kidney Dis.* II:223, 1982.
8. Hollingsworth, J. W., and Resnik, R. Rheumatologic and Connective Tissues Disorders in R. K. Creasy and R. Resnik (eds.), *Maternal-Fetal Medicine: Principles and Practice* (2nd ed.). Philadelphia: Saunders, 1989.
9. Kelton, J. Management of the pregnant patient with idiopathic thrombocytopenic purpura. *Ann. Intern. Med.* 99:796–800, 1983.
10. Lockshin, M. D., Druzin, M. L., and Qamar, T. Prednisone does not prevent recurrent fetal death in women with antiphospholipid antibody. *Am. J. Obstet. Gynecol.* 160:439, 1989.
11. Reece, E. A., et al. Recurrent adverse pregnancy outcome and antiphospholipid antibodies. *Am. J. Obstet. Gynecol.* 163(1):162, 1990.
12. Scott, J., et al. Fetal platelet counts in the obstetrical management of immunologic thrombocytopenic purpura. *Am. J. Obstet. Gynecol.* 136:495–499, 1980.

13. Singsen, B. H., et al. Congenital complete heart block and SSA antibodies: Obstetric implications. *Am. J. Obstet. Gynecol.* 152:655, 1985.
14. Syrop, C. H., and Varner, M. V. Systemic lupus erythematosus. *Clin. Obstet. Gynecol.* 26(3):547, 1983.
15. Territo, M., et al. Management of autoimmune thrombocytopenia in pregnancy and in the neonate. *Obstet. Gynecol.* 41:579–584, 1973.
16. Thurnau, G. R. Rheumatoid arthritis. *Clin. Obstet. Gynecol.* 26(3):558, 1983.

Selected Readings

Gabbe, S. G. Drug therapy in autoimmune diseases. *Clin. Obstet. Gynecol.* 26(3):635, 1983.

Harris, E. D. Rheumatoid arthritis: pathophysiology and implications for therapy. *N. Engl. J. Med.* 322(18):1277, 1990.

Hazes, J. M., et al. Reduction of the risk of rheumatoid arthritis among women who take oral contraceptives. *Arthritis Rheum.* 33(2):173, 1990.

Kitridou, R. C. Pregnancy in mixed connective tissue disease, poly/dermatomyositis and scleroderma. *Clin. Exp. Rheumatol.* 6(2):173, 1988.

Lockshin, M. D., et al. Lupus pregnancy: Case-control prospective study demonstrating absence of lupus exacerbation during or after pregnancy. *Am. J. Med.* 77:893, 1984.

Lockshin, M. D., et al. Pregnancy in systemic lupus erythematosus. *Exp. Rheumatol.* 7(Suppl. 3):S195, 1989.

Lockwood, C. J., et al. The prevalence and biologic significance of lupus anticoagulant and anticardiolipin antibodies in a general obstetric population. *Am. J. Obstet. Gynecol.* 161(2):369, 1989.

Loizou, S., et al. Association of quantitative anticardiolipin antibody levels with fetal loss and time of loss in systemic lupus erythematosus. *Q. J. Med.* 68(255):525, 1988.

Lubbe, W. F., et al. Lupus anticoagulant in pregnancy. *Br. J. Obstet. Gynecol.* 91:357, 1984.

Maymon, R., and Fejgin, M. Scleroderma in pregnancy. *Obstet. Gynecol. Surv.* 44(7):530, 1989.

Mintz, G., et al. Prospective study of pregnancy in systemic lupus erythematosus. *J. Rheumatol.* 13(4):732, 1986.

Nicholas, N. S., and Panayi, G. S. Rheumatoid arthritis and pregnancy. *Clin. Exp. Rheumatol.* 6(2):179, 1988.

Ostensen, M., Aune, B., and Husby, G. Effect of pregnancy and hormonal changes on the activity of rheumatoid arthritis. *Scand. J. Rheumatol.* 12:69, 1983.

Persellin, R. H. The effect of pregnancy on rheumatoid arthritis. *Bull. Rheum. Dis.* 27:922, 1977.

Petri, M., et al. Antinuclear antibody, lupus anticoagulant, and anticardiolipin antibody in women with idiopathic habitual abortion. *Arthritis Rheum.* 30(6):601, 1987.

Spector, T. D., and Silman, A. J. Is poor pregnancy outcome a risk factor in rheumatoid arthritis? *Ann. Rheum. Dis.* 49(1):12, 1990.

Tan, E. M., et al. Criteria for the classification of systemic lupus erythematosus. *Arthritis Rheum.* 25:53, 1982.

Unander, A. M., et al. Anticardiolipin antibodies and complement in ninety-nine women with habitual abortion. *Am. J. Obstet. Gynecol.* 156(1):114, 1987.

Varner, M. W., et al. Pregnancy in patients with systemic lupus erythematosus. *Am. J. Obstet. Gynecol.* 145(8):1025, 1983.

15 Thromboembolic Disease and Vascular Complications

Mark C. Williams

I. Vascular complications

A. Arterial disease

1. **Arterial aneurysms.** Arterial aneurysms are uncommon but potentially life-threatening complications of pregnancy. They may involve the aorta and other arteries, including the cranial, ovarian, renal, and splenic arteries. Aneurysmal dilation of arterial structures may be due to congenital metabolic defects or infection (syphilis, mycotic aneurysms), or associated with atherosclerotic vascular disease. Both coarctation of the aorta and adult polycystic renal disease are associated with an increased incidence of intracranial saccular (berry) aneurysms.

   a. **Aortic aneurysm.** Aortic aneurysms (AAs) commonly result from local trauma or underlying disease that disrupts the elastic properties of the aorta. Among women of reproductive age, underlying medical conditions and developmental abnormalities are often seen in association with AA. Coarctation of the aorta (more commonly in the abdominal aorta among women) and congenital AA reflect two developmental abnormalities predisposing to AA. Hereditary abnormalities affecting connective tissue strength that predispose to AA include Marfan's syndrome, Ehlers-Danlos syndrome, homocystinuria, osteogenesis imperfecta, pseudoxanthoma elasticum, and the mucopolysaccharidoses. Certain infections, such as syphilis aortitis, may cause dilatation of the aortic root.

   Aortic aneurysms **may result in either dissection of the intima or actual rupture.** In cases of dissection, rupture may soon follow. Rupture of the aorta is frequently catastrophic and has a very high associated mortality rate. If aneurysmal dilation of the aorta is noted before morbid events have occurred, surgical correction may be attempted.

   Pregnancy appears to have either a causative or a provocative role in AA disease. Women of reproductive age have disproportionately high rates of aneurysmal disease [23]. Up to 50% of aortic dissections in women of reproductive age occur in association with pregnancy, with most problems presenting in the third trimester or during parturition [40]. Known major valvular or aortic disease should be corrected surgically prior to the third trimester; abnormalities diagnosed in the third trimester may best be managed expectantly, with delivery by cesarean section followed by surgical management. Successful vaginal delivery after (traumatic) AA has been reported [27].

2. **Intracranial hemorrhage.** Subarachnoid hemorrhage (SAH) is the third most common nonobstetric cause of maternal death. Arteriovascular malformations (AVMs) and intracranial aneurysms are responsible for 50% of maternal deaths due to intracranial hemorrhage. The interval encompassing the third trimester and the initial six weeks post partum represents the greatest risk for SAH.

   a. **Diagnosis.** The sudden onset of an uncharacteristically severe headache, possibly accompanied by meningismus (positive Kernig's or Brudzinski's sign) or focal neurologic deficit, suggests intracranial hemorrhage or thromboembolism and should be carefully evaluated. Many patients have been noted to experience an initial "warning headache" approximately 10 days before subsequent intracranial hemorrhage. (See also Chap. 12, sec. **II.A.**)

Patients with such presentations should undergo a computed tomography (CT) scan of the head. An initial scan done without contrast media may identify accumulated blood in the subarachnoid space or within the ventricles. If no blood is identified, a contrast-enhanced CT scan should be obtained. The CT scanning will identify 95% of acute intracranial hemorrhages, but only 30% of SAH will be found if CT is performed 96 hours after the event. If no intracranial hemorrhage is documented by a CT scan, a lumbar puncture is recommended to further assess for blood within the cerebrospinal fluid, a finding that confirms SAH.

b. Management. Patients thought to have evidence of intracranial embolic disease should undergo **echocardiography** to assess for potential causes of cerebral embolism (valvular vegetations, atrioseptal defects, atrial myxoma, mitral valve prolapse). Findings indicating either intracranial aneurysm or arteriovenous malformations require neurosurgical consultation.

The recommended route of delivery and optimal timing of neurosurgical aneurysm correction remain controversial. **Both vaginal delivery and elective cesarean section have been advocated.** If vaginal delivery is attempted, the increased intracranial pressure associated with Valsalva and maternal expulsive efforts in the second stage of labor should be avoided. Assisted delivery and avoidance of pushing are recommended. Epidural anesthesia is likely to facilitate these goals. If general anesthesia is contemplated in such patients, care should be taken to avoid the transient hypertension often associated with intubation. Premedication with a suitable antihypertensive agent may be advisable.

Hypertension seems to play a significant role in aneurysm rupture, and these patients should be carefully followed for any evidence of hypertensive disorders during pregnancy.

Patients thought to be at high risk of intracranial hemorrhage from a newly diagnosed aneurysm may benefit from antepartum **surgical correction.** Elective aneurysm repair at the time of cesarean section has been reported [19].

3. **Arteriovenous malformations.** AVMs result from congenital developmental anomalies such as intracranial arteriovenous fistulae, which dilate and expand over time. They are more commonly seen in men (2:1 male preponderance) but occasionally complicate pregnancy. Familial clusters have been described. Saccular (berry) aneurysms are sometimes seen in association with AVMs.

   During pregnancy, AVMs are usually not amenable to surgical correction, but selective embolization of AVMs thought to be at increased risk of rupture is now sometimes possible. Appropriate neurosurgical evaluation is recommended.

   In pregnancy, AVMs tend to bleed during the mid-to-late second trimester and shortly before, during, or after labor, with an overall risk of bleeding during pregnancy of 87%.

4. **Berry aneurysms.** Round or saccular (berry) aneurysms are commonly found at bifurcations of major vessels composing the circle of Willis. Eighty-five percent of such anomalies are found anteriorly along divisions of the internal carotid artery. Multiple aneurysms are found in up to 20% of patients. Aneurysmal diameters less than 4 mm are usually stable; diameters greater than 5–7 mm are thought more likely to bleed.

   Berry aneurysms are more likely to rupture in the third trimester, or near the time of delivery. Maternal hypertension or preeclampsia appears to predispose to rupture [7].

5. **Raynaud's disease and phenomenon.** Raynaud's phenomenon consists of acutely decreased arterial perfusion of the peripheral extremities, usually the fingers and hands, as a result of exposure to cold or emotional shock. When such symptoms are noted without evidence of underlying disease process, it is termed **Raynaud's disease.** If it is due to underlying pathology, it is termed **Raynaud's phenomenon,** which is used in this section to refer globally to all presentations of Raynaud's type symptomatology.

a. Raynaud's phenomenon occurs much more commonly in women. The exact cause is not known, and a wide variety of causes have been identified. Among women of reproductive age, **a common underlying etiology is collagen-vascular disease.** Raynaud's phenomenon has been reported in association with a wide variety of collagen-vascular diseases, including rheumatoid arthritis, lupus erythematosus, and scleroderma.

b. Raynaud's phenomenon in pregnancy has a rather benign prognosis, but if an **associated connective tissue disorder** is present, it may significantly affect the pregnancy. Patients with Raynaud's phenomenon symptoms should be evaluated for connective tissue disease.

c. **Specific recommendations** for Raynaud's phenomenon include avoidance of exposure to cold by wearing warm clothing and gloves. All external surfaces should be protected from the cold, as reflex vasoconstriction in unexposed extremities has been reported. Among nonpregnant patients, nifedipine (10–20 mg, q 6–8 h) has been found to be helpful, but the use of calcium channel blockers in pregnancy is not currently recommended and may involve risk.

II. Arterial and venous thromboembolic disease

A. Thromboembolic disease. The risk of symptomatic thromboembolic disease (TED) in pregnancy is approximately 6 times greater than the nonpregnant state, with a quoted incidence of 3–12 occurrences per 1000 pregnancies. The true incidence of thrombosis may be significantly higher in the postpartum interval, as Friend [9] found 3% of postpartum patients showed evidence of thrombosis when ^{125}I-labeled fibrinogen scanning was performed.

1. **Risk factors** for TED include the following:
   a. Advanced maternal age (> 40 years)
   b. Blood group type other than type O
   c. Collagen-vascular disease (lupus erythematosus, presence of lupus anticoagulant)
   d. Estrogen. High estrogen states, as with oral contraceptives, pregnancy, and estrogenic lactation suppression
   e. Grand multiparity. More than four previous term pregnancies
   f. Hypercoagulable state (deficit of protein C or S, decreased production of antithrombin III [AT3], dysfibrinogenemia, paroxysmal nocturnal hemoglobinuria)
   g. History of previous thromboembolic disorder or vascular endothelial injury (as with trauma)
   h. Homocystinuria (predisposes to arterial and venous thrombosis)
   i. Nephrotic syndrome
   j. Operative delivery (cesarean section or instrumented delivery)
   k. Venous stasis (vascular stasis of pregnancy and as noted with prolonged bed rest)
2. In addition, **pregnancy-related alterations in the coagulation system** (elevation of fibrinogen, prothrombin, and coagulation factors VII, VIII, IX, and X; decreased production of AT3) may predispose to increased thrombosis. Patients in the immediate postpartum interval have been found to have levels of factors V, VII, and X that exceed those found prior to delivery.
3. Although a relatively strong correlation exists between historical risk factors and subsequent TED, no set of laboratory investigations has proved adequate to identify those patients at highest risk for TED. As a result, identification of predisposing risk factors and anticoagulant prophylaxis are the cornerstones of prevention.

B. Peripheral thrombophlebitis. Thrombophlebitis in the extremities may involve superficial or deep vascular systems. Although superficial venous thrombophlebitis (SVT) may cause significant discomfort, it has a generally favorable prognosis, as any thrombi generated are limited in size and are usually trapped by more distal venous structures prior to entry into the central circulation. Conversely, deep venous thrombosis may be life-threatening. Thrombi generated in deep venous structures may pass directly into the vena cava and obstruct the pulmonary arterial circulation. Unfortunately, the clinical differentiation between SVT from deep venous thrombophlebitis (DVT) based on physical findings is notoriously inaccurate. Because of the significant potential for morbidity with undiagnosed DVT, it is often necessary to use noninvasive tests such as impedance plethysmography, ultrasonic visualization of the involved area, or even venogram to differentiate between SVT and DVT.

1. **Superficial venous thrombophlebitis.** SVT is caused by thrombotic narrowing or blockage of the superficial venous system draining the lower extremities, resulting in inflammation, local swelling and edema, and superficial pain on palpation. It may develop after surgery or in extremities immobilized for significant periods of time.
   a. **Treatment** consists of warm packs, mild elevation of the involved extremity, and early initiation of ambulation. If the patient is unable to ambulate due to local pain and tenderness, physical therapy and range-of-motion exercises for the lower extremities should be instituted. If proper measures to treat SVT are not taken, DVT may also develop in adjacent deeper structures. **Anticoagulation is not necessary for SVT.**
2. **Deep venous thrombophlebitis.** DVT is caused by the partial or complete obstruction of the deep venous drainage of the lower extremity. It may occur after immobilization of the involved extremity or subsequent to prior trauma to the extremity (vascular endothelial injury). Symptomatic DVT is present in 1–3 per 1000 pregnancies prior to delivery and is 4–5 times more common in the postpartum period. DVT is more likely to occur in the left femoral vein as compared to the right. The timely diagnosis of DVT is very important, as up to 24% of patients with untreated DVT will develop pulmonary embolism (PE) with an associated mortality of 15%. Those treated with anticoagulation will experience embolic disease in only 5% of cases and associated mortality in only 1%.
   a. **Diagnosis.** Findings suggestive of DVT include local swelling, tenderness, and increased localized warmth to palpation, but the accuracy of the clinical exam in DVT is limited. An extremity diameter 2-cm greater than the opposite, uninvolved side is considered abnormal. Physical diagnosis has been found to be approximately 50% sensitive and 50% specific. For this reason, possible cases of DVT should be evaluated with more sensitive and specific diagnostic modalities.

      Evaluation may be performed with noninvasive modalities or radiologic dye studies (venography). **Noninvasive methods include impedance plethysmography, vascular Doppler ultrasound,** and **direct ultrasonic imaging** of the venous structures for the presence of clots. Techniques using physiologic proteins tagged to radioisotopes such as fibrinogen give excellent results among nonpregnant patients, but ^{125}I-labeled materials should not be used in pregnancy, due to the high potential of fetal radioiodine trapping and subsequent hypothyroidism. The optimal method of evaluation will depend to a large degree on the diagnostic capabilities available at a given institution.

      Current noninvasive testing modalities offer important advantages in diagnosis, as they are quite sensitive and specific, and are much safer than traditional radiographic venography (some dyes used in venography predispose to subsequent phlebitis due to local vascular irritation). In interpreting the findings of plethysmographic testing of the lower extremities, it is important to bear in mind that there are three venous outflow channels from the lower extremity distal to the knee, whereas only one channel is proximal to the knee. If one outflow tract distal to the knee remains open, a false-negative result for DVT may be obtained. As DVT may develop over time, if symptomatology persists, negative noninvasive tests should be repeated every four or five days, or should be further evaluated with contrast venography.
   b. **Treatment and prophylaxis.** Treatment for DVT in pregnancy centers on

anticoagulation. The reader is referred to sec. **III.** Other important aspects of DVT therapy include initial bed rest with the involved extremity elevated 8 in. above the level of the torso. Placing the bed in a mild Trendelenburg position rather than flexing the leg at the hip may promote venous drainage of the involved extremity. Warm packs should be frequently applied. The patient should be encouraged to frequently flex and extend the extremity. The provision of a foot board may facilitate this goal. Ambulation should be encouraged as soon as pain and inflammation have begun to resolve.

C. Arterial embolic occlusive disease. Transient ischemic attacks and PE, although infrequent, are significant causes of morbidity and mortality in pregnancy.

1. Conditions predisposing to arterial embolism include the following:

a. Anemia

b. Amniotic fluid embolism

c. Arteritis

(1) Collagen-vascular disease (polyarteritis, temporal arteritis, granulomatous arteritis, lupus erythematosus, Takayasu's disease)

(2) Syphilis, tuberculosis

d. Atherosclerosis

e. Hematologic disorders (hemoglobin SS and SC disease, polycythemia, thrombotic thrombocytopenic purpura)

f. Hypertensive disorders (hypertension, preeclampsia)

g. Inherited thrombotic predisposition (deficiency of AT3, protein C, protein S; dysfibrinogenemia)

h. Thrombotic disease (peripheral thrombosis, septic pelvic thrombophlebitis, ovarian vein thrombosis)

i. Trauma (fat or air embolism)

j. Valvular heart disease (congenital, postinfectious), mitral valve prolapse, artificial cardiac valves

2. Pulmonary embolism. In pregnancy, PE, the acute occlusion of the pulmonary artery, is most often due to embolization from thrombotic disease within the deep peripheral venous system. It occurs in up to 7 in 1000 pregnancies and is the second most frequent cause of maternal mortality. Additional causes of acute occlusion of the pulmonary artery include embolization with fat (associated with sickle cell disease), air, and amniotic fluid.

a. Presentation. Fifty percent of cases of fatal PE will have cardiovascular collapse (shock) as their initial presentation. Less severe cases may present with clinical findings such as acute-onset dyspnea, substernal or pleuritic chest pain, and tachypnea. On examination, patients may also be noted to have increased jugular venous distention, a parasternal cardiac heave, and an S_3 murmur.

(1) Laboratory findings include

(a) pulmonary vascular congestion (on chest x ray)

(b) hypoxia in the absence of hypercarbia ($pO_2 < 70$, pCO_2 nml)

(2) The differential diagnosis for acute cardiorespiratory collapse in pregnancy includes the following:

(a) Amniotic fluid embolism

(b) Internal hemorrhage (broad ligament hematoma; retroperitoneal hematoma; rupture of aneurysm, liver, or uterus)

(c) Medication overdosage (magnesium sulfate, narcotic analgesics)

(d) Myocardial infarction

(e) PE

(f) Tension pneumothorax

Of these events, PE is the most common. In circumstances of shock, it is often necessary to stabilize the patient prior to attempting to confirm the diagnosis. A scheme for evaluation of patients with possible PE follows.

b. Diagnosis. Arterial blood gases and ventilation/perfusion ($\dot{V}/\dot{Q}$) radioisotopic scanning is extremely useful in the diagnosis of PE. If a perfusion defect is noted in an area of normal ventilation (a $\dot{V}/\dot{Q}$ mismatch), a PE is very likely. In the case of significant preexisting pulmonary disease (e.g., pneumonia, emphysema), both ventilation and perfusion may be decreased (matching $\dot{V}/\dot{Q}$ defects) in certain portions of the lung. A chest x ray is helpful in determining the etiology of matching defects. If there is strong clinical suspicion of PE and a matching $\dot{V}/\dot{Q}$ abnormality is present, a pulmonary angiogram should be considered. If no definite evidence of PE is found, evaluation for venous thrombotic disease and other disease entities should be considered. See Fig. 15-1.

The evaluation of PE using $\dot{V}/\dot{Q}$ scanning and chest x rays requires the use of low amounts of radiation. It has been estimated that the diagnosis of DVT by radiographic means requires a fetal radiation exposure of approximately 0.5 rad, whereas the diagnosis of PE with $\dot{V}/\dot{Q}$ scanning requires a fetal exposure of 0.05 rad [10, 26]. It is estimated that in utero exposures in excess of 5.0 rad will predispose to some types of childhood malignancies. Neither $\dot{V}/\dot{Q}$ scanning nor chest x ray should be deferred if PE or DVT is thought possible, and noninvasive tests are inconclusive.

c. **Management.** Therapy for acute PE requires immediate anticoagulation and cardiorespiratory support. It will sometimes be necessary to initiate resuscitative measures prior to confirmation of the diagnosis.

Patients presenting with symptoms of **cardiovascular collapse** require aggressive resuscitative measures directed at maintaining oxygenation and circulation. **Hypotension** is best managed by initial fluid resuscitation. Persistent hypotension may then be corrected with pressor agents, such as dopamine, 200 μg/minute, or isoproterenol, 2–8 μg/minute. **Hypoxia** should be corrected by administration of oxygen. A pulmonary artery catheter should be in place if possible, to facilitate fluid and pressor therapy. Morphine, administered for analgesia, may also contribute a mild vasodilatory effect. An aminophylline infusion (loading dose of 4–5 mg/kg followed by 12–15 μg/kg/minute) may improve associated bronchospasm, if present. Patients not requiring immediate oxygen therapy should be monitored for incipient hypoxia with pulse oximetry or serial arterial blood gas determinations.

After initial stabilization and confirmation of diagnosis, **anticoagulation with heparin** should be begun. If a delay of more than three or four hours for confirmatory testing is anticipated, it may be reasonable to proceed with anticoagulation based on a provisional diagnosis of PE. Because heparin therapy does not promote thrombolysis, it should not obscure the diagnosis of PE. Conversely, early heparin therapy may prevent further (fatal) embolization. Careful heparinization in PE is only very rarely associated with hemorrhagic complications. In extreme circumstances, operative thrombectomy or thrombolytic therapy (streptokinase) should be considered.

The details of heparinization are discussed in sec. **V.**

3. **Transient ischemic attacks.** Among women of reproductive age, the incidences of stroke and transient ischemic attack (TIA) are estimated to be 2–11 and 4–5 per 100,000 women, respectively. Retrospective studies regarding the influence of pregnancy on stroke are equivocal. A population study involving stroke patients in Glasgow over 20 years [5] found that pregnant women were overrepresented by a factor of 3. More recently, Wiebers [39] was unable to find a predisposition attributable to pregnancy, but Johnson and Skre [16] found a possible association.

Cerebral arterial embolic occlusion is responsible for two-thirds of all nonhemorrhagic hemiplegias in pregnancy. A TIA, presenting as a focal neurologic deficit lasting less than 24 hours, may presage complete occlusion of the involved vessel. For this reason, focal neurologic abnormalities should be thoroughly investigated.

a. **Diagnosis.** The differential diagnosis for TIA includes migraine disorder and localized seizure disorder. Patients who have deficits persisting longer than several hours may have experienced some degree of ischemic neurologic injury (infarction). A history of recurring migratory polyneuropathies is suggestive of multiple sclerosis.

b. **Evaluation** for TIA includes a thorough history and physical examination.

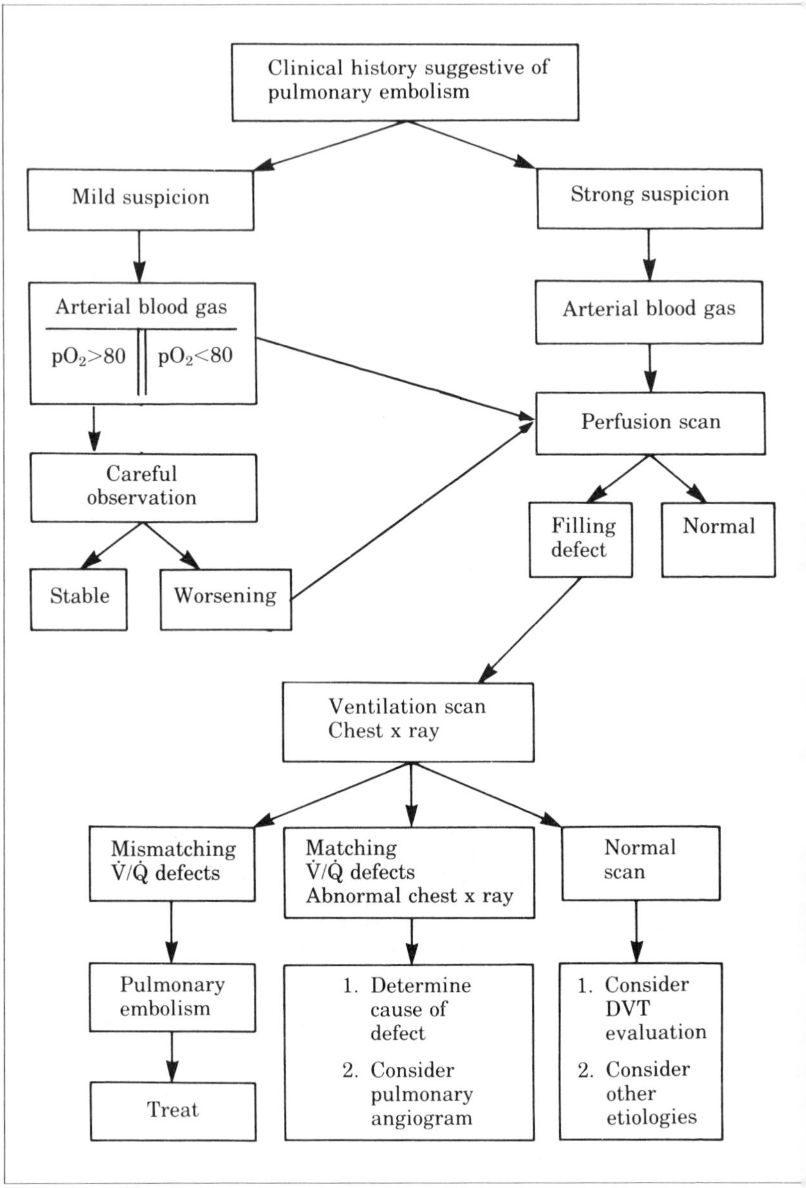

Fig. 15-1. Diagnosis of pulmonary embolism.

Historical features may point to a localizing tendency among neurologic manifestations suggestive of a certain cerebral region; an aura prior to symptoms is suggestive of a migraine disorder. The presence of a carotid bruit suggests possible carotid disease.

Laboratory evaluation of patients includes complete blood count, sedimentation rate, serum cholesterol and triglycerides, coagulation profile (prothrombin and partial thromboplastin time). Further evaluation with carotid ultrasound, echocardiogram, electroencephalogram, CT of the head to assess for intracranial mass-occupying lesions, and angiography or digital subtraction angiography should be considered in certain cases.

c. **Management.** The best treatment for TIAs is to remove the source of embolization, or (in rare circumstances) to attempt anticoagulation. Arterial disease not accessible to surgery may cause distal embolic phenomena and often requires anticoagulation. Neurologic or surgical consultation is recommended for difficult cases.

D. **Cerebral thrombosis.** Cerebral venous thrombosis (CVT) is a relatively rare complication of pregnancy with a case fatality rate of approximately 33%. It appears to occur more frequently in the postpartum interval. When presenting in the first trimester, it has usually occurred after miscarriage or elective termination. Presentations during pregnancy have frequently been associated with recurrences later in pregnancy or in the puerperium. The etiology of CVT is unknown but may be associated with underlying abnormalities of the clotting system.

1. **Diagnosis.** CVT may present with a variety of symptoms, including headache, vomiting, seizures, lethargy, and drowsiness. Findings may include papilledema; hemiplegia; and altered speech, vision, or sensation. Infrequently, bilateral cortical infarctions may result in visual field defects or blindness.

   The differential diagnosis for CVT includes intracranial hemorrhage, cerebral arterial embolism, tumor, seizure disorder, or migraine variant. Evaluation is the same as for suspected intracranial hemorrhage. A CT scan of the head may show compression of the ventricles or evidence of edema and infarction. Cerebral arteriography or digital subtraction angiography can be used to confirm the diagnosis.

2. **Management.** Acute management of CVT, focusing on anticoagulation and measures to reduce intracranial pressure, is controversial. If hemorrhage can be positively excluded from the differential diagnosis, anticoagulation may be indicated. This is especially so if the patient's condition begins to deteriorate rapidly. Steroid therapy, such as dexamethasone, 20 mg/day, is also recommended to attempt to reduce intracranial swelling. Mannitol infusions should also be considered. Neurologic consultation is advised.

   If the patient has a prior history of CVT, or if CVT has complicated a pregnancy, a thorough evaluation of the patient's clotting system should be done, looking for some predisposing factor for thrombosis. Given the high case fatality rate and tendency for recurrence, patients with a history of CVT may benefit from prophylactic anticoagulation, although this has not been assessed in a prospectively designed study.

   Patients with a history of CVT have **no contraindication to vaginal delivery.** Labor may be expectantly managed, although assisted vaginal delivery is advised. If thrombosis has occurred near term, some authors have advocated cesarean delivery.

E. **Ovarian vein thrombosis**

1. **Presentation.** Acute postpartum ovarian vein thrombosis has been reported to occur in 1 in 4000 pregnancies. It usually presents with fever and severe adnexal pain, occasionally with radiation to the flank. It frequently involves the right ovarian vein.

2. **Differential diagnosis.** The differential diagnosis includes septic pelvic thrombophlebitis (see sec. **IV**), adnexal torsion, and renal obstruction.

   Once an operative diagnosis, ultrasound and CT are now the preferred diagnostic techniques for ovarian vein thrombosis [2, 31].

3. **Management.** Ovarian vein thrombosis is best treated by anticoagulation. Initial heparin anticoagulation for four to five days should be followed by outpatient anticoagulation with either oral coumarin or subcutaneous heparin. If extension of the clot into the vena cava is evident, ligation of the ovarian vein should be considered.

III. Obstetric conditions requiring anticoagulation

A. Artificial heart valves. Patients with artificial heart valves have an extremely high risk of embolization. Among these patients, **coumarin** is the anticoagulant of choice. By comparison, heparin-treated patients have been much more likely to experience thromboembolic disease. "Heparin failures" among pregnant patients with prosthetic cardiac valves have been reported. Unfortunately, coumarin anticoagulation entails a significant degree of risk for the fetus.

1. Clearly patients with artificial cardiac valvular prostheses require some form of anticoagulation. The **dangers of cardiac valvular prosthesis in pregnancy** are well documented [1, 3, 4, 12–14, 18, 20, 24, 28, 29, 33]. If valve thrombosis occurs, the patient is at risk of severe complications. Massad [28] found that inadequate anticoagulation was responsible for 91% (10 in 11) of acutely thrombosed mitral valve prostheses from a series of 274 patients who had replacement surgery. The various considerations relative to the care of patients with prosthetic cardiac valves have been recently reviewed by McColgin [29]. Successful mitral valve replacement in pregnancy with postpartum oral anticoagulation has been reported by Vosa [38].
2. The best anticoagulation regimen, one capable of minimizing both maternal and fetal risks, has yet to be determined. Clinical regimens have been described by the following investigators: Ahmad [1], Ben-Ismail [3], Biale [4], Ibarra-Perez [12], Iturbe-Alessio [13], Javares [14], Lutz [24], and Sareli [33].
3. Strong evidence from **teratologic studies** suggests that coumarin derivatives are most teratogenic during the fourth through eighth weeks of gestation. Their use late in pregnancy seems to predispose to fetal intracranial hemorrhage.

   If coumarin use is felt necessary after cardiologic consultation, the best course of action is to convert the patient to adjusted-dose heparin anticoagulation from the beginning of pregnancy through the twelfth week of gestation (attempting to achieve 130–150% of baseline activated partial thromboplastin time [APTT], and then converting the patient to coumarin (maintaining a prothrombin time of 150–200% of control) for weeks 13–37. After 37 weeks of gestation, the patient should again be returned to adjusted-dose heparin anticoagulation. It is hoped that this approach will avoid the problems of inadequate anticoagulation noted with heparin and high teratogenicity and fetal wastage associated with continuous coumarin therapy in pregnancy.

   The reader is urged to review the cited articles and any more recent publications prior to establishing an anticoagulation plan for patients with artificial cardiac valve prostheses.

B. Hereditary thrombotic tendency. Within the body, various compounds act to control and mediate the clotting cascade. These substances include AT3, and proteins C and S. All are proteins produced within the liver. If adequate quantities of normally functioning versions of these proteins are not present, patients will be prone to thrombus formation. Additionally, abnormal variants of fibrinogen and plasminogen have been discovered, which predispose to thrombosis.

1. **Antithrombin III deficiency.** AT3 opposes the action of thrombin (factor IIa) and a number of other activated clotting factors, including factors IXa, Xa, XIa, XIIa, XIIIa, and activated Fletcher factor (kallikrein). In normal pregnancy, AT3 levels have been found by several investigators to be relatively unchanged.
   a. Both deficient production of AT3 and presence of abnormal AT3 variants have been reported among populations of patients demonstrating abnormal thrombotic tendencies. The **prevalence of AT3 deficiency** is estimated to be from 1 in 2000 to 1 in 20,000 population and has been found in 4–6% of young patients with unexplained venous thromboembolism. An autosomal dominant inheritance pattern has been observed, and 30–60% of heterozygote carriers suffer thrombosis [35]. Preeclampsia and other hypertensive disorders of pregnancy have been found to be frequently associated with significantly decreased AT3 levels, which usually normalize within three to five days post partum.
   b. Patients with deficient AT3 levels should receive **anticoagulation** for life.

Anticoagulation with agents such as coumarin is sometimes associated with increased AT3 production. Patients taking proper precautions against pregnancy may benefit from anticoagulation with oral coumarin derivatives. Estrogen-containing contraceptives have been reported to decrease AT3 production and are contraindicated in this condition. Patients not receiving adequate contraception, those interested in becoming pregnant, or those actually pregnant should be anticoagulated with a subcutaneous heparin regimen as described subsequently. Successful anticoagulation in pregnancy using heparin [6, 17] and coumarin, heparin, and peripartum AT3 infusion [8, 30] have been described. The use of AT3 concentrate to manage patients with AT3 deficiency during pregnancy has also been reported [35], although the value of such therapy has not yet been proved prospectively [30].

2. **Lupus erythematosus.** Patients who either suffer from lupus erythematosus or who have elevated titers of antiphospholipid antibodies (called **lupus anticoagulants)** have an increased tendency toward spontaneous arterial and venous thrombosis. The exact etiology of these disorders is unknown but is thought to be **related to autoimmune disease.** Antibodies present in these syndromes are "anti-self" antibodies. In vitro, they are responsible for disseminated microthrombi being generated throughout the body (at sites of antigen-antibody interaction and complement activation). In vitro, the antiphospholipid antibodies act to prolong the APTT coagulation test by interfering with a phospholipid compound integral to the test. These antibodies include those of the IgG class, which are capable of crossing the placenta and affecting fetal development.
   a. **Management.** Traditional management involves therapy with corticosteroids, such as prednisone, in an attempt to decrease immunoglobulin production. Recently, the utility of this therapy in pregnancy has been questioned by Lockshin [21], Stafford-Brady [36], and others. Lockwood [22] has suggested that a subpopulation with no prior negative obstetric history and antiphospholipid antibodies may not require steroid therapy. Acetylsalicylic acid is sometimes prescribed in order to decrease the possibility of thrombosis. There have been reports of alternate management strategies that centered on maternal heparin anticoagulation in pregnancy without steroid therapy. Successful experience with such a management plan was recently reported by Joffe [15] and Rosove [32].
3. **Protein C deficiency.** Protein C is a vitamin K–dependent anticoagulant. After activation by thrombomodulin, it works in conjunction with protein S to inhibit factors V and VIII. It has been reported in abnormally low quantities among 7–8% of patients with a first episode of thromboembolism prior to age 40, and also among patients with recurrent episodes of thrombosis. It has been reported to follow both autosomal dominant and recessive inheritance patterns. Infants homozygous for protein C deficiency may be predisposed to purpura fulminans neonatorum.

   In pregnancy, protein C levels appear to remain normal, or possibly rise slightly to 135% of prepregnancy levels. Patients with this disorder should receive lifelong anticoagulant therapy. While pregnant, a regimen of subcutaneous heparin is recommended.
4. **Deficient protein S and other abnormalities**
   a. **Protein S.** Protein S, vitamin K–dependent hepatic glycoprotein, acts as a cofactor for protein C by promoting the binding of protein C with the platelet surface membrane. Deficiency of protein S has been reported to predispose to thrombosis. Although not verified by all investigators, the levels of protein S have been found to fall significantly in pregnancy. It has been postulated that rising levels of protein C in pregnancy may help correct for falling levels of protein S and help to prevent thrombosis.
   b. **Others.** Certain hereditary abnormalities of fibrinogen and plasminogen have been found to predispose to thrombosis. Their effect on pregnancy is unknown.

C. **High risk for recurrent thromboembolic disease.** Certain groups of patients are at high risk for recurrent TED and would certainly benefit from prophylactic anticoagulation.

1. **Criteria.** Although experts disagree as to what exact criteria should be used to define this "high risk of recurrence" group, most would agree that this categorization should apply to patients with the following:
   a. Multiple prior episodes of DVT
   b. Known predisposition to thrombosis (e.g., AT3 deficiency, proteins C and S deficiencies)
   c. Possibly those with single prior episodes of severe complications of TED (e.g., previous PE or cerebral thrombosis)

   Patients who may also benefit from prophylaxis include those who have had a prior occurrence of TED either associated or not associated with pregnancy.
2. **Guidelines for individualization of therapy**
   a. **Patients judged at low risk** for recurrence of TED may be managed by regular evaluation, a regular program of exercise (e.g., walking), and avoidance of prolonged periods of venous stasis (e.g., sitting for intervals of more than one hour without standing and stretching legs or alternately flexing calves in place). Patients with proved prior DVT or other thrombotic phenomena should receive postpartum "mini-dose" prophylaxis of 5000 units SC for 4–6 weeks postpartum.
   b. Patients felt to be at **moderately increased risk** for recurrent TED may benefit from a fixed-dose heparin sulfate regimen (see sec. **V**).
   c. Patients thought to be at **very high risk** of recurrent TED may be treated with either fixed or adjusted-dose SC heparin therapy.

   (See sec. **V** for dose schedules.)

D. **Disseminated intravascular coagulopathy.** Disseminated intravascular coagulopathy (DIC) in obstetrics is usually seen in association with abruptio placentae or preeclampsia or as a result of depletion of coagulation factors due to massive hemorrhage. In many cases, the DIC seems to develop into a cycle of continuous thrombin activation and subsequent depletion of fibrinogen stores.

1. Although once thought to assist in the **management of obstetric DIC,** anticoagulation with heparin alone is not thought to be of value, and in some circumstances may worsen the hemorrhagic tendency seen with DIC. Recently, however, Maki [25] reported on the use of AT3 infusions in the management of DIC in obstetrics. Such therapy must still be considered experimental but does hold the hope of more successful therapy for DIC in the future. The reader is referred to Chap. 6 for further discussion of the modern management of DIC in obstetrics.

E. **Fetal demise with remaining viable fetus(es).** In the case of one or more fetuses dying in utero (either spontaneously or as a result of selective termination) while viable fetuses remain present, low-grade DIC has been reported to develop. (This is quite analogous to the mild DIC that often develops if a dead fetus is carried in utero for more than three or four weeks.) Heparin has been shown to control the mild DIC associated with this condition and to allow prolongation of the pregnancy until fetal lung maturity can be ensured.

If a patient is found to be carrying one or more dead fetuses in conjunction with other viable fetuses, she should be carefully followed for onset of DIC. **Hematologic studies should be evaluated** at four- to seven-day intervals **for thrombocytopenia,** a significant **elevation of baseline fibrin degradation products,** or a **drop in fibrinogen level.** If these phenomena occur remote from fetal viability, intravenous heparin therapy should be initiated. After several days, the patient should be converted to subcutaneous heparin therapy adequate to maintain a normal platelet count and to return the fibrin degradation products to normal baseline levels.

It is also important to follow the remaining fetuses for evidence of **complications arising from shared circulations.** If thromboplastic materials generated as a nonviable fetus degenerates are released into the circulation of a remaining viable fetus, significant damage to the remaining fetus is possible. The remaining fetus should be surveyed at one- to two-week intervals for evidence of focal infarctions (such as the onset of porencephalic cysts). Szymonowicz et al. [37] reported on a group of six monozygotic twin pairs in which one twin had died while the other remained in utero. In this small series, 100% of the surviving infants had central nervous system infarctions, and 50% had multisystem disease. If such findings develop, consideration should be given to expeditious delivery.

IV. Septic pelvic thrombophlebitis. Septic pelvic thrombophlebitis is a thrombophlebitic syndrome involving the pelvic vasculature associated with infections in the postoperative or postpartum/abortal state.

A. Diagnosis of septic pelvic thrombophlebitis requires high clinical acumen and is suggested by the following triad of clinical findings:

1. The patient has undergone recent pelvic surgery or has recently been pregnant, and has developed a pelvic infection.
2. The patient has received several days of antibiotic therapy with an adequate spectrum of aerobic and anaerobic "coverage."
3. Intermittent febrile episodes (> 38°C) persist and do not seem to be resolving.

B. Evaluation. Patients meeting these criteria should be examined carefully for the presence of other infectious processes. This should include a **pelvic examination** to assess for an infected broad-ligament hematoma or pelvic abscess. Other potential causes of these findings include ureteral obstruction and "drug" fever. **Renal ultrasound** or **intravenous pyelography** can be used to ascertain the status of the kidney. Changing antibiotics to an alternative regimen (with equivalent spectrum) will help eliminate medication reactions.

C. If no other cause for persistent fever can be identified, a presumptive diagnosis of septic pelvic thrombophlebitis should be made and a **trial of intravenous heparin anticoagulation** should be initiated. If defervescence occurs within 24–48 hours, the diagnosis is considered confirmed. Antibiotics should be continued until at least 48 hours after afebrility has been achieved. Heparin should be continued for 5–10 days and then an outpatient regimen of anticoagulation instituted for 4–6 weeks.

D. Patients who fail to defervesce should be carefully evaluated for alternate sources of fever. Pelvic or retroperitoneal abscesses may be present. On occasion, more obscure medical illness may be manifesting (e.g., malaria, leukemia, tuberculosis).

V. Anticoagulation. Medications available for the treatment of thrombotic disorders can (1) cause altered platelet adherence and aggregation; (2) interfere with the process of fibrin formation; and (3) accelerate the process of fibrinolysis. **In pregnancy, therapy is generally restricted to agents that inhibit fibrin formation.** Patients receiving anticoagulants **must be carefully managed.** Agents that alter other components of the coagulation system (such as aspirin affecting platelet function) should be avoided. Certain medications may alter circulating levels of anticoagulants. Finally, anticoagulated patients should not receive epidural anesthesia, and intramuscular injections should not be administered.

A. Heparin. Heparin has a molecular weight of 15,000 daltons. Because of its large molecular size and negative polarity, it does not cross into the placenta or breast milk. It prolongs most laboratory clotting parameters, including the thrombin time, the APTT, and (to a lesser degree) the prothrombin time. The APTT is most commonly used to monitor anticoagulation with heparin therapy.

Heparin has no intrinsic anticoagulant effect but acts by binding at a specific site on the molecule, causing dramatic increase in this molecule's biologic activity. AT3 neutralizes a wide variety of activated components of the clotting system, including Iia, Ixa, Xa, Xia, XIIa, XIIIa, and activated Fletcher factor (kallikrein). AT3 has also been observed to inhibit factor VII, but only in the presence of heparin. Finally, heparin can inactivate thrombin by acting in combination with heparin cofactor II to form irreversible thrombin complexes.

Long-term heparin therapy has been reported to cause osteoporosis and thrombocytopenia. Bleeding episodes are uncommon and tend to occur only if large doses of medication are administered, if other medications with potential effects on the clotting system (such as aspirin) are taken, with local trauma, or if intramuscular injections occur.

Heparin has a relatively short half-life (1.5 hour), and **heparin activity** should be essentially nondetectable six hours after discontinuation of intravenous infusion. If more acute reversal of heparin effect is required, protamine sulfate should be administered to directly complex with the heparin molecule and remove it from circulation. Protamine is a weakly basic, arginine-rich protein that neutralizes heparin. The effective dose for reversal is 1-mg protamine per 100 units of heparin. The protamine dose should be calculated from twice the amount of heparin infused over the previous hour. Alternatively, the amount of circulating heparin may be calculated if plasma heparin concentration is known. Protamine dosage is calculated as follows:

1. Protamine (mg) = 2 × (units heparin per hour)/100 **or**
2. Protamine (mg) = [plasma heparin (IU/ml)] × [(weight in kg) × (50 ml/kg)]/100, where 50 ml/kg represents approximate ml per kg conversion for maternal plasma volume in pregnancy. **This simplifies to:**
3. Protamine (mg) = [heparin (IU/ml)] × [weight (kg)]/2

Rapid administration of protamine can cause hypotension and anaphylactoid reactions. It should be slowly administered IV at a rate not to exceed 50 mg/10 minutes. Doses in excess of 100 mg are rarely indicated.

1. **Intravenous anticoagulation.** Patients presenting with acute thrombophlebitis or PE should be started on intravenous heparin therapy immediately. Prior to starting heparin, initial hemogram, platelet count, prothrombin time, and APTT should be obtained.
   a. Patients should receive an **initial IV loading dose** of 5000–10,000 units, followed by a continuous infusion of heparin in saline at a rate of approximately 1000 units/hour. If infusion pumps are not available, the medication should be administered by intermittent IV boluses q4–6h in doses sufficient to achieve 1000 units/hour. After six hours, the APTT should be evaluated and the dosage adjusted to attain an APTT time of 150–200% of control. The APTT should then be serially evaluated at 12- to 24-hour intervals as long as intravenous heparin is being administered.
   b. These guidelines should provide adequate anticoagulation for most patients. **In cases of massive PE,** Sasahara [34] has recommended a larger initial loading dose (10,000–15,000 units) followed by infusions of approximately 1800 units/hour to provide a total initial 24-hour heparin dose of 60,000 units. It has been suggested that these initially higher doses may relieve vasospasm. These findings have not yet been duplicated by other investigators.
   c. After initial anticoagulation, the patient should be **maintained** on this regimen for 7–14 days. Then the patient should be converted to either subcutaneous heparin or oral coumarin therapy (see sec. **B.1**). If the patient is to be converted to coumarin, at lest three days of combined therapy (heparin and coumarin) should take place before heparin is discontinued.
2. **Subcutaneous therapy.** Heparin for subcutaneous injection is provided in concentrations of 10,000 and 20,000 units/ml. The concentration chosen should allow accurate dose measurement and, if possible, reduce the volume of the injection.

   Little uniformity exists in recommendations for subcutaneous heparin therapy in pregnancy. Regimens for subcutaneous heparinization may be categorized as either fixed- or adjusted-dose regimens.
   a. **Fixed-dose** regimens generally use lower doses of heparin. These doses range from 5000–7500 units q8–12h, depending on the stage of pregnancy. A commonly used fixed-dose heparin regimen recommends administration of heparin at dosages of 7500 units SC q12h in the first two trimesters, and 7500 SC q8h in the third trimester. Patients receiving doses in excess of 15,000 units/day should have their APTT evaluated on a regular basis (weekly until stable, then every four weeks). This value may not necessarily deviate significantly from control and is obtained to prevent excessive anticoagulation. Fixed-dose schedules have the advantage of requiring only infrequent evaluation of coagulation parameters but the disadvantage of possibly providing inadequate anticoagulation for some patients. (The frequent inadequacy of

heparin subcutaneous anticoagulation among patients with prosthetic cardiac valves has been thought to be due to inadequate daily heparin dose.)

b. Adjusted-dose heparin uses an initial heparin dose of 5000 units q8h. This dose is then gradually increased until the patient's APTT is prolonged to 130–150% of her own personal control value (obtained prior to beginning therapy). The APTT should be evaluated weekly until stable, and then monthly. If doses greater than 23,000 units/day are employed, weekly APTT testing should be continued. Some patients may require relatively large doses of heparin (i.e., in excess of 30,000 units/day). If such large doses are necessary, the patient should be provided more concentrated heparin (20,000 units/ml, see before).

The **advantage of the adjusted-dose method** is its ability to provide a standardized, defined level of anticoagulation (within the limits of the APTT to measure anticoagulation). Although large doses of heparin may be used, if clotting parameters are properly monitored, the risk of hemorrhage is minimal. The disadvantage of this method is that it requires frequent (expensive) laboratory evaluation. Such large doses of heparin may be somewhat more prone to bleeding complications, in spite of the most assiduous care. Osteoporosis has also been reported in association with prolonged heparin administration.

c. Since neither method has been shown superior in randomized, prospective studies, it is **best to individualize care.** Patients who have sustained major life-threatening embolic disease may benefit from aggressive initial therapy (i.e., APTT 150% or more of control). After some time interval has passed, they may be anticoagulated to a lesser degree (goal of APTT of 130% of control).

B. Coumarin. Coumarin (bishydroxycoumarin) is an effective anticoagulant in humans. Warfarin sodium (Coumadin) is the most commonly used coumarin derivative.

Coumarin and its derivatives act as competitive inhibitors of vitamin K in the final metabolic step of hepatic biosynthesis of factors II, VII, IX, and X. Coumarin also interferes with the production of natural anticoagulants such as proteins C and S. These anticoagulant factors have a short half-life and are stored in small quantities. Their initial decrease with initiation of coumarin anticoagulation, prior to decreased activity of factors II, VII, IX, and X, may actually temporarily predispose to increased thrombosis. **This finding underscores the need for alternate anticoagulation during initiation of coumarin.**

If coumarin therapy is initiated in the setting of resolving (acute) thrombosis, the **initially administered intravenous heparin should be continued for three to four days,** allowing oral coumarin therapy to "overlap" heparin for that interval. In spite of apparently therapeutic prothrombin times, patients not provided alternate anticoagulation have suffered thrombotic episodes.

Coumarin derivatives rely on normal hepatic biosynthetic mechanisms to have a predictable effect. Patients with altered hepatic function, as with hepatitis, congestive heart failure, and a wide variety of other illnesses, may have unpredictable responses to coumarin anticoagulation. Similarly, a large number of medications, including nonsteroidal anti-inflammatory agents, thyroid preparations, and antibiotics, may alter normal response to coumarin. The mechanisms of potentiation vary. Antibiotics are thought to decrease indigenous bowel flora production of vitamin K; other medications affect hepatic microsomal function, or compete for protein binding sites (and thereby increase plasma-free coumarin).

1. Teratogenicity. Coumarin and its derivatives are well-documented human teratogens. When administered in the first trimester, they are associated with a rate of fetal wastage as high as 80% [24]. These fetuses are commonly noted to suffer from **chondrodysplasia punctata,** a syndrome involving multiple congenital anomalies, nasal cartilage hypoplasia, and stippling of the bones. The fourth through eighth weeks appear to be the most critical exposure interval. Infants exposed to coumarin later in pregnancy have a fetal loss rate approximating 11%, possibly due to a tendency toward intracranial hemorrhage.

Women of reproductive age should be treated with coumarin only if they have adequate contraception. **Under no circumstances should coumarin be employed in the first trimester.** In rare circumstances (artificial cardiac valve prostheses), coumarin may be successfully employed in the second and third trimesters. Such usage is not without some risk to the fetus and should only be considered if life-threatening maternal complications present that are not manageable by other means.

2. Dosage

a. The initial dose of coumarin is 10–15 mg PO/day until a prolongation of the prothrombin time of 150–200% (traditionally 250%) of control is achieved. In starting therapy, it should be remembered that a given dose will manifest its full effect at 48 hours after administration. For this reason, caution should be exercised in the initial two doses of coumarin.

b. Recent research by Hirsh [11] indicates that **a lower target for coumarin therapy may be reasonable.** It was found that prothrombin time elevations to 120–150% of control, as measured by current laboratory methodology, are adequate for prophylaxis and treatment of venous thromboembolism. Doses yielding prothrombin elevations of 150–200% were found adequate among patients with recurrent systemic embolism. No value was found for prothrombin prolongations in excess of 200%. It is not known if these findings can be safely extrapolated to the pregnant state.

c. Reversal. In the adult, coumarin has a physiologic clearance half-life of 44 hours. The fetal clearance is unknown but thought to be in the range of 3–14 days. If it is necessary to reverse coumarin anticoagulation, vitamin K (5 mg PO or SC) should be administered. This dose will begin to reverse anticoagulation within six to eight hours. More rapid reversal can be obtained by administration of larger doses of vitamin K (25–50 mg), but such large doses will render the patient refractory to further coumarin anticoagulation for up to two weeks. Alternatively, reversal may be accomplished by administration of fresh-frozen plasma.

3. Neonatal management. Infants born to mothers receiving coumarin anticoagulation should receive 1 mg of vitamin K at birth. Additionally, evidence exists that maternally administered vitamin K may, to a small degree, cross the placenta and correct the infant's clotting system.

Patients inadvertently receiving coumarin during the first trimester should be counseled regarding the high likelihood of teratogenesis and offered termination. It is unclear if similar counseling should apply to exposures exclusive of the first trimester.

References

1. Ahmad, R., et al. Dipyridamole in successful management of pregnant women with prosthetic valve. *Lancet* ii:1414–1415, 1976.
2. Angel, J. L., and Knuppel, R. A. Computed tomography in the diagnosis of puerperal ovarian vein thrombosis. *Obstet. Gynecol.* 63:61, 1984.
3. Ben-Ismail, M., et al. Cardiac valve prosthesis, anticoagulation, and pregnancy. *Br. Heart J.* 55:101–105, 1986.
4. Biale, Y., et al. The course of pregnancy in patients with artificial heart valves treated with dipyridamole. *Int. J. Gynaecol. Obstet.* 18:128–132, 1980.
5. Cross, J. N., Castro, P. O., Jennett, W. B. Cerebral strokes associated with pregnancy and the puerperium. *Br. Med. J.* 3:214–218, 1968.
6. Dahlman, T. C., Hellgren, M. S., and Blomback, M. Thrombosis prophylaxis in pregnancy with use of subcutaneous heparin adjusted by monitoring heparin concentration in plasma. *Am. J. Obstet. Gynecol.* 161(2):420–425, 1989.
7. de la Monte, S. M., et al. Risk factors for the development and rupture of intracranial berry aneurysms. *Am. J. Med.* 78:957–964, 1985.
8. De Stefano, V. et al. Management of pregnancy in women with antithrombin III congenital defect: Report of four cases. *Thromb. Haemost.* 59(2):193–196, 1988.

9. Friend, J. R., and Kakkar, V. V. The diagnosis of deep vein thrombosis in the puerperium. *J. Obstet. Gynecol. Br. Comm.* 77:820, 1970.
10. Ginsberg, J. S., et al. Risks to the fetus of radiologic procedures used in the diagnosis of maternal venous thromboembolic disease. *Throm. Haemost.* 61(2):189–196, 1989.
11. Hirsh, J. Is the dose of warfarin prescribed by American physicians unnecessarily high? *Arch. Intern. Med.* 147:769–771, 1987.
12. Ibarra-Perez, C., et al. The course of pregnancy in patients with artificial heart valves. *Am. J. Med.* 61:504–512, 1976.
13. Iturbe-Alessio, I., et al. Risks of anticoagulant therapy in patients with artificial heart valves. *N. Engl. J. Med.* 315:1390–1393, 1986.
14. Javares, T., et al. Pregnancy after heart valve replacement. *Int. J. Cardiol.* 5:731–739, 1985.
15. Joffe, A. M., et al. Anticoagulant therapy for prevention of spontaneous abortion in a patient with a lupus anticoagulant. *Am. J. Hematol.* 29(1):56–57, 1988.
16. Johnson, S. E., and Skre, H. Transient cerebral ischemic attacks in the young and middle aged: A population study. *Stroke* 17:662–666, 1986.
17. Leclerc, J. R., et al. Management of anti-thrombin III deficiency during pregnancy without administration of anti-thrombin III. *Thromb. Res.* 41(4):567–573, 1986.
18. Lee, P. K., et al. Combined use of warfarin and adjusted subcutaneous heparin during pregnancy in patients with artificial heart valve. *J. Am. Coll. Cardiol.* 8:221, 1986.
19. Lennon, R. L., Sundt, T. M., and Gronert, G. A. Combined cesarean section and clipping of intracerebral aneurysm. *Anaesthesiology* 60:240–242, 1984.
20. Limet, R., and Crondin, C. M. Cardiac valve prosthesis, anticoagulation, and pregnancy. *Ann. Thorac. Surg.* 23:337–431, 1970.
21. Lockshin, M. D., Druzin, M. L., and Qamar, T. Prednisone does not prevent fetal death in women with antiphospholipid antibody. *Am. J. Obstet. Gynecol.* 160:430–443, 1989.
22. Lockwood, C. J., et al. The prevalence and biologic significance of lupus anticoagulant and anticardiolipin antibodies in a general obstetric population. *Am. J. Obstet. Gynecol.* 161(2):369–373, 1989.
23. Locufier, J. L., et al. Aneurysm of the descending thoracic aorta in a young woman. *J. Cardiovasc. Surg.* (Torino) 30(3):499–502, 1989.
24. Lutz, D. J., et al. Pregnancy and its complications following cardiac valve prosthesis. *Am. J. Obstet. Gynecol.* 131:460–468, 1978.
25. Maki, M., et al. Clinical evaluation of antithrombin III concentrate (BI 6.013) for disseminated intravascular coagulation in obstetrics. Well-controlled multicenter trial. *Gynecol. Obstet. Invest.* 23(4):230–240, 1987.
26. Marcus, C. S., et al. Pulmonary imaging in pregnancy. Maternal risk and fetal dosimetry. *Clin. Nucl. Med.* 10(1):1–4, 1985.
27. Marks, F., Schweizer, W. E., and Young, B. K. Pregnancy after traumatic aortic aneurysm repair. *Am. J. Obstet. Gynecol.* 159(2):389–390, 1988.
28. Massad, M., et al. Thrombosed Bjork-Shiley standard disc mitral valve prosthesis. *J. Cardiovasc. Surg.* (Torino) 30(6):976–980, 1989.
29. McColgin, S. W., Martin, J. N., Jr., and Morrison, J. C. Pregnant women with prosthetic heart valves. *Clin. Obstet. Gynecol.* 32(1):76–88, 1989.
30. Michiels, J. J., et al. Prophylaxis of thrombosis in antithrombin III-deficient women during pregnancy and delivery. *Eur. J. Obstet. Gynecol. Reprod. Biol.* 18(3):149–153, 1984.
31. Munsick, R. A., and Gillanders, L. A. A review of the syndrome of puerperal ovarian vein thrombophlebitis. *Obstet. Gynecol. Surv.* 36:57, 1981.
32. Rosove, M. H., et al. Heparin therapy for prevention of fetal wastage in women with anticardiolipin antibodies and lupus anticoagulants. *Blood* 70:379, 1987.
33. Sareli, P., et al. Maternal and fetal sequelae of anticoagulation during pregnancy in patients with mechanical heart valve prostheses. *Am. J. Cardiol.* 63(20):1462–1465, 1989.

34. Sasahara, A. A., et al. Pulmonary thromboembolism. *J.A.M.A.* 249:2945, 1983
35. Schwartz, R. S., et al. Clinical experience with antithrombin III concentrate in treatment of congenital and acquired deficiency of antithrombin. The Antithrombin III Study Group. *Am. J. Med.* 87(3B):53S–60S, 1989.
36. Stafford-Brady, F. J., Gladman, D. D., and Urowitz, M. B. Successful pregnancy in systemic lupus erythematosus with an untreated lupus anticoagulant. *Arch Intern. Med.* 148(7):1647–1648, 1988.
37. Szymonowicz, W., Preston, H., and Yu, V. Y. The surviving monozygotic twin *Arch. Dis. Child.* 61(5):454–458, 1986.
38. Vosa, C., et al. Cardiac valve replacement during pregnancy. Report of two cases. *Ital. J. Surg. Sci.* 18(2):175—177, 1988.
39. Wiebers, D. O. Ischemic cerebrovascular complications of pregnancy. *Arch Neurol.* 42:1106–1113, 1985.
40. Williams, G. M., et al. Aortic disease associated with pregnancy. *J. Vasc. Surg* 8(4):470–475, 1988.

Selected Readings

Creasey, R. K. and Resnik, R. (eds.). *Maternal-Fetal Medicine: Principles and Practice* (2nd ed.). Philadelphia: Saunders, 1989.

De Swiet, M. (ed.). *Medical Disorders in Obstetric Practice* (2nd ed.). Oxford Blackwell, 1989.

Laros, R. K. (ed.). *Blood Disorders in Pregnancy*. Philadelphia: Lea & Febiger 1986.

Stern, B. J. Cerebrovascular Disease and Pregnancy. In P. J. Goldstein (ed.) *Neurological Disorders of Pregnancy*. Mt. Kisco, N.Y.: Futura, 1986. Pp. 19-40.

AORTIC ANEURYSM

Smith, V. C., et al. Marfan's syndrome, pregnancy, and the cardiac surgeon *Milit. Med.* 154(8):404–406, 1989.

Tilson, M. D. Histochemistry of aortic elastin in patients with nonspecific abdominal aneurysmal disease. *Arch. Surg.* 123(4):503–505, 1988.

THROMBOTIC PREDISPOSITION AND HEREDITARY THROMBOTIC TENDENCY

Baguley, E., MacLachlan, N., and Hughes, G. R. SLE and pregnancy. *Clin Exp. Rheumatol.* 6(2):183–185, 1988.

Bithell, T. C. Hereditary dysfibrinogenemia–the first 25 years. *Acta Haematol* (Basel) 71:145–149, 1984.

Brenner, B., et al. Cerebral thrombosis in a newborn with a congenital deficiency of antithrombin III. *Am. J. Hematol.* 27(3):209–211, 1988.

Brenner, B., et al. Hereditary protein C deficiency during pregnancy. *Am. J Obstet. Gynecol.* 157(5):1160–1161, 1987.

Caldwell, D. C., Williamson, R. A., and Goldsmith, J. C. Hereditary coagulopathies in pregnancy. *Clin. Obstet. Gynecol.* 28(1):53–72, 1985.

Comp, P. C., and Esmon, C. T. Recurrent venous thromboembolism in patients with a partial deficiency of protein S. *N. Engl. J. Med.* 311:1525–1528, 1984

de Boer, K., et al. Enhanced thrombin generation in normal and hypertensive pregnancy. *Am. J. Obstet. Gynecol.* 160(1):95–100, 1989.

De Swiet, M. Thromboembolism. *Clin. Haematol.* 14(3):643–660, 1985.

Delshammar, M., et al. Abnormal proteolysis (DIC)—successful treatment with antithrombin III concentrate and a concentrate containing F XIII and native von Willebrand factor. *J. Intern. Med.* 225(1):21–27, 1989.

Derksen, R. H., et al. Coagulation screen is more specific than the anticardiolipin antibody ELISA in defining a thrombotic subset of lupus patients. *Ann. Rheum. Dis.* 47(5):364–371, 1988.

Englert, H. J., et al. Pregnancy and lupus: prognostic indicators and response to treatment. *Q. J. Med.* 66(250):125–136, 1988.

Ezenagu, L. C., and Brandt, J. T. Laboratory determination of heparin cofactor II. *Arch. Pathol. Lab. Med.* 110(12):1149–1151, 1986.

Friedman, K. D., Borok, Z., and Owen, J. Heparin cofactor activity and antithrombin III antigen levels in preeclampsia. *Thromb. Res.* 43(4):409–416, 1986.

Gilabert, J., et al. Physiological coagulation inhibitors (protein S, protein C and antithrombin III) in severe preeclamptic states and in users of oral contraceptives. *Thromb. Res.* 49(3):319–329, 1988.

Gromnica-Ihle, E., and Ziemer, S. Treatment with AT III concentrates in hereditary and acquired AT III deficiency. *Folia Haematol.* (Leipz.) 115(3):307–313, 1988.

Hellgren, M., et al. Severe acquired antithrombin III deficiency in relation to hepatic and renal insufficiency and intrauterine fetal death in late pregnancy. *Gynecol. Obstet. Invest.* 16(2):107–118, 1983.

Henny, C. P., et al. Thrombosis prophylaxis in an AT III deficient pregnant woman: application of a low molecular weight heparinoid (letter). *Thromb. Haemost.* 55(2):301, 1986.

Hirsh, J., Piovella, F., and Pini, M. Congenital antithrombin III deficiency. Incidence and clinical features. *Am. J. Med.* 87(3B):34S–38S, 1989.

Horellou, M. H., et al. Congenital protein C deficiency and thrombotic disease in nine French families. *Br. Med. J.* 289:1285–1287, 1984.

Kobayashi, T., and Terao, T. Preeclampsia as chronic disseminated intravascular coagulation. Study of two parameters: thrombin-antithrombin III complex and D-dimers. *Gynecol. Obstet. Invest.* 24(3):170–178, 1987.

Kueh, Y. K., Radhakrishnan, U., and Han, P. Hereditary protein C deficiency—the first symptomatic family in Singapore. *Ann. Acad. Med. Singapore* 18(4):456–458, 1989.

Lao, T. T., Yuen, P. M., and Yin, J. A. Protein S and protein C levels in Chinese women during pregnancy, delivery and the puerperium. *Br. J. Obstet. Gynaecol.* 96(2):167–170, 1989.

Letsky, E., and de Swiet, M. Thromboembolism in pregnancy and its management. *Br. J. Haematol.* 57(4):543–552, 1984.

Lockshin, M. D. Pregnancy does not cause systemic lupus erythematosus to worsen. *Arthritis Rheum.* 32(6):665–670, 1989.

Malm, J., Laurell, M., and Dahlback, B. Changes in the plasma levels of vitamin K-dependent proteins C and S and of C4b-binding protein during pregnancy and oral contraception. *Br. J. Haematol.* 68(4):437–443, 1988.

McRoyan, D. K., et al. Constitutional hypofibrinogenemia associated with third trimester hemorrhage. *Ann. Clin. Lab. Sci.* 16(1):52–57, 1986.

Menache, D., et al. Evaluation of the safety, recovery, half-life, and clinical efficacy of antithrombin III (human) in patients with hereditary antithrombin III deficiency. Cooperative Study Group. *Blood* 75(1):33–39, 1990.

Morrison, A. E., Walker, I. D., and Black, W. P. Protein C deficiency presenting as deep venous thrombosis in pregnancy. Case report. *Br. J. Obstet. Gynaecol.* 95(10):1077–1080, 1988.

Nelson, D. M., Stempel, L. E., and Brandt, J. T. Hereditary antithrombin III deficiency and pregnancy: report of two cases and review of the literature. *Obstet. Gynecol.* 65(6):848–853, 1985.

Otoya, J., Nemcek, A. A., Jr., and Green, D. Venous thromboembolism (clinical conference). *Chest* 96(5):1169–1174, 1989.

Pinto, S., et al. Increased thrombin generation in normal pregnancy. *Acta Eur. Fertil.* 19(5):263–267, 1988.

Schwartz, M. E., Harrington, E. B., and Rand, J. H. Unusual venous thrombosis associated with protein C deficiency. *J. Vasc. Surg.* 7(3):443–445, 1988.

Sorin, J., et al. Plasminogen Paris 1: Congenital abnormal plasminogen and its incidence in thrombosis. *Thromb. Res.* 32:229–238, 1983.

Srum, Y., Handeland, G. F., and Abildgaard, U. On the clinical significance of acquired antithrombin deficiency. *Folia Haematol.* (Leipz.) 111(6):797–805 1984.

Tengborn, L., and Bengtsson, T. Antithrombin III concentrate. Thromboprophylaxis during pregnancy in a patient with congenital antithrombin III deficiency. *Acta Obstet. Gynecol. Scand.* 65(4):375–376, 1986.

Terao, T., et al. Pathological state of the coagulatory and fibrinolytic system in preeclampsia and the possibility of its treatment with AT III concentrate. *Asia Oceania J. Obstet. Gynaecol.* 15(1):25–32, 1989.

Vellenga, E., van Imhoff, G. W., and Aarnoudse, J. G. Effective prophylaxis with oral anticoagulants and low-dose heparin during pregnancy in an antithrombin III deficient woman (letter). *Lancet* 2(8343):224, 1983.

Vogel, J. J., de Moerloose, P. A., and Bounameaux, H. Protein C deficiency and pregnancy: a case report. *Obstet. Gynecol.* 73(3 Pt. 2):455–456, 1989.

Warwick, R., et al. Changes in protein C and free protein S during pregnancy and following hysterectomy. *J. R. Soc. Med.* 2(10):591–594, 1989.

Weenink, G. H., et al. Antithrombin III levels in normotensive and hypertensive pregnancy. *Gynecol. Obstet. Invest.* 16(4):230–242, 1983.

Thromboembolic Disease

Badaracco, M. A., and Vessey, M. Recurrence of venous thromboembolic disease and use of oral contraceptives. *Br. Med. J.* 1:215–217, 1974.

Barss, V. A., et al. Use of the subcutaneous heparin pump during pregnancy. *J. Reprod. Med.* 30(12):899–901, 1985.

Bergqvist, A., Bergqvist, D., and Hallbrook, T. Acute deep vein thrombosis (DVT) after cesarean section. *Acta Obstet. Gynecol. Scand.* [Suppl.] 58:473–476, 1979.

Bergqvist, A., Bergqvist, D., and Hallbrook, T. Deep vein thrombosis during pregnancy. A prospective study. *Acta Obstet. Gynecol. Scand.* 62:443–448, 1983.

Clarke-Pearson, D. L., and Jelovsek, F. R. Alterations of occlusive cuff impedance results in the obstetric patient. *Surgery* 89:594–598, 1981.

Davies, J. A. The pre-thrombotic state. *Clin. Sci.* 69:641–646, 1985.

Delclos, G. L., and Davila, F. Thrombolytic therapy for pulmonary embolism in pregnancy: A case report. *Am. J. Obstet. Gynecol.* 155(2):375–376, 1986.

Department of Health and Social Security Report on Confidential Enquiries into Maternal Deaths in England and Wales 1979–81. London: Her Majesty's Stationery Office, 1986.

Gallus, A. S. Venous Thromboembolism: Incidence and Clinical Risk Factors. In J. L. Madden and M. Hume (eds.), *Venous Thromboembolism*. New York: Appleton-Century-Crofts, 1976.

Hellgran, M., and Nygards, E. B. Long term therapy with subcutaneous heparin during pregnancy. *Gynecol. Obstet. Invest.* 13:76–89, 1981.

Hirsch, J., Cade, J. F., and O'Sullivan, E. F. Clinical experience with anticoagulant therapy during pregnancy. *Br. Med. J.* 1:270–273, 1970.

Howie, P. W. Anticoagulants in pregnancy. *Clin. Obstet. Gynaecol.* 13(2):349–363, 1986.

Huisman, M. V., et al. Serial impedance plethysmography for suspected deep venous thrombosis in outpatients. *N. Engl. J. Med.* 314:823–828, 1986.

Hull, R. D., et al. Diagnostic efficacy of impedance plethysmography for clinically suspected deep-vein thrombosis: a randomized trial. *Ann. Intern. Med.* 102:21–28, 1985.

Mogensen, K., et al. Thrombectomy of acute iliofemoral venous thrombosis during pregnancy. *Surg. Gynecol. Obstet.* 169(1):50–54, 1989.

Prevention of venous thrombosis and pulmonary embolism. NIH Consensus Development. *J.A.M.A.* 256(6):744–749, 1986.

Rutherford, S. E., and Phelan, J. P. Thromboembolic disease in pregnancy. *Clin. Perinatol.* 13(4):719–739, 1986.

Splinter, W. M., et al. Anaesthetic management of emergency cesarean section followed by pulmonary embolectomy. *Can. J. Anaesth.* 36(6):689–692, 1989.

Tlanc, D., Kakkar, V. V., and Clarke, M. B. Detection of venous thrombosis of the legs using ^{125}I labeled fibrinogen. *Br. J. Surg.* 55:742, 1968.

Treffers, P. E., et al. Epidemiological observations of thrombo-embolic disease during pregnancy and in the puerperium, in 56,022 women. *Int. J. Gynaecol. Obstet.* 21(4):327–331, 1983.

Walsh, J. J., Bonnar, J., and Wright, F. W. A study of pulmonary embolism and deep leg vein thrombosis after major gynecological surgery using labeled fibrinogen-phlebography and lung scanning. *Br. J. Obstet. Gynaecol.* 81:311, 1974.

White, R. H., et al. Diagnosis of deep vein thrombosis using duplex ultrasound. *Ann. Intern. Med.* 111(4):297–304, 1989.

Septic Pelvic Thrombophlebitis

Cohen, M. B., et al. Septic pelvic thrombophlebitis: An update. *Obstet. Gynecol.* 62:83, 1983.

Duff, R., and Gibbs, R. S. Pelvic vein thrombophlebitis: Diagnostic dilemma and therapeutic challenge. *Obstet. Gynecol. Surv.* 38:365, 1983.

Cerebrovascular Thromboembolic Disease

Banerjee, A. K., et al. Cerebrovascular disease in north-west India: A study of necropsy material. *J. Neurol. Neurosurg. Psychiatry* 52(4):512–515, 1989.

Bansal, B. C., Gupta, R. R., and Prakash, C. Stroke during pregnancy and puerperium in young females below the age of 40 years as a result of cerebral venous/venous sinus thrombosis. *Jap. Heart J.* 21:171–183, 1980.

Bousser, M. G., et al. Cerebral venous thrombosis—a review of 38 cases. *Stroke* 16:199–213, 1985.

Cerebral Embolism Study Group. Immediate anticoagulation of embolic stroke: Brain hemorrhage and management options. *Stroke* 15:779–789, 1984.

Estanol, B., et al. Intracranial venous thrombosis in young women. *Stroke* 10:680–684, 1979.

Imai, A., et al. Successful pregnancy in a patient with paroxysmal nocturnal hemoglobinuria: case report. *Arch. Gynecol. Obstet.* 246(2):121–124, 1989.

Lavin, P. J. M., et al. Intracranial venous thrombosis in the first trimester of pregnancy. *J. Neurol. Neurosurg. Psychiatry* 41:726–729, 1978.

Lavin, P. J. M., et al. Wernicke's encephalopathy: a predictable complication of hyperemesis gravidarum. *Obstet. Gynecol.* 62:135, 1983.

Levine, S. R., et al. Cerebral venous thrombosis with lupus anticoagulants. Report of two cases. *Stroke* 18(4):801–804, 1987.

Ockelford, P. Heparin 1986. Indications and effective use. *Drugs* 31(1):81–92, 1986.

Ravindran, R. S., and Zandstra, G. C. Cerebral venous thrombosis versus postlumbar puncture headache (letter; comment). *Anesthesiology* 71(3):478–479, 1989.

Ravindran, R. S., Zandstra, G. C., and Viegas, O. J. Postpartum headache following regional analgesia: A symptom of cerebral venous thrombosis. *Can. J. Anaesth.* 36(6):705–707, 1989.

Srinivasan, K. Cerebral venous and arterial thrombosis in pregnancy and puerperium: A study of 135 patients. *Angiology* 34:731–746, 1983.

Srinivasan, K. Puerperal cerebral venous and arterial thrombosis. *Semin. Neurol.* 8(3):222–225, 1988.

Tran, T. H., et al. Methodology and clinical significance of heparin cofactor II. Probable heparin cofactor II deficiency in a patient with cerebrovascular thrombosis. *Semin. Thromb. Hemost.* 11(4):342–346, 1985.

Wood, D. H. Cerebrovascular complications of sickle cell anemia. *Stroke* 9:73–75, 1978.

Younker, D., et al. Maternal cortical vein thrombosis and the obstetric anesthesiologist. *Anesth. Analg.* 65(10):1007–1012, 1986.

Intracranial Hemorrhage

Barno, A., and Freeman, D. W. Maternal deaths due to spontaneous subarachnoid hemorrhage. *Am. J. Obstet. Gynecol.* 125:384–392, 1976.

Robinson, J. L., Hall, C. S., and Sedzimir, C. B. Arteriovenous malformations, aneurysms, and pregnancy. *J. Neurosurg.* 41:63–70, 1974.

Tuttelman, R. M., and Gleicher, N. Central nervous system hemorrhage complicating pregnancy. *Obstet. Gynecol.* 58:651–657, 1981.

Wilkins, R. H. Natural history of intracranial vascular malformations: a review. *Neurosurgery* 16:421–430, 1985.

Young, D. C., Leveno, K. J., and Whalley, P. J. Induced delivery prior to surgery for ruptured cerebral aneurysm. *Obstet. Gynecol.* 61:749–752, 1983.

Artificial Heart Valves

Shaul, W. L., and Hall, J. G. Multiple congenital anomalies associated with anticoagulants. *Am. J. Obstet. Gynecol.* 127:191–198, 1977.

Anticoagulation

Ginsberg, J. S., et al. Risks to the fetus of anticoagulant therapy during pregnancy. *Thromb. Haemost.* 61:197–203, 1989.

Ginsberg, J. S., and Hirsh, J. Optimum use of anticoagulants in pregnancy. *Drugs* 36(4):505–512, 1989.

Ginsberg, J. S., and Hirsh, J. Use of anticoagulants in pregnancy. *Chest* 95(2):156S–160S, 1989.

Hall, J. G., Pauli, R. M., and Wilson, K. M. Maternal and fetal sequelae of anticoagulation during pregnancy. *Am. J. Med.* 68:122–140, 1980.

Hirsh, J., Deykin, D., and Poller, L. "Therapeutic range" for oral anticoagulant therapy. *Chest* 89(2):11s–15s, 1986.

Poller, L. Laboratory control of anticoagulant therapy. *Semin. Thromb. Hemost.* 12(1):13–19, 1986.

Stults, B. M., Dere, W. H., and Caine, T. H. Long-term anticoagulation. Indications and management. *West. J. Med.* 151(4):414–429, 1989.

16 Surgical and Gynecologic Complications

Gary S. Leiserowitz
and Lloyd H. Smith

Surgical Complications During Pregnancy

As noted by Sir Zachary Cope [15], pregnancy complicated by surgical disease "is always a source of special anxiety, both from the maternal and the fetal point of view. Exploratory operations are not lightly to be advised on account of the risk of abortion, and one therefore needs to be very sure of the indications of various acute diseases needing intervention before advising the abdomen to be opened." However, for approximately 2 in 1000 pregnancies complicated by such diseases, delay of diagnosis or of indicated surgical intervention will not be in the best interest of the mother or the fetus. In fact, the treatment for the pregnant patient is usually the same as for the nonpregnant patient, and the severity of the surgical disease, not the surgery itself, appears to be the more important factor in determining the risk of abortion, prematurity, and perinatal mortality.

I. General considerations

A. Surgical diagnosis in the pregnant patient

1. History and physical examination. Symptoms sometimes attributed to pregnancy alone (e.g., headache, syncope, nausea, vomiting, abdominal discomfort) should be interpreted with care as they may also be associated with intercurrent surgical illness. Conversely, it should be recognized that diastolic blood pressures in the fifties and a heart rate of 85–90 may be normal in pregnancy. Supine dyspnea and hypotension are concomitants of the aortocaval compression syndrome found in many normal pregnant women near term who assume a supine position. The relative hyperemia of the skin may, however, mask typical changes of hypotension and shock seen in nonpregnant patients. In addition, signs of surgical disease in the abdomen may be masked as the enlarging uterus displaces interperitoneal organs. Localization of tenderness by palpation or elicitation of abdominal reflexes such as guarding and rigidity may be obscured.

2. Laboratory and radiologic diagnosis. Radiologic tests appropriate for the nonpregnant patient should be employed in pregnancy if their omission would delay or adversely affect diagnosis. Use of the maximum x-ray exposure, avoidance of redundant studies, and shielding of the fetus are advisable. Pregnancy is accompanied by physiologic adaptations that may alter the normal ranges of commonly used laboratory tests. As summarized in Table 16-1, a relative state of anemia, mild leukocytosis, lower normal values for blood urea nitrogen and creatinine, and higher normal values for fibrinogen and erythrocyte sedimentation rate are characteristic.

B. Perioperative management

1. Preoperative management

a. Timing

b. Patient population. When possible, informed consent should be obtained from the patient when a procedure is anticipated. External fetal heart rate monitoring is appropriate for viable pregnancies before, after, and occasionally during surgery if not in the operating field. If the risk of premature

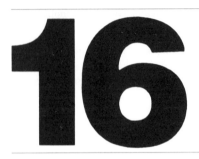

Table 16-1. Alterations in laboratory values in normal pregnancy

Laboratory test	Value in pregnancy
Hemoglobin and hematocrit levels	Lower limits at term: 10 gm/dl; 30%
White blood cell count	Late pregnancy: up to 15,000/μl Labor and puerperium: up to 25,000/μl
Fibrinogen level	Second and third trimesters: 250–600 mg/dl (100–300 mg/dl more than nonpregnant values); increases toward term
Erythrocyte sedimentation rate	Increases two- to sixfold over non-pregnant values
Blood urea nitrogen level	7.2–10.2 mg/dl
Creatinine level	0.4–1.0 mg/dl
Serum glucose level	Fasting decreased 10%
Serum albumin level	May decrease 1 gm/dl by term
Serum glutamic-oxaloacetic transaminase, serum glutamic-pyruvic transaminase, and bilirubin levels	Unchanged
Lactic acid dehydrogenase, creatine phosphokinase, and alkaline phosphatase levels	Increased
Urine evaluation	Glycosuria common; proteinuria common; urine porphyrins may be increased

delivery is significant, arrangements for neonatal intensive care services should be made. Adequate blood replacement should be available. Consideration of prophylaxis against venous thromboembolism is important for pregnant patients who are at high risk, which includes surgery greater than 30 minutes, age greater than 40, previous myocardial infarction, heart failure, previous venous thrombosis, previous pulmonary embolus, cancer, stroke, or major orthopedic surgery [34]. Prophylaxis can be with heparin, 5000 units SC, 2 hours prior to surgery, and then repeated q12h until the patient is ambulatory postoperatively. An alternative is to use intermittent pneumatic compression stockings both during the procedure and postoperatively [34].

2. Intraoperative and anesthetic considerations

a. Incision. The incision that will allow the most effective exposure should be selected. Handling of the uterus should be minimized to lessen the risk of abortion or premature labor.

b. Prevention of pulmonary aspiration. Pregnancy is accompanied by a delay in gastric emptying and an increased risk of aspiration pneumonitis in the anesthetized gravida. Preoperative administration of nonparticulate antacids, use of cricothyroid pressure during induction, and intraoperative nasogastric suctioning will decrease this risk.

c. Anesthetic considerations

(1) Teratogenesis and abortion. Some anesthetic agents have been shown to be teratogenic in animals, and female operating room employees experience an increased risk of spontaneous abortion and birth defects [9]. The first trimester is identified as the period of highest risk for teratogenesis because of organogenesis. Exposure to anesthesia is best delayed until the second trimester. However, studies have failed to show an increased risk of birth defects resulting from anesthesia exposure [18, 30]. An increased risk of spontaneous abortion has been shown to be associated with surgery under general anesthesia during the first or second trimester [20]. The use of time-related drugs in minimum effective doses that give maximum benefit is recommended.

(2) **Choice of anesthetic.** Regional anesthesia is preferred because local anesthetics are not associated with birth defects, and scant amounts of drug pass into the fetal circulation. Caution must be used to avoid maternal hypotension during spinal or epidural anesthesia by careful intravascular volume loading prior to induction. During general anesthesia, agents felt to be safe include thiopental, muscle relaxants, narcotics, nitrous oxides, and low-dose inhalational agents such as halothane, enflurane, and isoflurane [30]. Respiratory adaptations in pregnancy predispose the patient to overdosage of inhalation anesthetics and more rapid development of hypoxemia. Reversal of neuromuscular blockade with neostigmine must be done carefully since this agent may cause acetylcholine release in the myometrium, resulting in augmentation of uterine contractility.

d. **Prevention of fetal asphyxia.** Maternal hypotension and placental hypoperfusion as a result of vena caval compression are avoided by either left lateral tilt of the supine patient or lateral displacement of the uterine fundus. Increased inspired oxygen concentrations should be used and arterial blood gas measurements performed if prolonged general anesthesia is necessary. Hemoglobin measurements should be made frequently if blood loss is significant. Bladder catheterization is important to monitor maintenance of adequate urine production, which is reflective of an adequate intravascular volume, both intraoperatively and postoperatively.

3. **Postoperative management**

a. **Prevention of fetal asphyxia.** For fetuses beyond 25–26 weeks' gestation, a continuous fetal heart rate recording (though sometimes difficult to obtain) in the immediate postoperative period may allow for the early identification of uterine hypoperfusion as reflected by changes in the baseline fetal heart rate, beat-to-beat variability, or periodic decelerations. Such changes should lead to efforts to correct maternal hypovolemia or hypoxemia or to inhibit uterine contractions. Again, maternal hypotension is minimized by avoiding the flat supine position. Sufficient parenteral fluids should be administered to result in a urine output of at least 30 ml/hour. Arterial blood gas measurement should be done if hypoxemia is suspected, and when confirmed, appropriate measures should be taken. The maternal hematocrit should be maintained at 30% or higher, allowing some protection for subsequent blood loss or equilibration. Nasogastric suctioning and prophylactic heparin may be continued for their original indications.

b. **Prevention of premature labor.** As pregnancy approaches term, the gravid uterus becomes increasingly irritable, especially when traumatized, and the risk of premature labor increases accordingly. When possible, postoperative monitoring should be performed to detect premature labor in pregnancies past 20 weeks' gestation. The prophylactic use of tocolytic agents (e.g., magnesium sulfate or sympathomimetic agents) in the postoperative period may be justified for certain high-risk patients. The use of magnesium sulfate in this setting has advantages over beta-sympathomimetics, which cause maternal tachycardia, decreased diastolic blood pressure, and hemodilution, all of which may confound attempts to monitor for hypovolemia. Adequate sedation and analgesia may also reduce the risk of premature labor, as will the avoidance of hypoxemia and hypovolemia.

c. **Pain.** Meperidine and morphine use in pregnancy appears to be safe when given for short periods of time. Codeine has been associated with birth defects, and so should be limited to use after the first trimester. Controversy remains about the safety of acetylsalicylic acid in regard to birth defects, constriction of the ductus arteriosus in utero, and platelet dysfunction leading to a hemostatic disorder. Its use should be restricted to situations where its benefit outweighs the risk. Acetaminophen appears safe as an analgesic and antipyretic [3].

II. Management of shock in the pregnant patient. The obstetrician must be able to rapidly identify and treat shock. The pathophysiology of acute hypotension and shock are discussed in standard textbooks [10, 25].

A. Etiology. In all patients, potential causes include hypovolemia (due to hemorrhage or excessive fluid loss such as diarrhea), myocardial failure, circulatory obstruction (e.g., pulmonary embolus), redistribution of blood or fluid, or both, from the intravascular space (e.g., septic shock, burns), reduction of peripheral vasomotor tone (e.g., spinal or epidural anesthesia), as well as supine hypotension syndrome [10]. Signs and symptoms of shock may be masked early because of increased blood and plasma volume increases. Once the diagnosis of shock is made based on hypotension and tachycardia, a blood loss of 15–25% may be present. The risk of shock should be anticipated in patients with predisposing causes such as hemorrhage, sepsis, and burns. Shock may be the first manifestation of some catastrophic conditions such as pulmonary embolus or amniotic fluid embolus. The two most common causes of shock in obstetrics are discussed here.

1. **Hemorrhage.** Blood loss from vaginal delivery or cesarean section is notoriously underestimated. Compensatory mechanisms may provide a normal blood pressure until blood loss exceeds 1000–1500 ml. Blood loss can be concealed (e.g., placental abruption) and not appreciated until shock occurs. Patients at risk for obstetric hemorrhage (e.g., multiparity, placenta previa) should have large-bore intravenous lines in place and blood available.
2. **Septic shock.** Despite the frequent presence of infections in the upper and lower genital tracts, septic shock is distinctly uncommon. Because of the young age of most obstetric patients and their lack of underlying chronic disease, mortality from septic shock is rare [25]. A detailed discussion of the etiology of septic shock can be found elsewhere [7, 26]. As in hemorrhage, compensatory mechanisms may mask the severity of sepsis, and shock may occur suddenly when they are overcome. Adult respiratory distress syndrome and disseminated intravascular coagulation may accompany septic shock.

B. Diagnosis

1. **Clinical.** The appreciation of high-risk situations will often identify those patients at risk to develop shock. Low blood pressure associated with a flat supine position is physiologic because of decreased blood return due to uterine compression of the inferior vena cava. Symptoms of shock include fainting, light-headedness, nausea and vomiting, plus those specific to the underlying cause. Vital sign changes can be subtle until cardiovascular collapse, at which time hypotension, tachycardia, tachypnea, and occasionally hypothermia can be seen. The physical examination will often show the most likely etiology (such as blood loss or sepsis). Cardiogenic shock will have further associated findings such as jugular venous distention and pulmonary rales.
2. **Laboratory aids.** The most probable etiology for shock will determine what laboratory evaluation is needed for confirmation. In all patients, a complete blood count, serum electrolytes, blood type and cross-match, coagulation studies, arterial blood gases, and radiologic exams should be considered. Those patients with sepsis will need cultures of the suspected source.
3. **Hemodynamic assessment.** The presence of shock mandates critical care monitoring. A urinary catheter should be placed to measure urine output, a good indirect measure of response to resuscitation. A central line should be placed both for rapid administration of fluids and blood, as well as for hemodynamic monitoring. A Swan-Ganz catheter is helpful to evaluate fluid status and cardiac function. An arterial line provides access to direct blood pressure monitoring as well as frequent arterial blood gases. Consideration of transfer to an intensive care unit is important in order to provide careful monitoring and intensive nursing care. Normal hemodynamic values in pregnancy are noted:

heart rate, 60–100 beats/minute; central venous pressure, 5–10 mm Hg; pulmonary capillary wedge pressure, 6–12 mm Hg; mean arterial blood pressure, 80–85 mm Hg; and cardiac output, 6.2–6.4 liters/minute [1].

C. Principles of management

1. Initial management. Diagnostic and therapeutic measures are begun simultaneously as the morbidity and mortality from shock depend on its duration. If possible, the directly supine position is avoided in patients past the middle of the second trimester, or the fundus is laterally displaced to avoid vena caval compression. One or more large-gauge intravenous catheters are inserted, and rapid crystalloid administration is started. A central line is preferable both for fluids and for hemodynamic monitoring. At present, colloid solutions (albumin, fresh-frozen plasma) do not appear to have an advantage over crystalloids (e.g., Ringer's lactate) for initial fluid resuscitation. Further, volume replacement is based on specific need, e.g., blood transfusions for hemorrhage; crystalloids or colloids, or both, for septic shock. If blood pressure support is needed, then **dopamine** is preferable since at low doses it not only increases cardiac output and arterial blood pressure, but also improves renal perfusion. Dopamine may decrease uterine blood flow [27] and so should be used once demonstrated that volume replacement is insufficient. Ephedrine is valuable to counteract hypotension from epidural or spinal anesthesia if fluids are ineffective. Oxygen administration is given to prevent fetal hypoxemia. Ventilatory support is necessary if respiratory failure occurs.

2. Central venous catheter insertion

a. Subclavian technique. Both subclavian and internal jugular veins are commonly used for placement of central venous catheters. The choice of which to use is based on operator preference and experience as well as the specific clinical situation. Physicians with less experience should be supervised in the technique by another physician with specific training. A thorough understanding of the regional anatomy of the head and neck, precautions, contraindications, and potential complications should be obtained prior to starting. Once placed, the central line can be used to insert a Swan-Ganz pulmonary artery catheter. The technique is summarized here; a complete description can be found elsewhere [2].

(1) Position. The patient should lie in a mild (15-degree) Trendelenburg position with her face turned to the opposite shoulder (avoid the straight supine position). Using a sterile gloved technique, the clavicular area is prepared with antiseptic and is draped, and 2–3 ml of 1% lidocaine is injected into the skin, subcutaneous tissue, and periosteum at the inferior border of the clavicle's midpoint.

(2) Subclavian venipuncture. A 2-in., 14-gauge needle with attached syringe is inserted, bevel downward, just lateral to the clavicular midpoint and is advanced beneath the clavicle in a horizontal plane aimed at the anterior margin of the trachea at the suprasternal notch (Fig. 16-1). Gentle aspiration is continued until venipuncture occurs. The needle is slightly advanced into the vein; blood flow in and out of the syringe should be easily demonstrated.

(3) Catheter insertion. To prevent air embolism, the open end of the needle is covered as the syringe is removed, and if possible, the patient should perform the Valsalva maneuver as the catheter is inserted. A 16-gauge catheter is carefully inserted and threaded in approximately 8 in. **Never** withdraw the catheter through the needle as this may shear off the distal portion, which may embolize. If the catheter cannot be inserted, it should be removed with the needle **as one unit,** and another attempt should be made. After successful catheter placement, the needle and catheter are withdrawn **simultaneously** until the needle tip emerges from the skin. A protective guard is placed around the needle; guard and catheter are sutured to the skin, and a sterile dressing is placed.

(4) Seldinger wire technique. An alternative technique employs the use of a guide wire to mark the position of the vein that will be cannulated

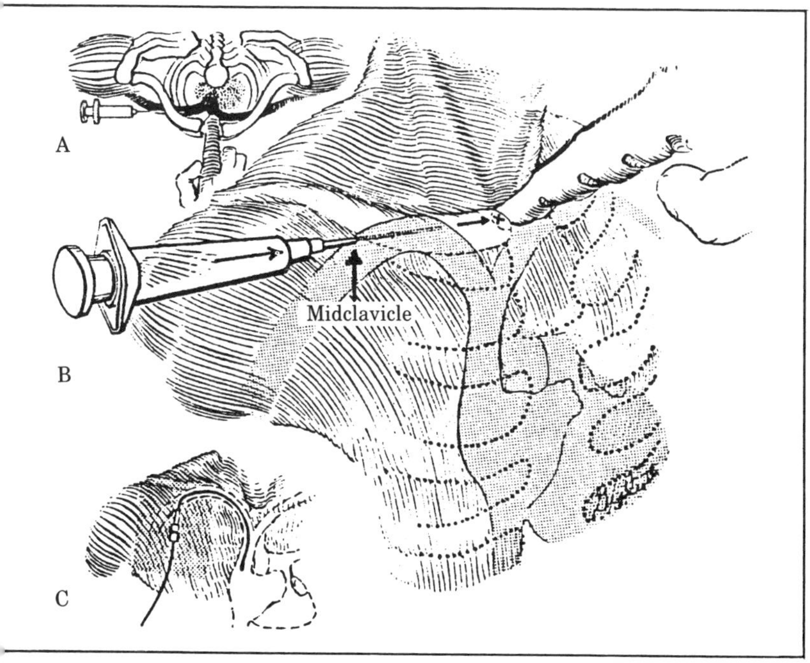

Fig. 16-1. Technique of percutaneous infraclavicular subclavian catheterization. The needle, inserted under the midclavicle and aimed in three dimensions at the top of the posterior aspect of the sternal manubrium (indicated by the fingertip in the suprasternal notch), lies in a plane parallel with the frontal plane of the patient and will enter the anterior wall of the subclavian vein. (From S. J. Dudrick, Intravenous hyperalimentation. *Med. Clin. North Am.* 54(3):577, 1970.)

The benefits include the elimination of risk of catheter-fragment embolus and the ability to reposition the needle or wire if the vein is not initially cannulated [2]. The vein position is identified with an 18-gauge thin-walled needle. Once venous blood is easily aspirated, a guide wire with a flexible J-tip is passed into the vein. Care is taken to keep the end of the guide wire outside of the guiding needle. If the wire does not easily pass into the vein, the wire is carefully removed and the guiding needle repositioned. The guide wire must never be forced into the vein, as perforation of the vein could result. Once the wire is successfully placed and advanced into the superior vena cava, the guiding needle is removed. The skin entrance is enlarged with a scalpel. A vein dilator is passed over the guide wire into the vein, and then removed. A central venous catheter or a catheter sheath is then passed over the guide wire, taking care to maintain a length of wire beyond the hub of the catheter. The wire is then removed and the catheter is flushed with heparinized saline and secured in place with suture. After chest x-ray examination, the catheter may be used for fluids, blood, hyperalimentation, or medications, or a Swan-Ganz catheter can be passed if a catheter sheath has been inserted.

(5) Confirm proper catheter placement. Aspiration of venous blood should be easily accomplished. A chest x ray must always be obtained after placement of a central line to ensure that the tip of the catheter is in the superior vena cava and to check for pneumothorax. Misplacement must be immediately corrected and another chest x ray performed to confirm position.

b. Contraindications and complications. Contraindications to subclavian central venous catheterization include apical bullous emphysema, previous clavicular fracture that distorted the anatomy, and prior radiotherapy in the area of placement. Coagulopathy is also a relative contraindication since venous laceration may lead to massive hemorrhage or hematoma formation in the neck or mediastinum, or both. In such circumstances, longer central venous lines are best placed via the brachial or femoral veins. Complications also arise from the close proximity of the pleura and subclavian artery. Subclavian artery puncture should be recognized promptly and lead to withdrawal and prolonged compression of the site. Although both hemothorax and hydrothorax may occur, pneumothorax is the most frequent complication and is usually self-limited. Chest roentgenograms should be obtained after all central venous catheterization attempts.

3. Blood replacement therapy is discussed in Chap. 6.

4. Adjuvant measures in the treatment of shock. Aside from definitive medical or surgical therapy to correct the cause of shock, several other therapeutic methods are available. Such adjuncts to therapy should be used with caution and only in cases of great need in the pregnant patient, as the effects on the fetus are largely unknown.

a. Hemorrhagic shock

(1) Administration of hyperosmotic electrolyte solution.

(2) External counterpressure. Anecdotal reports continue to suggest a benefit from the use of the military antishock trouser (MAST) apparatus with the obstetric hemorrhagic shock patient [42]. For example, the MAST apparatus has been employed in the management of shock associated with hepatic rupture during pregnancy, ruptured ectopic pregnancy, placenta previa, intraabdominal pregnancy, postpartum hemorrhage, and ischiorectal hematoma [43]. The beneficial effects of inflatable leg and abdominal compartments appear to be related to a shunting of blood (750–1000 ml) away from the legs and abdomen, with a resultant increase in blood pressure and central venous pressure, as well as an enhancement of mechanisms that seal vascular damage [43]. Other studies, however, suggest a much smaller shift of vascular fluid, accompanied by the potentially deleterious effects of reduced venous return and reduced cardiac output [29]. Nevertheless, when other modalities have failed, the MAST apparatus may allow temporary stabilization of the critically ill preoperative or postoperative patient. Contraindications include bleeding above the diaphragm, congestive heart failure, and cerebral or pulmonary edema. Guidelines for use of the MAST apparatus can be found elsewhere [42, 43].

(3) Blood substitute. The use of emulsions of oxygen-carrying perfluorocarbon (Fluosol-DA 20%) in postpartum hemorrhagic shock patients who, for religious reasons, refuse administration of blood products has been reported [31]. Although still experimental and associated with some side effects, the use of this substance may be lifesaving.

(4) Definitive therapy will involve directly or indirectly stopping the hemorrhage. Obstetric hemorrhage is the most common cause of shock. Other conditions such as maternal trauma are also responsible.

(a) Postpartum hemorrhage is managed conventionally with determination of the exact source of bleeding and then treatment specific to the cause (see Chap. 20).

(b) Surgical approaches are occasionally necessary for treatment of uterine bleeding when other therapy such as pitocin, Methergine, and prostaglandins is not sufficient. Manual exploration of the uterus to check for retained products of conception or uterine tears is done. Repair of obstetric injuries is necessary. If bleeding persists, then other measures must be undertaken.

(i) **Uterine artery ligation** (O'Leary method) can be used to control severe uterine bleeding [25]. Continued bleeding from collateral circulation can be controlled by bilateral ovarian artery ligation [16].

(ii) **Hypogastric artery ligation** can also be used to control hemorrhage by taking away the major source of blood supply to the uterus [21]. If this is ineffective, then the ovarian artery should also be ligated to control bleeding from collateral circulation [16].

(iii) **Hysterectomy** should be considered for grand multiparous women and those with placenta accreta, severe uterine injuries, or other uterine pathology. Since hypogastric artery ligation should not be done by the inexperienced operator, hysterectomy is often a safer method of definitive treatment of uncontrolled uterine bleeding [44].

(iv) **Selective pelvic artery embolization** has been utilized by interventional radiologists during arteriography for control of bleeding. Its greatest use in obstetrics/gynecology has been for treatment of hemorrhage from gynecologic cancers and pelvic trauma [25]. Less experience has been gained in obstetric hemorrhage but could be considered in institutions where such a service is offered.

b. **Septic shock.** Management involves support of circulation and blood pressure, aggressive search for the source of infection, early use of empiric antibiotics, and treatment of associated complications. Initial management was detailed before. Aggressive hemodynamic monitoring with a Swan-Ganz catheter and arterial line is indicated for the critically ill patient. Broad-spectrum antibiotics are employed early to cover the range of anaerobic and aerobic organisms common to polymicrobic infections of the pelvis, but other sources for infection such as urinary tract infections, pneumonia, endocarditis, or wounds may need more specific treatment. Corticosteroid use is still controversial, but at present the greatest support for their use is in patients with decreased adrenal reserve [25]. More recently, other treatment modalities have been used including prostaglandin synthetase inhibitors, antilipopolysaccharide immunoglobulin against endotoxin, and naloxone to reverse the hypotension associated with elevated beta-endorphin levels [25].

5. **Complications and sequelae of shock.** As the duration of shock increases, irreversible cellular damage may occur, and even when aggressively managed, shock may have serious sequelae including acidosis, intrauterine fetal demise, Sheehan's syndrome, disseminated intravascular coagulation, acute tubular necrosis, adult respiratory distress syndrome, and other manifestations of prolonged ischemia. Prevention of such complications is the goal of aggressive management, but these sequelae do occur. Detailed discussion of their treatment, however, is beyond the scope of this chapter.

III. **Trauma.** Accidents and trauma are the leading causes of death in reproductive-aged women, and they are also the leading cause of nonobstetric maternal death in many areas of the United States. Up to 7% of pregnant women may sustain injury, accounting for more than 200,000 injuries to pregnant women annually, although most victims do not require hospitalization. Motor vehicle accidents are responsible for an increasing fraction of maternal and fetal trauma [11]. For the critically injured gravida, rapid initiation of diagnostic and therapeutic efforts is essential and requires close cooperation between physicians of different specialties. Whenever possible, emergency room management of severely injured pregnant women should be done in the presence of appropriate members of the obstetric service.

A. **Initial management of the injured gravida.** Initial lifesaving efforts employing the basic principles of management of the nonpregnant trauma victim are made. Serious head, chest, and abdominal injuries are treated, with increasing concern for the fetus as the patient is successfully stabilized. Because medicolegal issues frequently accompany trauma in pregnancy, careful records should be kept to document initial and subsequent management. General principles of immediate management include the following:

1. **Airway.** Appropriate respiratory support is initiated if the airway is compromised or the patient apneic. Intubation is important in the unconscious victim to prevent aspiration and in the patient with significant thoracic trauma.
2. **Circulation.** Indications for cardiopulmonary resuscitation and open heart massage are the same as for the nonpregnant injured patient. In performing cardiopulmonary resuscitation, care should be taken to avoid unnecessary uterine trauma.
3. **Shock.** Treat shock as outlined in sec. **II.** Avoid vena caval compression by avoiding the directly supine position.
4. **Diagnostic efforts.** A review of the patient's medical history and a careful physical examination to reveal the extent of apparent injuries as well as initially nonapparent injuries should be done as soon as possible. Laboratory studies are submitted, and indicated radiologic studies are performed. Fractures are stabilized with splints. A bladder catheter may be helpful in allowing for retrograde radiologic studies if injury to the urinary tract is suspected. The presence of hemoperitoneum is assessed as described in sec. **B.2.a.** The abdomen is also examined to reveal fetal size, uterine tenderness, or contractions, and a pelvic examination is performed to check cervical status, determine fetal presentation, and assess vaginal bleeding or leaking amniotic fluid.
5. **Assessment of fetal status.** The presence or absence of fetal heart tones is important, but when possible, external fetal heart rate electronic monitoring is preferable beyond 25–26 weeks' gestation. Because of the expanded circulating blood volume, early maternal hypovolemia may be unrecognizable clinically. However, because of compensatory vasoconstriction, uterine blood flow may be markedly reduced and manifested only by signs of distress in the continuous fetal heart rate recording [23, 28]. Real-time ultrasonography may aid in estimating the gestational age and detecting placental pathology. Amniocentesis and rapid foam stability testing may be helpful in timing delivery where laparotomy is imminent. Tests for fetomaternal hemorrhage should be done on all seriously injured gravidas and in those with any abdominal trauma (see sec. **B.3.b).**
6. **Tetanus prophylaxis.** Because many women do not have tetanus booster shots every 10 years following initial immunization in childhood, 0.5 ml of tetanus toxoid should be administered to pregnant patients suffering significant abrasions, lacerations, or penetrating trauma. Those never immunized should be given 200–500 units IM of immune serum globulin and 0.5 ml of tetanus toxoid and be instructed to complete a series of three toxoid immunizations subsequently. When significant tissue necrosis is present, patients should receive 250–400 units of immune serum globulin in addition to tetanus toxoid, and with extensive necrosis, antibiotic prophylaxis has sometimes been recommended [11].
7. **Postmortem cesarean section.** In the face of certain or imminent maternal death, the question of fetal salvage arises. The causes of maternal mortality are shifting from chronic illnesses to acute situations such as motor vehicle accidents, pulmonary embolus, and anesthetic complications [25]. The potential for salvaging a viable fetus requires the readiness to deliver the mother once death is recognized. Much literature supports postmortem cesarean sections [25, 39, 47, 52]. Survival for the fetus depends on the timing of the operation; few surviving infants are delivered after 10 minutes of maternal death, and an intact fetus is best delivered within four to six minutes of total anoxia. There are also reports of maternal resuscitation following delivery of the infant. In the situation where maternal death has occurred, cardiopulmonary resuscitation should be continued while the cesarean section is performed. When the time of maternal death is uncertain, clinical judgment must be used to decide if fetal salvage is realistic. If the patient is critically unstable, a perimortem cesarean section should not be performed in anticipation of maternal cardiac arrest. Blood loss associated with a cesarean section will certainly contribute to a worse maternal outcome. If cardiopulmonary resuscitation is

successful, then the cesarean should not be performed since in utero resuscitation is likely.

B. Blunt abdominal trauma. The enlarging pregnant uterus is vulnerable to trauma. Although falls cause a large number of cases of minor blunt abdominal trauma, severe blunt abdominal injury in automobile accidents may cause significant maternal and fetal mortality [35].

1. Fetal injury. Fetal injury is unusual from blunt abdominal trauma early in pregnancy because of the cushioning effect of amniotic fluid. Fetal skull fractures, intracranial hemorrhage, and death may occur later in pregnancy when the fetal head is contained in the bony pelvis. In general, the risk of early spontaneous abortion is not increased by maternal trauma.

2. Maternal injury

a. Intraabdominal hemorrhage. Motor vehicle accidents may result in traumatic laceration of the liver, spleen, or great vessels and may lead to uncontrollable hemorrhage and death. Assessment of the pregnant patient who has sustained significant blunt abdominal trauma must include evaluation for hemoperitoneum. Culdocentesis may be feasible in early gestation, but later, peritoneal lavage via supraumbilical incision using the technique of Rothenberger and colleagues [45] may be more successful. Ringer's lactate, 1000 ml, is infused via a peritoneal dialysis catheter directed toward the pelvis. Based on criteria of the aspirated fluid as shown in Table 16-2, the test is positive, negative, or indeterminate, requiring repeat lavage.

Intraperitoneal hemorrhage requires immediate laparotomy via a long midline incision to control bleeding and repair damaged organs. Occasionally, cesarean section is required to achieve adequate exposure, but usually the pregnancy can be left undisturbed.

b. Uterine trauma. Uterine rupture occurs in less than 1% of pregnant women injured in motor vehicle accidents [32]. Direct uterine trauma may increase intrauterine pressure so abruptly and significantly as to result in rupture

Table 16-2. Criteria for interpretation of diagnostic peritoneal lavage

Positive[a]
Free aspiration of blood (> 10 ml)
Grossly bloody lavage fluid
Passage of lavage fluid through Foley catheter or chest tube
Red blood cell count > 100,000/μl
White blood cell count > 500/μl
Amylase > 175 units/dl
Indeterminate[b]
Red blood cell count > 50,000 but < 100,000/μl
White blood cell count > 100 but < 500/μl
Amylase > 75 but < 175 units/dl
Dialysis catheter fills with blood
Negative
Red blood cell count < 50,000/μl
White blood cell count < 100/μl
Amylase < 75 units/dl

[a]The presence of any criterion indicates a positive peritoneal lavage.
[b]Indeterminate lavages are repeated.
Source: From D. A. Rothenberger et al., Diagnostic peritoneal lavage for blunt trauma in pregnant women. *Am. J. Obstet. Gynecol.* 129:479, 1977.

as early as the third month of gestation. Massive hemorrhage requiring laparotomy may result, and if the damage is extensive or involves the uterine vessels, cesarean hysterectomy may be required. In the absence of uterine rupture, uterine trauma may precipitate spontaneous labor, rupture of the membranes, or placental injury.

3. **Placental injury**

   a. **Placental abruption.** Major maternal trauma is often accompanied by placental abruption (7–66% of cases) [39]. Automobile passengers who are pregnant should use seat belts (lap or three-point). Any small risk of uterine or placental trauma from a seat belt is far outweighed by the fact that maternal death (often a result of multiple injuries sustained on ejection) is the most common cause of fetal death [32]. Placental abruption may occur in patients with trauma remote from the abdomen; supine vena caval compression may increase its occurrence.

      Abruptio placentae should be suspected in the presence of vaginal bleeding, abdominal pain, and uterine irritability, but up to 20% of abruptions may not be accompanied by vaginal bleeding [35]. External fetal heart rate monitoring may reveal subtle signs of distress consistent with occult abruption [23]. Delayed placental abruption has been observed up to five days after major maternal trauma [28]. Severely injured gravidas should be continuously monitored for at least 48 hours. Plasma fibrinogen is elevated in pregnancy. Thus, a fibrinogen level below 250 mg/dl (the norm in a nonpregnant patient) may reflect an early abruption. Ultrasonic examination, while lacking sensitivity, may occasionally reveal a retroplacental hematoma. Management of placental abruption and intravascular coagulopathy are discussed in Chap. 20.

   b. **Fetomaternal hemorrhage.** Villous injury and subsequent leakage of fetal blood into the intervillous space (and thus into the maternal circulation) may be a significant consequence of blunt abdominal trauma, accompanied or unaccompanied by placental abruption [6]. Sequelae of fetomaternal hemorrhage include fetal or neonatal anemia, fetal distress, intrauterine fetal demise, and sensitization of the maternal immune system to Rh or other blood group antigens. A test for circulating fetal red blood cells in maternal blood (e.g., Kleihauer-Betke test) is useful to assess the severity of the abdominal injury and to allow proper dosing of $Rh_0(D)$ immunoglobulin to the injured Rh-negative gravida.

4. **Triage of pregnant women with blunt abdominal trauma.** Pregnant women who have sustained major trauma and are more than 25–26 weeks pregnant clearly require continuous external fetal heart rate monitoring and vigilant observation for placental abruption for at least 48 hours [28]. Those with abdominal trauma also require observation for abruption and fetomaternal hemorrhage, and probably deserve a longer period of external fetal heart rate monitoring than do those without direct abdominal trauma. A positive test for fetomaternal hemorrhage suggests more pronounced trauma and may warrant a longer observation period. Some have recommended the use of the contraction stress test if the fetus is beyond 25–26 weeks' gestation, especially when the nonstress test is nonreactive.

C. **Penetrating abdominal wounds**

1. **Visceral trauma.** The enlarged uterus protects other intraabdominal organs during penetrating trauma, and consequently, maternal mortality and visceral injury are unusual. With gunshot wounds of the pregnant abdomen, the incidence of injury to organs other than the uterus is only 19%, but the fetal injury rate (60–90%) and fetal mortality (40–70%) are high [35].

2. **Management.** Pregnant patients with penetrating abdominal wounds are stabilized as described in sec. **A.**

   a. **Gunshot wounds.** Because of the low incidence of visceral injury, there have been no maternal deaths reported since 1912 from gunshot wounds to the gravid uterus [12]. Laparotomy can be avoided and the patient managed conservatively if the entrance wound is below the uterine fundus, the bullet is radiographically within the uterus, and the fetus is dead [12]. Otherwise, or if signs of peritoneal inflammation develop during observation, laparotomy is performed. Uterine injury is managed conservatively, if possible, with ligatures to control bleeding. If the bullet has penetrated the uterus, fetal injury is likely. As long as the uterus does not interfere with exploration, and as long as the patient remains stable, cesarean section is not performed. Labor and delivery of a dead fetus in the postoperative period have no deleterious physical maternal effect, and subsequent development of amnionitis after penetrating trauma is unusual. If the fetus is still alive, cesarean section may be indicated after considering the relative risks of premature delivery versus subsequent intrauterine demise as a result of fetal injury.

b. **Stab wounds.** With stab wounds, if no peritoneal penetration has occurred as judged by examination and fistulogram, observation is appropriate [11]. Penetration in the lower abdomen may involve the uterus but carries a low risk of visceral injury, and in the absence of evidence of such injury or worsening clinical status, observation alone may be warranted [11]. Penetration of the upper abdomen warrants exploration.

D. **Fractures.** During pregnancy, management of fractures by internal fixation rather than prolonged traction is preferred because movement of the patient is necessary if labor ensues and because there is an increased risk of thromboembolism with pregnancy and immobilization.

1. **Vertebral fractures** usually involve the terminal thoracic or first three lumbar vertebrae and may require open reduction, spinal fusion, and a body spica cast if dislocated. Vaginal delivery is indicated for all but unstable vertebral fractures, for which the lithotomy position could result in spinal cord damage.
2. **Pelvic fractures** may be uncomplicated, requiring symptomatic therapy only, or may be severe, creating multiple complications such as massive retroperitoneal hematoma, distortion of the birth canal, and lacerations of the urethra or bladder. The acute management of severe pelvic fracture may include surgical intervention only when intractable shock continues. The superior gluteal artery may be damaged owing to its course and lack of soft tissue covering. The inaccessibility of this vessel makes hypogastric artery ligation the procedure of choice to control bleeding. However, this procedure may compromise fetal well-being, and therefore, if viable, the fetus should be delivered by cesarean section. Lower urinary tract injury occurs in 10–15% of cases of pelvic fracture. Bladder catheterization, retrograde radiographic studies, and repair of bladder lacerations may be indicated. Vaginal delivery in the presence of an unstable or displaced pelvic fracture may produce further trauma to the lower urinary tract, and consequently, cesarean section should be performed. The history of a previous pelvic fracture is not an indication for cesarean section unless x-ray pelvimetry demonstrates significant distortion. Most women with prior pelvic fractures have successful vaginal deliveries [37].

E. **Burns.** Of more than 2 million persons burned in the United States each year, approximately 4% are pregnant [49]. Initial management of burns includes careful assessment of the depth and extent of the burn, as prognosis is best determined from such estimates. Mortality data are as follows [49]:

Body burned (%)	**Maternal mortality (%)**	**Fetal mortality (%)**
< 40	3	17–27
50	25	53
> 80	100	100

The management of burns in pregnancy differs little compared to the nonpregnant state. It is divided into three components. First is the **acute management** requiring fluid and electrolyte support. Second is providing **hemodynamic and respiratory support.** Third is **evaluating fetal status.** For the fetus greater than 25–26 weeks, fetal monitoring and uterine activity monitoring are indicated. Tocolysis may be considered in the less severely burned patient, but expectant management is preferable in the near-term fetus or if the patient has suffered greater than 50% total surface burn. Active delivery of the fetus has been suggested for the patient who has greater than 50% burn. A more detailed discussion may be found elsewhere [25, 49].

IV. The acute abdomen

A. Diagnosis. Physiologic adaptations to pregnancy may alter a woman's response to intraabdominal disease, making diagnosis difficult. A careful history, physical examination, and review of laboratory data should lead to a working diagnosis and identification of those patients who require hospitalization or immediate surgical exploration. Some of the causes of abdominal pain in pregnancy are listed in Table 16-3. A more detailed description of the diagnostic features of many of these conditions may be found elsewhere in this manual. Surgical management of the more common or significant causes of acute abdominal pain in pregnancy is reviewed here.

B. Surgical management

1. Acute appendicitis. Because of changes in the location of the appendix as pregnancy progresses, signs and symptoms are less predictive than in the nonpregnant patient. As a result, the rate of gangrenous or perforated appendix is higher in the third (69%) than in the first or second (31%) trimesters [52]. Coupled with this, the higher perinatal mortality with perforated (28%), as opposed to unperforated (5%), appendicitis calls for aggressive management (i.e., laparotomy) when the diagnosis cannot be eliminated. Although in such cases 20–25% of patients will be found to have a normal appendix, with aggressive management the risk of maternal mortality has been greatly reduced historically from 40 to 0% in recent series [53]. Operation in the first trimester is best accomplished through a vertical midline incision since the incidence of misdiagnosis is high. Later in pregnancy, a muscle-splitting incision over the point of maximum tenderness is recommended. The appendix is excised whether inflamed or normal; after ligation, the stump may be safely left without inversion. Peritonitis and abscess formation may require peritoneal drainage, the use of broad-spectrum antibiotics, and, occasionally, cecostomy. In general, the uterus is not disturbed, but cesarean section may be desirable in the presence of a mature fetus and severe peritonitis. Cesarean hysterectomy is rarely indicated in the face of advanced gangrene. Complications of appendectomy include premature labor and wound infection; prophylactic tocolytic agents and delayed wound closure may be indicated.

2. Cholecystitis. After appendicitis, cholecystitis is the most common surgical condition in pregnancy. Nevertheless, gallstones will usually not cause sufficient problems to warrant a cholecystectomy during pregnancy. Of women undergoing routine obstetric ultrasound, 3.5% have demonstrated gallstones. In contrast, 0.3% of cholecystectomies performed in women 16–45 years of age were pregnant at the time of cholecystectomy [33]. The diagnosis of cholelithiasis and cholecystitis remains much the same as in the nonpregnant state. Pregnancy does not alter the pain or location, but other diseases can also have similar presentations acutely (e.g., appendicitis, peptic ulcer disease). The physical exam is also similar, except that pregnancy can obscure the severity of symptoms. Use of the ultrasound may supplant the need for radiologic or radionuclide studies in pregnancy.

Initial conservative management is recommended (nasogastric suctioning, intravenous fluids, analgesics), and this results in relief in the majority of patients. Failure to respond, repeated attacks, suspected perforation, uncontrolled diabetes, obstructive jaundice, or uncertain diagnosis are indications for surgical exploration [48]. Because of the risk of teratogenesis and spontaneous abortion in the first trimester, and of difficult exposure due to the enlarging uterus in the third trimester, less urgent cholecystectomy should ideally be performed in the second trimester.

3. Inflammatory bowel disease. Most acute episodes of ulcerative colitis in pregnancy can be controlled medically. Surgical intervention is indicated only for emergency management of fulminating disease, obstruction, unresponsive toxic megacolon, massive hemorrhage, peritonitis, or the appearance of strictures

Table 16-3. Differential diagnosis of abdominal pain in pregnancy (no. of cases/no. of pregnancies)

Intraabdominal disease
Acute gastroenteritis (common)
Appendicitis (1/800–2000)
Chronic inflammatory bowel disease (approximately 1/1000)
Cholecystitis-cholelithiasis (1/1000–2000)
Intestinal obstruction (1/3600–66,000)
Pancreatitis (1/3000–11,000)
Peptic ulcer disease (< 1/1000)
Hepatic rupture (rare)
Acute mesenteric adenitis (uncommon)

Urinary tract disease
Acute pyelonephritis (1/50–100)
Nephrolithiasis (1/1500)
Urethral obstruction (pathologic uterine retroversion) (rare)

Obstetric and gynecologic disease
Hyperemesis gravidarum (1/60–150)
Spontaneous abortion (1/6)
Round ligament syndrome (common)
Uterine contractions (common)
Degenerating uterine fibroid tumor (rare)
Ectopic pregnancy (1/40–250)
Adnexal torsion (rare)
Cyst rupture (rare)
Placental abruption (1/120)
Salpingitis (rare)
Chorioamnionitis (1/100–200)
Spontaneous uterine rupture (rare)

Medical disease
Diabetic ketoacidosis (uncommon)
Uremic syndrome (rare)
Henoch-Schönlein purpura (rare)
Acute porphyria (very rare)
Sickle cell anemia (1/600 blacks)
Lead poisoning (rare)
Black widow spider bite (rare)
Pleuritic disease (uncommon)
Spinal pathology (uncommon)
Herpes zoster (uncommon)

suggestive of malignancy [51]. A total proctocolectomy with ileostomy may be indicated; lesser operations may be beneficial temporarily. Surgery for a minority of Crohn's disease patients is indicated in pregnancy only after failure of exhaustive medical management for intractable disease, or for obstruction, abscess, or fistula formation. Preferred management consists of local resection and primary reanastomosis with prophylactic appendectomy [51].

4. **Intestinal obstruction.** Adhesions, volvulus, intussusception, and hernias, in order of decreasing incidence, are the most frequent causes of bowel obstruction in pregnant women. Preoperative management (nasogastric suctioning, correction of metabolic disturbance) should not delay definitive surgical therapy for long. At laparotomy, the obstruction is repaired and a thorough search made for other intraabdominal pathologic findings [17].
5. **Spontaneous hepatic rupture.** Spontaneous hepatic rupture is rare, is almost always associated with preeclampsia or eclampsia, and may be catastrophic [38]. Maternal mortality ranges from 33% for those that undergo surgery versus 60–96% for those treated conservatively. A subset of patients with subcapsular hematoma only have been treated conservatively and survived with close observation. If hepatic rupture with hemorrhage occurs, then immediate surgical management is potentially lifesaving. Surgery involves ligation of bleeding vessels, repair of lacerations with atraumatic needles, electrocoagulation, and placement of Gelfoam for hemostasis. Intractable hemorrhage has also been managed successfully using transcatheter embolotherapy directed angiographically [36]. Cesarean section is often performed to terminate the pregnancy (to salvage the fetus and help resolve the preeclampsia) and to provide better surgical exposure.

V. Other diseases in pregnancy

A. Heart disease. Some heart diseases are poorly tolerated during pregnancy and may result in high maternal mortality as follows: aortic stenosis, 10–20%; Eisenmenger's syndrome, 30–70%; and mitral valve stenosis with atrial fibrillation, 14–17% [50]. Prepregnancy counseling, contraception, and elective abortion are important components in managing these high-risk women. Surgery is reserved for those with severe cardiac disability not responding to medical management and for whom abortion is unacceptable [50].

B. Pulmonary disease. Surgery may be indicated in pregnant women with recurrent or persistent infection from bronchiectasis or in gravidas with a tumor for biopsy or therapy. If pulmonary function tests demonstrate adequate reserve, partial resection or pneumonectomy can be safely performed.

C. Vascular disease. Pregnancy in Marfan's syndrome may result in a maternal mortality of 25–50% [50]. Such women should be offered abortion and, if that is refused, managed with beta-blocker therapy and constant observation for dissecting aortic aneurysm.

Surgical therapy for recurrent, life-threatening thromboembolism involves, ultimately, interruption of the vena cava and ovarian veins. Patients with venous insufficiency should be prescribed support hose, and to those with symptomatic vulvar varices, compressive support should be recommended. Management of arterial aneurysms is discussed in Chap. 15. Surgically correctable hypertension is rare in pregnancy. Diagnosis and management of patients with pheochromocytoma is discussed in Chap. 10.

D. Esophageal bleeding and rupture. Massive bleeding from esophageal varices may lead rapidly to hypovolemic shock and fetal asphyxia. Management with blood replacement, esophageal balloon tamponade, and ice-water lavage may not be effective, and surgical therapy consisting of portal system shunting may be required. Operative mortality may be as high as 30%; pregnancy termination may be elected. Rupture of the esophagus during severe vomiting may present not with hematemesis but, rather, with chest pain, tachypnea, and subcutaneous emphysema. Prompt surgical repair, Levin tube decompression, antibiotics, and pleural drainage are indicated. Mortality ranges from 30–70%.

E. Urologic disease (See Chap. 5.)

F. Endocrine disease (See Chap. 10.)

G. Neurologic disease (See Chap. 12.)

VI. Cancer. Malignant diseases that occur in pregnancy, in order of decreasing frequency, are as follows: breast cancer, hematopoietic malignancy, melanoma, gynecologic cancer, and bone tumors.

A. Breast cancer. The incidence of breast cancer is approximately 1 in 3500–10,000 deliveries [5]. However, about 1.5–4.0% of breast cancers coexist with pregnancy, making it an uncommon, but not rare event [40]. The glandular hyperplasia of the breast that accompanies pregnancy makes the recognition of suspicious breast masses difficult. Therefore, breast cancer is often recognized at a later stage than would occur in the nonpregnant state. The diagnosis relies on the physical exam, since mammograms are not routinely obtained during pregnancy. The suspicious breast lump is evaluated the same as when the patient is not pregnant. Tissue diagnosis is obtained by fine-needle aspiration of fluid or tissue core, or by open biopsy. The role of x-ray mammography or xeromammography remains controversial [5, 13, 41]. The radiation dose is negligible and therefore could be used safely, especially after the first trimester. Debate continues about the best form of therapy in the nonpregnant state, but modified radical mastectomy appears to be the most common choice during pregnancy. Simple lumpectomy with radiation treatment is probably a poor consideration because of fetal radiation exposure. The role of adjuvant chemotherapy remains uncertain because of the unknown risks of fetal teratogenesis and mutagenesis and whether it is best postponed until after termination of the pregnancy. It has been suggested that breast cancer has a worse prognosis in pregnancy, but a less favorable outcome in pregnancy may be due to the advanced stage of cancer at the time of discovery or a higher proportion of high-grade and estrogen receptor–negative cancers. When matched for age and stage, survival rates are not different from the nonpregnant state. Survival is not improved by pregnancy termination. However, it may be recommended to avoid the risk of fetal exposure to either chemotherapy or radiation therapy.

B. Melanoma. Although pregnancy does not seem to increase the incidence of malignant melanoma, there is controversy as to whether the prognosis of this disease may be affected [5]. Because survival is inversely proportional to the depth of invasion, early recognition is essential and requires thorough prenatal examination. Wide excision may result in five-year survival for 80% of patients in the early stages of disease. However, if regional nodes are involved, survival drops to 20–30%. Superficial and deep regional lymphadenectomy may have both prognostic and therapeutic benefit in more advanced cases.

C. Bone tumors. Ewing's sarcoma, osteogenic sarcoma, and osteocystoma are the most common malignant bone tumors in young women. Recently, dramatic improvements in survival have been reported after radical surgery and aggressive chemotherapy. Consequently, termination of early pregnancy usually is recommended even though pregnancy itself seems to have no effect on the disease [5].

D. Hematopoietic malignancy. (See Chap. 6.)

E. Pelvic malignancy. (See the following sections.)

Gynecologic Disease During Pregnancy

I. External genitalia

A. Bartholin abscess. Although asymptomatic cysts need not be treated, abscesses of the Bartholin's gland usually cause significant pain and inflammation. Drainage via an incision on the mucosal side of the gland is appropriate when the area is fluctuant. Otherwise, sitz baths are recommended until the abscess is ready for drainage. Cultures are useful as gonococcus is often the etiologic agent, and when suspected, antibiotics are appropriate. Ideally, a Word catheter is placed for four weeks to allow adequate epithelialization of a drainage tract. Recurrent infection or development of recurrent symptomatic cysts warrants subsequent marsupialization.

B. Condylomata acuminata. The very common condylomata acuminata (genital warts) must be distinguished clinically from the rare wartlike growths of *condyloma latum* caused by *Treponema pallidum*. The human papillomaviruses cause genital warts that, during pregnancy, may rapidly enlarge, even to obstruct the vaginal canal. In addition, evidence is accumulating that human papillomavirus may be transmitted to the newborn, resulting in laryngeal papillomas. Consequently, treatment of condylomata acuminata during pregnancy appears to be warranted. Although podophyllin and other cytotoxic agents have been recommended in the past for treatment of genital warts during pregnancy, such methods are probably inadvisable. Anecdotal reports of both fetal and maternal toxicity after use of podophyllin have appeared. Outpatient treatment of genital warts during pregnancy can be achieved either by cryotherapy (liquid nitrogen application or nitrous oxide cryoprobe) or by carbon dioxide laser therapy. Cautery is an alternative that may require general anesthesia. Both cryotherapy [4] and carbon dioxide laser therapy [22, 46] appear to be highly effective in pregnancy; no significant fetal, neonatal, or maternal morbidity has been reported. The recurrence rate of genital warts appears to be lowest when they are treated in the third trimester.

C. Genital herpes simplex. (See Chap. 11.)

II. Vaginitis. Speculum examination and microscopic study are essential in the evaluation of pregnant women complaining of vaginal discharge [24]. Both physiologic secretions and occult rupture of the membranes may be misdiagnosed as vaginitis.

A. Candidiasis. Typical symptoms include itching, burning, an erythematous vulva, and cottage cheese-like discharge. Pregnant women, especially those previously infected, are at increased risk for candidal vulvovaginitis. The signs, symptoms, and method of diagnosis are the same as for the nonpregnant patient. Clotrimazole and miconazole nitrate are more effective than nystatin and require fewer treatment days. Since small amounts of these drugs may be absorbed from the vagina, they should be used in the first trimester with caution.

B. Trichomoniasis. Typical signs and symptoms of this venereally transmitted protozoan include an often malodorous, frothy yellow-green discharge accompanied by intense pruritus and dysuria. In 25% of cases, there may be red subepithelial abscesses giving the cervicovaginal epithelium a strawberry appearance. The diagnosis is confirmed microscopically. Treatment for the nonpregnant patient and her partner is metronidazole (Flagyl), either a single, 2-gm dose PO or 250 mg PO tid for 7–10 days. In the pregnant patient, local measures such as dilute providone-iodine (Betadine) douche or vaginal clotrimazole suppositories are sometimes helpful. If symptoms are severe, metronidazole is effective, though it should be avoided in early pregnancy.

C. *Gardnerella vaginalis.* This vaginitis was previously named for the presence of *G. vaginalis,* which is now understood to be a marker for a potpourri of anaerobic organisms. Typically, the discharge is described as having a fishy odor, and the microscopic finding of squamous cells studded with coccobacilli ("clue cells") suggests the diagnosis. Although ampicillin has been used with some success, the most effective therapy is metronidazole (given to patient and partner), but this drug should be avoided in the first trimester and used only for severe symptoms later in pregnancy.

III. Diseases of the cervix

A. Cervical intraepithelial neoplasia. Abnormal cervical cytology is seen in up to 3% of pregnancies. Carcinoma in situ or cervical intraepithelial neoplasia III is present in 1.3 in 1000 pregnancies. Invasive cervical carcinoma occurs in 0.45 in 1000 pregnancies [19]. Pregnancy represents an opportunity to screen a wide range of women for preinvasive disease who might otherwise not seek routine exams. The evaluation of abnormal cervical cytology differs little compared to the nonpregnant state. Eversion of the transformation zone makes colposcopy easier in many pregnant women. Directed biopsies must be done to rule out invasive cancer. An endocervical curettage is omitted to avoid the risk of miscarriage. Rarely, a cone biopsy is necessary if the full extent of the disease is not seen or if the directed biopsy shows microinvasion [5]. Otherwise cone biopsy should be avoided since it is associated with a significant risk of hemorrhage and spontaneous abortion. If the lesion can be confirmed to be no worse than cervical intraepithelial neoplasia, then it can be managed expectantly with periodic colposcopic examinations through the duration of the pregnancy. Any apparent progression in the lesion must be biopsied to rule out invasive cancer. **Microinvasion** (cancer that does not penetrate more than 3 mm below the basement membrane) can potentially be managed expectantly [5] with the consultation of a gynecologic oncologist. The patient must be carefully followed with repeated exams to ensure that progression of the lesion does not occur. Vaginal delivery can be expected, with cesarean section reserved for obstetric indications. Definitive treatment can be performed post partum.

B. Invasive carcinoma of the cervix

1. **Diagnosis.** Although invasive cervical carcinoma has become less prevalent as a result of cytologic screening and irradication of precursor lesions, a larger fraction of women with the disease are of reproductive age and 1 case may be expected among 2500 pregnancies [5]. Pregnancy does not affect the growth of cervical cancer, and stage-for-stage survival is the same as for nonpregnant women. The diagnosis is based on biopsy, either colposcopically directed or obtained directly from suspicious exophytic lesions. The diagnosis should be considered in any woman with unexplained vaginal bleeding, especially if the bleeding occurs after sexual intercourse.
2. **Recommendations for management.** Although little data substantiate an increased risk to the patient from vaginal delivery through a cervical carcinoma, theoretic considerations (risk of uncontrollable hemorrhage, spread of disease via lymphatic vessels) suggest such a risk. Treatment recommendations vary but depend on the stage of the disease and gestational age of the pregnancy [5]. A shallow cone biopsy is recommended to rule out deeper invasion when biopsies show only microinvasive disease, and may be curative. The route of delivery is determined by obstetric indications in these patients. For stage 1B or 2A disease up to 20 weeks, the patient can be treated with radiotherapy (which usually results in a spontaneous abortion), or primary radical hysterectomy with pelvic lymphadenectomy (with the fetus left in situ, or evacuated by hysterotomy prior to the hysterectomy). After 20 weeks, the fetus can be allowed to reach a viable gestational age and then delivered by cesarean section. This can then be followed by radical hysterectomy with pelvic lymphadenectomy or radiotherapy. For stage 2B to 3B disease, radiotherapy is recommended; after 24 weeks' gestation, cesarean section should be performed prior to starting radiotherapy.

IV. Diseases of the uterus

A. Abnormalities of position

1. **Anterior sacculation of the uterus.** Severe anteflexion of the uterus caused by poor abdominal muscle tone in the late third trimester may result in abnormal presentation and lack of engagement of the presenting part. This abnormality is seen almost exclusively in the grand multipara. Correction of the abnormal orientation of the fetus with abdominal pressure provided by a well-fitting girdle or other binding support may allow pushing in the second stage.
2. **Retroflexion.** Retrodisplacement of the uterus is common in early pregnancy, but the enlarging uterus nearly always assumes a more anteverted position by 12 weeks of pregnancy. Rarely, the retroflexed enlarging uterus may become incarcerated in the hollow of the sacrum, with resulting edema from venous obstruction, marked pain, and, notably, an inability to void because of urethral obstruction. Patients with this complication should be placed in the knee-chest position, and the anterior lip of the cervix should be grasped and pulled with a ring forceps. (The pregnant cervix is so friable that it may be torn if grasped with a tenaculum.) Simultaneously, the posterior surface of the uterus is pushed by exerting pressure through the posterior fornix. This procedure occasionally requires anesthesia.
3. **Prolapse.** Complete prolapse of the uterus is rare in pregnancy since fertility is minimized by difficulty with intercourse. With partial prolapse, a pessary may provide relief of symptoms. A Gellhorn pessary is especially useful. Attention to cleanliness is important to prevent infection.

B. Torsion of the uterus. This rare complication of pregnancy almost always is associated with a pathologic condition of the uterus (e.g., leiomyomas) or adhesions from previous uterine surgery. The clinical picture is that of an abdominal catastrophe (severe abdominal pain, or shock) and may be confused with the picture of abruptio placentae. The patient has acute surgical abdominal disease and requires laparotomy. Detorsion may be attempted in early pregnancy. Cesarean section followed by hysterectomy often is required near term. Fetal mortality is very high; maternal mortality is reportedly as high as 50%.

C. **Leiomyoma uteri.** Uterine fibroid tumors are usually asymptomatic in pregnancy but may interfere with conception and may cause early spontaneous abortion. Later, they may predispose the fetus to abnormal presentation, obstruct labor, and occasionally lead to placental separation or postpartum hemorrhage. Infarction may occur, leading to acute abdominal pain, fever, leukocytosis, and uterine tenderness. Treatment is bed rest and analgesics; laparotomy is avoided unless the diagnosis is uncertain. Fibroid tumors that obstruct labor may necessitate cesarean section and, because the uterine incision may be difficult or impossible to repair in the presence of massive leiomyomas, cesarean hysterectomy is occasionally indicated. Hysterectomy may also be indicated for intractable postpartum hemorrhage owing to submucous leiomyomas.

V. Diseases of the fallopian tubes

A. **Acute salpingitis.** Coexistent acute or chronic pelvic inflammatory disease is rare in pregnancy. The diagnosis is difficult to make and easily confused with other entities such as appendicitis, torsion of the adnexa, threatened abortion, and ectopic pregnancy. In fact, these other conditions are far more common and should be considered prior to entertaining a diagnosis of pelvic inflammatory disease. In many cases, it may have been present prior to conception. One theory holds that pathogenic organisms may be able to ascend from the cervix to the upper tract early in pregnancy, contrary to the thought that the conceptus acts as a barrier to the development of salpingitis [8]. The presence of gonococcus or chlamydia should be confirmed by cervical culture. Because it is distinctly uncommon, laparoscopy should be considered to rule out the other potential etiologies as noted before. Treatment is the same as in the nonpregnant patient. Fetal wastage is high and septic abortion may occur [8]. In subclinical disease, vaginal delivery puts the fetus at risk for contracting gonococcal or chlamydial ophthalmia, or chlamydial pneumonia if the mother is not treated beforehand.

B. **Torsion of the fallopian tube** has been described in pregnancy and so should be included in the differential diagnosis of abdominal pain during pregnancy [14]. Presentation may be varied. The only consistent feature is pain, generally sudden in onset, located in the quadrant of the involved tube and perhaps radiating to the flank or thigh. Tenderness usually is present, but signs of peritoneal irritation are variable. Other symptoms include nausea, vomiting, and bladder or bowel irritability. Temperature, white blood cell count, and erythrocyte sedimentation rate usually are normal or slightly elevated. Differential diagnosis includes torsion or degeneration of an ovarian cyst or uterine leiomyomas, ureteral or renal colic, acute appendicitis, placental abruption, inflammatory peritoneal processes, and intraperitoneal bleeding. Therapy is surgical. If the affected tube is beyond recovery, it is excised. There is no reason to remove a normal ovary. If torsion is incomplete or recent and if tissue distal to the torsion remains viable, conservation of the tube with stabilization by suture may be considered.

VI. Diseases of the ovaries

A. **The pelvic mass in pregnancy.** The most important issue in any woman with a pelvic mass is the possibility of malignant ovarian neoplasia. The differential diagnosis includes functional cysts, which should be less than 8 cm in diameter and should resolve spontaneously by the beginning of the second trimester. Cystic masses of 8 cm or larger, smaller masses that increase in size or persist, or solid adnexal masses all require surgical exploration in the early second trimester. Adnexal masses of any kind may precipitate torsion of the mass or the entire adnexa, resulting in acute symptoms and signs, which may be intermittent but may necessitate exploration either during pregnancy or in the puerperium. Ovarian masses may also obstruct labor, making cesarean section necessary.

B. Ovarian cancer. A malignant ovarian neoplasm is encountered once for every 9000–25,000 deliveries. Epithelial cancers (especially borderline tumors) predominate and are usually asymptomatic. Thorough surgical staging of the disease is desirable, followed by operative therapy. Unilateral salpingo-oophorectomy in women who desire to bear more children appears to be justified if the tumor is unilateral and localized (stage 1A). Further adjuvant therapy may be required for stage 1A malignant germ cell tumors, and unilateral pelvic and periaortic lymphadenectomy is recommended for correct evaluation of apparently stage 1A dysgerminomas because of their propensity for lymphatic dissemination. When ovarian cancer is suspected in the third trimester, therapy may be delayed until fetal pulmonary maturity is demonstrated. Cesarean section then is performed along with definitive surgery for the neoplasm. Cancers other than stage 1A are treated as in the nonpregnant patient.

References

1. American College of Obstetricians and Gynecologists. Invasive hemodynamic monitoring in obstetrics and gynecology. *ACOG Tech. Bull.* No. 121, October, 1988.
2. American Heart Association. Intravenous Techniques. In *Textbook of Advanced Cardiac Life Support.* Dallas: American Heart Association, 1987.
3. Barron, W. M. Medical evaluation of the pregnant patient requiring nonobstetric surgery. *Clin. Perinatol.* 12:481, 1985.
4. Bergman, A., Matsunaga, J., and Bhatia, N. N. Cervical cryotherapy for condylomata acuminata during pregnancy. *Obstet. Gynecol.* 69:47, 1987.
5. Berman, M. L., and DiSaia, P. J. Pelvic Malignancies, Gestational Trophoblastic Neoplasia, and Nonpelvic Malignancies. In R. K. Creasy and R. Resnik (eds.), *Maternal-Fetal Medicine: Principles and Practice.* Philadelphia: Saunders, 1989.
6. Bickers, R. G., and Wenberg, R. P. Fetomaternal transfusion following trauma. *Obstet. Gynecol.* 61:258, 1983.
7. Blaisdell, F. W., and Holcroft, J. W. Septic shock. *Prob. Gen. Surg.* 1:639, 1984.
8. Blanchard, A. C., Pastorek, J. G., II, and Weeks, T. Pelvic inflammatory disease during pregnancy. *South. Med. J.* 80:1363, 1987.
9. Brodsky, J. B. Anesthesia and surgery during early pregnancy and fetal outcome. *Clin. Obstet. Gynecol.* 26:449, 1983.
10. Braunwald, E., and Williams, G. H. Alterations in Arterial Pressure and the Shock Syndrome. In E. Braunwald et al. (eds.), *Harrison's Principles of Medicine* (11th ed.). New York: McGraw-Hill, 1987.
11. Buchsbaum, H. J. *Trauma in Pregnancy.* Philadelphia: Saunders, 1979.
12. Buchsbaum, H. J., and Staples, P. P., Jr. Self-inflicted gunshot wounds to the pregnant uterus: Report of two cases. *Obstet. Gynecol.* 65(Suppl.):32, 1985.
13. Canter, J. W., Oliver, G. C., and Zaloudek, C. J. Surgical diseases of the breast during pregnancy. *Clin. Obstet. Gynecol.* 26:853, 1983.
14. Chambers, J. T., et al. Torsion of the normal fallopian tube in pregnancy. *Obstet. Gynecol.* 54:487, 1979.
15. Cope, Z. *Cope's Early Diagnosis of the Acute Abdomen* (revised by W. Silen). Oxford: Oxford University Press, 1979.
16. Cruikshank, S. H., and Stoelk, E. M. Surgical control of pelvic hemorrhage: Bilateral hypogastric artery ligation and method of ovarian artery ligation. *South. Med. J.* 78:539, 1985.
17. Davis, M. R., and Bohon, C. J. Intestinal obstruction in pregnancy. *Clin. Obstet. Gynecol.* 26:832, 1983.
18. Delaney, A. G. Anesthesia in the pregnant woman. *Clin. Obstet. Gynecol.* 26:795, 1983.
19. DePetrillo, A. D. Non-Invasive Carcinoma of the Cervix. In H. H. Allen and J. A. Nisker, (eds.), *Cancer in Pregnancy.* Mt. Kisco, N.Y.: Futura, 1986.

20. Duncan, P. G., et al. Fetal risk of anesthesia and surgery during pregnancy. *Anesthesiology* 64:790, 1986.
21. Evans, S., and McShane, P. The efficacy of internal iliac artery ligation in obstetrical hemorrhage. *Surg. Gynecol. Obstet.* 160:250, 1985.
22. Ferenczy, A. HPV-associated lesions in pregnancy and their clinical implications. *Clin. Obstet. Gynecol.* 32:191, 1989.
23. Freeman, R. K., and Garite, T. J. *Fetal Heart Rate Monitoring.* Baltimore: Williams & Wilkins, 1981.
24. Friedrich, E. G., Jr. *Vulvar Disease* (2nd ed.). Philadelphia: Saunders, 1983.
25. Gonik, B. Intensive Care Monitoring of the Critically Ill Pregnancy Patient. In R. K. Creasy and R. Resnik (eds.), *Maternal-Fetal Medicine: Principles and Practice.* Philadelphia: Saunders, 1989.
26. Gonik, B. Septic shock in obstetrics. *Clin. Perinatol.* 13:741, 1986.
27. Gonik, B. Septic Shock in Obstetrics. In S. L. Clark, J. P. Phelan, and D. B. Cotton (eds.), *Critical Care Obstetrics.* Oradell, N.J.: Medical Economics, 1987.
28. Higgins, S. D., and Garite, T. J. Late abruptio placenta in trauma patients: Implications for monitoring. *Obstet. Gynecol.* 63(Suppl.):10, 1984.
29. Holcroft, J. W. Impairment of venous return in hemorrhagic shock. *Surg. Clin. North Am.* 62:17, 1982.
30. James, F. M., III. Anesthesia for nonobstetric surgery during pregnancy. *Clin. Obstet. Gynecol.* 30:621, 1987.
31. Karn, K. E., et al. Use of a whole blood substitute, Fluosol-DA 20%, after massive postpartum hemorrhage. *Obstet. Gynecol.* 65:281, 1985.
32. Katz, M. Maternal Trauma During Pregnancy. In R. K. Creasy and R. Resnik (eds.), *Maternal-Fetal Medicine: Principles and Practice.* Philadelphia: Saunders, 1984.
33. Key, T. C. Gastrointestinal Diseases. In R. K. Creasy and R. Resnik (eds.), *Maternal-Fetal Medicine: Principles and Practice.* Philadelphia: Saunders, 1989.
34. Laros, R. K. Thromboembolic Disease. In R. K. Laros (ed.), *Blood Disorders in Pregnancy.* Philadelphia: Lea & Febiger, 1986.
35. Lavin, J. P., Jr., and Polsky, S. S. Abdominal trauma during pregnancy. *Clin. Perinatol.* 10:423, 1983.
36. Loevinger, E. H., et al. Hepatic rupture associated with pregnancy: Treatment with transcatheter embolotherapy. *Obstet. Gynecol.* 65:281, 1985.
37. Madsen, L. V., et al. Parturition and pelvic fracture: Follow-up of 34 obstetric patients with a history of pelvic fracture. *Acta Obstet. Gynecol. Scand.* 62:620, 1983.
38. Neerhof, M. G., Zelman, W., and Sullivan, T. Hepatic rupture in pregnancy. *Obstet. Gynecol. Surv.* 44:407, 1989.
39. Neufeld, J. D. G., et al. Trauma in pregnancy. *Emerg. Med. Clin. North Am.* 5:623, 1987.
40. Nugent, P., and O'Connell, T. X. Breast cancer and pregnancy. *Arch. Surg.* 120:1221, 1985.
41. Parente, J. T., et al. Breast cancer associated with pregnancy. *Obstet. Gynecol.* 71:861, 1988.
42. Pearse, C. S., et al. Use of MAST suit in obstetrics and gynecology. *Obstet. Gynecol. Surv.* 39:416, 1984.
43. Pelligra, R., and Sandberg, E. C. Control of intractable abdominal bleeding by external counterpressure. *J.A.M.A.* 241:708, 1979.
44. Plauche, W. C. Cesarean hysterectomy: Indications, techniques, and complications. *Clin. Obstet. Gynecol.* 29:318, 1986.
45. Rothenberger, D. A., et al. Diagnostic peritoneal lavage for blunt trauma in pregnant women. *Am. J. Obstet. Gynecol.* 129:479, 1977.
46. Schwartz, D. B., et al. The management of genital condylomas in pregnant women. *Obstet. Gynecol. Clin. North Am.* 14:589, 1987.
47. Sherer, D. M., and Schenker, J. G. Accidental injury during pregnancy. *Obstet. Gynecol. Surv.* 44:330, 1989.
48. Simon, J. A. Biliary tract disease and related surgical disorders during pregnancy. *Clin. Obstet. Gynecol.* 26:810, 1983.

49. Smith, B. K., et al. Burns and pregnancy. *Clin. Perinatol.* 10:383, 1983.
50. Uleland, K. Cardiac Diseases. In R. K. Creasy and R. Resnik (eds.), *Maternal-Fetal Medicine: Principles and Practice*. Philadelphia: Saunders, 1984.
51. Warsof, S. L. Medical and surgical treatment of inflammatory bowel disease in pregnancy. *Clin. Obstet. Gynecol.* 26:822, 1983.
52. Weber, C. E. Postmortem cesarean section: Review of the literature and case reports. *Am. J. Obstet. Gynecol.* 110:158, 1971.
53. Weingold, A. B. Appendicitis in pregnancy. *Clin. Obstet. Gynecol.* 26:801, 1983.

17 Spontaneous Abortion

Peter T. Rogge

Abortion is the termination of pregnancy, by any means, resulting in the expulsion of an immature, nonviable fetus. The difficult question of when viability begins, underscored by recent advances in neonatal intensive care of very small infants, generally is dispensed with by convention: A fetus of less than 20 weeks' gestation, counting from the first day of the last menstrual period, or a fetus weighing less than 500 gm, is considered an abortus. The term **miscarriage** has been used for all pregnancy losses. Although imprecise, its use is preferred in discussions with patients, as the word **abortion,** for many, has undesirable connotations.

The incidence of spontaneous abortion generally is believed to be 15–20% of all pregnancies. Substantial numbers of abortions, however, are unreported or are very early and subclinical; some have estimated the true incidence to be as high as 50–78% [13]. Most early abortuses are morphologically abnormal, with chromosome anomalies found in as many as 60% in some series [2]. First-trimester spontaneous abortion is an instrument of natural selection, a natural function that effectively improves the quality of fetuses eventually reaching term.

Management of abortion relies on accurate clinical classification. Depending on the patient's signs and symptoms, abortions are stated to be **threatened, inevitable, incomplete, complete, missed, septic,** or **habitual. Induced abortions,** probably the largest class numerically in the United States today, are discussed in Chap. 1.

I. Threatened abortion

A. Diagnosis. The diagnosis of threatened abortion should be strongly considered when vaginal bleeding with or without menstruallike cramps occurs in the first 20 weeks of pregnancy. No history of passage of tissue or rupture of membranes is elicited. Symptoms of pregnancy (nausea and vomiting, fatigue, breast tenderness, urinary frequency) may be present. On physical examination, the patient is afebrile and abdominal findings are minimal. Speculum examination reveals blood coming from the cervical os without amniotic fluid or tissue seen in the vaginal vault or endocervical canal. On bimanual examination, the **internal** cervical os is closed, the uterus is soft and enlarged appropriate to gestational age, and uterine tenderness is absent or mild.

B. Differential diagnosis

1. **Benign and malignant lesions of the genital tract.** Careful speculum examination will reveal bleeding caused by vaginal and cervical lesions. During pregnancy, the highly vascular and friable cervix often bleeds from an ectropion. To achieve hemostasis, apply pressure for several minutes with a large swab; if this fails, cautery with silver nitrate sticks often is successful. Atypical cervical lesions should be evaluated with colposcopy or biopsy.
2. **Anovulatory bleeding** with an antecedent period of amenorrhea may be confused with threatened abortion. Here, the early symptoms of pregnancy are absent, and no history of a positive pregnancy test is obtained. The uterus, on bimanual examination, is of normal size and is not softened; the cervix is firm and not cyanotic; and Hegar's sign—easy compressibility of the isthmus—is absent. A history of previous similar episodes may be elicited.
3. **Disorders of pregnancy**
   a. **Hydatidiform mole** may present with bleeding during early pregnancy and be mistaken for threatened abortion; the diagnosis often is made later as symptoms evolve. The passage of grapelike vesicles certainly should arouse suspicion. In only 50% of cases is the uterus enlarged beyond the size ex-

pected from the patient's dates. No heart tones are heard with the Doppler apparatus (generally after 12 weeks' gestation, they are detectable in viable gestations by pocket Doppler instruments). Hyperemesis, preeclampsia, or hyperthyroidism may be present. Large theca lutein cysts may be palpable in the adnexal regions. Ultrasonography confirms the diagnosis.

b. **Ectopic pregnancy** should be considered in every patient who bleeds in the first trimester and has pain. The pain may be unilateral or generalized. Orthostatic light-headedness or syncope (hypovolemia), rectal or urinary pressure, or shoulder pain (diaphragmatic irritation) may occur. On abdominal examination, tenderness with or without rebound (often minimal) is noted. Pelvic examination usually reveals cervical motion tenderness. This sign must be elicited cautiously, as the clumsy, rough examiner often will produce a false-positive result. The cul-de-sac may bulge (hemoperitoneum), and an adnexal mass (50% of the time) is helpful if present. Often, fullness rather than a mass is appreciated, and exquisite tenderness may preclude an adequate examination. The traditional pregnancy test is positive in only 50% of cases. Radioimmunoassay for beta-human chorionic gonadotropin (β-HCG) generally is positive. A high index of suspicion is necessary since classic presentations are uncommon.

c. **Other type of abortion.** (See the sections that follow.)

C. Laboratory tests

1. **Blood count** (if bleeding has been heavy).
2. **Serum β-HCG level** (if pregnancy is undocumented). Positive tests may occur in nonviable gestations since β-HCG may persist in the serum for several weeks after fetal death [15].
3. **Ultrasonography.** In experienced hands, this may be helpful. At 7½ weeks' gestation or greater, fetal heart motion normally is detectable. In one study, absence of fetal heart motion in gestations 9 weeks or greater predicted nonviable fetuses 100% of the time; 92% of patients with fetal heart motion continued the pregnancy to term [1]. If dates are uncertain, repeat ultrasonography may be required. Persistent failure to detect fetal heart motion past 9 weeks' gestation should prompt serious consideration of curettage.

D. Treatment. As most fetuses destined to abort in the first trimester are grossly malformed, with fetal death occurring two to six weeks before expulsion, all forms of treatment must be regarded with suspicion.

1. **Medication.** Progestational agents should not be given; an increased incidence of missed abortion as well as occasional masculinization of female fetuses that were successfully carried to term have been reported. The traditional treatment is bed rest with sedation and abstinence from intercourse. Controlled studies, however, are lacking, and this regimen may well provide needless hardship, economic and otherwise [1]. Furthermore, medications given during the period of organogenesis (days 18–55 after conception) subject the fetus to possible teratogenic effects.
2. **Other measures.** A regimen of bed rest and abstinence from sexual intercourse seems more rational for **late** threatened abortions (after 12 weeks' gestation), as these measures occasionally are successful in averting premature labor in more advanced gestations; abortuses after 12 weeks are unlikely to be anomalous.
3. **Psychological aspects.** Essential in approaching these patients is a sympathetic attitude and a willingness to inform. The physician, truthfully, has little to offer as a healer but much as an educator and a lender of emotional support. The patient is reassured that bleeding during early pregnancy is very common and that the prognosis for a normal child in those who do not abort is excellent. (Some studies have reported an increase in abruptio placentae, placenta previa, prematurity and its complications, and a slight increase in anomalies. Perinatal mortality is not much affected.) In early threatened abortion without cramping, the chances are 50–75% that the pregnancy will continue successfully.

4. **Recurring symptoms.** Threatened abortion is best managed on an outpatient basis. The patient should be told to report increased bleeding (greater than a normal menses) or cramping (increased probability of inevitable or incomplete abortion), passage of tissue, or fever. Tissue passed should be saved for examination.

II. Inevitable abortion

A. Diagnosis. This diagnosis is made when the patient with the symptoms of threatened abortion is found to have a dilated **internal** cervical os. Amniotic fluid may be seen in the vaginal vault, or there may be fluid leaking from the cervix. The patient usually complains of menstruallike cramps.

B. Differential diagnosis

1. **Incomplete abortion.** With incomplete abortion, tissue already has passed. On examination, tissue may be seen in the vagina or the endocervical canal. A history of tissue passage may be elicited. This differential diagnosis often is difficult to make clinically.
2. **Threatened abortion.** With threatened abortions, the internal os is closed (i.e., it will not admit a fingertip or a standard-size ring forceps). The cotton-swab test—attempting to pass a cotton swab through the internal os—is of value only if negative, as commonly the normal undilated cervix will admit a swab.
3. **Incompetent cervix.** Caution must be exercised in instrumentation of the cervix, partly because of the possibility of incompetent cervix. This treatable condition (see sec. **VII.B.1**) has as a feature dilatation of the cervix without cramps early in the disease process.

C. Management. Surgical evacuation of the uterus is advised in nearly all cases (see sec. **III**). Generally, progression to incomplete abortion will occur in a few hours or days. Placental tissue is most likely to be retained in gestations of 8–14 weeks. Rh_o(D) immunoglobulin (RhoGAM) is administered to Rh-negative, unsensitized patients for isoimmunization prophylaxis. Prior to 13 weeks' gestation, give RhoGAM, 50 μg IM; for gestations of 13 weeks or more, give 300 μg IM.

III. Incomplete abortion

A. Signs and symptoms. These patients complain of cramping and bleeding and may report the passage of tissue. (**Caution:** Organized clots may be mistaken for tissue by the patient as well as by the physician.) Speculum examination reveals a dilated internal os with tissue present in the vagina or endocervical canal. Bleeding may be profuse, and initial evaluation should include inquiry about orthostatic dizziness and syncope and examination for postural pulse and blood pressure changes.

2. **Laboratory tests**
   - a. Blood count (if bleeding has been heavy; the blood count may not reflect blood loss if recent).
   - b. Rh typing.
   - c. Consider blood typing and cross-matching if bleeding is heavy or if postural changes are present.

B. Treatment

1. **Stabilization.** If the patient has signs and symptoms of heavy bleeding, at least one intravenous line with a large-bore catheter suitable for blood transfusion is started immediately. Ringer's lactate or normal saline with 30 units oxytocin/1000 ml is appropriate for intravenous use at 200 ml/hour or greater (the uterus is less sensitive to oxytocin in early pregnancy than in late pregnancy). Such doses may depress urine output because of the antidiuretic hormone–like activity of oxytocin and should be discontinued as soon as appropriate. With a ring forceps, products of conception should quickly be removed from the endocervical canal and uterus; this maneuver often will dramatically decrease the bleeding. Curettage is performed after the patient's vital signs have stabilized.
2. **Curettage**
   - a. **Procedure.** The patient is placed in a dorsal lithotomy position in stir-

rups and suitably prepped, draped (as for vaginal delivery), and sedated. If general anesthesia is not available or not elected, the following analgesia often is satisfactory: meperidine hydrochloride (Demerol), 35–50 mg IV over 3–5 minutes. The goal is a drowsy patient, not one who is asleep with depressed respirations. Naloxone hydrochloride (Narcan), 0.4 mg IV push, to antagonize narcotic-induced depression of respirations, as well as facilities for resuscitation, must be available.

A weighted speculum is placed intravaginally, and the vagina and cervix are scrubbed with provide-iodine solution. Paracervical block is performed—chloroprocaine hydrochloride 1% (Nesacaine), 12 ml total, divided into equal doses submucosally into the lateral vaginal fornices, with a 20-gauge spinal needle at 2 and 4 o'clock (6 ml) and 8 and 10 o'clock (6 ml). Beware of inadvertent intravenous placement of the needle tip; aspirate for blood prior to injection. Bimanual examination confirms the position and size of the uterus and the direction of the endocervical canal. Uterine sounding is performed only to confirm the direction of the endocervical canal. Mechanical dilatation usually is not needed, but if necessary, it may be completed with Hegar or Pratt dilators. The amount of dilatation (in millimeters) required for a given gestation is equal to the gestational age in weeks (e.g., dilate to No. 9 Hegar for a 9-week pregnancy). Curettage is performed carefully but systematically, with a suction instrument. A single-tooth tenaculum or a ring forceps placed on the anterior cervical lip is used for counteraction. Vacuum curettage may be faster and result in less blood loss with advanced gestations. Use of vacuum curet that is 1 mm smaller than the measured cervical dilatation. To decrease perforation risk, advance the tip of the curet no farther than the middle of the uterine cavity. Sharp curettage and exploration with polyp or ring forceps should always follow vacuum aspiration to ensure completeness.

b. **Perforation.** Great care must be used, especially in gestations greater than 12–14 weeks, to avoid perforation of the uterus. If perforation is suspected, treatment depends on its location (midline perforations are less likely to damage large blood vessels), on the presence or absence of signs of intraperitoneal bleeding, on whether the perforation has occurred with the suction curet (increased chance of bowel or bladder injury), and on whether the abortion has been completed. Perforation with a suction curet usually demands laparotomy to assess possible bowel or bladder injury. **A midline perforation** with a sound, dilator, or sharp curet without obvious bleeding may require only observation for 24–48 hours for evidence of bleeding or peritonitis. Laparoscopy is indicated for **lateral perforations** to detect possible laceration of the uteroovarian vessels and their branches. If the abortion is incomplete at the time of the perforation, only an experienced operator should complete the procedure; completion under direct vision of the uterus through a laparoscope is advisable [3]. Alternatively, ultrasound guidance may be employed [4]. Intravenous oxytocin or intramuscular methylergonovine maleate (0.2 mg q4h) will decrease the size of the uterus and make repeat curettage safer.

c. **Anomalies.** During curettage, the uterine cavity should be explored for septa and other anomalies that may be related to abortion (see sec. **VII**).

3. **Postcurettage.** After curettage, the patient is observed for several hours. Repeat blood count is ordered if bleeding has been excessive. If the vital signs are stable, the patient is discharged with instructions to avoid coitus, douching, or the use of tampons for two weeks (owing to risk of infection with an open cervical os). Oral ferrous sulfate is prescribed if blood loss has been significant. Analgesics other than ibuprofen rarely are required. Rh-negative, unsensitized patients are given intramuscular RhoGAM (see sec. **II.C**). Methylergonovine (0.2 mg PO q4h for 6 doses) may be prescribed if moderate bleeding continues. A return office appointment is made for

two weeks, and the patient is instructed to call if bleeding becomes excessive, if cramps are severe, or if fever greater than 100.4°F occurs. The pathologic findings are reviewed when she returns.

4. **Psychological aspects.** Again, a sympathetic, understanding approach is stressed. It is helpful to suggest to the patient that it may be better to lose an abnormal pregnancy early than to carry it to term. Many women believe they are inadequate as childbearers or feel they have done something that caused the gestation to abort. Guilt and depression often are present, and the patient should be allowed to express her feelings. The role of abortion as a beneficial, natural (if unpleasant) function may be suggested.

IV. Complete abortion

A. Diagnosis. This diagnosis is considered when the passage of products of conception appears to be complete. The uterus, on bimanual examination, is well contracted and much smaller than the duration of pregnancy would indicate; the cervical os may be closed.

B. Differential diagnosis

1. **Incomplete abortion.**
2. **Ectopic pregnancy** with passage of decidual cast, masquerading as products of conception. All suspected products of conception should be examined grossly and submitted to the pathology laboratory for examination. If no fetal tissue or villi are recognized grossly, and even if the patient is asymptomatic and has a normal pelvic examination, ectopic pregnancy must be suspected. At the very least, she should be warned about the symptoms of ectopic pregnancy and followed closely.

C. Management. Between 8 and 14 weeks, curettage is advised because of the high risk that the abortion is truly incomplete. Outside these limits, the patient is given the option of being followed as an outpatient without surgical intervention. Appropriate warnings regarding increased bleeding and fever are given. RhoGAM is administered to Rh-negative unsensitized patients (see sec. **II.C**). β-HCG levels should be obtained weekly until they reach zero. Suspect incomplete abortion if levels plateau or fail to reach zero within four weeks.

V. Missed abortion

A. Diagnosis. Missed abortion is defined as the retention of products of conception well after the fetus is known to have expired; a two-month time period conventionally is used in the definition. If the pregnancy products are retained for four weeks or more, the development of a severe coagulation defect with consequent bleeding must be considered. The diagnosis of missed abortion is suspected when the pregnant uterus fails to grow as expected, when the symptoms and signs of pregnancy regress, or when fetal heart tones disappear. Amenorrhea may persist, or intermittent vaginal bleeding, spotting, or brown discharge may occur. Ultrasonography is essential in confirming the diagnosis. With prompt, appropriate use of ultrasound (uterine size $<$ dates, significant bleeding, inability to detect fetal heart tones when expected), the textbook definition for missed abortion is rarely met [12].

B. Management

1. **Laboratory tests.** A baseline complete blood count (CBC) with determination of platelet count, fibrinogen level, and partial thromboplastin time, and ABO blood typing and antibody screen (to facilitate blood availability should transfusion be necessary) are obtained.
2. **Evacuation.** Because of the psychological implications of carrying a dead fetus, as well as the risk of coagulopathy, evacuation of the uterus is advised as soon as a firm diagnosis of fetal death has been made. Suction curettage is suitable when the uterus is less than 12–14 weeks' gestational size, but in advanced gestations special skills and instruments are required. Other methods of emptying the second-trimester uterus are high-dose intravenous oxytocin administration, intraamniotic prostaglandin

$F_{2\alpha}$, and intravaginal prostaglandin E_2 suppositories. Curettage should follow expulsion of the fetus in these latter three methods. Regardless of the method of termination chosen, it is helpful in achieving atraumatic dilatation of the cervix to insert as many Laminaria tents as possible into the cervix the night before evacuation.

a. **Dilatation and evacuation.** This probably is the best method for an **experienced** operator. The largest available suction curet should be used. If fetal parts are encountered that are of excessive size, crushing and extraction with Bier or Sopher forceps is necessary, taking care to work in the center of the uterine cavity. General anesthesia may be required, and continuous sonographic guidance is recommended to reduce perforation risk and to confirm completeness of the procedure.

b. **Oxytocin induction**

(1) **Procedure.** Oxytocin, 40 units, is added to 1000 ml of 5% dextrose in Ringer's lactate. The solution is infused at 1 μ/milliunits and the rate is doubled every 20–30 minutes until adequate contractions are produced. When labor is established, the membranes are ruptured.

(2) **Risk.** Water intoxication may result because of the antidiuretic hormone–like effect of oxytocin. Fluid intake and output must be monitored carefully and the administration of large amounts of hypotonic fluids avoided.

(3) This method may fail to induce labor.

c. **Intraamniotic prostaglandin $F_{2\alpha}$**

(1) **Procedure.** The technique is similar to that recommended for second-trimester amniocentesis. After the intraamniotic placement of the needle has been ensured, a test dose of 1 ml (approximately 6 mg) of the prostaglandin is injected, and the patient is observed for adverse reaction. The remainder of the 40-mg vial is infused slowly, aspirating occasionally to ensure intraamniotic location of the needle tip.

(2) **Risks.** Possible adverse effects are nausea and vomiting, diarrhea, hyperpyrexia, bronchospasm, bradycardia, and cervical rupture. Prostaglandin is relatively contraindicated in asthmatic patients and in patients with hypertension.

(3) The clinician may be unable to inject the prostaglandin. Intraamniotic injections are technically difficult because of the often scant amount of amniotic fluid. Ultrasonic guidance is helpful.

d. **Prostaglandin E_2 vaginal suppositories**

(1) **Procedure.** These are placed intravaginally q3h until adequate contractions are obtained.

(2) **Risks.** The adverse effects of prostaglandins listed in sec. **c.(2)** above are more common with this route of administration because of substantial systemic absorption of prostaglandin when given intravaginally.

Regardless of how prostaglandins are administered, the patient's cervix should be inspected carefully postabortion for lacerations and fistulas.

3. **RhoGAM** is administered to Rh-negative, unsensitized patients (see sec. **II.C**).

VI. **Septic abortion** and its complications—septic shock, renal failure, and disseminated intravascular coagulation—were a source of considerable maternal morbidity and mortality during the 1950s and early 1960s. Perhaps because of improved contraceptive methods and the availability of legal induced abortion, these complications are seen less commonly today.

A. **Diagnosis.** The diagnosis of septic abortion is made when a temperature of at least 100.4°F (38°C) exists in the presence of signs and symptoms of abortion in any stage, assuming other sources of fever have been excluded. Septic abortion generally is seen in the context of prolonged, neglected ruptured membranes, in the presence of intrauterine pregnancy with an intrauterine device in place, or with a history of criminal attempts to terminate the pregnancy (usually either by mechanical means, such as intrauterine catheters, or by injection of soaps or phenolics). History of criminal instrumentation may be difficult to elicit but should always be considered. Physical examination, depending on the extent of the infection and whether the uterus has been perforated, may reveal abdominal tenderness, with or without guarding or rebound, purulent drainage from the cervical os, and uterine and adnexal tenderness. The extent of infection may be staged as follows [10]: stage 1 = endometrial-myometrial involvement; stage 2 = adnexal spread; stage 3 = generalized peritonitis. Approximately 6% of septic abortions are complicated by endotoxic shock.

B. Management. These patients should be evaluated rapidly but thoroughly, with attention to estimating the seriousness of the infection and detecting the previously mentioned complications. Associated with a less favorable prognosis and the need for aggressive treatment are high spiking fever, hypotension, oliguria, advanced gestational age of pregnancy, and signs of infection beyond the uterus [10].

1. In seriously ill patients, the following measures should be initiated:
   - **a. Closely monitor** vital signs and urine output (indwelling Foley catheter).
   - **b.** Obtain a CBC, urinalysis, serum electrolytes, blood urea nitrogen, creatinine, blood type and Rh factor, cross-match, platelet count, prothrombin time, partial thromboplastin time, fibrinogen, fibrin split products, and arterial blood gases. Hemolytic studies are performed (e.g., plasma free hemoglobin) if *Clostridium perfringens* infection is suspected. (A gross test of hemolysis is provided by centrifugation of a blood sample and observation of the serum for a pink tinge.)
   - **c.** Take **cultures** of blood, urine, endometrium, and products of conception—aerobic and anaerobic. Perform a Gram's stain of products of conception, obtained by endometrial swab; gram-positive rods with swollen ends suggest *C. perfringens* infection. If bulging of the cul-de-sac is detected, aspirate pus by gently lifting the posterior cervix with a tenaculum and inserting a 20-gauge spinal needle 1–2 cm through the cul-de-sac between the uterosacral ligaments. Culture the aspirate and perform a Gram's stain.
   - **d.** Obtain **roentgenograms** of the chest (for possible septic emboli; air under the diaphragm implies uterine perforation), and anteroposterior supine and upright films of the abdomen (for foreign bodies; intramyometrial gas ["onionskin" pattern] implies *C. perfringes* infection).
   - **e.** Give **tetanus toxoid,** 0.5 ml SC, to immunized patients with a history of instrumentation.
   - **f.** Administer **intravenous fluids** (normal saline) through at least one large-bore catheter. Fluids are given at a rate such that urinary output of at least 30 ml/hour is maintained. The intravascular space often expands dramatically in septic shock, necessitating vigorous fluid replacement. Pulmonary edema secondary to fluid overload, however, must be avoided. In critically ill patients or in the presence of significant pulmonary or cardiac disease, placement of a Swan-Ganz catheter with monitoring of pulmonary wedge pressures is indicated. These patients should be in an intensive care unit.
   - **g. Whole blood** is given to maintain hematocrit between 30 and 35%.
   - **h. Antibiotics** for seriously ill patients include the following:
     - **(1) Penicillin G** sodium, 4–8 million units IV q4h, **or ampicillin,** 1–2 gm IV q4h.
     - **(2) In addition, gentamicin sulfate,** 1.5 mg/kg/dose, slowly IV q8h, with careful monitoring of renal and eighth cranial nerve function. Serum gentamicin levels—peak (one-half hour after dose is given) and trough (just before dose is given)—should be ordered and dosage adjusted as necessary. If possible, the use of nephrotoxic drugs on oliguric patients should be avoided [6].

(3) In addition, **clindamycin,** 600 mg IV q6h.
(4) Alternatively, for less seriously ill patients, **cefoxitin,** 2 gm IV q6h, may be used. If chlamydia is suspected, add **doxycycline,** 100 mg IV q12h.

i. **Operative intervention,** from curettage to total abdominal hysterectomy and bilateral salpingo-oophorectomy, as well as its timing, continues to be controversial. Operative intervention offers the promise of removing infected tissue and hence averting the complications of endotoxic shock from gram-negative organisms and intravascular hemolysis (which can lead to renal failure) from *C. perfringens* toxin. However, it places the patient at risk for dissemination of the infection intraoperatively. An increased incidence postoperatively of sepsis and hypotension has been reported when curettage is performed on febrile patients [10].

2. **Low-risk patients.** Treatment should be individualized and strict regimens abandoned. Patients at low risk (i.e., those with a fever lower than 103°F, a small uterus, localized infection only, and no indications of shock) probably are best managed with intensive antibiotics; late curettage should be done only if needed, **unless** the uterus is believed to contain substantial amounts of necrotic material or unless bleeding is excessive. Incomplete abortions should be evacuated as soon as effective circulating antibiotic levels have been achieved. Profuse hemorrhage obviously demands rapid curettage.

3. **High-risk patients.** Patients at high risk (i.e., those with a significantly enlarged uterus, infection beyond the uterus, fever above 103°F, evidence of *C. perfringens* infection, a history of instrumentation, or evidence of shock) are candidates for aggressive intervention when antibiotics have been started. The operative procedure may vary from curettage to total abdominal hysterectomy and bilateral salpingo-oophorectomy in extremely ill patients. Laparotomy should be reserved for patients with evidence of massive uterine infection (i.e., onionskin pattern on roentgenogram), pelvic abscesses, uterine perforation, or failure of conservative management [8].

C. Septic shock

1. **Signs.** Septic shock is suggested by the following signs:
   a. Oliguria
   b. Hypotension
   c. Tachypnea
   d. Mental confusion
   e. Warmth and dryness of the extremities (low peripheral resistance) or cold and cyanotic extremities (increased resistance)

2. **Management.** Acidosis in this setting generally is secondary to hypoperfusion. If severe (i.e., pH < 7.2, persisting despite volume replacement), it should be corrected with intravenous sodium bicarbonate; rapid or complete correction may be dangerous. Sympathomimetic agents occasionally may be necessary to maintain perfusion of vital organs; dopamine hydrochloride is therapeutic and does not decrease renal blood flow at usual therapeutic doses. High-dose corticosteroids (e.g., methylprednisolone, 30 mg/kg, followed by 100–200 mg IV q4–6h for 48–72 hours) often are recommended, although their efficacy has not been firmly established. Digitalis is given for congestive heart failure. Internal medicine consultation is advised.
   a. **Renal failure.** If renal failure ensues, preparation for peritoneal dialysis should be made. Careful intake and output determinations and daily weights are ordered. Serum electrolytes are followed carefully. Penicillin G sodium should be used in these patients, and the dosages of all medications are reduced commensurate with the degree of renal failure. Nephrology consultation is advised.
   b. **Disseminated intravascular coagulation** should be vigorously treated

with volume replacement (fresh whole blood). Successful treatment of shock is of primary importance in reversing the coagulopathy. Early curettage to remove the source of thromboplastins is mandatory. Heparin is not advised. Hematology consultation is helpful.

c. **The cornerstones of therapy** of septic shock are

(1) Fluid and whole blood resuscitation

(2) Respiratory support—from airway maintenance and administration of oxygen by nasal cannula as a minimal treatment, to endotracheal intubation with assisted ventilation, as necessary

(3) A decrease in the endotoxin load with antibiotics directed against the infecting organisms

(4) Surgical removal of necrotic tissue where indicated.

VII. Habitual abortion

A. **Diagnosis.** This is defined most commonly as the occurrence of three or more consecutive spontaneous abortions. Habitual abortion comprises approximately 5% of all spontaneous abortions [5]. It seems likely that many cases, but not all, occur by chance. Cytogenetic studies of abortion specimens have demonstrated chromosomal anomalies in 20–60% of abortuses. Approximately 95% of chromosomally abnormal fetuses are of less than 8 weeks' developmental age although they often are retained for excessive periods of time [2]. Among abortuses past 12 weeks of development, chromosomal anomalies are uncommon.

B. **Management.** All abortuses should be submitted for pathologic examination. Couples who have had repeated losses of early developmental-age fetuses have an increased chance of having chromosomal disorders, so chromosomal studies using banding techniques are recommended for both the male and female partner. The incidence of chromosomal anomalies in habitual aborters (including losses of fetuses of all developmental ages) is estimated at 6.2% [5]. Genetic counseling is indicated if abnormalities are found.

Patients with repeated abortions at greater than 12 weeks' gestation should be investigated for known maternal causes of abortion.

1. Patients with an **incompetent cervix** present with a history of repeated midtrimester losses with painless cervical dilatation. Contractions that expel the fetus occur when dilatation is advanced. Patients may complain of lower abdominal pressure symptoms or urinary frequency and urgency prior to aborting [18]. A past history of cervical operations, such as dilatation and curettage, may be elicited, and cervical incompetence is believed, in many cases, to arise from trauma at such procedures. Maternal diethylstilbestrol exposure occasionally is associated with cervical incompetence. Treatment is by cerclage* at 14–16 weeks, but the operation is contraindicated if there is uterine bleeding, cramping, or dilatation of the cervix greater than 4 cm.
2. **Anatomic uterine defects** occasionally are responsible for repeated late abortions. A double uterus, a separate uterus, Asherman's syndrome, endometrial polyps, and leiomyomas that infringe on the endometrial cavity have all been implicated as causes. Hysterosalpingography or hysteroscopy may be necessary for the diagnosis. Treatment is surgical, by a reunification procedure for congenital uterine anomalies, or polypectomy or myomectomy where appropriate. If a subsequent pregnancy occurs, delivery by cesarean section is indicated if the surgical procedure resulted in an endomyometrial scar.
3. **Lupus anticoagulant/anticardiolipin antibodies** are uncommon, but when present are associated with high fetal loss rates secondary to diffuse pla-

*The effectiveness of cerclage in prolonging pregnancy is in serious doubt as a result of two randomized clinical trials, both of which have failed to reveal any prolongation of pregnancy or improved fetal survival with cervical cerclage [7, 14]. This almost irrefutable evidence will probably have an impact on the frequency with which cerclage is employed.

cental thrombosis and infarction [9]. Preliminary experience suggests that **low-dose aspirin** (75 mg/day) and **prednisone** (20–60 mg/day) greatly improve outcome.

4. **Other causes** of habitual abortion are less well documented.
   a. Hypothyroidism and hyperthyroidism occasionally are found, and appropriate studies to rule these out are indicated if the prior workup has been negative.
   b. Endometrial cultures for *Toxoplasma gondii* and *Ureaplasma urealyticum,* with specific antimicrobial treatment, have been advised by some [16] but remain unproved.
   c. Luteal phase insufficiency has been described as a cause of habitual abortion, though considerable controversy exists concerning this theory, as well as the diagnosis and treatment of the condition. At this writing, the recommended diagnosis is by appropriately timed (2–3 days prior to expected menses) endometrial biopsy. A positive diagnosis requires demonstration during two cycles of histologic dating that is delayed more than 2 days from cycle dating, as established by the onset of subsequent menses. Treatment is clomiphene citrate (Clomid), 50 mg/day PO for 5 days, beginning on day 5 of the cycle. Alternatively, progesterone vaginal suppositories, 25 mg bid, during the luteal phase and continued through 8 weeks' gestation (10 menstrual weeks), have been recommended.
   d. Maternal-fetal HLA antigen (major histocompatibility complex) sharing has been associated with habitual abortion in some studies, but other investigators have found no relationship. As of this writing, attempts at immunotherapy remain experimental.

C. **Chance of successful subsequent pregnancy.** Following spontaneous abortion, the patient often will inquire regarding her chance of successfully carrying a subsequent pregnancy to term. She can be told that after one abortion, the chance of a fetal loss in the next pregnancy is not increased. After two consecutive abortions, the risk of a third rises somewhat. After three losses, the chance of a fourth is approximately 25–50%. Following two or three consecutive losses, the patient should be evaluated. If the history is not helpful and physical examination does not suggest any of the previously discussed disorders, investigation probably should begin with hysterosalpingography and chromosomal studies. If the completed investigation fails to reveal a cause for recurrent pregnancy loss, the couple may be counseled that the chances for a successful subsequent pregnancy are approximately 80% [17].

References

1. Eriksen, P. S., and Philipsen, T. Prognosis in threatened abortion evaluated by hormonal assays and ultrasound scanning. *Obstet. Gynecol.* 55:435, 1980.
2. Fabricant, J. D., Boullie, J., and Boullie, A. Genetic studies on spontaneous abortion. *Contemp. Obstet. Gynecol.* 11:73, 1978.
3. Freiman, S. M., and Wulff, G. J. L. Management of uterine perforation following elective abortion. *Obstet. Gynecol.* 50:647, 1977.
4. Kaali, S. G., et al. The frequency and management of uterine perforations during first-trimester abortions. *Am. J. Obstet. Gynecol.* 161:407, 1989.
5. Khuda, G. Cytogenics of habitual abortion. *Obstet. Gynecol. Surv.* 29:229, 1974.
6. Knuppel, R. D., Rao, P. S., and Cavanaugh, D. Septic shock in obstetrics. *Clin. Obstet. Gynecol.* 27:3, 1984.
7. Lazar, P., et al. Multicentred controlled trial of cervical cerclage in women at moderate risk of preterm delivery. *Br. J. Obstet. Gynaecol.* 91:731, 1984.
8. Ledger, W. L. *Infection in the Female.* Philadelphia: Lea & Febiger, 1977.
9. Lubbe, W. F., and Liggins, G. C. Lupus anticoagulant and pregnancy. *Am. J. Obstet. Gynecol.* 153:322, 1988.

10. Neuwirth, R. S., and Friedman, E. A. Septic abortion. *Am. J. Gynecol.* 85:24, 1963.
11. Poland, B. J., et al. Reproductive counseling in patients who have had a spontaneous abortion. *Am. J. Obstet. Gynecol.* 127:685, 1977.
12. Pridjian, G., and Moawad, A. Missed abortion: still appropriate terminology? *Am. J. Obstet. Gynecol.* 161:261, 1989.
13. Roberts, C. J., and Lowe, C. R. Where have all the conceptions gone? *Lancet* 1:498, 1975.
14. Rush, R., and Toaff, M. E. Diagnosis of impending late abortion. *Obstet. Gynecol.* 91:724, 1984.
15. Steier, J. D., Bergsjo, P., and Myking, D. L. Human chorionic gonadotropin in maternal plasma after induced abortion, spontaneous abortion, and removed ectopic pregnancy. *Obstet. Gynecol.* 64:391, 1984.
16. Stray-Pederson, B., and Stray-Pederson, S. Etiologic factors and subsequent reproductive performance in 195 couples with a prior history of habitual abortion. *Am. J. Obstet. Gynecol.* 148:140, 1984.
17. Taylor, E. S. Prognosis of subsequent pregnancy after recurrent spontaneous abortions in first trimester: Editorial comment. *Obstet. Gynecol. Surv.* 43:91, 1988.
18. Toaff, R., and Toaff, M. E. Diagnosis of impending late abortion. *Obstet. Gynecol.* 43:756, 1974.

Selected Readings

Gant, N. F. Recurrent Spontaneous Abortion. In *Williams Obstetrics (Suppl.)* New York: Simon & Shuster, 1989.

Reid, D. E., and Benirschke, K. Abortion. In D. E. Reid et al. (eds.), *Principles and Management of Human Reproduction.* Philadelphia: Saunders, 1972.

Rock, J. A., and Zacur, H. A. The clinical management of repeated early pregnancy wastage. *Fertil. Steril.* 39:123, 1983.

18 Ectopic Pregnancy

Leslie Andrews and
Silverio T. Chavez

I. **Definition.** In an ectopic pregnancy, the fertilized ovum implants at any site other than the endometrial cavity. The fallopian tube is the most common site, accounting for more than 95% of ectopic pregnancies, but other implantation sites include the cervix, abdominal cavity including the broad ligament, and the ovary. One vaginal pregnancy has been reported.

II. **Incidence.** The incidence of ectopic pregnancy in the United States nearly tripled in the 1970s and continued to rise during the 1980s [3]. Currently, approximately 1.4% of reported pregnancies are ectopic [19]. Ectopic pregnancy is the leading cause of first-trimester maternal death. The risk of ectopic pregnancy increases by age and is highest for women ages 35–44 years old. The relative risk of death from ectopic pregnancy is approximately 10 times greater than that from childbirth and more than 50 times greater than that from legal induced abortion [8].

III. **Etiology.** The following conditions have been implicated as possible causes of ectopic pregnancy:

A. **Conditions preventing or retarding the passage of the fertilized ovum** into the uterine cavity.

1. **Salpingitis.** Acute salpingitis has been shown to cause a sevenfold increase in the risk of ectopic pregnancy [32]. Salpingitis causes narrowing of the tubal lumen resulting from agglutination of the arborescent folds of the tubal mucosa. Chlamydial salpingitis is a suspected cause of the increase in tubal pregnancies because it is less likely to cause complete tubal blockage than gonorrheal pelvic inflammatory disease and may further contribute to abnormal egg transfer by damage to tubal cilia.
2. **Developmental abnormalities** of the tube such as diverticula, accessory ostia, and hypoplasia. Diethylstilbestrol exposure is associated with a 4–5 times greater risk of ectopic pregnancy [31].
3. **Peritubal adhesions** following postabortal or puerperal infections, appendicitis, or endometriosis.
4. **Tumors** that may exert extrinsic pressure on the tube.
5. **Tubal surgery,** including tubal ligation, conservative surgery for ectopic pregnancy, and infertility tubal surgery. In pregnancies after laparoscopic tubal coagulations, the incidence of ectopics has been shown to be up to 50% [18]. A 15–20% recurrence of ectopic pregnancy in patients undergoing salpingostomy for ectopics is generally cited [7].
6. The **use of intrauterine devices** has been suggested as a causative factor. Current studies suggest this may not be true with available nonhormonal devices [31].
7. **Hormonal effects** caused by the morning-after pill, progesterone-only pills, and progesterone-containing intrauterine devices have been suggested as etiologic agents in tubal pregnancy due to inhibited tubal motility or inefficient cilial currents [31].

B. **Conditions that increase the receptiveness of foreign tissue**

1. A **change in the physiology of the tube** may occur involving abnormal peristalsis or abnormal cilial activity.

C. **Transmigration.** Migration of the egg from one ovary to the opposite tube may be the etiology of some ectopic pregnancies. This delay may encourage an ectopic location for implantation. The corpus luteum is in the contralateral ovary in 30–50% of ectopics [31].

D. Conditions associated with multiple embryos

1. In vitro fertilization with transfer of multiple fertilized ova is associated with a greater risk of ectopic gestation, particularly heterotopic pregnancies [16]. The incidence of combined gestations with intrauterine and extrauterine pregnancy in the absence of ovarian stimulation is generally estimated at about 1 in 30,000 pregnancies.

IV. Pathogenesis. Since most ectopic pregnancies are in the fallopian tube, the pathologic process there will be presented. Ovarian, cervical, and abdominal pregnancies will be discussed separately in sec. **VII.**

The fertilized ovum that implants in the epithelium of the tube penetrates the mucosa much as it does in the endometrium. Early nidation changes are similar to those seen in an intrauterine pregnancy, including softening of the cervix and isthmus and some increase in uterine size. The erosive action of trophoblast into the tubal muscularis with invasion of the maternal blood supply results in bleeding that may be intraluminal or may dissect through submucosal tissue planes. Bleeding may precede tubal rupture. The decidual changes with ectopic pregnancy are less pronounced than with intrauterine pregnancy. Since the tube provides inadequate room for growth, the pregnancy is extruded through the fimbriated end or the tube ruptures, generally between the sixth and twelfth gestational weeks.

A. Ampulla. Eighty percent of ectopic pregnancies occur in this portion of the fallopian tube, where more growth of the embryo can occur prior to disruption. Rupture is most commonly noted at approximately 12 weeks and may take place through the serosal surface with extrusion into the abdominal cavity, or the pregnancy may abort out through the fimbriated end of the tube. This extrusion may be the etiology of some fimbrial, ovarian, or abdominal pregnancies.

B. Isthmus. Approximately 13% of ectopic pregnancies occur in the isthmus of the tube. Erosion and rupture in this narrow portion take place early and usually include rupture through the serosal surface into the peritoneal cavity. Occasionally rupture may occur along the line of attachment of the mesosalpinx; the embryo escapes between the folds of the broad ligament and continues to develop as a ligament pregnancy.

C. Interstitium. Pregnancy in this location accounts for approximately 2% of all tubal gestations. Because of the greater distensibility of the myometrium, rupture is likely to occur later in the pregnancy, even up to the fourth month. Bleeding is more severe and may be rapidly fatal. Hysterectomy is occasionally necessary with a large uterine defect.

D. Fimbria. Implantation occurs on the fimbria in approximately 5% of tubal pregnancies.

V. Diagnosis. The diagnosis of ectopic pregnancy is not always obvious; incorrect initial diagnoses are common. Women with ectopic pregnancy may present catastrophically in shock or may have vague lower abdominal pain and minimal vaginal bleeding. They key to the diagnosis is the maintenance of a high index of suspicion in the evaluation of any woman in the reproductive-age group who presents with lower abdominal pain.

The early pain from an ectopic pregnancy is usually colicky in nature and is believed to be a result of tubular distention. The growing pregnancy occasionally can be palpated as an adnexal or cul-de-sac fullness, although corpus luteum cysts may be confused with a tubal mass. With the production of hormones, the endometrium undergoes decidual change, and the uterus may enlarge slightly and soften, giving the impression of an early intrauterine pregnancy. When the embryo dies, hormonal support of the endometrium is lost. This gives rise to vaginal bleeding, which may be mistaken for menses or miscarriage. A decidual cast may be sloughed and confused with products of conception; any tissue brought in by a patient should be inspected microscopically.

Aggressive diagnostic evaluation of the patient with a suspected ectopic pregnancy is essential. A ruptured ectopic pregnancy represents a major surgical emergency. If the patient undergoes the operation before shock intervenes, morbidity approaches zero, compared with 16–30% with delayed surgery. Diagnosis before rupture is also associated with improved fertility rates.

A. Diagnosis of the catastrophic presentation. Little diagnostic acumen is required.

The patient is in shock and has a surgical abdomen with rigidity, tenderness, and signs of peritoneal irritation. Fever is usually absent. Pelvic examintion may reveal a full or doughy mass in the cul-de-sac caused by intraperitoneal blood. Culdocentesis (see sec. **VI.B.1**) at the time of speculum examination can be done rapidly to confirm hemoperitoneum. The clinical picture usually demands that the patient be taken to the operating room. Conditions that may present similarly are few but may include ruptured corpus luteum cyst and ruptured spleen.

B. Diagnosis of the subtly presenting ectopic pregnancy

1. The classic triad of symptoms and signs of ectopic pregnancy includes (1) history of missed menstrual period followed by abnormal vaginal bleeding, (2) abdominal or pelvic pain, and (3) an adnexal mass. This triad is noted in less than half of patients with ectopic pregnancy. Cervical motion tenderness is an abnormal finding of substantial importance.
   a. **Missed menses** is reported in 74–98% of patients [1, 10]; 15% have a normal menstrual history [15]. Vaginal bleeding is reported in 50–94% of patients with ectopic pregnancies [1, 6, 10]. Various degrees may occur, with mild to moderate bleeding associated with ectopic pregnancy, and heavy vaginal bleeding more indicative of threatened or incomplete abortion.
   b. **Abdominal or pelvic pain** is reported in 90–100% of patients with ectopic pregnancies [1, 6, 10, 15]. The pain is often localized initially and is unilateral in 25% or more patients in some series.
   c. **A palpable mass in the adnexae** or cul-de-sac is reported in approximately 40% of cases [1, 10]. The absence of a mass even during examination under anesthesia does not rule out ectopic pregnancy. Conversely a corpus luteum cyst may cause an adnexal mass.
2. **Physical examination** shows abdominal or pelvic tenderness in 97% of cases [1]. The tenderness is generalized in 45%, in the bilateral lower quadrants in 25%, and in a unilateral lower quadrant in 30%. Rebound tenderness may or may not be present, depending on the amount of peritoneal irritation. Cervical motion tenderness, if elicited with gentleness, suggests adnexal pathology, which in the absence of infection or a twisted ovarian cyst strongly suggests tubal pregnancy. Vigorous cervical motion will cause discomfort in most patients regardless of the condition of the adnexae.
3. **Other signs and symptoms**
   a. **Shoulder pain** may accompany a ruptured ectopic pregnancy and is believed to be secondary to diaphragmatic irritation from hemoperitoneum. Approximately 15% of patients present with this symptom.
   b. **A soft and slightly enlarged uterus** is palpable in most patients if the pelvic organs can be adequately evaluated.
   c. **Cullen's sign** (periumbilical ecchymosis from intraperitoneal bleeding) is a very rare finding not noted in recent studies.
   d. **A low-grade temperature** is present in less than 10% of women with ectopic pregnancies [31].
4. **Differential diagnosis.** In attempting to diagnose ectopic pregnancy in a stable patient, one must consider the following possibilities:
   a. **Salpingitis** is the disease most commonly mistaken for a tubal pregnancy. Abdominal pain, abnormal vaginal bleeding, and cervical motion tenderness may all by present, although bleeding is unusual. Fever is common and is usually greater than 38°C. The leukocyte count is higher than with ectopic pregnancy. Adnexal tenderness may be unilateral. A pregnancy test is negative.
   b. **Threatened abortion** may present with similar symptoms. Bleeding is usually more profuse, pain is usually in the lower midline abdominal area, and cervical motion tenderness is usually absent. A corpus luteum cyst may cause a confusing adnexal mass.
   c. **Appendicitis,** like ectopic pregnancy, frequently presents with widely varying clinical pictures. Persistent right lower quadrant pain and tenderness, usually with fever and gastrointestinal symptoms, suggest this diagnosis. A rectal exam may show pain posterior to the uterus and adnexal area.
   d. **Many other diagnoses** can cause pelvic pain or vaginal bleeding to the extent

that a patient will present to the emergency room. Dysfunctional uterine bleeding is usually painless and heavier than with ectopic pregnancy. A persistent corpus luteum or corpus luteum cyst may cause abdominal pain and an adnexal mass. A ruptured corpus luteum or follicular cyst with intraperitoneal bleeding may present the same clinical picture as ruptured ectopic pregnancy. Torsion of an ovarian cyst usually presents with abdominal pain and an adnexal mass but without a history of amenorrhea or abnormal vaginal bleeding. A pregnancy test will be discriminatory. Patients occasionally present with severe dysmenorrhea or pain from an intrauterine device; pain is usually midline and the pregnancy test is negative. In early pregnancy, gastroenteritis or a pathologic condition of the urinary tract such as infection or colic from a calculus may also mimic ectopic pregnancy. In this case intravenous pyelography or fetal sonogram is indicated. Informed consent is necessary for the x-ray exposure if a viable intrauterine pregnancy is in question.

C. Laboratory tests

1. With **catastrophic presentation** routine laboratory work should be obtained at the same time blood is drawn for ABO typing and cross-matching. Appropriate surgical intervention should not be delayed while awaiting laboratory results.
2. **Subtle presentation**
   a. A **complete blood count** should be obtained as a baseline. A significantly elevated leukocyte count suggests an infectious process. Hemoglobin and hematocrit determinations are necessary for follow-up to rule out intraabdominal bleeding.

   b. **Urinalysis** is necessary when the presence of a urinary tract infection or renal calculus has not been ruled out.

   c. **Pregnancy test.** Enzyme-linked immunoabsorbent assay urine pregnancy tests are generally sensitive to 50 mIU/ml. They are available within 30 minutes and can be run on random urine specimens if not excessively dilute. The reaction is very specific and no cross-reactivity is noted with urine protein. The results can also be semiquantitative based on the depth of color change.

   For **discrimination of ectopic or other abnormal pregnancies from normal** intrauterine pregnancies, the most sensitive test is the serum beta-human chorionic gonadotrophic (HCG) radioimmunoassay. A qualitative test will usually be positive to 25 mIU/ml. Quantitative beta-HCG testing is positive to 5 mIU and allows determination of doubling time, which has been reported to range from 1.4–1.5 days in early pregnancy, to 3.3–3.5 days in 6- to 7-week gestations. Approximately 85% of normal pregnancies will be within these limits [12].

   Ectopic pregnancies are generally associated with lower beta-HCG levels than intrauterine pregnancies. An exact correlation with the last menstrual period is difficult to determine due to the uncertainty of the onset of the last menstrual period in many patients. Abnormal doubling time allows differentiation of an abnormal from a normal pregnancy but does not specify the location of the pregnancy.

   d. **Progesterone.** A recent study using direct radioimmunoassays to compare ectopic with early intrauterine (3½–7½ weeks post last menstrual period) pregnancies found no normal gestations with progesterone levels below 20. The highest level in an ectopic gestation was 12.9 [17]. Not all studies have shown as clear-cut a delineation, and serum progesterone drops in the first trimester, reaching a nadir at about nine weeks. Low levels also occur with early spontaneous abortion. Taking these factors into account as well as the individual variation between labs, the increasing availability of rapid serum progesterone assays may be a useful method of differentiating viable from nonviable early pregnancies.

   e. A recent report suggested that **human chorionic somatomammotropin** may be a sensitive predictor of impending tubal rupture in medically treated patients [4].

f. Ultrasound. Abdominal ultrasound will generally show an intrauterine gestational sac with beta-HCG levels of 6000–6500 mIU/ml (or greater). An absence of a gestational sac with a beta-HCG at or above this level is diagnostic of ectopic pregnancy in about 86% of cases [11]. Unfortunately only 25–40% of ectopic pregnancies present with beta-HCG concentrations greater than or equal to 6000 mIU/ml at the initial evaluation. An ultrasonographically detected complex adnexal mass may be suggestive of an ectopic pregnancy, especially when associated with free peritoneal fluid.

(1) Transvaginal ultrasound has recently become available with improved resolution over abdominal scanning. It also has the advantage of not requiring a full bladder, resulting in less patient discomfort and less technical difficulty. In one series intrauterine pregnancies were identifiable 35 days from the last menstrual period, approximately 7 days earlier than could be achieved with abdominal ultrasound [27]. Some studies have suggested that an intrauterine pregnancy should be visualized with beta-HCG levels as low as 2500 mIU/ml. The gestational sac is visualized within five weeks of the last menstrual period, with the embryonic sac seen at about five-and-a-half weeks. A pseudogestational sac caused by a decidual cast may occur in 10–20% of patients with ectopic pregnancies [20, 25]. A **double-lined sac** was correlated with an intrauterine pregnancy in 98.3% of patients studied in one review [20], making this finding extremely helpful in identifying an early intrauterine pregnancy. The fetal pole will be visualized a few days later, and fetal heart motion may be detected as early as five-and-a-half weeks after the last menstrual period and is almost always seen by the end of the sixth week [27].

Ultrasound is most useful when an early intrauterine pregnancy can definitely be diagnosed or if fetal heart tones are visible in the adnexae. The information is otherwise only suggestive, not diagnostic.

VI. Treatment

A. Catastrophic presentation. The patient presenting in shock with a surgical abdomen should be taken directly to the operating room.

1. In preparation for operation, resuscitation with intravenous fluids should be started immediately. After vital signs are obtained and prior to completing the history and physical, two large-bore intravenous cannulas should be placed and fluid replacement begun with balanced salt solution (Ringer's lactate). A **Foley catheter** should be inserted into the bladder and urine output maintained at 30–50 ml/hour. Central venous monitoring is generally superfluous to the patient's care and time should not be spent placing one. **Blood should be drawn** for routine preoperative tests and for ABO typing and cross-matching of at least 4 units of packed cells. **History** from the patient or accompanying family and friends should be obtained as quickly as possible and a **general physical and pelvic examination** should be performed. As with other acute surgical emergencies involving substantial blood loss, **control of the blood loss is critical.** It may be necessary in some patients to proceed to laparotomy to stop the bleeding while fluid resuscitation is continued rather than spending time with attempts at stabilization. Mortality can be the result of overly vigorous crystalloid resuscitation without replacement of needed blood products or surgical stabilization. This may cause inadequate oxygen transport, pulmonary edema, or coagulopathy.

2. Operative procedure. The indicated procedure is the one that will control the hemorrhage in the shortest period of time. Either a low midline or Pfannenstiel's incision may be made, depending on the relative certainty of the etiology of the patient's condition. On entering the peritoneal cavity, one may encounter a significant hemoperitoneum. Since most ectopic pregnancies are tubal in location, the site of rupture can generally be localized by rapid digital exploration of the pelvis. The site should be mobilized into the wound where hemostasis can be obtained quickly by clamping the pedicle. With the bleeding under control, full resuscitation with fluids, including blood if necessary, should rapidly stabilize the patient. The treatment of choice is partial or complete salpingectomy. The ipsilateral ovary should only be removed if involved or diseased. With a ruptured interstitial or cornual pregnancy, hysterectomy may be required. In any other case, hysterectomy has no place in the treatment of the patient with a catastrophic presentation.

B. **Subtle presentation.** In a patient with an unruptured ectopic pregnancy in whom blood loss is not great enough to produce a catastrophic picture, a significant diagnostic and therapeutic challenge is presented to minimize the patient's morbidity and preserve future fertility, if desired.

1. **Culdocentesis** is a practical way to make the diagnosis of hemoperitoneum in a woman because of the dependent position of the pouch of Douglas.
   a. **Technique** (Fig. 18-1)
      (1) With the woman in the lithotomy position, **the cervix is visualized** with a bivalve speculum. A semi-Fowler's position, if possible, will improve the pooling of blood in the cul-de-sac.
      (2) **The vagina is swabbed** in an appropriate antiseptic.
      (3) **The posterior lip of the cervix is grasped** with a single-toothed tenaculum and pulled anteriorly and caudally. A local anesthetic may be used if desired.
      (4) **Puncture of the posterior fornix is performed** sharply with an 18- or 20-gauge spinal needle attached to a 10-ml syringe. Local anesthetic, again, may reduce patient discomfort. A pop is usually felt, followed by the sensation of being in an empty space as the peri-

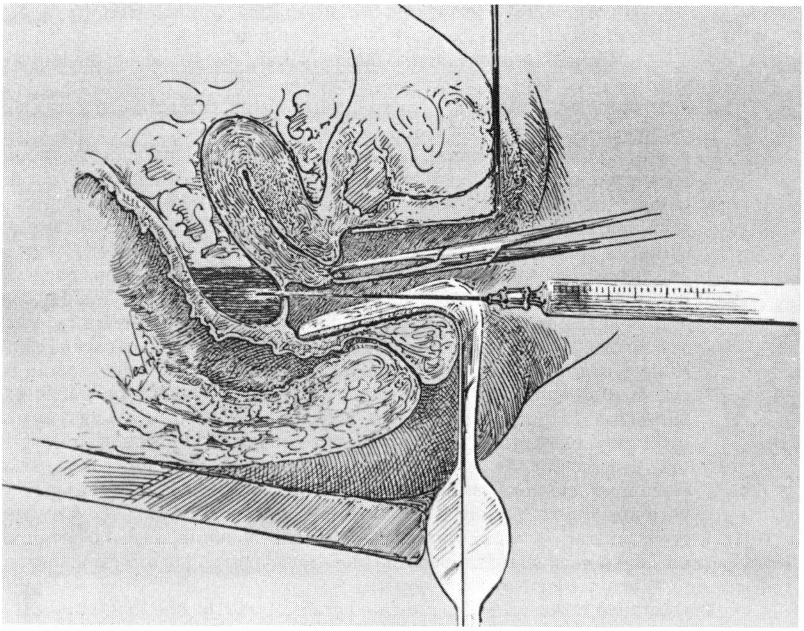

Fig. 18-1. Technique of culdocentesis. (From V. Capraro, J. Chuang, and C. Randall, Cul-de-sac aspiration and other diagnostic aids for ectopic pregnancy. *Int. Surg.* 52:254, 1970.)

toneum is perforated and the cul-de-sac is entered. A loss of resistance technique may also be used to confirm entry.

(5) **The syringe is used to aspirate** as the needle is withdrawn.

b. **Results**

(1) **Positive.** Nonclotting blood greater than 5 ml indicates a hemoperitoneum.

(2) **Negative**

(a) **Clear fluid** from the peritoneal cavity may be normal or may indicate a leaking or ruptured ovarian cyst. Fluid may also be serosanguinous.

(b) **Purulent aspirate** strongly suggests pelvic inflammatory disease or possibly a ruptured appendix as the cause of the symptoms. The fluid may be sent for culture.

(3) **Equivocal (nondiagnostic)**

(a) **No fluid** may indicate that no hemoperitoneum is present, that the area is walled off by adhesions, or that the needle has not penetrated the cul-de-sac.

(b) **Clotting blood** usually means that the needle has punctured a blood vessel. Rarely, bleeding into the peritoneal cavity can be so rapid that blood obtained by culdocentesis will be clotted. Culdocentesis is not usually needed in such cases because the patient is in significant shock.

c. **Success rates.** False-positive culdocentesis results can be caused by ruptured ovarian cysts, retrograde menses, or incomplete abortion. False-negatives are generally a result of technical difficulty. The false-negative rate for culdocentesis is 11–14%. False-positive rates are not commonly reported in the literature. Approximately 15% of culdocenteses are nondiagnostic [31].

d. **Complications** of culdocentesis are unusual but include the following:

(1) **Accidental amniocentesis.**

(2) **A loop of small bowel held in the cul-de-sac by adhesions may be perforated.** No significant sequelae have been reported.

(3) **A rectal serosal hematoma** from culdocentesis has been reported [2].

e. **Usefulness.** Culdocentesis is helpful in the diagnosis of ectopic pregnancy if its limitations are known and understood. If the clinical picture is suggestive of an ectopic pregnancy and one obtains a positive culdocentesis, one should proceed to laparotomy or operative laparoscopy without further delay to minimize morbidity and maximize chances of preserving fertility. One study [6] noted a positive culdocentesis with 65% of unruptured and 85% of ruptured ectopic pregnancies. However, it must be remembered that a positive result only confirms the presence of hemoperitoneum and not the presence of ectopic pregnancy. An equivocal tap is not helpful. A negative result does not definitely rule out an unruptured ectopic pregnancy. Therefore, a negative or equivocal result requires continued diagnostic procedures or careful observation, or both.

2. **Operative approach.** Procedures for direct visualization of the pelvis may be done on an outpatient or short-stay basis if these options are available in a full-service hospital. Scheduling diagnostic procedures for an ectopic pregnancy at an ambulatory clinic or a surgical center not capable of handling major procedures is not recommended. All procedures should be performed under general anesthesia for optimal visualization with the laparoscope.

a. **Examination under anesthesia.** The patient should be gently examined bimanually under general anesthesia to minimize chances of rupturing the ectopic pregnancy. Pain and tenderness during the initial examination without anesthesia may have prevented the recognition of a pelvic mass.

b. Dilatation and curettage can be performed prior to laparoscopy in those patients desiring pregnancy termination in the event that the pregnancy is intrauterine. The presence of chorionic villi on a frozen section confirms intrauterine pregnancy. As mentioned before, combined intrauterine and extrauterine pregnancies can occur, but in the absence of ovarian stimulation are very rare. The absence of villi, especially with decidual changes or Arias-Stella reaction, strongly suggests an ectopic pregnancy. This reaction (marked cellular atypism, glandular proliferation, and evidence of hypersecretory endometrium) is noted in approximately 25% of pregnancies at any site and is a manifestation of marked progesterone stimulation of the endometrium.

c. Laparoscopy is an extremely valuable tool in the diagnosis and treatment of ectopic pregnancy, especially when the fallopian tube is unruptured. General anesthesia is usually required for adequate insufflation of the peritoneal cavity with carbon dioxide to allow visualization of the entire pelvis. Problems with visualization may occur in the patient with postoperative adhesions or with a history of severe pelvic inflammatory disease. A manipulating probe is required and is inserted through a second suprapubic incision. Rarely, the pelvic organs and cul-de-sac cannot be visualized adequately and a minilaparotomy is required for exposure. In those patients with a history of multiple abdominal or pelvic procedures or possible adhesive disease, an open laparoscopic technique may be employed to minimize the risk of bowel injury.

If a significant hemoperitoneum is noted on initial inspection of the peritoneal cavity, one should terminate the laparoscopic procedure and proceed to laparotomy. Otherwise, a fusiform enlarged blue fallopian tube on one side suggests an ectopic pregnancy. If only a unilateral ovarian cyst is noted, the patient's symptoms may be attributable to this. If both tubes in their entirety, the ovaries, the broad ligament, and the cul-de-sac can all be visualized with no apparent abnormality, the results of the laparoscopy are negative. It is possible to perform laparoscopy at such an early gestation that a very early ectopic pregnancy can be missed. Thus, all patients with negative findings should be followed closely postoperatively until an intrauterine pregnancy can be confirmed.

In addition to being valuable in the diagnosis and treatment of ectopic pregnancy, laparoscopy is **safe and cost-effective** in terms of hospital stay. The current estimated maternal mortality from laparoscopy is approximately 5 in 100,000. The false-positive rate for laparoscopy is approximately 5% and the false-negative rate is 3–4% [31].

(1) Surgical findings at laparoscopy with prognostic significance for fertility should be described. These include adhesions, the condition of the ovaries and contralateral tube, the site and size of the ectopic, the location of the corpus luteum, and the length of the remaining tube [31].

d. Operative laparoscopy is desirable for the removal of a small unruptured isthmic or ampullary gestation.

(1) Selection. Most authors consider a diameter of 3 cm or less for removal through the laparoscope. With overly large gestations, it is difficult to remove the tissue from the abdomen, and an increased risk of hemorrhage from the ectopic site postoperatively exists. Ruptured ectopic gestation is generally considered a contraindication to laparoscopic approach with all but extremely experienced operators. Cornual gestations, whether ruptured or unruptured, should never be treated laparoscopically because of the high risk of uncontrollable hemorrhage [30].

(2) Technique

(a) Salpingostomy. Either a double- or a triple-puncture technique is used. With a **double-puncture technique,** a 10- or 11-mm operative laparoscope is introduced through the primary incision inferior to the umbilicus and a 5-mm accessory trocar is used through the suprapubic puncture site. A **triple-puncture technique** allows more flexibility. A smaller (5 or 7 mm) primary puncture is used for a nonoperative panoramic laparoscope and a 5-mm trocar is inserted on the side contralateral to the operative site. The suprapubic site is used for the introduction of atraumatic grasping forceps through a third puncture for stabilization of the tube. The operative instruments are inserted through the lateral puncture site.

The hemoperitoneum is aspirated. Next, atraumatic forceps are introduced through the suprapubic site and used to stabilize the tube close to the ectopic site. The antimesenteric border of the ectopic is incised using a fine-needle electrode or an operative laser, and the incision is extended 1–2 cm over the gestation with hook scissors. The products of conception usually extrude spontaneously but may be removed with fine forceps. The site should be irrigated carefully with Ringer's lactate using a suction irrigation device, and any remaining tissue should be removed. Tissue should be sent for microscopic analysis, both to confirm the diagnosis and because true trophoblastic disease has been reported in tubal pregnancies, as well as triploidy (partial moles) [22].

(i) Hemostasis is accomplished using coagulation with electrocautery or laser. The salpingostomy may be left open or closed using endosutures or extracorporeal knots; in animal models no significant differences were found in subsequent pregnancy rates or adhesions.

Vasopressin (5 IU in 20 ml normal saline) can be injected into the mesosalpinx or tubal wall prophylactically or for persistent bleeding. A spinal needle can be used to inject through the abdominal wall. If these measures fail to provide hemostasis, laparotomy should be performed.

(b) Salpingectomy. Laparoscopic segmental resection can be accomplished for ruptured isthmic or ampullary gestation. After aspiration of the hemoperitoneum, the segment of tube containing the gestation is elevated. The tube is coagulated with bipolar forceps proximal and distal to the ectopic and then divided with scissors or laser. The mesosalpinx is coagulated and cut in a similar fashion. The segment can be removed entirely or in pieces through a 10-mm sleeve.

e. Laparotomy. Again, in the patient without a catastrophic presentation, a conservative procedure can be considered. Operations include salpingostomy, salpingotomy, partial salpingectomy, and expression of tubal abortion. In the patient desirous of future fertility, atraumatic techniques should be used. These include meticulous hemostasis, minimal handling of the tubes, copious irrigation with a balanced salt solution, and atraumatic instruments and sutures [31].

More radical procedures for patients not interested in fertility include salpingectomy and salpingo-oophorectomy. In the absence of cornual pregnancy with uncontrollable bleeding, hysterectomy is not recommended.

(1) Conservative methods

(a) Salpingostomy can be performed as described before. After the linear incision is made in the antimesenteric border of the tube, the products of conception can be removed with forceps, suction, or scalpel handle. The tube is then thoroughly irrigated with Ringer's lactate. This can be conveniently done using the cannulas from two large-bore angiocaths and 10-ml syringes. Further bleeding points are identified and coagulated. If bleeding continues, vasopressin can be injected into the mesosalpinx as described before, or the mesenteric vessels underneath the tube can be ligated with a 4-0 or 5-0 suture. Alternatively, compression of the mesosalpinx below the operative site for five minutes may control the bleeding. If bleeding persists despite these measures, a segmental resection of the tube should be performed. Tubal closure is not necessary as discussed before. Tubal contents should be verified pathologically. The technique of salpingostomy is shown in Fig. 18-2.

Linear salpingostomy or salpingotomy seems to result in a higher rate of subsequent intrauterine pregnancy than either total or partial salpingectomy [30]. However, the more favorable reproductive outcome may, in part, reflect selection bias, as linear

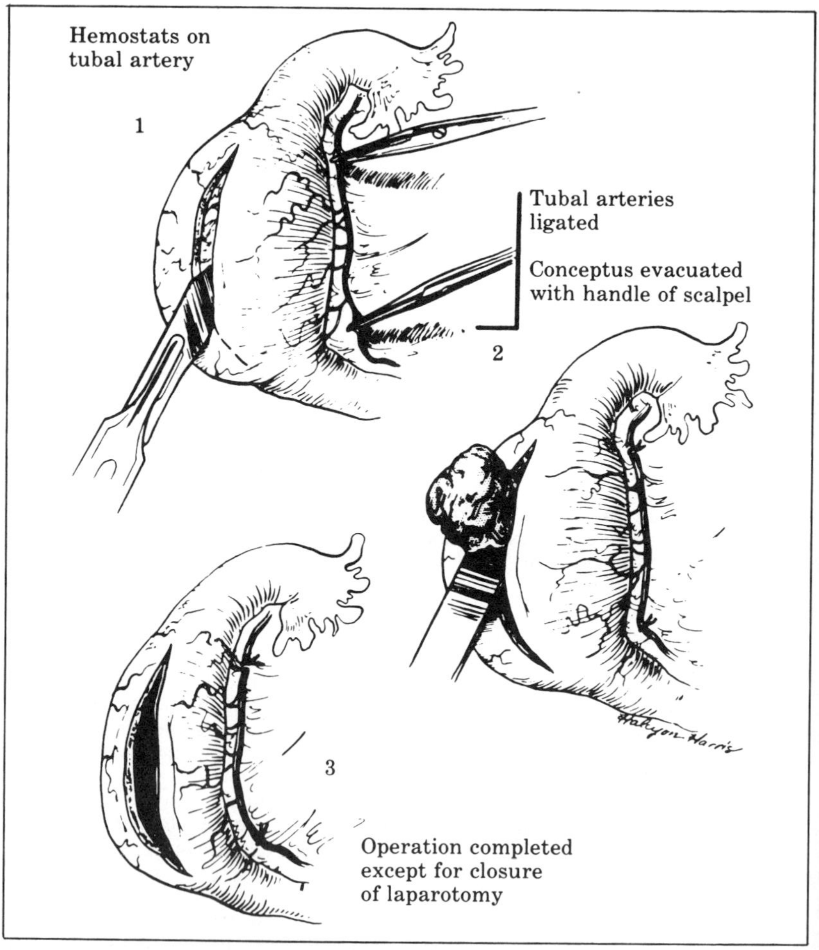

Fig. 18-2. Conservative management of unruptured tubal pregnancy by salpingostomy. (From P. Tompkins, Preservation of fertility by conversative surgery for ectopic pregnancy: Principles and report of a case. *Fertil. Steril.* 7:448, 1956. Reproduced by permission of The American Fertility Society.)

salpingostomies are generally reserved for small, unruptured gestations. Viable pregnancy rates are reported as 50–60% with a repeat ectopic rate of approximately 20%. The overall subsequent conception rate in women with ectopic pregnancy is approximately 60%, with only half of these resulting in live births [30].

(b) Partial salpingectomy has the theoretic advantage of preserving the tube for future reanastamosis and can be performed through a minilaparotomy incision. In patients not desirous of future fertility, it also has the further advantage of eliminating the possibility of residual trophoblastic tissue.

(c) Expression of tubal abortion ("milking"). Fimbrial evacuation is the easiest procedure but is also associated in most studies with the most complications [30]. The risk of recurrence may be more than double the risk reported for radical surgery. However, in one study with carefully selected patients, the subsequent intrauterine pregnancy rate was 92%. This method is not currently recommended by most authors.

(2) Definitive surgery

(a) Salpingectomy and salpingo-oophorectomy were formerly the most common procedures for the treatment of tubal pregnancy. The risk of recurrence in the contralateral tube has been reported as up to 33% [31]. Salpingo-oophorectomy has no advantage over salpingectomy alone since data indicate that fertility after either procedure is almost the same [31].

(b) Hysterectomy was previously considered for patients with pelvic inflammatory disease or recurrent ectopics with destruction of both tubes. With the current status of in vitro fertilization, this is no longer advisable for patients who desire future fertility. Hysterectomy has also been advocated for patients with large symptomatic leiomyomas or malignant ovarian tumors. It is not advisable for the patient with previous tubal ligation or desire for sterilization due to the increased morbidity of surgery and risk of further blood loss with the need for transfusion. Hysterectomy eliminates the risk of recurrent ectopic pregnancy, although pregnancy in the tubal remnant after hysterectomy has been reported [26]. The risk of subsequent uterine pathology is eliminated.

If hysterectomy is considered, the patient should have had a normal Pap smear within the last six months and no excessive intraperitoneal blood loss. Hysterectomy for sterilization is not possible in most states. An emergency hysterectomy for ruptured interstitial pregnancy does not fall under these sterilization restrictions.

f. Postoperative management. With the increasing popularity of conservative surgery for ectopic pregnancy, it is not always possible to guarantee complete removal of all trophoblastic tissue. Residual functional tissue may result in continued growth and delayed hemorrhage. Patients with conservative surgery should be followed with quantitative beta-HCG levels. With fairly complete removal of trophoblast, levels should be 20% or less of intraoperative levels 48–72 hours after surgery [24]. **Symptomatic patients** with rising beta-HCG levels require repeat surgery. **Asymptomatic patients** have been managed with reoperation, or observation if persistent levels are below 200 [30]. **Methotrexate therapy** also shows promise in treatment of these patients [23].

Patients undergoing **conservative tubal surgery** are generally advised to use contraception for a minimum of one month after their surgery to allow resolution of edema and inflammation. Patients scheduled for secondary surgery or reanastomosis should use contraception until the time of the second operation. There is a risk of repeat ectopic in the residual stump. **Hysterosalpingogram or second-look laparoscopy** should be considered if conception has not occurred by six months after the procedure.

Rh immunization is possible after ectopic pregnancy, and a microdose of RhoGAM immunoglobulin should be given to any Rh-negative–unsensitized patient. Although the risk of Rh sensitization is small, the safety of the immunoglobulin argues for reducing this risk to near zero.

VII. Unusual locations. Ectopic pregnancy may develop in locations other than the fallopian tube.

A. A true ovarian pregnancy is one in which the sperm fertilized the ovum prior to ovulation, following which the zygote implanted within the ovarian tissue. Specific criteria were established by Spiegelberg [26a]:

1. The tube on the affected side is intact.
2. The fetal sac occupies the position of the ovary.
3. The ovary is connected to the uterus by the utero-ovarian ligament.
4. Definite ovarian tissue is present in the gestational sac wall.

It is known that the egg undergoes myosis in the follicle and is ready for fertilization before ovulation. Many authorities believe that ovarian pregnancies result from implantation of a fertilized ovum into the ovary. Treatment is cystectomy or wedge resection; oophorectomy is rarely necessary.

B. Cervical pregnancy occurs when the zygote bypasses the endometrium and implants into the cervical mucosa, eventually embedding in the connective tissue structure of the cervix. The incidence is approximately 0.1%. Examination shows a **large tumor separate from the uterine fundus.** Products of conception may extrude from the external os and may mimic an incomplete abortion, with the external os open, but the internal os closed. The uterus may take on an **hour-glass shape** on ultrasound. The **primary symptom is bleeding,** which may be so serious as to require termination of the pregnancy before 20 weeks.

Most cervical pregnancies present during the second trimester. Maintenance of the pregnancy to viability is rarely reported, and previous maternal mortality rates were as high as 45%. Prior treatment was termination by abdominal hysterectomy, but successful treatment with methotrexate allowing conservation of fertility has recently been reported [21, 28].

C. Abdominal pregnancy. Abdominal pregnancies are pregnancies implanted on a peritoneal surface. They account for approximately 0.003% of all ectopic gestations. An abdominal pregnancy may result from a tubal pregnancy that aborts out the fimbriated end of the tube, reimplants on a peritoneal surface, and survives. Exceedingly rare cases have been reported of abdominal pregnancy after extrusion of an intrauterine pregnancy through a myometrial defect into the broad ligament. Some cases may implant primarily in the abdominal cavity. An abdominal pregnancy without mechanical growth restrictions may rarely progress to term. Risks include hemorrhage from placental abruption, especially with surgical manipulation, and injury to other organs.

1. **Diagnosis.** The patient may give a history consistent with tubal abortion (vaginal bleeding, mild abdominal pain). Physical examination may show a very easily palpated fetus and a separate small uterine fundus. A cross-table lateral x ray of the maternal abdomen showing the fetal skeleton overlaying the maternal vertebrae is strong evidence of an abdominal pregnancy. Ultrasound can be diagnostic.
2. **Treatment.** Once the diagnosis is made, intervention is usually advised due to the risk of placental accident. Fetal survival without intervention is approximately 20%. Preparations for laparotomy should include a well-hydrated patient and at least 6–8 units of packed cells, typed, crossed, and readily available. Excessive bleeding should be expected. Expert anesthetic support is essential. Exposure should be excellent and technique atraumatic.

The fetus is generally easily delivered. The placenta should be left in situ as profuse hemorrhage can occur with attempted manipulation unless the blood supply can be isolated and ligated. Most placentas will resorb without sequelae, but possible risks include infection, adhesions, bowel obstruction, and sepsis. The risks associated with leaving the placenta in place are generally felt to be less serious than the risk of fatal hemorrhage or injury to vital structures associated with removal.

VIII. Medical management

A. Expectant management has been reported since 1955. Surgical reoperation is necessary in up to 50% and inflammation with dense adhesions is reported. Survival of chorionic villi with tubal destruction has been reported up to 15 months after the demise of the pregnancy [30]. It has been suggested that the probability of spontaneous resolution is highest for patients with serum beta-HCG levels less than 1000 who are without pain [9].

With increasingly sensitive pregnancy hormone assays and careful surveillance of patients undergoing infertility evaluation, more patients with early ectopic pregnancy or possible tubal abortion are likely to be encountered. Prognostic signs for observation include a negative culdocentesis, an asymptomatic patient, and low and dropping levels of beta-HCG.

B. Methotrexate has been used in the treatment of ectopic gestations [29]. Initial reports were in cases of abdominal pregnancy, but good results have also been demonstrated in patients with small unruptured tubal gestations. It is contraindicated if cardiac activity is seen in the tube on ultrasound due to the risk of severe hemorrhage [29]. Subsequent intrauterine and recurrent ectopic pregnancy rates have not been determined. The availability of laparoscopic treatment and the need for laparoscopic diagnosis of ectopic pregnancy make this method less desirable except when necessary for preservation of fertility as in cornual or cervical pregnancies [13, 21, 28]. It has also been used for a patient with ovarian hyperstimulation syndrome [5].

C. RU-486. Although this antiprogesterone is an effective abortifacient in an early intrauterine pregnancy, some attempts have failed because a tubal gestation was later discovered. Initial attempts at use for ectopic pregnancy have not been successful, possibly due to abnormal progesterone levels in ectopic gestations [14, 30].

References

1. Alsuleiman, S. A., and Grimes, E. M. Ectopic pregnancy: A review of 147 cases. *J. Reprod. Med.* 27:101, 1982.
2. Anasti, J., et al. Rectal serosal hematoma: An unusual complication of culdocentesis. *Obstet. Gynecol.* 65:725, 1985.
3. Barnes, A. B., Wennberg, C. N., and Barnes, B. A. Ectopic pregnancy: Incidence and review of determinant factors. *Obstet. Gynecol. Surv.* 38:345, 1983.
4. Carson, S. A., et al. Rising human chorionic somatomammotropin predicts ectopic pregnancy rupture following methotrexate therapy. *Fertil. Steril.* 51:593, 1989.
5. Chotiner, H. C. Nonsurgical management of ectopic pregnancy associated with severe hyperstimulation syndrome. *Obstet. Gynecol.* 66:740, 1985.
6. DeCherney, A. H., and Mayheux, R. Modern management of tubal pregnancy. *Curr. Probl. Obstet. Gynecol.* 6:4, 1983.
7. DeCherney, A. H., Maheaux, R., and Naftolin, F. Salpingostomy for ectopic pregnancy in the sole patent oviduct: Reproductive outcome. *Fertil. Steril.* 37:619, 1982.
8. Dorfman, S. F., et al. Ectopic pregnancy mortality in the United States, 1979 to 1980: Clinical aspects. *Obstet. Gynecol.* 64(3):386, 1984.
9. Fernandez, H., et al. Spontaneous resolution of ectopic pregnancy. *Obstet. Gynecol.* 71:171, 1988.

10. Gonzalez, F. A., and Waxman, M. Ectopic pregnancy: A retrospective study of 501 consecutive patients. *Diagn. Gynecol. Obstet.* 3:181, 1981.
11. Kadar, N., DeVore, G., and Romero, R. Discriminatory hCG zone: Its use in the sonographic evaluation for ectopic pregnancy. *Obstet. Gynecol.* 58:156, 1981.
12. Kadar, N., and Romero, R. Observations on the log human chorionic gonadotropin-time relationship in early pregnancy and its practical implications. *Am. J. Obstet. Gynecol.* 157:73, 1987.
13. Kaplan, E. R., et al. Successful treatment of a live cervical pregnancy with methotrexate and folinic acid: A case report. *J. Reprod. Med.* 34:10, 1989.
14. Leach, R. E., and Ory, S. J. Modern management of ectopic pregnancy. *J. Reprod. Med.* 34:324, 1989.
15. Lucas, C. Place of culdocentesis in the diagnosis of ectopic pregnancy. *Br. Med. J.* 1:200, 1970.
16. Lund, P. R., Fielaff, G. W., and Aiman, E. J. In vitro fertilization patient presenting in hemorrhagic shock caused by an unsuspected heterotopic pregnancy. *Am. J. Emerg. Med.* 7:49, 1989.
17. Matthews, C. P., Coulson, P. B., and Wild, R. A. Serum progesterone levels as an aid in the diagnosis of ectopic pregnancy. *Obstet. Gynecol.* 68:390, 1986.
18. McCausland, A. High rate of ectopic pregnancy following laparoscopic tubal coagulation failures. *Am. J. Obstet. Gynecol.* 136:97, 1980.
19. U.S. Dept. of Health and Human Services. Ectopic pregnancy: United States, 1986. *M.M.W.R.* 38:1, 1989.
20. Nyberg, D. A., et al. Ultrasonographic differentiation of the gestational sac of early intrauterine pregnancy from the pseudogestational sac of ectopic pregnancy. *Radiology* 146:755, 1983.
21. Oyer, R., et al. Treatment of cervical pregnancy with methotrexate. *Obstet. Gynecol.* 71:469, 1988.
22. Parmley, T. H. The histopathology of tubal pregnancy. *Clin. Obstet. Gynecol.* 30:119, 1987.
23. Patsner, B., and Kenigsberg, D. Successful treatment of persistent ectopic pregnancy with oral methotrexate therapy. *Fertil. Steril.* 50:982, 1988.
24. Pittaway, D. E. Beta HCG dynamics in ectopic pregnancy. *Clin. Obstet. Gynecol.* 30:129, 1987.
25. Reece, E. A., et al. Combined intrauterine and extrauterine gestations: A review. *Am. J. Obstet. Gynecol.* 146:323, 1983.
26. Reese, W. A. et al. Tubal pregnancy after total vaginal hysterectomy. *Ann. Emerg. Med.* 18:1107, 1989.
26a. Spiegelberg, O. Zur Cosuistik der ovarial schwangerschaft. *Arch. Gynaekol.* 13:73, 1878.
27. Steinkampf, M. P. Transvaginal sonography. *J. Reprod. Med.* 33:12, 1988.
28. Stovall, T. G., et al. Successful nonsurgical treatment of cervical pregnancy with methotrexate. *Fertil. Steril.* 50:672, 1988.
29. Stovall, T. G., Ling, F. W., and Buster, J. E. Outpatient chemotherapy of unruptured ectopic pregnancy. *Fertil. Steril.* 51:3, 1989.
30. Vermesh, M. Conservative management of ectopic gestation. *Fertil. Steril.* 51:559, 1989.
31. Weckstein, L. N. Current perspective on ectopic pregnancy. *Obstet. Gynecol. Surv.* 40:259, 1985.
32. Westrom, L., Bengtsson, L. P., and Mardh, P. A. Incidence, trends and risks of ectopic pregnancy in a population of women. *Br. Med. J.* 282:15, 1981.

19 Hypertensive Disorders

Helayne M. Silver

In recent years, the terminology and classifications used to describe the hypertensive disorders found in association with pregnancy have become increasingly confusing and misleading. Although the issue may sometimes appear to be one of semantics, the distinction between hypertension preceding pregnancy versus that induced by pregnancy is critical. The pathophysiology of these entities is distinct, the prognosis for mother and fetus is different, and therefore management is different. Chronic hypertension and preeclampsia will be discussed separately, but it must be kept in mind that these entities can, and fairly frequently do, coexist.

I. Classification*

A. Preeclampsia. Onset of hypertension with proteinuria, edema, or both, at greater than 20 weeks' gestational age. **Hypertension** is defined as a rise in systolic blood pressure of greater than 30 mm Hg or diastolic blood pressure greater than 15 mm Hg over baseline (nonpregnant or first trimester) or a blood pressure greater than 140/90 mm Hg on more than two occasions greater than six hours apart.

1. Eclampsia. The occurrence of seizures in a patient with preeclampsia.

2. Severe preeclampsia is diagnosed when one of the following criteria is met:

a. Blood pressure greater than 160 mm Hg systolic or 110 mm Hg diastolic on two occasions more than six hours apart.

b. Proteinuria greater than 5 gm/24 hours or 3–4+ on dipstick.

c. Oliguria less than 400 ml/24 hours.

d. Cerebral or visual disturbances.

e. Pulmonary edema or cyanosis.

B. Chronic hypertension may be diagnosed prospectively when the prepregnant blood pressure is known to be greater than 140/90 mm Hg or is detected prior to 20 weeks' gestation. When hypertension persists beyond six weeks' post partum, a diagnosis of chronic hypertension can be made retrospectively.

C. Chronic hypertension with superimposed preeclampsia. Preeclampsia is said to be superimposed on chronic hypertension when there is an exacerbation of hypertension of greater than 30 mm Hg systolic or 15 mm Hg diastolic, plus the appearance of significant proteinuria.

D. Late or transient hypertension. The development of hypertension during pregnancy without other signs of preeclampsia.

II. Preeclampsia

A. Epidemiology

1. Incidence. Preeclampsia occurs in 5–10% of pregnancies and is severe in less than 1%. Eclampsia occurs in approximately 0.1%.

2. Risk factors

a. Parity. Two-thirds of patients are nulliparous.

b. Family history of preeclampsia.

c. Medical problems. Higher incidence in patients with diabetes, chronic hypertension, and renal disease.

d. Extremes of age. In younger group, related to low parity. In older group, related to higher frequency of associated medical problems, such as chronic hypertension.

*As recommended by the American College of Obstetricians and Gynecologists (ACOG).

e. **Obstetric problems.** Higher incidence in patients with twins, hydatidiform mole, and hydrops fetalis.

3. **Predictive tests**

a. **Elevated second-trimester blood pressure.** Mean arterial blood pressure ([diastolic × 2 + systolic] ÷ 3) in the second trimester greater than 90 mm Hg has been said to predict subsequent development of preeclampsia. However, predictive ability of this test has varied widely.

b. **Angiotensin II infusion test.** Women who subsequently develop preeclampsia do not demonstrate the normal pregnancy-related refractoriness to the vasopressor effect of angiotensin II infusion. A large number of false-positives occur with this test, and the test is difficult to perform, which limits the clinical usefulness.

c. **Supine pressor test.** An increase in diastolic blood pressure of at least 20 mm Hg when turned from recumbent to supine when tested at 28–32 weeks has been said to be predictive of subsequent development of preeclampsia. Unfortunately, a high incidence of false-positives results, up to 90%.

d. The use of **screening laboratory studies** such as plasma fibronectin, atrial natriuretic factor, and urinary calcium excretion to predict the patient at risk for preeclampsia has been reported often, but unfortunately, none has proved to be clinically useful.

B. Diagnosis

1. **Hypertension.** Hypertension results from vasospasm and hyperdynamic circulation.

a. **Criteria. Significant hypertension** is defined as a rise of 30 mm Hg systolic or 15 mm Hg diastolic over baseline blood pressure either prepregnant or in the first trimester, or a blood pressure of 140/90 mm Hg after 20 weeks. The timing of the baseline blood pressure is critical, as blood pressure normally declines in the second trimester. Forty percent of severe chronic hypertensives will be normotensive in the midtrimester; therefore, a subsequent rise back to baseline in the third trimester may be misinterpreted as preeclampsia [3].

b. **Errors.** Common errors in measurement of blood pressure include the following:

(1) **Incorrect cuff size.** Too small a cuff size will result in falsely elevated and too large will result in falsely lowered blood pressure.

(2) **Position** is important to standardize, with the cuffed arm at the level of the heart. A frequent error is to repeat an elevated measurement with the patient in left lateral recumbency, with the cuff on the upper arm. Due to elevation of the arm above the level of the heart, this will falsely lower the blood pressure by 10–20 mm Hg. The best position for measurement is sitting, with the cuffed arm resting on the desk, at approximately heart level.

(3) **Korotoff's phase.** During pregnancy, the diastolic blood pressure measured at phase V (disappearance of sound) may be unusually low. To standardize measurements, use of phase IV (muffling of sound) is preferable.

(4) **Patient anxiety, exercise.** Wait 10 minutes after arrival to measure resting blood pressure.

2. **Proteinuria** is due to glomerular damage, resulting in increased basement membrane permeability, with protein loss of low selectivity.

a. **Criteria**

(1) **Significant proteinuria** is usually defined as greater than 1+ on dipstick or greater than 500 mg/dl in a 24-hour collection.

b. **Errors**

(1) **False-positive results** most commonly occur because of contamination with vaginal secretions, strenuous exercise, urinary tract infection, or dehydration.

(2) **False-negative results** may result from dilution.

(3) It is important to remember that preeclampsia can occur in the absence

of proteinuria; the kidney is only one of many target organs. In fact, in Chesley's [2] large series of eclamptic patients, 13% did not have significant proteinuria.

3. **Edema.** Edema results from the lowering of the serum colloid oncotic pressure secondary to albuminuria and loss of integrity of capillary endothelial cells leading to increased permeability. Both of these factors contribute to loss of fluid from the intravascular space into the extracellular space, clinically manifested by edema.
   a. **Criteria**
      (1) Significant edema is nondependent (face and hands) and is frequently associated with a rapid weight gain of greater than 5 lb in one week.
   b. **Errors**
      (1) Significant edema is found in many nonpreeclamptic patients, as high as 30% [19].
      (2) Significant edema is absent in many preeclamptics (40% of eclamptics in one institution) [19].

C. Complications of severe preeclampsia

1. **Maternal**
   a. **Central nervous system**
      (1) **Eclamptic seizure** occurs in 1% of preeclamptic patients. Computed tomography scans suggest the seizures of preeclampsia are the result of vasogenic cerebral edema [8]. The etiology is most likely endothelial permeability defects that result from the loss of protective vasospasm of cerebral autoregulation. The mean arterial pressure (MAP) at which this occurs varies individually, depending on the patient's normal baseline blood pressure. The normal MAP limits for cerebral autoregulation are 60–150 mm Hg, but in a young patient whose normal MAP may be 70–80 mm Hg, a MAP of 120–130 mm Hg may result in a loss of autoregulation [5]. This explains the frequently observed uncertain relationship between the severity of hypertension and the occurrence of eclampsia, and the importance of adequate blood pressure control.
      (2) **Intracerebral hemorrhage.** Although this is a rare complication of preeclampsia, it is a common finding on autopsy studies of patients with fatal preeclampsia [6]. In previously normotensive animals, a diastolic blood pressure of 120 mm Hg is associated with a risk of intracerebral hemorrhage [5], hence the common clinical practice of reserving antihypertensive therapy for treatment of diastolic blood pressures greater than 110 mm Hg.
      (3) **Blindness** may be secondary to retinal or cerebral edema or arterial spasm. This is a rare complication.
   b. **Renal**
      (1) **Acute tubular necrosis** results from underperfusion of the kidneys. Pregnancy appears to predispose to ischemic renal insults. Renal vasoconstriction and hypovolemia are common components of severe preeclampsia. Many severe preeclamptics will demonstrate oliguria; however, aberrations so severe as to result in acute tubular necrosis are uncommon.
      (2) **Acute cortical necrosis.** When renal ischemia is prolonged or extremely intense, destruction of glomeruli may result. Unlike acute tubular necrosis, this lesion is not reversible.
   c. **Hepatic**
      (1) **Subcapsular hematoma.** Hepatic ischemia may result in subcapsular hematoma. Hemorrhage may be extensive and on rare occasion results in hepatic rupture.
   d. **Cardiac**
      (1) **Cardiac failure.** The acute increase in afterload seen in severe preeclampsia may culminate in left ventricular failure. Initially, the heart will compensate by dilatation, making use of the Frank-Starling mechanism. When the heart dilates to such a degree that further stretching of the myocardial fibers offers no further mechanical benefit, and wall tension

increases, compromising coronary perfusion and increasing myocardial oxygen consumption, the **limit of preload reserve** is said to have been reached [16]. With a further increase in afterload, an increase in the inotropic state will be required. This is accomplished with an increase in sympathetic drive, which will further increase the afterload, and thus a vicious cycle may begin, culminating in left ventricular failure. This in turn will compromise other organ systems, leading to further complications.

e. Respiratory

(1) Pulmonary edema. Pure cardiogenic pulmonary edema will begin to manifest clinical symptoms at a pulmonary capillary wedge pressure of approximately 20–25 mm Hg. If the patient also has a low colloid oncotic pressure, or increased capillary permeability, as is common with severe preeclampsia, pulmonary edema may manifest earlier. When pulmonary edema occurs in preeclampsia, each of the abnormalities mentioned usually makes some contribution.

f. Coagulation

(1) Consumptive coagulopathy. Thrombocytopenia complicates severe preeclampsia in approximately 10% of cases [15]. Although the mechanism of platelet consumption is not completely understood, it is felt to be intravascular consumption secondary to excessive thrombin activity, which in turn results from endothelial damage. Generally, this is associated with elevated fibrin degradation products. The findings are more consistent with a chronic rather than an acute process. A compensatory increase in fibrinogen occurs beyond that normally found in association with pregnancy, and the prothrombin and partial thromboplastin times are usually normal.

(2) Acute disseminated intravascular coagulopathy. Abruptio placentae may occur in severe preeclampsia. In these cases there may be an acute coagulopathy secondary to the release of procoagulants such as thromboplastin.

2. Fetal

a. Intrauterine growth retardation. Growth retardation is a frequent complication of severe preeclampsia; in one series it occurred in 56% of patients [10]. In the placental site vessels of women with preeclampsia, the normal physiologic changes of loss of endothelium and smooth muscle do not occur. Histologic studies reveal decidual vascular lesions similar to the lesions seen in the vessels of rejected transplanted kidneys. Grossly, placental infarctions are frequently seen. These changes result in reduced placental perfusion and, subsequently, intrauterine growth retardation.

b. Prematurity. With severe preeclampsia, the requirement for delivery results in a prematurity rate of approximately 40% [1].

c. Perinatal mortality. Perinatal mortality is greatly increased secondary to the high incidence of prematurity and abruptio placentae. The rate in one series was 8 times higher than in the general population [1].

D. Evaluation

1. History. Symptoms of preeclampsia may relate to any organ system.

a. Central nervous system

(1) Headache.

(2) Somnolence.

b. Visual symptoms due to retinal artery spasm and retinal edema

(1) Blurry vision.

(2) Scotomata.

(3) Blindness.

c. Renal

(1) Decreased urine output.

(2) Hematuria.

d. Gastrointestinal

(1) Epigastric or right upper quadrant pain due to hepatic capsular distention.

(2) Nausea and vomiting.

- **e. Respiratory**
  - **(1) Dyspnea** due to pulmonary edema (cardiogenic or noncardiogenic).
- **f. Fetoplacental**
  - **(1) Constant abdominal pain** secondary to abruptio placentae.
  - **(2) Absent fetal movement** due to intrauterine demise.
  - **(3) Premature labor.**

2. Physical findings

- **a. Neurologic**
  - **(1) Hyperreflexia.** This finding should not be overemphasized. It is **not** predictive of increased risk for seizure activity [22].
- **b. Fundoscopic exam**
  - **(1) Retinal vascular spasm,** usually segmental.
- **c. Abdominal exam**
  - **(1) Hepatic enlargement,** right upper quadrant tenderness.
  - **(2) Uterine tetany** or tenderness secondary to abruptio placentae.
- **d. Cardiovascular**
  - **(1) Hypertension.**
  - **(2) Signs of cardiac failure:** Gallop, jugular venous distention, bibasilar rales.
  - **(3) Peripheral and facial edema.**

3. Laboratory findings

- **a. Renal function tests**
  - **(1) Uric acid.** A value greater than 5 mg/dl is considered abnormal in pregnancy. This test can be helpful in distinguishing preeclampsia from uncomplicated chronic hypertension, where a normal result can be expected. Tubular secretion of uric acid is decreased as a result of the decrease in renal plasma flow found in preeclampsia.
  - **(2) Blood urea nitrogen and creatinine.** Blood urea nitrogen greater than 10 mg/dl and creatinine greater than 1.0 mg/dl are considered abnormal during pregnancy. Although creatinine clearance is frequently abnormal in preeclampsia, this is not reflected in the serum blood urea nitrogen and creatinine except in severe cases with significant renal involvement.
  - **(3) Fractional excretion of calcium.** Twenty-four-hour urinary calcium excretion is markedly reduced in patients with preeclampsia, a finding frequently noted in patients with early renal disease. Preliminary studies suggest that hypocalciuria may distinguish preeclamptics from patients with uncomplicated chronic hypertension [23].
- **b. Liver function tests**
  - **(1) Liver enzymes.** Mild elevations of serum glutamic-oxaloacetic transaminase and serum glutamic-pyruvic transaminase may be seen in patients with severe preeclampsia, most likely related to hepatic edema and ischemia. Higher elevations are found in patients with subcapsular hematoma. Elevated alkaline phosphatase is a routine finding in pregnancy consequent to placental production of this enzyme and therefore is not a useful clinical study.
- **c. Coagulation tests**
  - **(1) Platelets.** As noted previously, thrombocytopenia complicates approximately 10% of cases of severe preeclampsia. When followed serially in patients destined to develop preeclampsia, platelet counts have been found to decline long before the clinical appearance of disease [13].
  - **(2) Fibrinogen** is usually normal or elevated. In cases associated with abruptio placentae, there may be an acute coagulopathy and therefore decrease in fibrinogen.
  - **(3) Prothrombin and partial thromboplastin times** are usually normal except in cases associated with abruptio placentae or another cause of acute coagulopathy.
  - **(4) Fibrin degradation products** are frequently positive due to chronic coagulopathy.

E. Management

1. Antepartum

a. Mild preeclampsia usually occurs at term. As preeclampsia may continue to worsen, but will not resolve prior to delivery, **hastening delivery is the most prudent course with fetal maturity.** However, in the patient with mild preeclampsia earlier in gestation, conservative management is indicated. The patient may be hospitalized for bed rest or, if reliable, may be instructed to rest at home. Once suspicion of preeclampsia is raised, the patient should be reevaluated shortly thereafter to evaluate the rapidity of progression of disease. If the disease appears to be stable, visits may be decreased to twice weekly. Each evaluation should include blood pressure, urinalysis, and weight. Laboratory studies such as platelet count, liver enzymes, uric acid, and quantitation of proteinuria are tested initially and repeated when clinically indicated by signs of worsening disease. Fetal monitoring is usually performed weekly to twice weekly (see Chap. 22). Assessment of fetal growth by ultrasound is appropriate. Delivery is indicated when fetal maturity is achieved, with evidence of fetal compromise, or when the disease worsens to severe preeclampsia.

b. Severe preeclampsia. Once the diagnosis of severe preeclampsia is established, the usual course of action is to expedite delivery irrespective of fetal maturity. Inpatient conservative management of severe preeclampsia remote from term has been attempted, but large series indicate that perinatal mortality is not improved due to inability to significantly prolong the pregnancy, and maternal morbidity is unacceptably high [21]. The one exception to this rule is the patient whose preeclampsia is judged severe solely on the basis of proteinuria. In these patients, if remote from term, conservative management is acceptable; however, delivery is mandated by development of other criteria suggesting severe disease.

2. Intrapartum

a. Seizure prophylaxis. In the United States, the standard is to medicate all preeclamptics during the acute phase of illness, intrapartum, and during the first 12–48 hours post partum to prevent convulsions. Approximately 50% of seizures occur antepartum, 25% intrapartum, and 25% post partum [2]. Clinically, it is not possible to predict patients at higher risk for seizure [2]. Many patients will require prophylaxis to prevent this complication, so the drug used must prove to be very safe both for the mother and fetus. **Magnesium sulfate** has been used for this indication for many years. An initial IV bolus of 4–6 gm is given slowly. The maintenance dose is determined by serum levels, as renal clearance is highly variable. Usual doses are 1–3 gm/hour. Toxicity encountered with magnesium sulfate is the result of overdosage; therefore, serum levels need to be repeated every six hours during the infusion. Therapeutic and toxic doses are shown in Table 19-1. Although a transient, mild decrease in blood pressure may be seen after magnesium sulfate therapy is initiated, a common misconception is that this is an effective antihypertensive agent. Adverse neonatal effects are also related to overdosage, with no correla-

Table 19-1. Therapeutic and toxic effects of magnesium sulfate

Effect	mEq/liter	mg/dl
Antiseizure	4–7	4.8–8.4
Loss of deep tendon reflexes	10	12
Respiratory arrest	15	18
General anesthesia	15	18
Cardiac arrest	> 30	> 36

tion between serum levels and Apgar scores when levels are in the therapeutic range [12]. Even though magnesium sulfate has proved to be both an effective prophylactic and therapeutic anticonvulsant, treatment failures with documented therapeutic levels have occurred. In these cases addition of a second agent such as **diazepam,** 5–10 mg, or **pentobarbital,** 125 mg, is recommended. Magnesium sulfate overdosage is treated by administration of calcium gluconate, 1 gm IV push, and respiratory and other support as required.

b. Antihypertensive therapy. Chronic therapy of moderate hypertension does not delay progression of the disease or decrease maternal or perinatal morbidity, and therefore is not recommended. Antihypertensive therapy is reserved for the acute treatment of severe preeclampsia. The most appropriate medications are those with a rapid onset of action, easily titrated to the patient's blood pressure, and having no adverse effects on the fetus or uteroplacental perfusion. Generally, antihypertensive therapy is given for a diastolic blood pressure of greater than 110 mm Hg. The therapeutic goal is a diastolic blood pressure between 90 and 105 mm Hg. As many of these patients are relatively hypovolemic, decreasing diastolic blood pressure below 90 mm Hg may compromise uterine perfusion, due to loss of pressure head. Hypovolemia will also cause the patient to be exquisitely sensitive to vasodilators, and too rapid a decline in blood pressure with overzealous administration will frequently result in signs of fetal distress. It is therefore judicious to **treat slowly,** with simultaneous adequate hydration as judged by the adequacy of urine output. Therapeutic choices will be discussed next. The pharmacology of the acceptable antihypertensive agents is shown in Table 19-2.

(1) Hydralazine. This vasodilator is the agent of choice for treatment of acute hypertensive crisis during pregnancy.

(a) Advantages

(i) Ease of administration. Given in boluses, does not require intraarterial blood pressure monitoring.

(ii) Effect primarily on resistance, not capacitance vessels. Advantageous in a hypovolemic patient.

(iii) Effect on uterine blood flow more favorable than other vasodilators.

(iv) More experience with use during pregnancy than other antihypertensive agents.

(b) Disadvantages

(i) Relatively slow onset and long duration of action make it relatively difficult to titrate the dose to the patient's blood pressure.

(ii) Reflex tachycardia will increase myocardial oxygen consumption.

Table 19-2. Antihypertensive agents for use in hypertensive emergencies during pregnancy

	Initial dose	Maximum effect	Duration
Direct vasodilators			
Hydralazine	5 mg	20 min	2–6 hr
Nitroprusside	0.25 μg/kg/min	2 min	3–5 min
Nitroglycerin	10–25 μg/min	2 min	2–5 min
Nifedipine	10 mg	15 min	3–5 hr
Diazoxide	30 mg	2–5 min	4–24 hr
Sympatholytic vasodilators			
Labetalol	20 mg	10 min	2–8 hr
Clonidine	0.2 mg	2–4 hr	6–12 hr

(2) **Nitroprusside**

(a) **Advantages**

(i) **Rapid onset and short duration of action** allow easy titration to patient's blood pressure response.

(ii) **Extremely potent vasodilator** that works when other agents will not.

(b) **Disadvantages**

(i) Because of fine control of blood pressure, requires **intraarterial blood pressure monitoring.**

(ii) **Potential cyanide toxicity** is a concern with large doses over prolonged infusions. Toxicity has not been reported in mothers or fetuses at the doses required for therapy of preeclampsia. However, animal studies have raised concerns, limiting the use in obstetrics.

(3) **Nitroglycerin**

(a) **Advantages**

(i) **Rapid onset and short duration** of action allow easy titration to patient's blood pressure response.

(ii) **Effect primarily on capacitance,** not resistance vessels. This is advantageous in a patient with pulmonary edema.

(b) **Disadvantages**

(i) Because of fine control of blood pressure, **requires intraarterial blood pressure monitoring.**

(ii) **Effect primarily on capacitance vessels.** May not be an effective antihypertensive agent in a well-hydrated patient.

(iii) **Increases cerebral blood flow;** therefore, increases intracranial pressure.

c. The following antihypertensive agents are used less commonly in the treatment of severe preeclampsia.

(1) **Nifedipine**

(a) **Advantages**

(i) **Easily administered** sublingually.

(ii) **Effect greater on resistance** than capacitance vessels.

(iii) **Induced decrease in blood pressure** is proportional to the baseline blood pressure. Hypotension is rare.

(iv) **Dilates coronary arteries** and increases subendocardial blood flow.

(b) **Disadvantages**

(i) **Relatively slow onset and long duration of action.**

(ii) **Increases cerebral blood flow;** therefore, increases intracranial pressure.

(iii) **Causes uterine relaxation.**

(iv) Animal studies have shown development of **fetal acidosis** unrelated to maternal hypotension with use of similar calcium channel blockers. This has not been reported in humans.

(v) **Concurrent use with magnesium sulfate contraindicated;** both agents are calcium antagonists.

(2) **Diazoxide**

(a) **Advantages**

(i) **Easily administered in boluses.**

(ii) **Effect primarily on resistance vessels.**

(b) **Disadvantages**

(i) Standard doses frequently precipitate **maternal hypotension** and **fetal distress.** Must give in mini-boluses, as in Table 19-2.

(ii) **Long duration of action.**

(iii) **Mild maternal and fetal hyperglycemia.**

(iv) **Decreases uterine activity.**

(3) **Labetalol** is a mixed alpha-1- and beta-1-antagonist and beta-2-agonist.

(a) **Advantages**

(i) **Easily administered in boluses.**

(ii) **No reflex tachycardia** (beta-1-antagonist).

(iii) Appears to have **better preservation of uterine blood flow** than many of the vasodilators.

(b) **Disadvantages**

(i) **Long duration of action.**

(ii) **Variable efficacy.**

(4) **Clonidine.** Rarely used for acute blood pressure control in the antepartum patient. Useful in the immediate postpartum period.

d. **Fluid management** is an area of controversy. Preeclamptic patients are frequently hypovolemic due to loss of fluid to the interstitial spaces (low serum oncotic pressure, increased capillary permeability). Therefore, some believe these patients should not be fluid restricted, but maintained at approximately 125 ml/hour. Conversely, due to the risk for development of pulmonary edema, others believe in fluid restriction to approximately 75 ml/hour. The hazards of fluid restriction include extreme sensitivity to vasodilators with subsequent fetal distress, and decrease in organ perfusion, most specifically the kidneys. With fluid restriction, the patients frequently will develop oliguria, leading to the necessity for invasive interventions. With fluid restriction, the patient cannot receive epidural anesthesia (vasodilatation secondary to sympathetic blockade) and will require a general anesthetic for operative procedures, therefore incurring increased maternal and fetal risks. Conversely, this approach has been practiced with apparent good results for many years at Parkland Memorial Hospital at the University of Texas Southwestern Medical School, one of the largest delivery hospitals in the nation [11].

(1) **Oliguria** is defined as urine output less than 30 ml/hour sustained over a 2- to 3-hour period. Initial therapy consists of a crystalloid fluid bolus of 300–500 ml. With no response, this may be repeated once. With still no response, a pulmonary artery catheter should be placed for further guidance of therapy.

(2) **Pulmonary edema.** As described in sec. **C.1.e.(1),** pulmonary edema may be cardiogenic or noncardiogenic; therefore, a pulmonary artery catheter is required to guide therapy.

(3) **Postpartum management.** In the postpartum period, abnormalities begin to correct. Generally, the patient enters a diuretic phase 12–48 hours after delivery. Magnesium sulfate infusion is usually continued until the patient enters this phase, as there is still a risk of eclamptic seizure. If the patient is requiring continued boluses of an antihypertensive agent, she may be started on **clonidine,** 0.1–0.2 mg bid, for smoother blood pressure control.

III. Chronic hypertension

A. Complications

1. Maternal

a. **Superimposed preeclampsia.** This complication develops in 10–40% of patients with chronic hypertension, with the incidence reported highly dependent on the definition of superimposition. The diagnosis may be difficult to confirm in the patient with underlying renal disease, who may already exhibit proteinuria. Serum uric acid may help, as this value is usually normal with uncomplicated chronic hypertension, and will rise with superimposed preeclampsia. When preeclampsia superimposes, it frequently occurs in the late second or early third trimester.

b. **Other maternal morbidity.** Morbid events may occur in the pregnant chronic hypertensive as in the nonpregnant hypertensive if there are extreme elevations in blood pressure. Pregnancy does not predispose to these events. However, with superimposed preeclampsia, the maternal morbidity and mortality is higher than in the preeclamptic patient with no history of chronic hypertension.

2. Fetal

a. **Intrauterine growth retardation.** In patients with mild (diastolic blood pressure < 110 mm Hg), uncomplicated (no superimposed preeclampsia) chronic hypertension, the incidence of fetal growth retardation is the same as in the general population. However, with superimposed preeclampsia, the incidence rises to 30–40% [9, 20].

b. **Prematurity.** The rate of prematurity is increased over the general population with reported rates between 20 and 30% [9, 20]. How much of this increase can be accounted for by patients with superimposed preeclampsia is not clear in the reports.

c. **Perinatal mortality.** Perinatal mortality is comparable to the rate found in a general high-risk population [9, 20].

B. Evaluation

1. Laboratory studies

a. **Renal function tests.** A baseline 24-hour urine should be collected for creatinine clearance and total protein. Baseline blood urea nitrogen, creatinine, and uric acid should be determined. If normal, no repeat tests are needed unless the patient develops signs of superimposed preeclampsia.

b. **Ultrasound.** A baseline study should be ordered to confirm dates for later comparison should the patient develop preeclampsia and signs of intrauterine growth retardation.

C. Management

1. **Antihypertensive therapy.** For the patient with mild hypertension (blood pressure < 160/100 mm Hg), the use of antihypertensive agents is controversial. Randomized studies show no significant benefit [14, 24]. Therapy does not decrease the rate of superimposed preeclampsia, the source of maternal morbidity and fetal intrauterine growth retardation. Therapy does not decrease the perinatal mortality rate. Conversely, although the majority of antihypertensive agents are felt to be safe during pregnancy, with the exception of α-methyldopa, experience is limited. Therefore, with the threat of unknown adverse fetal effects, and inability to document benefit, the most prudent course probably is to defer therapy of mild hypertension during the 10 months of pregnancy. In patients with severe hypertension, therapy should not be denied, since the potential for maternal morbidity remains. This potential for morbidity occurs at a diastolic blood pressure of 110 mm Hg; however, to leave a margin of safety, it is reasonable to begin therapy for a diastolic blood pressure of 105 mm Hg. The more commonly used antihypertensive agents are discussed here.

a. **α-Methyldopa** is the antihypertensive agent of choice for use during pregnancy. It has been studied more completely during pregnancy than any other agent. Studies by Redman and colleagues [13] extend to a seven-year follow-up on two cohorts of children of mothers with moderate hypertension [4]. Mothers were randomly assigned to α-methyldopa versus no therapy. At birth and at 6 months, head circumference was smaller in the treated group. On further analysis this was associated with entry into the trial at 16–20 weeks' gestation. This difference persisted at 7 years only in this subset of male children. This difference is probably a statistical artifact and of no clinical significance. No differences in growth, development, or behavior were noted. The usual starting dose is 250 mg bid, with a maximum dose of 3 gm/day.

b. **Clonidine.** One study suggests prenatal exposure to clonidine results in **sleep disturbances** during childhood [7]. No other adverse findings have been reported.

c. **Hydralazine.** Although there have been no adverse findings noted, this is not an effective single chronic agent due to the development of **tachyphylaxis** after several days of therapy. It is useful as a **second agent.**

d. **Propranolol.** Most retrospective studies have shown an association between this drug and **intrauterine growth retardation,** but most prospective studies have not [18]. Retrospective studies have also noted an association with neonatal hypoglycemia, bradycardia, and delayed onset of sustained respiration. When other choices are available, it is preferable to avoid use of propranolol during pregnancy.

e. **Labetalol.** Most studies do not report an excess of small-for-gestational-age babies, neonatal hypotension, hypoglycemia, or impairment of stress response. This is an acceptable alternative for the patient unresponsive to α-methyldopa. The usual starting dose is 100 mg bid, with a maximum dose of 2400 mg/day.

f. **Captopril and enalapril** are clearly **contraindicated** during pregnancy. Multiple cases of prolonged, severe neonatal hypotension and neonatal renal failure have been reported [17].

g. **Thiazide diuretics.** There have been isolated reports of neonatal thrombocytopenia; however, these mothers had ingested multiple drugs. Thiazide diuretics do interfere with maternal plasma volume expansion and, therefore, cannot be recommended.

h. **Calcium channel blockers.** As mentioned in the discussion of acute antihypertensive agents, some concerns raised by animal data limit the usefulness of these agents (see sec. **II.E.2.c.[1][b][iv]**).

2. **Obstetric**

a. **Fetal surveillance** should include **serial ultrasound examinations** if there is clinical suspicion of intrauterine growth retardation or evidence of superimposing preeclampsia, and fetoplacental testing beginning at 32–34 weeks' gestation.

b. **Induction of labor.** The patient with uncomplicated mild hypertension may be allowed to continue pregnancy to 42 weeks if no signs of fetal compromise are evident. In the severely hypertensive patient requiring medication, induction at 40 weeks is the usual management protocol.

References

1. Benedetti, T. J., Benedetti, J. K., and Stenchever, M. A. Severe preeclampsia—maternal and fetal outcome. *Clin. Exper. Hypertens.* B1:401, 1982.
2. Chesley, L. C. *Hypertensive Disorders in Pregnancy.* New York: Appleton-Century-Crofts, 1978.
3. Chesley, L. C., and Annito, J. E. Pregnancy in the patient with hypertensive disease. *Am. J. Obstet. Gynecol.* 53:372, 1947.
4. Cockburn, J., et al. Final report of study on hypertension during pregnancy: The effects of specific treatment on the growth and development of the children. *Lancet* i:647, 1982.
5. Donaldson, J. O. *Neurology of Pregnancy.* Philadelphia: Saunders, 1984.
6. Govan, A. D. T. The pathogenesis of eclamptic lesions. *Pathol. Microbiol.* 24:561 1961.
7. Huisjes, H. J., Hadder-Algra, M., and Touwen, B. C. L. Is clonidine a behavioral teratogen in the human? *Early Hum. Dev.* 14:43, 1986.
8. Kirby, J. C., and Jaindl, J. J. Cerebral CT findings in toxemia of pregnancy. *Radiology* 151:114, 1984.
9. Mabie, W. C., Pernoll, M. L., and Biswas, M. K. Chronic hypertension in pregnancy. *Obstet. Gynecol.* 67:197, 1986.
10. Martin, T. R., and Tupper, W. R. C. The management of severe toxemia in patients at less than 36 weeks' gestation. *Obstet. Gynecol.* 54:602, 1979.
11. Pritchard, J. A., and Pritchard, S. A. Standardized treatment of 154 consecutive cases of eclampsia. *Am. J. Obstet. Gynecol.* 123:543, 1975.
12. Pritchard, J. A., and Stone, S. R. Clinical and laboratory observations on eclampsia. *Am. J. Obstet. Gynecol.* 99:754, 1967.
13. Redman, C. W. G., Bonnar, J., and Beilin, L. Early platelet consumption in pre-eclampsia. *Br. Med. J.* 1:467, 1978.
14. Redman, C. W. G., et al. Fetal outcome in trial of antihypertensive treatment in pregnancy. *Lancet* ii:753, 1976.
15. Roberts, J. M., and May, W. J. Consumptive coagulopathy in severe preeclampsia. *Obstet. Gynecol.* 48:163, 1976.
16. Ross, J. Afterload mismatch and preload reserve: A conceptual framework for the analysis of ventricular function. *Prog. Cardiovasc. Dis.* 18:255, 1976.

17. Rothberg, A. D., and Lorenz, R. Can captopril cause fetal and neonatal renal failure? *Pediatr. Pharmacol.* 4:189, 1984.
18. Rubin, P. C. Beta-blockers in pregnancy. *N. Engl. J. Med.* 305:1323, 1981.
19. Sibai, B. M. Pitfalls in the diagnosis and management of preeclampsia. *Am. J. Obstet. Gynecol.* 159:1, 1988.
20. Sibai, B. M., Abdella, T. N., and Anderson, G. D. Pregnancy outcome in 211 patients with mild chronic hypertension. *Obstet. Gynecol.* 61:571, 1983.
21. Sibai, B. M., et al. Maternal and perinatal outcome of conservative management of severe preeclampsia in midtrimester. *Am. J. Obstet. Gynecol.* 152:32, 1985.
22. Sibai, B. M., et al. Reassessment of intravenous $MgSO_4$ therapy in preeclampsia-eclampsia. *Obstet. Gynecol.* 57:199, 1981.
23. Taufield, P. A., et al. Hypocalciuria in preeclampsia. *N. Engl. J. Med.* 316:715, 1987.
24. Welt, S., et al. The effect of prophylactic management and therapeutics on hypertensive disease in pregnancy: Preliminary studies. *Obstet. Gynecol.* 57:557, 1981.

20 Third-Trimester Bleeding

Carolyn C. LoBue

Late-pregnancy bleeding complicates 2–5% of all pregnancies. The differential diagnosis for late-pregnancy bleeding is complex, as illustrated by Table 20-1. Although in many cases no obvious source of bleeding will be identified, placenta previa and placental abruption must be ruled out because of the increased maternal and fetal morbidity and mortality associated with these complications.

I. Overall approach to the patient with late-pregnancy bleeding

A. History. The following information is essential:

1. Is there any history of trauma?
2. What is the amount and character of the bleeding?
3. Is the patient experiencing pain?
4. Is there a history of bleeding earlier during the pregnancy?

B. Evaluation of patient's general condition

1. Obtain maternal and fetal vital signs.
2. Perform a physical examination, **excluding** digital pelvic examination, with or without gentle speculum examination.*

C. Initial laboratory data and therapy

1. Hemoglobin or hematocrit determinations (or both) should be checked in all patients with late-pregnancy bleeding.
2. Coagulation studies—prothrombin time, partial thromboplastin time, platelet count, fibrinogen level, and fibrin split products—should be performed if there is any possibility of placental abruption.
3. Urinalysis should be obtained to check for hematuria and albuminuria.
4. Blood should be typed and cross-matched as indicated.
5. Unless bleeding is minimal, an intravenous fluid line should be started.
6. If the patient is in labor, an Apt test should be performed to determine whether bleeding is maternal or fetal. (Mix vaginal blood with an equal part of 0.25% sodium hydroxide. Blood of fetal origin will not change color. Maternal blood will turn light brown.)
7. Obtain Kleihauer-Betke test as indicated.

II. Placental abruption (also known as abruptio placentae, premature separation, ablatio placentae, and accidental hemorrhage)

A. Definition. Placental abruption occurs when a normally implanted placenta separates from the decidua basalis after the twentieth week of gestation and prior to the third stage of labor (Fig. 20-1).

B. Incidence. This occurs in approximately 1 in 100 deliveries.

C. Classification. A variety of systems have been employed in attempting to classify the severity of placental abruption; the following scheme is a combination of several systems and is useful in considering the management of this condition:

1. Mild

a. Vaginal bleeding is absent or slight (< 100 ml).

*The use of a gentle speculum examination to evaluate the patient with late-pregnancy bleeding is controversial. Most clinicians believe that the information to be gained outweighs the slight risk of initiating or aggravating bleeding. If performed, however, the examination must be gentle to minimize the risk of increased bleeding from a placenta previa.

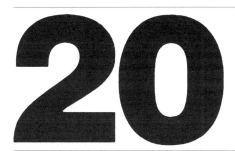

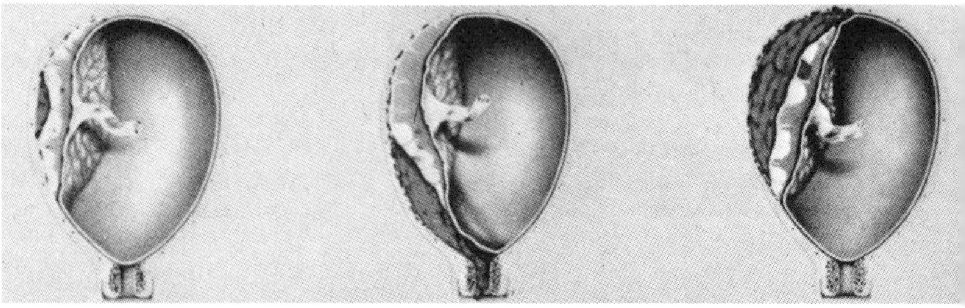

Fig. 20-1. Types of placental abruption. (From *Abnormalities of the Placenta*. Clinical Education Aid, No. 12. Columbus, OH: Ross Laboratories, 1972.)

b. Uterine reactivity may be slightly increased, but no fetal heart rate abnormalities are present.
c. There is no evidence of shock or coagulopathy.

2. **Moderate**
   a. External bleeding may be absent to moderate (100–500 ml).
   b. Uterine tone may be increased; the uterus usually is hypersensitive.
   c. Mild shock may be present.
   d. Fetal heart tones may be present or absent.
   e. If fetal heart tones are present, monitoring may show evidence of fetal distress.
3. **Severe**
   a. External bleeding may be moderate to excessive (greater than 500 ml) but can be completely concealed.
   b. The uterus is tetanic and very reactive to palpation.
   c. Moderate or profound shock may be present.
   d. Fetal demise is frequent.
   e. Coagulopathy also is frequent.

(If there is any doubt about the category of abruption, the patient should be treated as if she has the more severe form.

D. Etiology and associations. The actual cause of placental abruption is unknown. It generally is believed that a defective placental vasculature may be a contributing factor in many cases of placental abruption. In a number of conditions, the incidence of placental abruption is increased:

1. Preeclampsia and other hypertensive disorders, particularly in the severe forms of abruptio placentae
2. Prior history of placental abruption (recurrence rate is approximately 10%)
3. High multiparity
4. Increasing maternal age
5. Shortness of the umbilical cord
6. Supine hypotensive syndrome
7. Trauma
8. Association with folic acid deficiency (questionable)
9. Amniocentesis (rarely)
10. Cigarette smoking
11. Illicit drugs including cocaine and (met)amphetamine may lead to abruptio placentae
12. Excessive alcohol consumption

E. Diagnosis

1. The diagnosis usually is made on clinical grounds; ultrasonography may be helpful in certain cases.
   a. Retroplacental and preplacental hemorrhage have increased risk of fetal death compared to subchorionic hemorrhage [7].

b. Larger hemorrhage increases the risk of fetal death as does hemorrhage detaching 50% or more of the placenta [7].

2. Bleeding is present vaginally in 80% of cases; it is concealed in 20% of cases.
3. Pain is present in most cases of placental abruption, but not all, and it usually is of sudden onset, constant, and localized to the uterus and lower back.
4. Uterine tenderness usually is found with the more severe forms of placental abruption; tenderness may be localized or generalized.
5. Uterine hypertonicity generally is present, especially in the more severe forms of placental abruption.
6. An increase in uterine size may occur with placental abruption, particularly when most of the hemorrhage is concealed.
7. Amniotic fluid may be bloody, classically considered to have the color of port wine.
8. Shock is variably present.
9. Fetal compromise is variably present.
10. Proteinuria may occur, particularly with the more severe forms of placental abruption.
11. Consumptive coagulopathy may occur.
    a. Placental abruption is the most common cause of consumptive coagulopathy in pregnancy.
    b. Coagulation occurs intravascularly as well as retroplacentally; the intravascular component is the significant one in terms of altered coagulation factors.
    c. Secondary fibrinolysis occurs.
    d. Fibrinogen levels, as well as prothrombin, factor V, factor VIII, and platelets are decreased; fibrin degradation products are increased and they exert an anticoagulant effect of their own.
    e. Placental separation precedes the onset of the coagulopathy; the coagulopathy is progressive as long as the uterus remains unevacuated.
    f. If hypofibrinogenemia occurs, it generally does so within eight hours of the initial separation.
    g. Placental abruption may cause premature labor.

F. Management

1. **Mild placental abruption.** The only indication for expectant management of the patient with placental abruption is a mild abruption with an immature fetus. If expectant management is elected, the fetus must be monitored by standard antepartum fetal activity testing. The value of such tests in these cases remains to be established, however. Serial ultrasonic examinations probably are worthwhile in an attempt to monitor the size of the abruption as well as to evaluate possible intrauterine growth retardation [7, 8]. Serial hemoglobin or hematocrit determinations should be ordered. If bleeding continues, delivery should be accomplished once fetal maturity has been documented. In the patient with mild abruption and a term fetus, delivery is expedited as discussed in sec. **G.**
2. **Moderate to severe abruption**
    a. Careful monitoring of the gravida with abruption is essential if long-term complications are to be minimized. The fetus, if viable, must also be monitored carefully.
    b. If shock is present, the patient must be treated vigorously, as outlined in sec. **V.**
    c. Coagulopathy
        (1) In the presence of coagulopathy, fresh whole blood, if available, should be used to replace blood loss.
        (2) If hypofibrinogenemia or disseminated intravascular coagulation (DIC) is present, clotting factors may be replaced using cryoprecipitate or fresh-frozen plasma. One unit of fresh-frozen plasma will increase fibrinogen concentration approximately 10 mg/dl; cryoprecipitate contains an average of 250 mg of fibrinogen/bag.
        (3) Platelet transfusion may be required if the platelet count is less than 50,000/μl.

(4) The coagulation defects resolve once delivery occurs; coagulation factors return to normal in 24 hours and platelets return to normal in two to four days.
(5) The use of heparin in DIC-associated placental abruption is mentioned only to condemn it.

G. Mode and timing of delivery

1. An attempt should be made to expedite delivery in all cases of placental abruption other than the very mild ones.
2. In the past, arbitrary time limits for delivery were employed, the most common one being six hours. Recent work, however, indicates that the time interval to delivery is not as significant as prompt and adequate replacement of maternal blood loss.
3. Once the diagnosis of placental abruption has been made, amniotomy should be performed, since it may facilitate labor and decrease thromboplastin entry into the circulation.
4. Oxytocin augmentation may be instituted as needed.
5. Vaginal delivery is preferred. The use of forceps or a vacuum extractor to shorten the second stage of labor is controversial; the risk of prolonging labor must be weighed against the risk of trauma with the forceps or vacuum extractor.
6. Cesarean section is indicated in the following cases:
   a. When fetal distress develops and vaginal delivery is not imminent.
   b. In cases of severe abruption with a viable fetus.
   c. When hemorrhage is severe enough to jeopardize the life of the mother.
   d. In patients who have failed a trial of labor.

H. Complications. The following are the major complications of placental abruption. Their frequency is a function of the severity and duration of abruption.

1. Hemorrhagic shock.
2. Consumptive coagulopathy.
3. Couvelaire uterus (hemorrhage into the myometrium resulting in a poorly contractile uterus).
4. Ischemic necrosis of distant organs, the most frequently involved being the kidney and the anterior pituitary. Damage to the kidney may be caused by either acute tubular necrosis or cortical necrosis or both (see Chap. 5). The management of renal failure and panhypopituitarism is beyond the scope of this discussion.

I. Prognosis. Placental abruption is one of the gravest of obstetric complications. Perinatal mortality is approximately 35%, whereas maternal mortality should be less than 1%.

III. Placenta previa

A. Definition and classification. Placenta previa occurs when any part of the placenta implants in the lower uterine segment (Fig. 20-2). Placenta previa is classified as **marginal, partial,** or **total,** depending on the relationship of the placenta to the internal cervical os. In the partial form, the os is partially covered. In the total form, the os is completely covered. As the cervix dilates, the degree of placenta previa may change.

B. Incidence. Placenta previa occurs in approximately 1 in 200 pregnancies. The marginal form accounts for 24% of all cases, the partial form for 29%, and the total form for the remaining 47% [3].

C. Etiology. The cause of placenta previa is unknown. Theoretic considerations include deficient decidual vasculature.

D. Associated conditions. The following conditions are associated with an increased incidence of placenta previa:

1. Increasing age. Placenta previa is 3 times as frequent at age 35 as at age 25.
2. Increasing parity, regardless of age. Age, however, probably is a more significant factor than parity.
3. Prior uterine scar.

E. Signs and symptoms. Bleeding from placenta previa may occur at any time during pregnancy. As a general rule, the greater the degree of placenta previa,

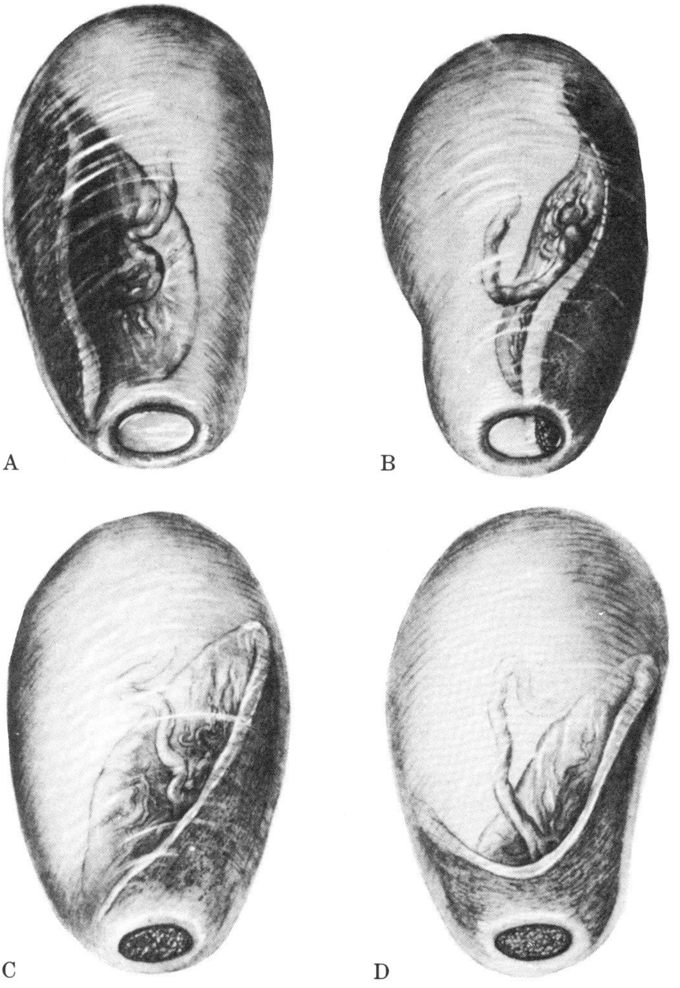

Fig. 20-2. Types of placenta previa. **A.** Low-lying placenta. **B.** Marginal placenta previa. **C** and **D.** Varieties of complete placenta previa. (From J. R. Willson, *Atlas of Obstetric Technic* [2nd ed.]. St. Louis: Mosby, 1969. Daisy Stilwell, medical illustrator.)

the earlier the appearance of bleeding. Initial bleeding may be slight or profuse; the initial bleeding generally will cease spontaneously in the absence of pelvic examination. Bleeding usually is painless and bright red in color. If labor is present, the uterus should relax between contractions. An abnormal presentation occurs in one-third of cases.

F. Diagnosis. A number of diagnostic techniques have been used in an attempt to localize the placenta. Ultrasonic scanning is preferred because of its accuracy and safety. Ultrasonography should be 95–98% accurate in the diagnosis of placenta previa. A placenta previa diagnosed in the second trimester of pregnancy in an asymptomatic patient has only a 2–10% chance of persisting at delivery [6].

G. Management of placenta previa depends on gestational age and the extent of bleeding.

1. Immediate delivery

a. In a pregnancy of 37 weeks or greater, or with documented fetal maturity, the patient should be delivered by cesarean section unless there is only a minimal degree of placenta previa.

b. If there is doubt about the diagnosis, a double setup examination—that is, an examination for diagnostic purposes but with all preparations for cesarean section already accomplished—should be performed. A double setup must be performed in an operating room.

c. In the case of anterior placenta previa, many clinicians advocate low vertical uterine incision.

d. If bleeding is sufficient to jeopardize the mother or the fetus, immediate delivery by cesarean section is indicated.

2. Expectant management

a. This approach is employed only when the bleeding is not excessive and there are significant risks of prematurity to the fetus.

b. The patient must be hospitalized or in a location where rapid transportation to the hospital is available.

c. Physical activity should be restricted.

d. Intercourse and douching are not permitted.

e. The hematocrit should be maintained at 30% or greater.

f. Pelvic examination is performed **only** in the operating room.

g. Once the patient has attained a gestational age of 36–38 weeks, or fetal maturity has been documented, the patient is readied for elective double setup examination to lessen the risk of maternal hemorrhage with the onset of labor.

h. It is possible to treat expectantly approximately 70% of patients with a premature fetus. Tocolytic agents may be employed in selected cases. Betamimetic agents may be the preferred tocolytic [2]. Von Friesen [9] and Arias [1] have advocated the use of cerclage to treat placenta previa. This therapy may prolong pregnancy complicated by placenta previa, but this remains controversial.

H. Maternal mortality from placenta previa should approach zero. **Perinatal mortality** in recent studies is reported to be approximately 8%, and this is caused by prematurity [4].

I. Complications. The major maternal complication associated with placenta previa is hemorrhagic shock. Other complications are those associated with transfusion therapy and cesarean section.

J. Precaution. Patients with placenta previa who are managed expectantly should be watched carefully for evidence of growth retardation and congenital malformations.

IV. Bleeding not caused by placenta previa or abruptio placentae. As indicated by Table 20-1, late-pregnancy bleeding may be a result of many causes other than abruptio placentae or placenta previa. Some of the more common causes and their management will be considered in this section [5].

A. Cervical bleeding

1. Cytologic sampling is mandatory when cervical bleeding occurs.

2. Control of bleeding with cauterization or packing is preferred. Attempts at suturing may only result in further bleeding.

3. Cultures for various vaginal pathogens may be indicated.

B. Bleeding caused by cervical polyps

1. Bleeding usually is self-limited.

2. Trauma should be avoided.

3. Polypectomy may be performed to control the bleeding and for tissue diagnosis.

4. Cytologic sampling is mandatory.

C. Vasa previa

1. An Apt test will indicate fetal source for bleeding.

Table 20-1. Late-pregnancy bleeding

Cause	Number	Percentage
Cause undetermined —probable "marginal sinus rupture" in many cases	236	58.6
Probable show	86	21.3
Cervicitis and cervical erosion	34	8.4
Trauma	22	5.5
Low-lying placenta	15	3.7
Vulvovaginal varicosities	2	0.5
Genital infections	2	0.5
Hematuria	2	0.5
Genital tumor	2	0.5
Other	2	0.5

Source: R. G. Douglas and W. B. Stromme, *Operative Obstetrics* (4th ed.). New York: Appleton-Century-Crofts, 1982. P. 347.

2. Fetal monitoring should be instituted, and preparations for possible cesarean section should be accomplished.

D. Show. This is a diagnosis of exclusion. The patient should show cervical changes. Blood usually is mixed with mucus.

E. Vulvovaginal trauma

1. The patient's history should provide a clue.

2. Careful pelvic examination should be performed using analgesia and anesthesia as necessary.

3. Penetration of the cul-de-sac necessitates exploratory laparotomy.

4. All foreign bodies must be removed.

5. Wounds should be debrided and closed, if clean.

6. Hematomas should be evacuated and bleeding points ligated. Drains should be placed.

7. Tetanus prophylaxis is indicated.

F. Uterine rupture. The diagnosis and management of this condition is considered in Chap. 30.

V. Management of hemorrhagic shock

A. Management of the patient in shock requires extremely careful monitoring.

1. Vital signs should be monitored and recorded on a flow sheet.

2. Urine output must be monitored through an indwelling Foley catheter and should be maintained at 25–30 ml/hour.

3. A means of hemodynamic monitoring should be instituted.

a. A central venous pressure line may be used if left ventricular function is believed to be normal.

b. If left ventricular function is abnormal, hemodynamic measurement is best performed by a Swan-Ganz catheter. The central venous pressure should be maintained in the range of 5–15 cm H_2O. Pulmonary artery occlusive pressure should be between 6 and 18 mm Hg.

c. Supplemental oxygen should be administered to all patients in shock.

B. For the patient in shock, adequate replacement of blood loss is mandatory. When a coagulopathy is present, the blood should be as fresh as possible. While waiting for blood, blood loss should be replaced by colloid or crystalloid (3 ml of crystalloid for every ml of blood lost).

C. In monitoring blood replacement, it should be remembered that a decrease in hematocrit is **not** a sensitive indicator of acute blood loss, since hemodilution is only one-half complete at eight hours.

D. Electrolytes, calcium, oxygenation, and acid base status should be carefully monitored in the patient with shock.

E. Vasopressors probably have no role in the management of hemorrhagic shock (see Chap. 16).

References

1. Arias, F. Cervical cerclage for the temporary treatment of patients with placenta previa. *Obstet. Gynecol.* 71:545, 1988.
2. Chesnut, D. H., et al. Does the intravenous infusion of ritodrine or magnesium sulfate alter the hemodynamic response in gravid ewes? *Am. J. Obstet. Gynecol.* 159:1467, 1988.
3. Cotton, D., et al. The conservative aggressive management of placenta previa. *Am. J. Obstet. Gynecol.* 137:687, 1980.
4. Crenshaw, C., Darnell Jones, D., and Parker, R. T. Placenta previa: A survey of twenty years' experience with improved perinatal survival by expectant therapy and cesarean delivery. *Obstet. Gynecol. Surv.* 28:461, 1973.
5. Harris, B. A. Peripheral placental separation: A review. *Obstet. Gynecol. Surv.* 43:577, 1988.
6. Newton, E. R., et al. The epidemiology and clinical history of asymptomatic mid-trimester placenta previa. *Am. J. Obstet. Gynecol.* 93:148, 1982.
7. Nyberg, D. A., et al. Placental abruption and placental hemorrhage: Correlation of sonographic findings with fetal outcome. *Radiology* 164:357, 1987.
8. Rivera-Alsina, M. E., et al. The use of ultrasound in the expectant management of abruptio placentae. *Am. J. Obstet. Gynecol.* 146:924, 1983.
9. Von Friesen, B. Encircling suture of the cervix in placenta previa. *Obstet. Gynecol. Surv.* 28:104, 1974.

Selected Readings

Abdella, T. N., et al. Relationship of hypertensive disease to abruptio placentae. *Obstet. Gynecol.* 63:365, 1984.

Angelo, L. J., and Irwin, L. F. Conservative management of placenta previa: A cost-benefit analysis. *Am. J. Obstet. Gynecol.* 149:320, 1984.

Brenner, W. E., Edelman, D. A., and Hendricks, C. H. Characteristics of patients with placenta previa and results of "expectant management." *Am. J. Obstet. Gynecol.* 132:180, 1978.

Green-Thompson, R. W. Antepartum hemorrhage. *Clin. Obstet. Gynecol.* December 1980, 479.

Hord, W. W., et al. Selective management of abruptio placentae: A prospective study. *Obstet. Gynecol.* 61:467, 1983.

Nevi, A., et al. Placenta previa and growth retardation. *Isr. J. Med. Sci.* 16:429, 1980.

Pritchard, J. A., and Brekken, A. L. Clinical and laboratory studies on severe abruptio placentae. *Am. J. Obstet. Gynecol.* 97:681, 1967.

The Fetus

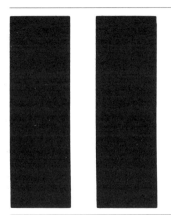

21 Fetal Growth Abnormalities

Michael P. Nageotte

I. **Intrauterine growth retardation.** Low-birth-weight infants were defined in 1961 by the Expert Committee on Maternal and Child Health as those weighing less than 2500 gm, regardless of gestational age [14]. However, these infants should be further divided into three categories: (1) neonates delivered preterm (before 37 weeks) but of appropriate size for dates; (2) neonates delivered preterm and small for dates; and (3) neonates delivered at term or beyond who are small for gestational age. Infants in the latter two categories constitute the entity of intrauterine growth retardation (IUGR). With an incidence of 3–7% of all deliveries, IUGR as a diagnosis is applicable to the fetus suspected to weigh below the tenth percentile for gestational age.

An additional approach to attempt identification of the undergrown infant is with the use of the *ponderal index*. Although this measure can be applied to all newborns, it is of value in identifying the infant who, although weighing over 2500 gm at birth, is still undergrown. The ponderal index (PI) is a ratio of the weight (gm) times 100 and the length (cm) cubed.

$$PI = \frac{\text{Weight (gm)} \times 100}{\text{Length (cm)}^3}$$

A. **Classification.** IUGR is an obstetric diagnosis applied to those pregnancies with a suspected significant fetal growth lag. Attempts have been made to classify IUGR, but they are often of limited value. IUGR has been classified as symmetric (type I) and asymmetric (type II). Essentially, asymmetric IUGR is suspected with an apparent growth lag of the fetal abdomen but not of the head or long bones. This is the most frequent type of IUGR. Symmetric IUGR occurs with growth lag of all fetal parameters and is more rarely observed.

B. **Etiologies.** Various causes of abnormal fetal growth have been proposed. Normal growth involves essentially three phases as described by Winick [13]. During the first 16 weeks of pregnancy, the cell number rapidly increases. This rate slows until 32 weeks, at which point minimal further increase occurs. This is called the phase of **cellular hyperplasia.** From 16–32 weeks, the rate of cell hyperplasia decreases and cell size increases. This is called the **concomitant hyperplasia** and **hypertrophy** phase. From 32 weeks until term is the **cellular hypertrophy** phase, during which cell size increases.

1. **Growth abnormalities.** Depending on the timing of the insult, different types of growth abnormalities may result. Symmetric IUGR results from certain chromosomal, infectious, and environmental influences early in gestation. Asymmetric IUGR results from different problems leading to uteroplacental insufficiency. Frequently, the etiology of suspected IUGR cannot be identified. Further, often a growth lag is suspected, but the fetal measurements do not allow easy assignment of the IUGR to type I or II.

C. **Diagnosis.** Clinical suspicion supported by the use of real-time ultrasound is the means by which IUGR is identified. A multitude of ratios, formulas, and graphs have evolved along with rapid improvements in ultrasound technology in the search for the most reliable means of accurately identifying true fetal growth lag. However, the most important consideration in the clinical evaluation of fetal growth is the establishment of accurate menstrual history. Only with reliable clinical dating can meaningful data be derived from ultrasound measurements.

1. **Measurements.** Probably the most reliable single discriminatory measure of fetal growth is the **abdominal circumference** measurement. Other routine measurements include the fetal **biparietal diameter,** the **head circumference,** and the **femur length.** Elevated ratios of **head circumference** to **abdominal circumference** and **femur length** to **abdominal circumference** have been used to help identify the fetus with suspected asymmetric IUGR. However, caution must be exercised in that although ultrasound is highly sensitive in the ruling out of IUGR, it is not very specific (i.e., many false-positive results). Consistency of these parameters is of critical value in improving the diagnostic accuracy of growth lag.

D. Management of suspected IUGR.

1. **Antepartum testing.** The fetus affected with IUGR is at increased risk for antenatal demise. Further, if the growth lag is resulting from some degree of chronic uteroplacental insufficiency, identification of that fetus with antepartum testing allows for early treatment, including delivery.

   Various biochemical tests that have been used to monitor the high-risk fetus essentially have been replaced with fetal heart rate testing and real-time ultrasound. The most frequent forms of antepartum surveillance used include the contraction stress test, the nonstress test, the biophysical profile, and umbilical and uterine artery velocimetry [2, 7, 9, 10]. Depending on physician choice, all these parameters have been used to monitor patients with suspected IUGR along with serial ultrasound.

   When IUGR is suspected, some form of antepartum surveillance program is indicated. Frequent testing in addition to serial ultrasounds, looking at fetal growth parameters as well as amniotic fluid volume, is critical if one chooses to allow a pregnancy with suspected IUGR to continue undelivered.

2. **Timing of delivery.** One area of controversy regards timing of delivery in pregnancies with suspected IUGR. With reassuring antepartum surveillance and continued fetal growth, premature intervention does not appear to be indicated. Delivery with documented fetal lung maturity at or beyond 37 weeks of gestation is a reasonable goal in most cases of suspected IUGR. However, in cases without adequate interval growth, severe oligohydramnios, and nonreassuring fetal heart rate testing, premature intervention may be indicated. Individualization of management decisions is very important in improving outcome in pregnancies thought to be complicated by IUGR.

E. Treatment of suspected IUGR. Various treatments for suspected IUGR have been suggested. Since no proved therapy for most infectious etiologies and all chromosomal abnormalities exists, little can be offered to these patients. For patients with idiopathic IUGR, bed rest is perhaps the best form of treatment. Appropriate management of abnormal medical conditions (e.g., hypertension) is indicated during any pregnancy, even in the absence of suspected IUGR. A great deal of time and effort have been expended toward improving or altering the maternal diet. However, few data support the claim that dietary insufficiency is the cause of the vast majority of growth-retarded fetuses. Additionally, dietary supplementation is rarely of therapeutic value. Use of other agents such as heparin, plasma volume expanders, abdominal decompression, and beta-mimetic therapy plays no role in the treatment of this pregnancy complication.

F. Management of labor. Timing of delivery is very important in the management of IUGR. The route of delivery is determined by fetal presentation, inducibility of the cervix, and tolerance of the fetus to contractions. Pregnancies with suspected IUGR and abnormal antepartum surveillance (i.e., nonreactive nonstress test, positive contraction stress test, oligohydramnios) have a very high incidence of fetal distress in labor. Cesarean section is frequently indicated because of fetal intolerance to labor. Vaginal delivery can often be achieved, however, by positioning the patient on her side during labor and employing prophylactic amnioinfusion when oligohydramnios is discovered. A pediatrician available at the time of delivery is recommended. Preparation for **meconium aspiration prevention** should also be made since frequently meconium is passed prior to or during the intrapartum and antepartum period of pregnancies complicated by IUGR.

Temperature control, avoidance of hypoglycemia, awareness for the development of hyperbilirubinemia, as well as confirmation of diagnosis are all critical issues in the immediate neonatal period.

II. Fetal macrosomia

A. Definition. Fetal macrosomia has been defined in many different ways. The most frequent definitions are birth weight of greater than 4000 gm or greater than 4500 gm, or when the birth weight is above the ninetieth percentile for gestational age. As with growth retardation, macrosomia is really a pediatric diagnosis. However, because of significant obstetric issues related to this diagnosis, the ability to accurately identify and manage pregnancies complicated by fetal macrosomia is of critical importance.

B. Etiology. Whatever definition is used, the causes of fetal macrosomia are multiple. Perhaps the most frequently cited etiology is maternal diabetes, usually gestational. Actually, diabetes is causally related to macrosomia in the minority of cases. Other potential causes include genetic (e.g., large parents), fetal gigantism (Beckwith-Wiedemann syndrome), and maternal obesity. The incidence of infants weighing over 4000 gm at birth has increased in the United States at a rate greater than the change in mean newborn birth weight.

C. Diagnosis. The various modalities employed in attempting to correctly identify the macrosomic fetus include a high degree of clinical suspicion in conjunction with careful ultrasound evaluation. Maternal weight, height, previous obstetric history, fundal height, and the presence of gestational diabetes should be individually and collectively evaluated in each patient. Formulae have been used to estimate fetal weight based on ultrasound measurements [3, 6, 12]. Unfortunately, a large margin of error is found in these estimates. Further, the applicability of the various ultrasound formulae may be very dependent on the specific maternal risk factor for macrosomia.

Since one of the main concerns with delivery of a macrosomic fetus is the development of a shoulder dystocia, measurement of the difference between fetal head size and chest size has also been used, particularly in the pregnancy complicated by diabetes [4]. Unfortunately, this measure is not highly predictive of macrosomia (birth weight over 4000 gm) unless the difference between the head and chest is great [8].

D. Management of delivery. In addition to shoulder dystocia, other forms of birth injury to both mother and fetus are increased in macrosomic infants. If the estimated fetal weight is greater than 4500 gm in the nondiabetic or greater than 4000 gm in the diabetic patient, delivery by cesarean section is indicated. Liberal use of cesarean delivery and avoidance of instrumented vaginal delivery (i.e., forceps or vacuum) are also recommended in pregnancies complicated by suspected macrosomia [1].

If a shoulder dystocia occurs, employment of McRobert's maneuver (marked hip flexion) should be done immediately [5]. If the shoulder remains impacted anteriorly, cutting an episioproctotomy and delivery of the posterior arm are the next steps. In almost all instances, one or both of these procedures will result in a successful and minimally traumatic delivery. An alternative procedure occasionally reported is the Zavanelli maneuver [11]. This entails replacement of the fetal lead into the vaginal canal and delivery by emergency cesarean section.

References

1. Benedetti, T. J., and Gabbe, S. G. Shoulder dystocia: A complication of fetal macrosomia and prolonged second stage of labor with midpelvic delivery. *Obstet. Gynecol.* 52:526, 1978.
2. Bras, H. S. The use of Doppler ultrasound to assess intrauterine growth retardation in the fetus. *Semin. Perinatol.* 12:40, 1988.
3. Deter, R. L., et al. Longitudinal studies of fetal growth with the use of dynamic image ultrasonography. *Am. J. Obstet. Gynecol.* 143:545–554, 1982.
4. Elliot, J. P., et al. Ultrasonic prediction of fetal macrosomia in diabetic patients. *Obstet. Gynecol.* 60:159, 1982.

5. Gonick, B., Stringer, C. A., and Held, B. An alternative maneuver for management of shoulder dystocia. *Am. J. Obstet. Gynecol.* 145:882, 1983.
6. Hadlock, F. P., et al. Sonographic estimation of fetal weight. *Radiology* 150:535–540, 1984.
7. Lin, C., et al. Oxytocin challenge test and intrauterine growth retardation. *Am. J. Obstet. Gynecol.* 140:282, 1981.
8. Nageotte, M. P. Biparietal diameter–chest diameter difference as a predictor for macrosomia in pregnancies complicated by diabetes. Paper presented at the annual meeting of the American College of Obstetricians and Gynecologists, San Francisco, May, 1990.
9. Phelan, J. P. The nonstress test: A review of 3,000 tests. *Am. J. Obstet. Gynecol.* 139:7, 1981.
10. Platt, L. D., et al. Further experience with the biophysical profile. *Obstet. Gynecol.* 61:480, 1983.
11. Sandberg, E. The Zavanelli maneuver. *Am. J. Obstet. Gynecol.* 152:479, 1985.
12. Shepard, M. J., et al. An evaluation of two equations for predicting fetal weight by ultrasound. *Am. J. Obstet. Gynecol.* 142:47–54, 1982.
13. Winick, M. Cellular changes during placental and fetal growth. *Am. J. Obstet. Gynecol.* 109:166, 1971.
14. World Health Organization. Public health aspects of low birth weight. Third report of the Expert Committee on Maternal and Child Health. *W.H.O. Tech. Rep. Ser.* 217:3–16, 1961.

22

Fetal Heart Rate Monitoring

Manuel Porto and
Michael P. Nageotte

Although fetal heart tones were described in the seventeenth century, doubt about the value of auscultation lasted through the early 1800s. In 1848, Killian proposed that the fetal heart rate (FHR) might be used to diagnose fetal distress and thereby allow prompt intervention [11]. By 1893, it was generally agreed that signs of fetal distress included tachycardia (heart rate > 160 beats/minute [bpm]), bradycardia (heart rate < 100 bpm), irregularity of the heart rate, passage of meconium, and gross alteration of fetal movements. However in 1968, Benson and colleagues [1] suggested that these clinical signs were unreliable.

The earliest preliminary report of FHR monitoring was released in 1958 by Hon [16]. Subsequently Hon [15], Caldeyro-Barcia and colleagues [6], and Hammacher [14] reported their empiric observations on various heart rate patterns associated with fetal distress. The electronic fetal monitors that allowed these studies were developed commercially in the late 1960s, permitting a continuous beat-to-beat record of the FHR and a record of uterine activity. Since then, the technique of electronic intrapartum FHR monitoring has advanced and been popularized to the extent that it is now considered mandatory for high-risk pregnancies. In fact today many hospitals routinely monitor **all** patients in labor.

I. Regulators of fetal heart rate. As in the adult, FHR is primarily controlled by the autonomic nervous system: sympathetic (cardio-accelerator) and parasympathetic or vagal (cardio-decelerator). It is generally accepted that progressive vagal dominance occurs as the fetus approaches term.

Almost any stressful situation in the fetus evokes the baroreceptor reflex, which elicits selective peripheral vasoconstriction and hypertension with a resultant fetal bradycardia. This vasoconstriction spares the fetus's brain, heart, adrenal glands, and placenta from decreased blood flow. The same cardiovascular response occurs following a variety of fetal stimuli including hypoxia, uterine contractions, fetal head compression, and perhaps fetal grunting or defecation. Conversely, stimulation of the fetus's midbrain results in acceleration of the FHR and hypertension. This FHR acceleration response is often associated with fetal movements. Fetal tachycardia can also occur during maternal anxiety (catecholamines), maternal fever, and after drug intake (e.g., atropine). Whereas the etiology of many FHR changes is complex and unknown, those changes of FHR associated with fetal asphyxia, cord compression, and head compression are fairly well defined [12].

II. Instrumentation. An electronic monitor receives signals from both the fetus and the mother in order to identify FHR and to record the occurrence and intensity of uterine contractions. The FHR signals are obtained either by an **electrode** or by a **transducer,** and these signals are converted into usable electric analog signals for further processing. With amplification, the fetal heart signal is converted into a **pulse.** The interval between successive pulses is measured and converted into an **instantaneous FHR.** Commercial fetal monitors contain logic circuitry to eliminate signal noise and control signal strength. These internal controls allow monitors to express, in simple fashion, the FHR on a beat-to-beat basis; however, artifacts of recording can and do occur frequently.

A. Direct (internal) fetal electrocardiogram (FECG). The FHR tracing derived from the FECG is obtained by attaching a transcervical bipolar electrode to the fetal scalp or buttocks. The FHR is defined by the interval between R waves. The monitor performs a calculation of the instantaneous heart rate based on the

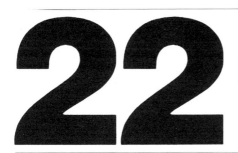

R-R interval. Thus, the direct FECG system can show the small rate differences between heart beats referred to as the beat-to-beat (or short-term) variability, which Doppler ultrasound systems are unable to measure [18]. The main disadvantage is that the fetal membranes must be ruptured to allow FECG monitoring.

B. Indirect (external) FHR monitoring

1. **Doppler ultrasound monitoring** is the most common method used when direct FECG is not possible or desirable. The method is based on the principle that an ultrasonic sound wave reflecting off a moving interface will undergo a frequency change (Doppler shift). A transducer placed on the abdomen directs an ultrasonic signal toward the fetal heart. The signal is reflected back by the moving organ to the transducer in either the systolic or diastolic interval, producing two major components in each cardiac cycle. Although the noninvasive nature of ultrasound monitoring is clearly advantageous, the system has several disadvantages as well. Loss of signal, as a result of maternal or fetal movement, may necessitate frequent transducer adjustments to maintain a continuous tracing. Short-term variability is not interpretable on standard monitors. The apparent variability in the tracing may be artifactually increased by (1) the internal logic system (FHR computed as the average of the previous four cycles) and (2) ultrasound beam recording heart wall or valve motion in different locations with successive beats (rather than the R-R interval of ECG). New-generation monitors have depth-directed Doppler systems or autocorrelation, which appear to yield a more reliable pattern of true variability [5]. Ultrasound monitoring has the further disadvantage of making fetal arrhythmias difficult to interpret. In addition, the simultaneous monitoring of twins usually requires transducers of different frequencies to avoid signal cancellation.
2. **Abdominal FECG.** Techniques for obtaining the FHR with the abdominal electrocardiogram (ECG) are fraught with difficulty owing to interference by signals generated by maternal muscle activity and maternal ECG complexes. In preterm fetuses, the signal is often lost and is difficult to use if the patient is moving her abdominal muscles (i.e., during labor). However, it does have the advantage that FHR short-term variability can be interpreted accurately [29].
3. **Phonocardiography.** This method relies on the sounds produced by fetal heart value closure. The signal results in less artifact than results from the Doppler signal, but ambient noise—such as maternal bowel sounds, microphone motion, or fetal motion—will interfere with recording. Phonocardiography is less satisfactory than the abdominal FECG or Doppler method for antepartum monitoring and is rarely used today.

C. Uterine contraction monitors. Two techniques are available for monitoring uterine contractions: direct intrauterine pressure measurement and external tokodynamometry.

1. **Intrauterine pressure monitoring** is achieved by transcervical insertion into the amniotic space of a fluid-filled catheter. The catheter is attached to a pressure transducer, which allows measurement of pressure at the open end of the catheter. The pressure within the uterine cavity is proportional to the tension in the uterine wall and inversely proportional to the uterine diameter at any given tension. Usually, pressure observed in the pregnant uterus during active labor at term ranges from 50–100 mm Hg at the peak of a contraction, with a baseline tone of 5–20 mm Hg.
2. **External tokodynamometry.** When membranes are intact, qualitative measurement of uterine activity can be performed by placement of a pressure transducer on the maternal abdomen over the uterine fundus. The technique does not allow quantitative measurement of the intrauterine pressure but is able to determine contraction frequency and duration. The advantage of this method compared to intrauterine monitoring is that it is noninvasive, less expensive, and carries no risk of intraamniotic infection.

D. Commercial instrumentation. Commercial FHR monitoring recorders have been standardized so that the FHR is recorded on paper at speeds of 1, 2, or 3 cm/minute, with a vertical scale varying from 20–30 bpm/cm. Uterine activity is represented either on a scale of 0–+4 or as 0–100 mm Hg. During monitoring, the paper usually should be run at 3 cm/minute.

III. Fetal monitoring terminology and basic FHR pattern recognition

A. The baseline FHR is that recorded between episodes of fetal stimulation or uterine contractions. The normal baseline FHR range is between 120 and 160 bpm. Changes of the FHR of greater than 15 minutes' duration are considered baseline changes. The baseline FHR is elevated by sympathetic activity and decreased by vagal activity. In the more mature fetus, there is increased vagal activity and a lower baseline rate. The baseline rate is elevated with maternal anxiety (catecholamines), maternal fever, or immaturity of the fetus.

1. **Tachycardia** is defined as a baseline rate greater than 160 bpm. There is usually an associated decrease in FHR variability. Known etiologic factors include fetal hypoxia; maternal fever; parasympatholytic drugs such as atropine, hydroxyzine pamoate (Vistaril), or phenothiazines; maternal hyperthyroidism; fetal tachyarrhythmia; and sympathomimetic drugs. Many investigators consider FHR in the upper 150s to represent "relative tachycardia" in the postterm fetus [10].
2. **Bradycardia** is defined as a baseline rate less than 120 bpm. It generally is benign if the associated beat-to-beat variability is normal. Congenital complete heart block may produce bradycardia with a rate less than 70 bpm and absent variability [31]. There is a strong association between maternal systemic lupus erythematosus (positive ANA, SS-A) and fetal heart block. FHR in the 100- to 120-bpm range is common in prolonged pregnancy.
3. **Variability** of the baseline FHR represents the most clinically significant indicator of fetal status. While variability is controlled to a large extent by the autonomic nervous system, recent studies suggest a more complex regulatory mechanism is involved [8, 22]. Variability consists of two components:
   a. **Short-term variability** is controlled primarily by the sympathetic and parasympathetic components of the nervous system and is the beat-to-beat irregularity between electrical cycles. The normal range is between 5 and 10 bpm. Increased variability may be seen with mild hypoxia. Decreased variability may have multiple causes, including fetal central nervous system depression due to hypoxia or asphyxia, drugs such as central nervous system depressants or parasympatholytic agents, fetal sleep cycles, congenital anomalies, extreme prematurity, or fetal tachycardia. With rare exception, when FHR variability is normal or increased, the fetal pH is also normal. However, loss of variability in a fetus with a nonreassuring FHR pattern (e.g., late decelerations) is associated with a high incidence of fetal acidosis and low Apgar scores [31].
   b. **Long-term variability** has a frequency of 3–10 cycles/minute, amplitude of 10–25 bpm, and is reflected in the waviness of the FHR tracing. Its significance is similar to that of short-term variability. Fetal sleep cycles (20–30 minutes) are associated with decreased variability. Increased variability (saltatory pattern) may be an early sign of mild fetal hypoxia or umbilical cord compression.

B. Periodic FHR changes may be either accelerations or decelerations.

1. **Decelerations**
   a. **Early decelerations** have a uniform shape, with a slow onset followed by a slow return to the baseline, and occur coincidentally with uterine contractions (Fig. 22-1). The amplitude is usually less than 20–30 bpm below the baseline. The decelerations generally are seen in early active labor and are associated with fetal head compression. Although these vagally mediated decelerations are not associated with fetal distress, they must be carefully differentiated from the potentially ominous late decelerations.
   b. **Late decelerations** have an appearance similar to early decelerations but are characterized by a latency period between the onset of the uterine contraction and the beginning of the deceleration (Fig. 22-2). Moreover, the descent and return are gradual and smooth; there are no associated accelerations. The magnitude of the deceleration is usually less than 10–20 bpm.

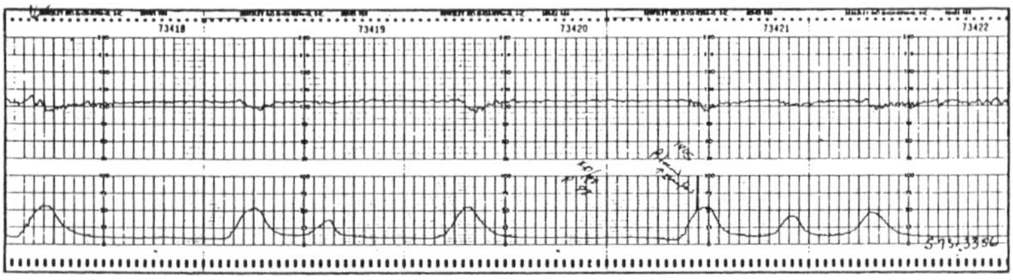

Fig. 22-1. Early decelerations during fetal heart monitoring. (From J. T. Parer, O. L. Puttler, Jr., and R. K. Freeman, *A Clinical Approach to Fetal Monitoring*. San Leandro, CA: Berkeley Bio-Engineering, 1974.)

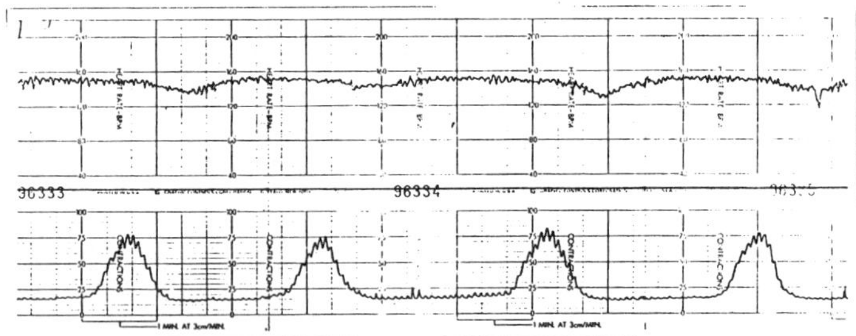

Fig. 22-2. Late decelerations during external monitoring. Note the latency period in contrast to the similarly shaped early decelerations in Fig. 22-1. (From J. T. Parer, O. L. Puttler, Jr., and R. K. Freeman, *A Clinical Approach to Fetal Monitoring*. San Leandro, CA: Berkeley Bio-Engineering, 1974.)

Late decelerations are caused by fetal hypoxia, whether mediated by the chemoceptor reflex or direct myocardial depression. Therefore, they are always considered potentially ominous, regardless of the depth of the deceleration. The presence of an associated fetal tachycardia, loss of variability, or a short latency period (< 45 seconds) correlates with progressive acidosis and neonatal depression [3].

c. **Variable decelerations** constitute the most frequently seen FHR deceleration pattern during labor (Figs. 22-3 and 22-4). The pattern is reflex in origin, in response to umbilical cord compression or certain other events and may be modified by sympathetic and parasympathetic blockage. Compression of the umbilical artery results in increased vascular resistance with a resulting baroreceptor response to slow the heart rate. Umbilical vein compression with reduction of oxygenated blood flow to the fetus can also cause a chemoreceptor response to slow the heart rate. These decelerations are characteristically variable in duration, intensity, and timing, but often coincide with uterine contractions. They are abrupt in onset and return to the baseline, and they often are preceded and followed by small abrupt accelerations. Such accelerations generally indicate a nonhypoxic fetus.
Fetal compromise is proportional to the preexisting adequacy of placental function. Frequent and repetitive cord compression can result in progressive oxygen debt with consequent metabolic as well as respiratory acidosis. Variable decelerations can be graded according to the criteria of Kubli and colleagues [19]. Associated features suggesting hypoxia include loss of beat-to-beat variability, tachycardia, **gradual** rather than abrupt return of the

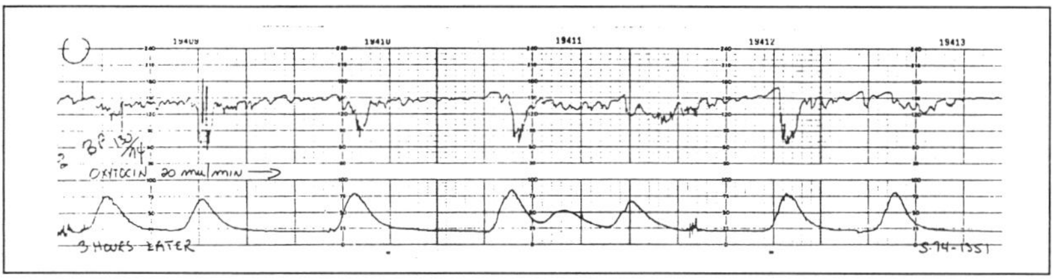

Fig. 22-3. Mild to moderate variable decelerations. Baseline heart rate and variability are normal. (From R. K. Freeman and T. J. Garite, *Fetal Heart Rate Monitoring*. Baltimore: Williams & Wilkins, 1981. P. 71.)

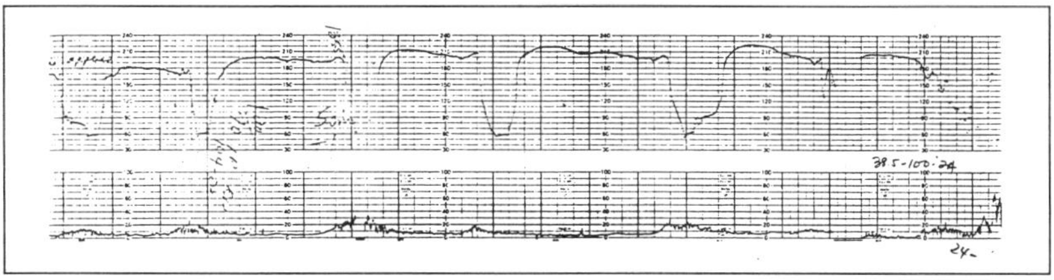

Fig. 22-4. Severe variable decelerations with baseline tachycardia, absent variability, and "overshoot." This is an ominous pattern; a premature baby was delivered by cesarean section with Apgars of 1 and 2 at 1 and 5 minutes, respectively. (From R. K. Freeman and T. J. Garite, *Fetal Heart Rate Monitoring*. Baltimore: Williams & Wilkins, 1981. P. 73.)

decelerations to the baseline, late decelerations, or a blunt acceleration ("overshoot") occurring after severe variable decelerations (Fig. 22-4) [13]. The evolution of the FHR tracing to one that contains these ominous features might warrant expeditious delivery [30].

d. **Prolonged decelerations.** Isolated decelerations of greater than two minutes' duration can be seen in many conditions including the following:

Maternal
Convulsion (eclampsia)
Supine hypotension
Maternal respiratory arrest
Obstetric
Tetanic contraction (spontaneous or oxytocin-induced)
Prolapsed umbilical cord
Prolonged umbilical cord compression, often associated with rapid fetal descent during expulsion
Iatrogenic
Vaginal examination
Application of internal fetal scalp electrode
Fetal scalp blood sampling
Paracervical block
Epidural block

e. Late in the course of severe variable decelerations, a prolonged deceleration may occur immediately prior to fetal death [30].

2. **Accelerations** of the FHR typically are abrupt in onset and generally are elevated to 15–25 bpm above the baseline. They occur in response to fetal movement or contractions and partial umbilical cord occlusion. Their presence generally is reassuring.

C. Unusual FHR patterns

1. **The sinusoidal pattern** is rarely seen and its significance is somewhat controversial. It consists of a smooth, undulating sine wave pattern with absent short-term variability and a cycle frequency of 4–8/minute (Fig. 22-5). It occurs most often in association with severe fetal anemia from a variety of sources (e.g., Rh isoimmunization, vasa praevia, fetal-maternal bleeding) and is generally an ominous finding requiring fetal intervention [26]. The pattern has been observed with alphaprodine hydrochloride (Nisentil) analgesia with no untoward fetal outcome. It is most important to differentiate "pseudosinusoidal" FHR from its true form; the former usually lacks uniformity in the wave pattern, short-term variability is present, and no fetal intervention is needed (Fig. 22-6).
2. **Fetal arrhythmias** are seen in approximately 5% of antepartum FHR tracings [31]. Most commonly these irregular rhythms are the result of premature atrial contractions; premature ventricular contractions are rare. These patterns have little clinical significance although an underlying cardiac lesion must be ruled out. Often these patterns are confused with monitoring artifact.
   Supraventricular tachycardia and atrial flutter/fibrillation have important fetal implications, including a greater frequency of cardiac anomalies and the potential for fetal congestive failure [2]. Detailed fetal echocardiography is required for management.

IV. Fetal acid-base determination is accomplished most commonly through the clinical technique of fetal scalp blood sampling (FSBS). In the presence of an abnormal FHR pattern, the patient is placed in either a lateral recumbent or a dorsal lithotomy position, and an endoscope is inserted through the cervix to allow visualization of the fetal scalp. A standard fetal scalp blade is used to make a 2-mm deep incision in the fetal scalp. Blood is withdrawn into a heparinized pipette for analysis. The FSBS values usually fall between those of the umbilical artery and vein (Table 22-1) [24].

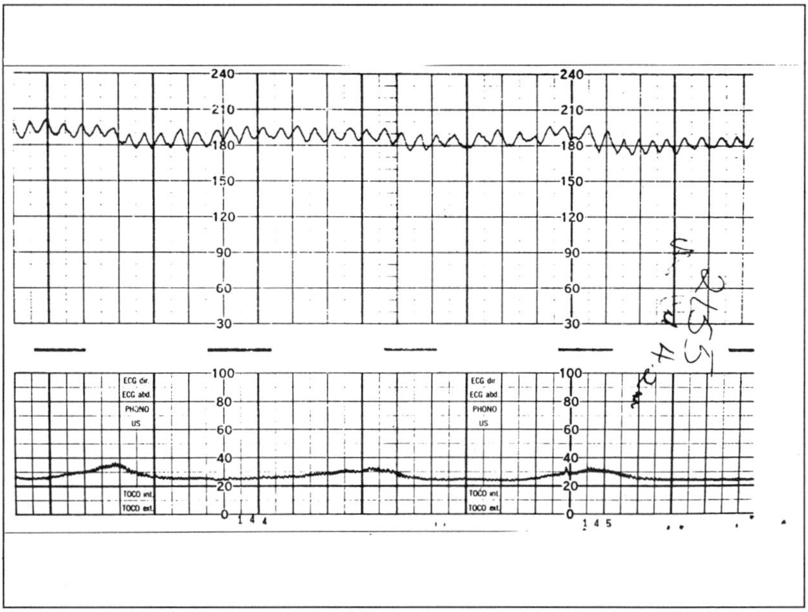

Fig. 22-5. Sinusoidal pattern during fetal heart rate monitoring. Note repetitive late decelerations hidden within the pattern.

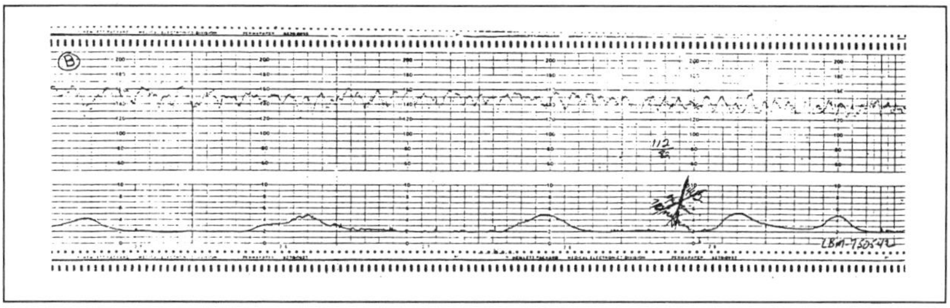

Fig. 22-6. The presence of short-term variability within the pattern distinguishes this as a "pseudosinusoidal" pattern. (From R. K. Freeman and T. J. Garite, *Fetal Heart Rate Monitoring*. Baltimore: Williams & Wilkins, 1981. P. 82.)

Table 22-1. Fetal acid-base determination by fetal scalp blood sampling

Acid-base status	Normal values	Values in metabolic acidosis	Values in respiratory acidosis
pH	7.25–7.35	< 7.25	< 7.25
pCO_2	40–50 mm Hg	45–55 mm Hg	> 50 mm Hg
pO_2	20–30 mm Hg	< 20 mm Hg	Variable
Base deficit	< 10 mEq/L	> 10 mEq/L	< 10 mEq/L

Source: R. K. Freeman and T. J. Garite, *Fetal Heart Rate Monitoring*. Baltimore: Williams & Wilkins, 1981.

Currently, there is disagreement about the indications for FSBS. It probably should be limited to patients with FHR tracings suggestive of hypoxia, as in the following situations:

A. In the presence of a confusing FHR pattern with elements suggesting hypoxia.

B. With a sustained flat FHR but no ominous periodic changes.

C. In the presence of a nonreassuring pattern where vaginal delivery is anticipated within 60 minutes. If the pH is greater than 7.25, observation should be continued and resampling may be indicated depending on the FHR pattern. A pH between 7.20 and 7.25 should be rechecked within a few minutes to determine a trend. If blood gas values indicate a metabolic component (Table 22-1), operative delivery is indicated in a patient with an initial pH below 7.20.

D. Most recently, the introduction of the scalp stimulation test [7] has reduced the need for many scalp samplings. FHR acceleration (15 bpm lasting 25 seconds) in response to digital or mechanical pressure applied to the fetal vertex correlated well with a nonacidotic pH (>7.20). This appears to be an appropriate first step in clinical situations where scalp sampling is contraindicated (e.g., fetal thrombocytopenia, hemophilia, or von Willebrand's disease).

V. Management of fetal distress

A. Whenever an abnormal FHR pattern occurs, the following usually are indicated:

1. **The patient should be turned off her back onto one side or the other.** Turning the patient onto her side may either relieve umbilical cord compression or alleviate poor return of blood to the maternal heart caused by occlusions of the maternal aorta or the inferior vena cava by the uterus. A good rule in the labor room is that no patient should be supine but should rather be in a semilateral position.
2. **Oxytocin infusion should be discontinued,** since excessive uterine activity may be the cause of the abnormal FHR response.
3. **Oxygen (100%) should be administered to the mother by face mask.**

4. **A vaginal examination should be done to rule out cord prolapse or imminent delivery.**
5. **Any hypotension should be corrected** by position change, intravenous hydration, or vasopressor treatment (ephedrine) if severe hypotension due to conduction anesthesia occurs.

Persistent late decelerations unresponsive to this therapy are an indication for expeditious (operative) delivery. Where FHR variability is normal and delivery is expected within 60 minutes, sequential scalp sampling may be used as long as the pH remains above 7.25. Any downward trend or worsening FHR pattern is an indication for immediate delivery. Persistent variable decelerations must be managed with greater individualism than late decelerations. Reassuring criteria can be defined, and if these are exceeded, management and intervention should be based on a consideration of proximity to vaginal delivery and other clinical data available. Generally, the greater the duration of decelerations, the greater the likelihood of fetal hypoxia and compromise.

Some studies [25, 28] suggest a role for saline amnioinfusion in patients with moderate to severe variable decelerations. Both the frequency and intensity of variable decelerations can be decreased with the infusion of saline solution through an intrauterine pressure catheter, often avoiding the need for cesarean section.

B. Criteria for reassuring variable decelerations

1. FHR deceleration of less than 30–45 seconds' duration on a repetitive basis.
2. Abrupt return of FHR to baseline; no "late component" as manifested by a slow return or a late deceleration after the return.
3. Stable baseline FHR (i.e., not increasing)
4. Good short- and long-term FHR variability.
5. Short, abrupt accelerations preceding and immediately following the deceleration.

Prolonged decelerations have a number of etiologies (see sec. **III.B.1.d**). If a correctable situation exists, labor should be allowed to continue, provided recovery occurs and the clinical situation warrants. If no obvious etiology can be determined, the patient should be observed for recovery while preparations are being made for an immediate cesarean section (amnioinfusion may play a role in such situations) [25]. If recovery occurs, 10–15 minutes' delay should be allowed for intrauterine resuscitation prior to proceeding with operative delivery.

VI. Antepartum monitoring. Although considerable controversy remains over which surveillance technique is preferable in the patient at risk for uteroplacental insufficiency, antepartum FHR monitoring is an integral part of the management of high-risk pregnancies. Current methods include the contraction stress test (CST), the nonstress test (NST), and most recently the biophysical profile (BPP).

A. The CST or oxytocin challenge test is a "pretest" of labor. Spontaneous or induced uterine contractions are recorded and the FHR observed for the presence of late decelerations, an *early* warning sign in fetal hypoxia and uteroplacental insufficiency [27]. Recently, breast (nipple) stimulation has been used to induce contractions and, thereby, avoid the need for intravenous oxytocin [17].

1. **Indications for testing.** Testing should be started when intervention (i.e., delivery) would be performed if the result clearly is abnormal. Generally accepted indications are listed in Table 22-2.
2. **Performing the CST.** A Doppler ultrasound transducer and an external tokodynamometer are most often used.
   a. The patient is placed in a lateral or semi-Fowler position to avoid supine hypotension.
   b. Baseline blood pressure is recorded at the start and every 15 minutes thereafter for the duration of the test.
   c. Baseline contractions and FHR are recorded for 20 minutes.
   d. If there are three contractions (each ≥ 40 seconds in duration) within 10 minutes during the baseline period and FHR recording is adequate, the test is concluded.
   e. If baseline uterine activity is insufficient, a warm, moist washcloth is placed on both breasts for several minutes. The patient then massages or rolls her

Table 22-2. Indications for antepartum fetal heart rate testing

Indication	When to start test
Preclampsia or eclampsia	When diagnosed after 26 wk
Chronic hypertension	34 wk
Collagen-vascular disease	34 wk
Diabetes mellitus	
Class A (uncomplicated)	40 wk
Class A with prior stillbirth, abnormal fasting blood glucose, or hypertension	34 wk
Class B, C, D	32–34 wk
Class F, R	26 wk
Severe anemia or hemoglobinopathy	34 wk
Severe Rh isoimmunization	26–34 wk
Hypertension	34 wk
Hyperthyroidism	34 wk
Cyanotic heart disease	34 wk
Prolonged pregnancy	41–42 wk
Previous stillbirth	34 wk
Suspected intrauterine growth retardation	26 wk or when suspected
Advanced maternal age (> 35 years)	If intrauterine growth retardation is suspected
Decreased fetal movement	26 wk or when suspected
Discordant twins	26 wk or when suspected

Source: Adapted from R. K. Freeman and T. J. Garite, *Fetal Heart Rate Monitoring*. Baltimore: Williams & Wilkins, 1981.

nipple for 10 minutes on one breast. If the contraction pattern remains unsatisfactory, bilateral breast stimulation is attempted. Once contractions begin, nipples are stimulated intermittently as needed. Approximately 75% of patients will have adequate CSTs with breast stimulation.

f. If breast stimulation fails, oxytocin is begun by IV infusion pump at 0.5 mU/minute, and the rate is increased at 15-minute intervals until three contractions lasting 40–60 seconds occur in a 10-minute period. The maximum dose of oxytocin is 32 mU/minute.

g. The frequency and duration of the contractions are used as the objective measurement of adequate stress.

h. If there are persistent late decelerations before adequate contraction frequency is obtained, the test is considered positive and may be stopped.

i. In either case, the patient is monitored until contractions have returned to baseline frequency.

3. Interpreting the CST

a. Negative. The absence of late decelerations with adequate frequency and duration of contractions, and a continuously interpretable FHR tracing.

b. Positive. Persistent late decelerations with the majority of contractions, in the absence of excessive uterine activity (hyperstimulation).

c. Equivocal tests

(1) Suspicious—the presence of **any** nonpersistent late decelerations.

(2) Hyperstimulation—decelerations associated with excessive uterine activity as defined by greater than five contractions in 10 minutes or a contraction duration greater than 90 seconds.

d. Unsatisfactory. Inadequate contraction frequency or inadequate recording of the FHR.

e. **Variable decelerations** on a CST may be suggestive of oligohydramnios, particularly if persistent. It may be an ominous pattern if associated with nonreactivity (intrauterine growth retardation, prolonged pregnancy).

4. **Patient management.** CSTs are graded as to reactivity as well (reactive if at least one acceleration of 15 bpm lasting 15 seconds occurs).
   a. **Reactive negative.** Very reassuring; repeat in one week unless maternal compromise occurs (e.g., diabetes out of control).
   b. **Nonreactive negative.** Unusual pattern; consider fetal central nervous system or cardiac anomaly, especially if associated with fetal bradycardia. Drug therapy (i.e., methadone, propranolol) may be implicated.
   c. **Reactive positive.** Fifty percent false-positive; generally associated with good outcome. If mature (i.e., term or documented fetal lung maturity), delivery should be accomplished with careful FHR monitoring (preferably internal). If immature, monitor with daily biophysical testing or continuous FHR monitoring, or both.
   d. **Nonreactive positive.** Ominous; rarely false-positive if ≥32 weeks; deliver by cesarean section regardless of fetal maturity status. Less than 32 weeks: there may be a role for daily biophysical profile testing with continuous FHR monitoring in selected cases [23].
   e. **Equivocal tests.** Approximately 20% of CSTs are equivocal. The test cannot be used to assure fetal health for one week as can a negative test; therefore, the CST must be repeated the next day.

5. **Contraindications** to contraction stress testing arise from the possible risk of oxytocin administration and subsequent contractions. These include
   a. Premature rupture of the membranes
   b. Previous classic cesarean section
   c. Placenta previa
   d. Multiple gestation } Relative contraindication
   e. Incompetent cervix } Relative contraindication
   f. History of premature labor } Relative contraindication

B. **Nonstress testing.** NST is based on the observation that FHR accelerations in association with fetal movement correlate with fetal well-being.

1. **Indications** are the same as for contraction stress testing with the advantage that the NST can be used where contraindications to a CST exist.

2. **Performing the NST**
   a. The patient is placed in a semi-Fowler position.
   b. Blood pressure is recorded.
   c. External monitors are applied.
   d. A recording is made for 20 minutes.
   e. Reactive NST. The presence of two accelerations of FHR in association with fetal movement, each lasting ≥ 15 bpm above baseline in a 20-minute span. Although the recommended test interval has been one week, recent studies suggest that twice-weekly NSTs effectively reduce antepartum stillbirth rates to levels approaching those for weekly CSTs [4, 9].
   f. If insufficient accelerations (0 or 1) occur in 20 minutes, the fetus is stimulated by 1 minute of manual manipulation and another 20-minute period is recorded.
   g. Should less than two accelerations occur subsequently, the test is interpreted as nonreactive (nonreassuring) and a CST must be performed.
   h. The CST may be discontinued at any point when the FHR becomes reactive.
   i. All accelerations probably have the same significance and are counted as such whether they occur in response to fetal movement, uterine contractions or spontaneously.

3. **Interpreting the NST.** The primary indication for use of the NST is as a screening test for fetal well-being. Approximately 10–35% of tests require a subsequent CST because of nonreactivity. Generally, the CST is preferred in critical high-risk situations, such as diabetes, preeclampsia, growth retardation, and postterm pregnancies. One should always critically evaluate the FHR response

to spontaneous contractions during an NST. Late or variable decelerations indicate a need for CST or ultrasound examination, or both.

C. Biophysical profile. Recent advances in real-time ultrasound technology provide the opportunity to image the fetus in motion and with remarkable detail. Qualitative assessment of amniotic fluid volume (AFV) by ultrasound is positively correlated with fetal outcome. The profile combines assessment of fetal breathing, fetal tone, gross body movements, AFV, and an NST. Several investigators have reported favorable outcomes in large series using the BPP for primary surveillance [20].

1. BPP scoring

a. NST: reactive—2 points.

b. Fetal breathing: 30 seconds of sustained breathing movement within a 30-minute observation period—2 points.

c. Fetal tone: one episode of extremity extension with a return to flexion (e.g., open and close fist)—2 points.

d. Gross body movements: three episodes of body movements (e.g., truncal or extremity) within 30 minutes—2 points.

e. AFV: at least one pocket of fluid more than 2 cm in depth—2 points.

2. Management protocol. See Table 22-3.

Although the BPP is an exciting addition to our armamentarium of surveillance techniques, **caution must be exercised** in adopting it as the primary mode of antepartum testing. A recent randomized trial found no difference in perinatal outcome when weekly BPPs were compared with NSTs [21]. The entire issue of which technique is preferable is controversial [32]; it remains our bias to use the CST, a potentially **earlier** sign of fetal jeopardy for primary fetal surveillance [9, 27].

Table 22-3. Biophysical profile (BPP) management protocol

Score	Interpretation	Recommended management
10	Normal infant, low risk for chronic asphyxia	Repeat testing at weekly intervals; repeat twice weekly in diabetic patients and patients ≥ 42 wk
8	Normal infant, low risk for chronic asphyxia	Repeat testing at weekly intervals; repeat twice weekly in diabetic patients and in patients ≥ 42 wk; indication for delivery—oligohydramnios
6	Suspected chronic asphyxia	Repeat testing within 24 hr; deliver patient if repeat test is 6 or less or if oligohydramnios is present
4	Suspected chronic asphyxia	≥ 36 weeks and favorable cervix, delivery; if < 36 wk and lecithin/sphingomyelin ratio <2.0, repeat test in 24 hr; indication for delivery: repeat score ≤ 6 or oligohydramnios
0–2	Strong suspicion of chronic asphyxia	Extend testing time to 120 min; indication for delivery—persistent score ≤ 4, regardless of gestational age

Source: Adapted from F. A. Manning. Assessment of fetal condition and risk analysis of single and combined biophysical variable monitoring. *Semin. Perinatol.* 9(no. 4):168–188, 1985.

References

1. Benson, R. C., et al. Fetal heart rate as a predictor of fetal distress: A report from the collaborative project. *Obstet. Gynecol.* 32:529, 1968.
2. Bergmans, M. G. M., Jonker, G. J., and Kock, H. C. L. U. Fetal supraventricular tachycardia. Review of literature. *Obstet. Gynecol. Surv.* 40:61, 1985.
3. Bisonette, J. M., Johnson, K., and Toomey, C. The role of a trial of labor with a positive oxytocin challenge test. *Am. J. Obstet. Gynecol.* 135:292, 1979.
4. Boehm, F. H., et al. Improved outcome of twice weekly nonstress testing. *Obstet. Gynecol.* 67:566, 1986.
5. Boehm, F. H., et al. The indirectly obtained fetal heart rate: Comparison of first and second generation electronic fetal monitors. *Am. J. Obstet. Gynecol.* 155:10, 1986.
6. Caldeyro-Barcia, R., et al. Control of Human Fetal Heart Rate During Labor. In D. Carsels (ed.), *The Heart and Circulation in the Newborn Infant.* New York: Grune & Stratton, 1966.
7. Clark, S., Gimovsky, M. L., and Miller, F. C. The scalp stimulation test. A clinical alternative to fetal scalp blood sampling. *Am. J. Obstet. Gynecol.* 148:272, 1984.
8. Dalton, K. J., Dawes, G. S., and Patrick, J. E. The autonomic nervous system and fetal heart rate variability. *Am. J. Obstet. Gynecol.* 146:456, 1983.
9. Freeman, R. K., Anderson, G., and Dorchester, W. A prospective multiinstitutional study of antepartum fetal heart rate monitoring. II. Contraction stress test versus nonstress test for primary surveillance. *Am. J. Obstet. Gynecol.* 143:1982.
10. Gimovsky, M. L., and Bruce, S. L. Aspects of FHR tracings as warning signals. *Clin. Obstet. Gynecol.* 29:55, 1986.
11. Goodlin, R. History of fetal monitoring. *Am. J. Obstet. Gynecol.* 133:325, 1979.
12. Goodlin, R. C., and Haesslein, H. C. Fetal reacting bradycardia. *Am. J. Obstet. Gynecol.* 129:845, 1977.
13. Goodlin, R. C., and Lowe, E. W. A functional umbilical cord occlusion heart rate pattern: The significance of overshoot. *Obstet. Gynecol.* 42:22, 1974.
14. Hammacher, K. In O. Kaser and V. Friedberg (eds.), *Gynakologie v. Gerburtshilfe BD II.* Stuttgart: Theime, 1967.
15. Hon, E. H. Observation on "pathologic" fetal bradycardia. *Am. J. Obstet. Gynecol.* 77:1084, 1959.
16. Hon, E. H. The electronic evaluation of the fetal heart rate. *Am. J. Obstet. Gynecol.* 75:1215, 1958.
17. Huddleston, J. F., Sutliff, G., and Robinson, D. Contraction stress test by intermittent nipple stimulation. *Obstet. Gynecol.* 63(5):669, 1984.
18. Klapholtz, H., et al. Role of maternal artifact in fetal heart rate pattern interpretation. *Obstet. Gynecol.* 44:373, 1974.
19. Kubli, F. W., et al. Observations on heart rate and pH in the human fetus during labor. *Am. J. Obstet. Gynecol.* 104:1190, 1969.
20. Manning, F. A., et al. Fetal assessment based on fetal biophysical profile scoring: Experience in 12,620 referred high-risk pregnancies. *Am. J. Obstet. Gynecol.* 151:343, 1985.
21. Manning, F. A., et al. Fetal biophysical profile score and the nonstress test: A comparative trial. *Obstet. Gynecol.* 64:326, 1984.
22. Martin, C. B. Physiology and clinical use of fetal heart rate variability. *Clin. Perinatol.* 9:339, 1982.
23. Merrill, P. A., et al. Evaluation of the non-reactive positive contraction stress test prior to 32 weeks—The role of the biophysical profile. Presented at 6th annual meeting, Society of Perinatal Obstetrics, San Antonio, #61, 1986.
24. Miller, F. C. Prediction of acid-base values from intrapartum fetal heart rate data and their correlation with scalp and funic values. *Clin. Perinatol.* 9:353, 1982.
25. Miyazaki, F. S., and Taylor, N. A. Saline amnioinfusion for relief of variable or prolonged decelerations. *Am. J. Obstet. Gynecol.* 146:670, 1983.

26. Modanlou, H. D., and Freeman, R. K. Sinusoidal fetal heart rate pattern: Its definition and clinical significance. *Am. J. Obstet. Gynecol.* 142:1033, 1981.
27. Murata, Y., et al. Fetal heart rate accelerations and late decelerations during the course of intrauterine death in chronically catheterized rhesus monkey. *Am. J. Obstet. Gynecol.* 144:218, 1982.
28. Nageotte, M. P., et al. Prophylactic intrapartum amnioinfusion in patients with preterm premature rupture of membranes. *Am. J. Obstet. Gynecol.* 153:557, 1985.
29. Nageotte, M. P., et al. Short-term variability assessment from abdominal electrocardiograms during the antepartum period. *Am. J. Obstet. Gynecol.* 145:566, 1983.
30. Schneider, E. P., and Tropper, P. J. The variable deceleration and sinusoidal fetal heart rate. *Clin. Obstet. Gynecol.* 29:64, 1986.
31. Shenker, L. Fetal cardiac arrhythmias. *Obstet. Gynecol. Surv.* 34:561, 1979.
32. Thacker, S. B., and Berkelman, S. B. Assessing the diagnostic accuracy and efficacy of selected antepartum fetal surveillance techniques. *Obstet. Gynecol. Surv.* 41:121, 1986.

Bibliography

Freeman, R. K., and Garite, T. J. *Fetal Heart Rate Monitoring.* Baltimore: Williams & Wilkins, 1981.

Parer, J. T. *Handbook of Fetal Heart Rate Monitoring.* Philadelphia: Saunders, 1983.

23 Isoimmunization

Robert Nathan Slotnick

Isoimmunization (maternal blood group immunization), a disease of genetic predisposition, has been a focus of concern for obstetricians for centuries. Fifty years ago, Landsteiner and Weiner [8] first described their classic experiment in which Rhesus monkey red-cell antisera was mixed with blood samples from a selected human population. Levine and colleagues [9] subsequently demonstrated that the Rh-immune response in an Rh-negative woman was the primary etiology for hemolytic disease in the newborn. The identification of the Rhesus antigen and its description in these classic works are a cornerstone of modern immunohematology. Improving technologies and the elucidation of the complexities of the Rh blood group system have led to the development of sensitive screening tests for blood group antibodies. The maternal isoimmunized patient and her caregiver now have choices for both prevention and management of this historically difficult problem.

I. Rh system

A. D antigen. Although the Rh antigens are grouped in three pairs (Dd, Cc, Ee), the presence of the D antigen determines that the individual is Rh-positive. The Rh-positive individual will be found to be homozygous for D (i.e., DD) approximately 45% of the time. This results from having inherited D-containing sets of alleles from both parents. The remainder of Rh-positive individuals will be heterozygous for the D locus (Dd). A homozygous partner of an Rh-negative woman can produce only Rh-positive offspring; a heterozygous partner can produce either Rh-positive or Rh-negative offspring with equal frequency in each pregnancy. Rh isoimmunization can occur only in the pregnancy where an Rh-positive fetus resides, and only that fetus will be affected by the maternally produced Rh antibody.

B. Other Rh antigens. A long list of other antibodies have been described than delineate other Rh antigens and argue for a hugely more complex system that the Cc-Dd-Ee antigen loci might suggest. **Hemolytic disease of the newborn and fetal erythroblastosis are much less common with these antigens (D^u, C^w),** which were first described in Tippett and Sanger's [14] classic article. The proteolipid Rh antigen chemically described by Brown and colleagues [4] in 1983 is an essential component of the red blood cell membrane.

C. Population distribution. The absence of the proteolipid Rh antigen (Rh-negativity) seems to be **an exclusively white trait.** In predominantly white national groups, approximately 15–16% of the population has been identified as Rh-negative. The distribution is not homogeneous, however. It appears that the Basque population of Spain has an incidence of 30–32% Rh-negativity. The frequency of Rh-negativity in Asian, Native American, and black populations is significantly lower. Approximately 8% of American blacks are Rh-negative; African blacks are significantly less likely to be Rh-negative. These population statistics argue that Rh-negativity was originally confined to the Basque population, and that initially all of the races were entirely Rh-positive.

II. Etiology. Blood group isoimmunization generally arises from one of two pathogenetic incidents: incompatible blood transfusion or fetal-maternal hemorrhage.

A. Incompatible blood transfusion. Although still the most common cause of non-Rhesus blood group immunization, transfusion isoimmunization generally is related to development of atypical blood group antibodies. Although the majority of atypical antibodies are of little clinical consequence, hemolytic disease of the fetus and newborn can be related to a few atypical antibodies (Table 23-1).

Table 23-1. Atypical maternal blood group antibodies and associated risk of fetal/neonatal hemolytic disease

Antibody	Relative hemolytic disease risk
c	Common
Kell	
E	
Fy^a	
e	Uncommon
C	
Ce	
Kp^a	
Kp^b	
cE	
k	
s	
S	Very rare
U	
M	
Fy^b	
N	
Do^a	
Co^a	
Di^a	
Di^b	
Lu^a	
Yt^a	
Jk^a	
Jk^b	
Le^a	None
Le^b	
P	

As demonstrated in 1986 by Bowman and colleagues [3], 75% of pregnancies have some evidence of transplacental hemorrhage during gestation or at delivery. As measured by the sensitive test developed by Kleihauer et al. [7] in 1957, the amount of fetal blood in maternal circulation is most frequently less than 0.1 ml. Antepartum hemorrhage, pregnancy-induced hypertension, manual removal of the placenta, cesarean section, and external version are all related to larger volumes of transplacental hemorrhage, however. Amniocentesis, for genetic or other indications, has also been associated with increased risk of maternal sensitization, particularly if the placenta is transversed during the amniocentesis process. A 5–25% incidence of fetal-maternal hemorrhage has been identified following abortion, both spontaneous and therapeutic.

B. Fetal-maternal hemorrhage. Maternal response to the introduction of Rh-positive fetal cells into maternal circulation is a two-step phenomenon. The first, primary Rh-immune response, is frequently slow and weak in its development. This may be related to the compromised immune response seen in the pregnant patient. The identification of immunoglobulin M (IgM) anti-D is often not seen before eight to nine weeks after exposure; six months may elapse before this primary response is seen. The pregnant patient then frequently switches rapidly to the production of IgG anti-D, which does cross the placenta. After the establishment of the primary response, a second exposure with a very small inoculum generally produces a rapid and profound increase in IgG anti-D.

III. Incidence. Although Rh immunization incidence appears dose dependent, a small inoculum may be sufficient to generate immunization. Zipursky and Israels [16] and Woodrow [15] have produced data that indicate that 50% of patients would become immunized with an inoculum of 50–75 ml of Rh-positive cells. The secondary response, however, can be provoked by as little as 0.1 ml of red cells.

A. ABO incompatibility. Empirically derived risk figures argue that the risk that Rh immunization will develop as the result of a first ABO-compatible, Rh-positive pregnancy to an Rh-negative woman is approximately 16%. If not immunized by a first pregnancy, the risk appears approximately the same for a second pregnancy. Although subsequent pregnancy risk for nonresponding patients decreases, a patient undergoing five Rh-positive ABO-compatible pregnancies has a 50% likelihood of becoming Rh immunized. An ancillary consideration in the evaluation of the Rh-negative woman is the consideration of ABO incompatibility. Conferring partial protection, ABO incompatibility decreases immunization risk markedly. Woodrow [15] has calculated empiric risk figures such that the risk of an Rh immunization after an ABO-incompatible Rh-positive pregnancy is approximately 2%. As Bowman and Pollock [2] have indicated, as many as 2% of Rh-negative unimmunized women become Rh immunized during pregnancy after 28 weeks' gestation. This represents 12% of all the Rh-negative women who would become Rh immunized as a result of Rh-positive pregnancies and has led to recommendation for administration of RhoGAM at approximately 28 weeks of gestation.

B. Risk factors. Although the numbers are equivocal, it appears that approximately 2% of women having spontaneous or therapeutic abortions are at risk of becoming Rh immunized. This risk grows by two-and-a-half–fold after 20 weeks of gestation. It is suggested that early abortion (six to eight weeks) provides a much lower risk than a later abortion. The diagnosis and management of the Rh-immunized pregnancy depends on the early initial evaluation and identification of patients at risk. As part of that evaluation, a blood sample should be taken from every woman at her first antenatal visit for Rh blood grouping and antibody screening. This test should be universal and should be carried out independent of parity and independent of reported results of prior screening tests. The Rh-positive woman with no demonstrable blood group antibodies should be rescreened at 34–38 weeks of gestation to identify the possibility of a significant atypical antibody developing late in pregnancy.

C. Paternal Rh status. The Rh-negative gravida should be further studied to assess her ABO Group and the Rh status and ABO group of her partner. If he is Rh-negative, the conceptus should be Rh-negative and the mother should not be at risk for Rh immunization. This patient should be rescreened at 34 weeks' gestation; extramarital pregnancies do occur. If the father is Rh-positive and his ABO group is known, the Rh phenotype can be calculated and the risk of Rh immunization can be calculated as well (Table 23-2).

IV. Management. It is incumbent on the practitioner to follow this pregnancy closely.

A. Antibody screening. Further antibody screening should be performed as the pregnancy progresses. A second test at 18–20 weeks' gestation and monthly tests thereafter are prudent. Rarely does the primary or secondary immune response become visible prior to 20 weeks of gestation.

B. RhoGAM should be administered at 28 weeks of gestation in those patients where immunization has not occurred previously. If the patient is a candidate for amniocentesis for genetic or nongenetic indications, consideration of RhoGAM administration should be foremost in the mind of the practitioner. Delivery route and its management can affect the quantity of fetal-maternal inoculation, and quantitation of RhoGAM dosage subsequent to delivery should be made through a Kleihauer-Betke test.

C. Progressive involvement. There are two classic patterns that allow prediction of the severity of the Rh-hemolytic disease in the isoimmunized gravida. It seems equally probable that the degree of the disease would remain the same from baby to baby as it would be likely to become progressively worse with each succeeding pregnancy. The risk of hydrops in the first sensitized pregnancy is approximately

Table 23-2. Approximate risk of Rh isoimmunization

Partner	Fetus	Risk (%)
D (−)	D (−)	0
D (+) homozygous, ABO compatible	D (+)	16
D (+) homozygous, ABO incompatible	D (+), ABO incompatible	2
D (+) heterozygous, ABO compatible	Rh unknown	8
D (+) heterozygous, ABO incompatible	ABO, Rh unknown	3.5

10%. Unfortunately there is no way to predict when, during a subsequent pregnancy, a fetus would become hydropic. Bowman and Pollock [2] have argued convincingly that proper management of the Rh-negative mother requires more than simple Rh-antibody titer testing during the pregnancy.

D. Liley graph. In an effort to more accurately predict a clinical course for an immunized pregnancy, and as a means to allow comparison of measurements from different laboratories, Liley [11] in 1961 described a method of **amniocentesis and amniotic fluid spectrophotometric analysis.**

1. The optical density reading at 450 nm (the Delta OD 450 reading) is directly related to the severity of hemolytic disease. By plotting Delta OD 450 versus gestational age, in his original study Liley was able to evaluate the degree of hemolytic disease in 101 Rh-immunized pregnancies.
2. This initial work performed on gestations after 28 weeks allowed prediction of the clinical course based on the arbitrary **division of the patients into three zones.** Severe hemolytic disease, fetal hydrops, and fetal death were temporally related to readings in the upper zone (zone 3). Mild or no hemolytic disease was identified in zone 1. Empiric data and evolving prognostic accuracy have allowed the evolution of the associated chart (Fig. 23-1). The method of measurement used, however, seems less important than the judgment and experience of the person reviewing amniotic fluid results.

E. Delivery. Those 50–60% of pregnancies immunized for the Rh antigen in which either amniocentesis has not been required or Delta OD 450 measurements have been measured to fall within mid zone 2 or lower should be allowed to deliver spontaneously. The patient in whom elevation to upper zone 2 is measured by amniocentesis at 35–37 weeks of gestation should be encouraged to deliver at 37–38 weeks of gestation, provided that lung maturity can be demonstrated. Pregnancies in which hydrops is noted after 34 weeks of gestation represent 20% of all pregnancies where hydrops is seen. Such patients should be promptly delivered if the Delta OD 450 measurement rises to upper zone 2 or zone 3. Although evidence of pulmonary maturity is preferable, corticosteroid administration may be considered 48 hours prior to delivery.

V. Treatment. In those pregnancies where prematurity is problematic and where neonatal morbidity and mortality rates are elevated, **intrauterine treatment** becomes the therapeutic mode of choice.

A. Transfusion. The original **intrauterine fetal transfusion,** an intraperitoneal transfusion technique, was first described by Liley [10] in 1963. With increasing sonographic sophistication, intravascular transfusion, providing more immediate diagnostic and therapeutic endeavors to be employed, was described by Rodeck and colleagues [13] in 1981 (via fetoscope) and via needle by Bang and colleagues [1] in 1982. These procedures, either intraperitoneal transfusion or intravenous transfusion, should only be attempted by those skilled at ultrasound interpre-

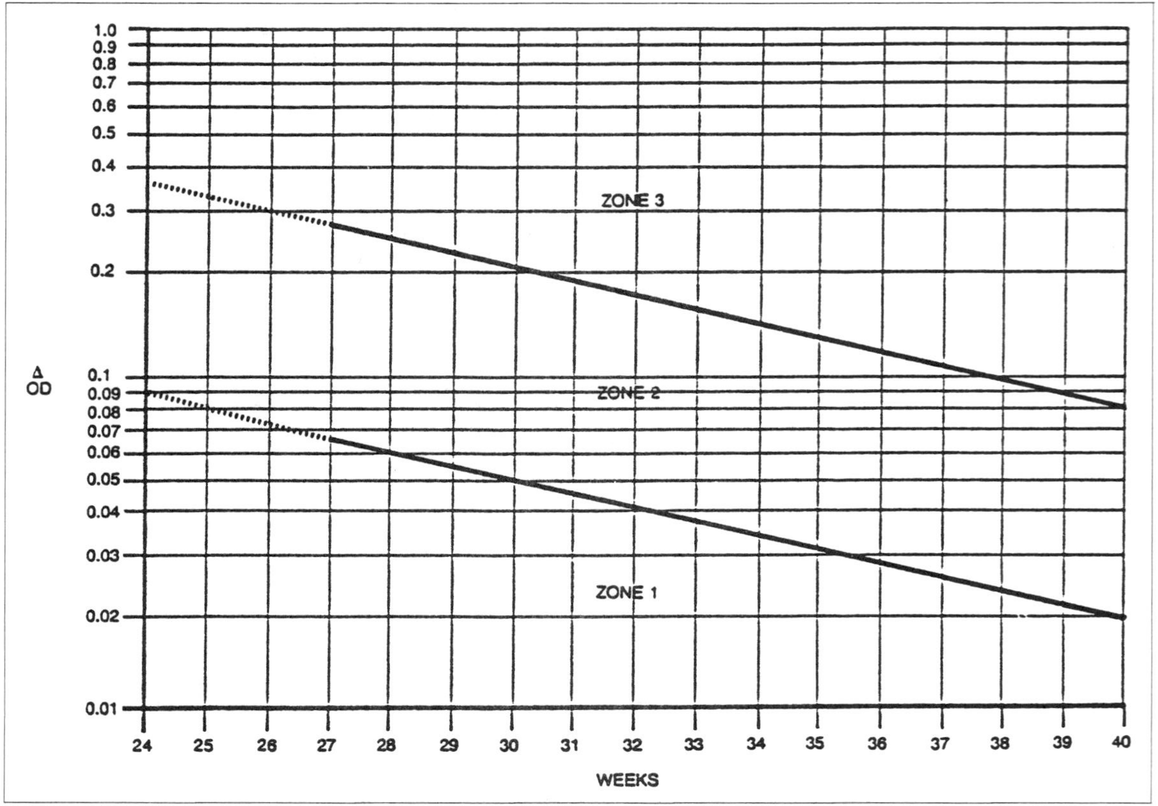

Fig. 23-1. Modified Liley graph used to depict degrees of sensitization. The dotted line represents a linear extrapolation from the original Liley data (solid line). (From the American College of Obstetricians and Gynecologists, *Management of Isoimmunization in Pregnancy*. ACOG Technical Bulletin no. 90, January 1986. Reprinted by permission of *Am. J. Obstet. Gynecol*. St. Louis: Mosby.)

Table 23-3. Intrauterine transfusion risks

Fetal
Exsanguination
Overtransfusion
Cardiac tamponade (intraperitoneal transfusion, primarily)
Infection
Labor induction
Umbilical vein compression (intrauterine transfusion, primarily)
Maternal
Infection
Tissue trauma
Fetal-maternal
Further transplacental hemorrhage

tation and cordocentesis since intrauterine transfusion carries distinct risks for the fetus (Table 23-3).

Frigoletto and colleagues [5] and Hamilton [6] argue convincingly that intrauterine transfusion is a legitimate therapeutic modality. When indicated premature deliveries are removed from statistical consideration, the **physical and intellectual development in most fetal transfusion survivors appears normal.** Although suppression of Rh immunization by various different modalities (promethazine, plasmophoresis, intravenous immune serum globulin) remains equivocal, it is quite obvious that prevention of Rh immunization altogether is a largely attainable goal.

B. Postpartum RhoGAM. Present recommendations indicate administration of Rhesus immunoglobulin (RhoGAM, RhIg) to the mother as soon after delivery as cord blood findings indicate the baby to be Rh-positive and the mother to be at risk. Adherence to the dictum that it is preferable to treat a woman unnecessarily than to fail to treat a woman who then becomes Rh sensitized is sensible. A woman at risk is inadvertently **not** given RhIg within 72 hours after delivery should still receive prophylaxis at least up to two weeks after delivery. If prophylaxis is delayed, it should be understood that it may not be effective.

1. If there is any question about **the amount of RhIg to be administered after delivery,** a Kleihauer-Betke test should be performed and a calculation of quantity of transplacental hemorrhage made. Current recommendations indicate that one vial (300 μg) of RhIg should be administered if the transplacental hemorrhage is 25 ml of blood or less, two vials (600 μg) if the transplacental hemorrhage is between 25–50 ml, and so forth.

References

1. Bang, J., Bock, J. E., and Trolle, D. Ultra-sound guided fetal intravenous transfusion for severe rhesus haemolytic disease. *Br. Med. J.* 284:373, 1982.
2. Bowman, J. M., and Pollock, J. M. Antenatal Rh prophylaxis: 28 week gestation service program. *Can. Med. Assoc. J.* 18:627, 1978.
3. Bowman, J. M., Pollock, J. M., and Penston, L. E. Fetomaternal transplacental hemorrhage during pregnancy and after delivery. *Vox Sang.* 51:117, 1986.
4. Brown, P. J., et al. The Rhesus D antigen. A dicyclohexylcarbodiimide-binding proteo-lipid. *Am. J. Pathol.* 110:127, 1983.
5. Frigoletto, F. D., et al. Intrauterine fetal transfusion in 365 fetuses during fifteen years. *Am. J. Obstet. Gynecol.* 139:781, 1981.
6. Hamilton, E. T. Intrauterine transfusion. Safeguard or peril. *Obstet. Gynecol.* 50:255, 1977.
7. Kleihauer, E., Braun, H., and Betke, K. Demonstration von Fetalem Haemoglobin in den Erythrozyten eines Blutrasstriches. *Klin. Wochenschr.* 35:637, 1957.

8. Landsteiner, K., and Weiner, A. S. An agglutinable factor in human blood recognized by immune sera for Rhesus blood. *Proc. Soc. Exp. Biol. Med.* 43:223, 1940.
9. Levine, P., Katzin, E. M., and Burnham, L. Isoimmunization in pregnancy: Its possible bearing on the etiology of erythroblastosis fetalis. *J.A.M.A.* 116:825, 1941.
10. Liley, A. W. Intrauterine transfusion of fetus in hemolytic disease. *Br. Med. J.* 2:1107, 1963.
11. Liley, A. W. Liquor amnii analysis in management of pregnancy complicated by rhesus immunization. *Am. J. Obstet. Gynecol.* 82:1359, 1961.
12. Mattison, D. R., et al. Effects of drugs and chemicals on the fetus. Parts 1–3. *Contemp. Obstet. Gynecol.* 34:97–110; 131–145; 163–176, 1989.
13. Rodeck, C. H., et al. Direct intravascular fetal blood transfusion by fetoscopy in severe rhesus isoimmunisation. *Lancet* 1:652, 1981.
14. Tippett, P., and Sanger, R. Observations on subdivisions of the Rh antigen D. *Vox Sang.* 7:9, 1962.
15. Woodrow, J. C. Rh Immunization and Its Prevention. In *Series Hematologia*, Vol. III. Copenhagen: Munksgaard, 1970.
16. Zipursky, A., and Israels, L. G. The pathogenesis and prevention of Rh immunization. *Can. Med. Assoc. J.* 97:1245, 1967.

24 Genetic Diseases

Frances R. Tennant

I. **Normal versus abnormal.** The most important skill of the practitioner (obstetrician, pediatrician, or family practitioner), and one that is absolutely essential to the detection and identification of birth defects, is a primary understanding and recognition of what is normal. This permits identification of the unusual and abnormal. In human babies, there are wide variations within the normal range. Not all unusual babies are abnormal or have pathologic disease. When a physician becomes concerned about the unusual appearance of an infant, perhaps the most useful first step is for him or her to compare the infant with other normal members of the infant's family (i.e., the parents and siblings). For example, the bulbous nose, those wide-set eyes, and the somewhat peculiar toes may be family traits and of no apparent significance for general health and prognosis.

A. **Differentiation.** When the physician is faced with something unusual that may be significant, the task of differentiation is paramount. The condition may be serious and of immediate concern, relatively unimportant, or of no urgency. The diagnosis may be simple, requiring no outside help, or it may be very complex, requiring special tests and assistance from medical specialists. Family counseling and proper management likewise may be simple or complex.

B. **Birth defects.** The emphasis here will be mainly on birth defects of a genetic nature as opposed to abnormalities caused by injury, infection, and so on. Obstetricians often are the first people to see newborn babies, and birth defects are some of the most common problems facing them. Two percent of the babies born in the United States will have some kind of defect detectable at birth. By age 1 year, 4–5% of the children will show some sort of defect; this doubling is attributable to defects not apparent at birth.

Since the advent of better delivery techniques, relatively fewer birth abnormalities are caused by birth injuries, and thus a higher proportion are caused by genetic factors. Approximately 25% of birth defects are caused primarily by genetic factors, 15% primarily by environmental effects, 30% by a combination, and 30% are of unknown cause. It would be advantageous to be able to tell which were caused by genetic factors and, thus, which kinds of tests to order (e.g., chromosome complements or metabolic studies) and how to interpret the results of these tests. This knowledge would also be helpful in making the decision of whether to refer the patient to a genetic counselor.

II. **General guidelines in differentiating genetic from environmental defects**

A. **Most genetic defects are congenital.** There are exceptions, however. Environmental factors such as excess x radiation, certain drugs, and rubella infection in early pregnancy can produce different kinds of congenital defects, whereas some genetic (mostly metabolic) problems, such as galactosemia, phenylketonuria, and Tay-Sachs disease, do not show the first clinical signs or symptoms until some days, weeks, or months after birth. Some genetic conditions, such as diabetes mellitus and Huntington' s chorea, usually do not appear until adulthood.

B. **Most genetic defects are familial.** They occur in the family in a particular pattern of inheritance. (How it runs in the family is very important—whether there are more affected male than female members, whether parents are normal or affected, and whether or not the defect skips generations.) There are exceptions to this too. There may be several cases of an infectious disease in a family and nutritional deficiencies that may involve different members of a family. These are familial but certainly not genetic. It may be very difficult to ascertain whether the defect is familial. We know albinism is genetic, but we usually do not find more than one case in a family, because of small family size, dispersion of families all over the country, and the fact that family members may have little or no knowledge of relatives elsewhere. New cases of genetic disorders spring up now and then because of fresh mutations and the bringing together of previously hidden recessive genes.

C. Many genetic defects are **metabolic** and show a progression of severity with time. (Many of these metabolic defects are autosomal recessive and show a typical autosomal recessive pattern of inheritance.) There are, of course, exceptions to this too. Porphyria can be part of both dominantly and recessively inherited conditions, or it can result from lead poisoning.

D. Many genetic defects are **chromosomal,** but not necessarily heritable. In fact, many of them are lethal, and many persons with chromosomal defects are sterile.

E. Twin studies may show some defects to be genetic. For example, if one identical twin has epilepsy, in 67% of cases the other twin has it too. If one nonidentical twin has epilepsy, in 3% of cases the other twin also will be epileptic. Obviously, there is a genetic influence operating, but the fact that both identical twins do not always get epilepsy suggests that it is not totally genetic; there may be different causes for epilepsy or there may be some unrecognized protective environmental factors affecting one twin and not the other.

F. Consanguinity (inbreeding) is present more frequently in parents of persons with genetic defects. Consanguinity increases the chance of both parents having the same hidden recessive gene, since they have a recent common ancestor. First cousins, for example, have one-eighth of their genes in common with each other. In this country, approximately 10% of albinos, for instance, have parents who are related, whereas the consanguinity rate in the general population is less than 1%. Thus, the presence of consanguinity in the parents of a defective or abnormal child makes one suspicious that the condition may be inherited by an autosomal recessive gene. The rarer the recessive, the more likely the parents are to be related. Alkaptonuria occurs in 1 in 1 million births, and 30% of alkaptonuric patients have parents who are related.

G. Animal studies may be helpful in identifying human genetic defects. For example, albinism is an autosomal recessive gene disorder in rabbits and mice, just as it is in humans.

III. Human chromosome analysis. The appropriate use of chromosome studies represents one of the most important advances of the past two decades with regard to the diagnosis of birth defects.

A. Incidence of chromosomal abnormalities. Approximately 1 in 150 liveborn babies has a detectable chromosomal abnormality. These irregularities are about equally divided between abnormalities of the sex chromosomes and alterations in the remaining chromosomes (autosomes). Approximately one in six recognized pregnancies ends in spontaneous abortion. Approximately one-half of these abortions are associated with detectable chromosomal abnormalities. Thus, nearly 10% of all recognized conceptions are accompanied by an identifiable chromosomal abnormality. Intelligent use of chromosome analysis as an investigative tool is essential if we are to understand and prevent the major causes of human wastage and congenital anomalies.

B. Indications for performing chromosome studies. An increase in a practitioner's index of suspicion regarding what sorts of abnormalities might be associated with chromosomal aberrations and in his or her understanding of local services available for chromosome analysis will help in making diagnoses, determining prognoses, and providing effective counseling.

Some indications that chromosome studies should be done include

1. Any obvious suspected chromosomal abnormality (e.g., Down's syndrome or infant Turner's syndrome) to verify the diagnosis and to distinguish unusual translocation and mosaic forms of the conditions.
2. Odd-looking children with some other problem; children who do not look like their parents or their normal siblings and who have some other anomaly such

as unexplained mental retardation; multiple anomalies—checking mainly for duplication and deletion abnormalities of the chromosomes.

3. Individuals in whom it is difficult to tell whether they are male or female—mainly for possible aberrations of the sex chromosomes.
4. Individuals with fertility problems—mainly for possible aberrations of the sex chromosomes.
5. Repeated miscarriages. Chromosome studies should be done on the fetal material (including the placenta) if available. If fetal material is not accessible, studies should be carried out on the normal parents, looking for a possible balanced translocation that could be transmitted to a child in an unbalanced form, causing abnormalities.
6. Individuals suspected of having myelogenous leukemia. Look for the presence of the "Philadelphia chromosome," a translocation of part of the long arm of one of the small number 22 chromosomes to chromosome 9. (An increasing number of cancerous conditions are found to have associated chromosome changes that can aid in diagnosis and prognosis.)
7. Individuals with a rare dominant syndrome not previously reported to have normal-appearing chromosomes.
8. Certain immunodeficiency disorders and history of drug ingestion. Look for chromosomal breakage and other aberrations.
9. Moderate retardation that fits an X-linked pattern in a family. Look for a fragile X chromosome.

IV. Genetic amniocentesis. Prenatal detection of a number of serious birth defects and genetic disorders now is possible and practical by amniotic fluid sampling. Amniocentesis is accomplished by inserting a needle into the amniotic cavity, usually with ultrasonic guidance, to withdraw fluid. The fluid can be used for diagnostic tests directly, or it can be centrifuged and incubated to grow the embryonic cells it contains for chromosome analysis (Fig. 24-1). This procedure usually is performed at approximately 12–20 weeks from the last menstrual period. Before that time, there is insufficient fluid (or cells in the fluid), and later, insufficient time will elapse between the harvest of the cells (2–3 weeks) and the 23-week gestational age usually considered the upper limit for an indicated abortion.

The following are indications for amniocentesis:

A. Maternal age of 35 or more. The risk that a woman will have a mentally retarded Down's syndrome baby (mongolism) increases from 1 in 2000 births for women in their twenties, to 1 in 350 births at age 35, 1 in 100 at age 40, and 1 in 40 at age 45. Failure to inform a woman of this increased risk and the fact that there are tests to identify this syndrome early enough to offer interruption of pregnancy has led to catastrophic lawsuits.

B. Previous delivery of a chromosomally abnormal child. A gravida who has previously delivered an infant affected with trisomy 21, Down's syndrome, or other chromosome trisomy has a moderate (1–2%) risk for repeat.

C. Other heritable chromosomal abnormalities. When one of the parents is a carrier of a balanced translocation, the chance for an abnormal fetus can be as high as 1 in 2. This condition may be signaled by repeated abortions.

D. When the gravida is a carrier. If the mother is a carrier of a serious sex-linked (X-linked) disease, such as hemophilia or muscular dystrophy, amniocentesis or chorionic villus sampling is indicated for sex determination. Many of these conditions can then be specifically diagnosed with gene probes. Male fetuses have a 50% risk of being affected, and female fetuses, although they may be carriers, will not be affected.

E. Family history of a neural tube defect. If a previous child of a mother has had a defect such as open spina bifida or anencephaly, abnormally elevated alpha fetoprotein (AFP) levels in the amniotic fluid will be seen with an abnormal fetus. The risk for a second child is 1 in 25 with each subsequent pregnancy. Even siblings of patients with neural tube defects have an increased risk of producing a child with a neural tube defect (approximately 0.8%). Aunts and uncles of a patient have a 0.4% risk of having affected children (first cousins of the patient). These elevations will not occur with closed neural tube defects.

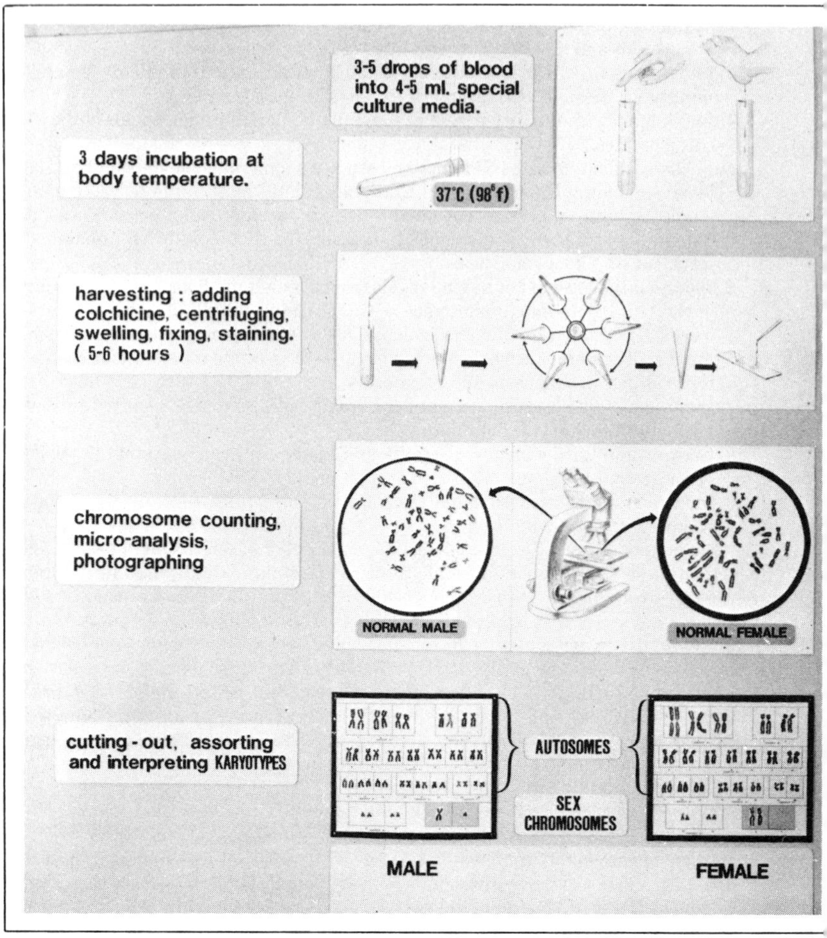

Fig. 24-1. Methodology used for karyotype determination by the micromethod. (Many laboratories now use heparinized venous blood rather than capillary blood.)

F. **If both parents are carriers.** When both parents are carriers of certain selected genetic (mostly autosomal recessive) metabolic disorders, the risk for an affected fetus is 25%. Carrier tests are available for some disorders (e.g., Tay-Sachs disease), or a family history may reveal a person to be a carrier.

G. **If the gravida is diabetic.** There is a tenfold increase in the frequency of neural tube defects in the progeny of diabetic mothers compared to nondiabetic mothers. This is 20 in 1000 births (2%), in contrast to the expected 1 or 2 in 1000 in routine pregnancies.

H. **Repeated miscarriages, usually three or more.** Since one-half of spontaneous abortions are associated with detectable chromosomal abnormalities, a woman with repeated miscarriages is at increased risk of producing a chromosomally abnormal child.

V. Other methods of prenatal diagnosis

A. **Maternal serum alpha fetoprotein testing.** In many states, levels of AFP in maternal serum can be determined for all pregnant women. This screening test identifies pregnancies at risk for neural tube defects. To really impact on conditions such as neural tube defects, for which 95% of affected individuals are born to parents without apparent risk factors, all pregnancies must be screened. The incidence of neural tube defects is approximately 1–2 in 1000 live births. In an initial screening, the serum AFP level will be elevated in approximately 50 in 1000 women. If the test is repeated in this group, AFP levels will still be elevated in 30 of the 50; the other 20 cases represent transient elevations. Ultrasonography will rule out incorrect dates (AFP levels vary with gestational age), multiple gestations, and fetal demise as reasons for an elevated AFP level, yet 17–18 of the original 50 presumptive positive results will remain as unexplained elevations. The patients whose AFP elevations remain unexplained after all these steps will require referral for amniotic fluid levels of AFP and the presence or absence of acetylcholinesterase to rule out a neural tube defect. Other structural defects, such as ventral wall defects and cystic hygroma can elevate maternal serum AFP. These would not be positive for acetylcholinesterase. These last few patients, although their fetuses may not have neural tube defects, do represent higher-risk pregnancies for prematurity and other factors. Patients with low levels of serum AFP are at increased risk of having a fetus with a chromosome abnormality. The precise risk will also depend on the patient's age, weight, and ethnic background.

B. Chorionic villus biopsy. An earlier and very promising new method of prenatal diagnosis uses a sample of the chorionic villus to determine chromosomal and metabolic abnormalities in a fetus. This sampling is done from 9–11 weeks' gestation, when termination of the pregnancy with a suspected adverse outcome could be done by the suction method rather than prostaglandin. Using a rapidly dividing tissue should eliminate the time delay caused by the tissue culturing needed for amniotic fluid cells. Unfortunately, spontaneous fetal loss at this early point in pregnancy is high. Pregnancy loss rates after the procedure are correspondingly high relative to amniocentesis loss rates. There has also been some doubt cast on the reliability of this procedure as sometimes unusual chromosomal complements found in the chorionic villus (mostly mosaic cell lines) do not show up later in fetal cells (from amniocentesis or at delivery).

VI. The goals of genetic counseling include the following:

A. To communicate to the family or individual the **problems** associated with the disorder, the **risk** of occurrence or recurrence, the **implications** of the risk to the family, and the **options** available for dealing with the risk

B. To communicate information on the availability of methods to determine the carrier state in order that arrangements can be made for **testing** of other family members when appropriate

C. To explore the medical, genetic, and social **aspects** of the disease and its impact on the family

D. To refer the parents to **agencies** that can help them manage the child

E. Perhaps, by prenatal diagnosis, to inform the parents whether the child they are expecting has a defect

F. To **assess** comprehension of counseling and the state of adjustment of the family by follow-up interview with the family or patient

G. To follow up with **written material** in simple lay language to enhance optimal counseling results

Selected Readings

Fraser-Roberts, J. A., and Pembry, M. E. *An Introduction to Medical Genetics* (7th ed.). New York: Oxford University Press, 1978.

Hirschhorn, K. Human genetics. *J.A.M.A.* 224:597, 1973.

McKusick, V. A. *Mendelian Inheritance in Man* (5th ed.). Baltimore: Johns Hopkins University Press, 1978.

Smith, D. W. Recognizable Patterns of Human Malformation. In M. Markowitz (ed.), *Major Problems in Clinical Pediatrics* (3rd ed.). Philadelphia: Saunders, 1982.

Stern, C. *Human Genetics*. San Francisco: Freeman, 1973.

Thompson, J. S., and Thompson, M. W. *Genetics in Medicine*. Philadelphia: Saunders, 1980.

25 Drugs, Chemicals, and Teratogens in Pregnancy

Carolyn C. LoBue

I. General considerations. It has been estimated that the average pregnant woman takes 3.8 drugs during her pregnancy. The estimated usage of different drug classes is indicated in Table 25-1. In addition to prescription and over-the-counter drugs, illicit drug use is estimated to occur in at least 10% of all pregnancies in the United States. To a greater or lesser extent, almost all of these drugs reach the fetus. The ultimate concentration in the fetus is influenced by maternal, placental, and fetal factors.

II. Evaluation of drug effects on the fetus

A. The effect of a drug on the fetus will depend on the fetal drug concentration, the gestational age of the embryo or fetus, and other modifying environmental influences. Table 25-2 summarizes teratogenicity during embryogenesis.

B. Little information is available on the effects of most drugs on the human fetus. Few if any drugs are known to be "safe" for the developing embryo.

C. Only 35 definite teratogens are known in the human (Table 25-3). Drugs are currently believed to account for 4–5% of malformations (Table 25-4). In addition, infectious agents, chemicals, and physical, nutritional, and other factors may also be teratogenic (see Table 25-3).

D. Data derived from animal studies may be irrelevant to the human fetus.

Table 25-1. Estimated usage of different drug classes during pregnancy

Drug class	Estimated percentage of women using class of drug during pregnancy
Analgesics and antipyretics	67
Narcotic analgesics	13
Nonaddicting analgesics	65
Antimicrobials and antiparasitic agents	35
Immunizing agents	45
Antinauseants, antihistamines, and phenothiazines	29
Sedatives, tranquilizers, and antidepressants	28
Drugs affecting the autonomic nervous system	25
Anesthetics, anticonvulsants, muscle relaxants, and stimulants	14
Caffeine and other xanthine derivatives	27
Cardiovascular drugs and diuretics	32
Drugs taken for gastrointestinal disorders	3
Hormones, hormone antagonists, and contraceptives	7
Inorganic compounds	20
Diagnostic aids	0.6

Source: Adapted from O. Heinonen et al., *Birth Defects and Drugs in Pregnancy*. Littleton, MA: Publishing Sciences Group, 1977.

Table 25-2. Teratogenicity during embryogenesis

Days of gestation	Cell differentiation and teratogenic effect
15	No differentiation of cells (germ layers formed). Embryo can be killed if enough cells are killed; otherwise, no teratogenic effects are seen
15–25	Central nervous system differentiation occurs
20–30	Precursors to axial skeleton and musculature occur and limb buds make appearance
25–40	Major differentiation of eyes, heart, and lower limbs
60	Organ differentiation well underway and in many areas completed
90	Differentiation complete and maturation occurring
90	Little susceptibility to the occurrence of congenital malformations

Source: E. T. Herfindal, *Clinical Pharmacy and Therapeutics*. Baltimore: Williams & Wilkins, 1975.

E. A slight increase in congenital malformations caused by a drug will be detected only when a large number of cases have been evaluated.

F. The effects of a drug may not be apparent immediately, as the diethylstilbestrol story demonstrates.

G. For most drugs implicated as teratogens, the increase in adverse effects is small.

H. Beyond the tenth postconceptual week, physiologic deficits and growth delay may result from exposure to teratogenic agents.

I. In 1980, the Food and Drug Administration defined the following drug categories based on the risk posed to the fetus by various agents.

1. **Category A.** Controlled studies in women have failed to demonstrate a risk to the fetus in the first trimester (and there is no evidence of a risk in later trimesters), and the possibility of fetal harm appears remote. An example is potassium chloride.
2. **Category B.** Animal reproduction studies have not demonstrated a fetal risk, or animal reproduction studies have shown an adverse effect that was not demonstrated in women in their first trimester. An example is insulin.
3. **Category C.** Either studies in animals have revealed adverse effects on the fetus and there are no controlled studies in women, or studies in women and animals are not available. An example from this category is isoniazid.
4. **Category D.** There is positive evidence of human risk, but the benefits from use in pregnant women may be acceptable despite this risk. Diazepam is an example of a category D drug.
5. **Category X.** Studies in animals or human beings have demonstrated fetal abnormalities, or there is evidence of fetal risk based on human or animal experience, or both. The risk of using in the drug in pregnancy clearly outweighs any possible benefit. The drug is contraindicated in women who are or who may become pregnant. An example from this category is isotretinoin.

III. Effects of maternal ingestion of drugs on the fetus or neonate. Table 25-5 includes the reported effects of maternal ingestion of drugs on the fetus or neonate. Some reports involve only a few cases, and other drugs have been studied incompletely. In prescribing any drug to a pregnant woman, the risk-benefit ratio should obviously be considered.

IV. Teratogen registries have become available in many communities recently. A physician (or, indeed, anyone) can call such a registry to inquire about the effect of a particular drug on pregnancy. One such organization is the California Teratogen Registry in San Diego, which has a toll-free telephone number.

Table 25-3. Teratogenic agents in humans

Radiation
Therapeutic
Radioiodine
Atomic weapons
Infections
Rubella virus
Cytomegalovirus
Herpes simplex virus I and II
Toxoplasmosis
Venezuelan equine encephalitis virus
Syphilis
Maternal metabolic imbalance
Endemic cretinism
Diabetes
Phenylketonuria
Virilizing tumors and metabolic conditions
Alcoholism
Hyperthermia
Connective tissue disease
Drugs and environmental chemicals
Androgenic hormones
Aminopterin and methylaminopterin
Cyclophosphamide
Busulfan
Thalidomide
Mercury, organic
Chlorobiphenyls
Diethylstilbestrol
Diphenylhydantoin
Trimethadione and paramethadione
Coumarin anticoagulants
Penicillamine (possibly)
Valproic acid
Goitrogens and antithyroid drugs
Tetracyclines
13-*cis*-retinoic acid (isotretinoin, Accutane)
Lithium
Methimazole

Source: From T. H. Shepherd. Human teratology. *Adv. Pediatr.* 33:225, 1986.

Table 25-4. Causes of human malformation (%)

Known genetic transmission	20
Chromosome anomalies	5
Environmental factors	10
Irradiation (< 1%)	
Infections (2–3%)	
(rubella, cytomegalovirus, toxoplasmosis, syphilis)	
Maternal disorders (1–2%)	
(diabetes, phenylketonuria, virilizing tumors)	
Drugs and chemicals (4–5%)	
Multifactorial/unknown	65
(e.g., most congenital heart disease, neural tube defects, facial cleft)	

Source: Adapted from J. G. Wilson, Environmental Effects of Development: Teratology. In N. S. Assali (ed.), *Pathophysiology of Gestation*, vol. 2. Orlando: Academic Press, 1972.

Table 25-5. Effects of maternal drug ingestion on fetus or neonate

Agent	Significance or effect	Stage of pregnancy during which effects occur	Documentation	Category
Analgesic agents				
Acetaminophen	No reported adverse effects; analgesic of choice during pregnancy	First trimester	More documentation needed	B
Heroin (diacetylmorphine)	SGA; chromosomal aberration	Throughout pregnancy	Fairly well documented	B
	Withdrawal symptoms; respiratory depression	Near term[a]	Fairly well documented	
Meperidine hydrochloride (Demerol)	Loss of beat-to-beat variability; decreased neonatal respiration	Near term	Fairly well documented	B
	Late depressive effects in the newborn	Neonatal period	Fairly well documented	
Methadone hydrochloride	Possible chromosomal rearrangement; SGA	Throughout	More studies needed	B
	Prolonged withdrawal	Near term	Fairly well documented	
Morphine	SGA	Throughout	Fairly well documented	B
	Depressed newborn; neonatal death	Neonatal period	More studies needed	
Nonsteroidal anti-inflammatory drugs such as ibuprofen, naproxen	No documented teratogenic effects; drugs in this category may prolong pregnancy and inhibit labor; the ductus arteriosus may constrict in utero, resulting in PPHN; blood clotting and hyperbilirubinemia reported in neonates	Labor and delivery	More studies needed; probably best avoided near term	B
Pentazocine (Talwin)	Withdrawal	Near term	Fairly well documented	B

Propoxyphene	Questionable weak association with major and minor defects	First trimester	More studies needed	C
	Neonatal withdrawal syndrome	Near term	More studies needed	D (if used for prolonged periods)
Salicylates	Neonatal bleeding; coagulation defects; premature closing of ductus arteriosus; diminished factor XII; toxicity (hypertonicity) with excessive maternal ingestion; may prolong pregnancy; may cause slightly increased risk of cardiac defects	Near term	Fairly well documented	C
Anesthetic agents				
Cyclopropane	Infant depression from narcosis	Near term	Established	
Ether	Infant depression from narcosis	Near term	Established	
Halothane	Uterine relaxation; possible abortion in exposed operating room personnel; animal studies show possible renal damage	Abortion—early; relaxation—near term	More studies needed; uterine relaxation well established	
Muscle relaxants	One case of fetal curarization	Near term	Rare effect	
Nitrous oxide	Questionable fetal anomalies	Early	More studies needed	
Anesthetic agents, local				
Bupivacaine hydrochloride (Marcaine)	Bradycardia; stillborn with PCB	Labor	More studies needed with lower drug concentrations	
Chloroprocaine hydrochloride (Nesacaine)	Possible bradycardia with PCB; little transfer to fetus; probably safest local anesthetic for fetus; possible maternal neurologic effects	Labor	More studies needed	

Table 25-5. (continued)

Agent	Significance or effect	Stage of pregnancy during which effects occur	Documentation	Category
Lidocaine	Fetal bradycardia; may cause CNS depression in newborn	Labor and neonatal period	More studies needed	
Mepivacaine hydrochloride (Carbocaine)	Fetal bradycardia; stillborn with PCB; substandard motor nerve response and poor muscle tone in fetus	Labor and neonatal period	More studies needed	
Prilocaine hydrochloride	Less bradycardia than with lidocaine or mepivacaine, but metabolite causes methemoglobinemia	Labor	More studies needed	
Procaine hydrochloride; tetracaine	May depress fetus by direct effect or via maternal hypotension	Labor and delivery	More studies needed	
Antibiotic agents				
Ciprofloxin	Arthropathy in immature animals	Throughout	More studies needed	C
Norfloxin	Possible embryonic loss	First trimester	More studies needed	C
Antidiabetic agents				
Chlorpropamide (Diabinese)	Teratogenic effects suspected	Early	More studies needed	D
	Respiratory distress; neonatal hypoglycemia; neonatal thrombocytopenia	Near term	More studies needed	
Insulin	Possible caudal regression syndrome	First trimester	More studies needed	B
Tolbutamide (Orinase)	Possibly teratogenic; neonatal hypoglycemia; neonatal thrombocytopenia	First trimester; throughout	More studies needed	D

Anti-infective agents				
Acyclovir (Zovirax)	No documented fetal effects; at high dose may cause chromosomal breakage	Throughout	Few human studies	C
Amphotericin B	No documented fetal effects		More studies needed	B
Ampicillin	No known adverse effects; may not reach therapeutic effects in utero			B
Cephalosporins	No reported adverse effects; high dose may be required to achieve therapeutic level in fetus			B
Chloramphenicol	Fetal levels equal maternal levels; "gray baby" syndrome	Near term	Fairly well documented	C
Chloroquine	Fetal CNS damage, particularly to auditory nerve; possible abnormal retinal pigmentation; congenital deafness	Throughout	More studies needed	D
Clindamycin	Concentrates in fetal liver; no adverse effects on fetus yet reported			B
Erythromycin	Crosses placenta only at high maternal dose; fetal level 25% of maternal; no adverse effects demonstrated			B
Ethambutol hydrochloride	Limited fetal damage			B
Gentamicin sulfate	Possible ototoxicity; fetal levels well below toxic adult levels; if maternal levels therapeutic, probably adequate for bacterial control in fetus	Near term		C
Griseofulvin	No known adverse fetal effects, but embryotoxic and teratogenic in some animal species			C

Table 25-5. (continued)

Agent	Significance or effect	Stage of pregnancy during which effects occur	Documentation	Category
Isoniazid	Embryotoxic in animals; possible psychomotor retardation	First trimester; throughout	More studies needed	C
Kanamycin sulfate	Fetal concentration 40% of maternal; probably ototoxic	Throughout	More studies needed	D
Lincomycin hydrochloride monohydrate	Fetal levels approximately 25% of maternal; no known adverse effects			B
Metronidazole (Flagyl)	Not recommended in first trimester; mutagenic in bacteria; questionably embryotoxic	First trimester	More studies needed	C
Nitrofurantoin (Furadantin, Macrodantin)	Hemolytic anemia in mother or fetus with G-6-PD deficiency	Near term	More studies needed	B
Novobiocin	Hyperbilirubinemia	Near term	More studies needed	C
Penicillin	Fetal levels 20–50% of maternal; no adverse effects reported			B
Primaquine phosphate	Hemolytic anemia in patients with G-6-PD deficiency	Near term	More studied needed	C
Pyrimethamine	May impair morphogenesis	First trimester	More studies needed	C
Ribavirin	Teratogenic and/or embryo-lethal in nearly all animals tested	Early	Few human studies; not recommended for use in pregnancy	X
Rifampin	Fetal serum concentration less than maternal; possible increase in fetal anomalies, including limb reduction defects and CNS		More studies needed	C

	lesions; possible neonatal hypoprothrombinemia or bleeding tendency			
Streptomycin sulfate	Eighth nerve damage; micromelia; slight danger of multiple skeletal anomalies	Throughout	More studies needed	D
Sulfonamides	Hyperbilirubinemia; kernicterus; thrombocytopenia; possibility of hemolysis in G-6-PD deficiency	Near term	Fairly well documented	B (D if administered near term)
Tetracycline	Inhibition of bone growth; discoloration of teeth	Second and third trimesters	Fairly well documented	D
	Possible micromelia; syndactyly, hypospadias, and inguinal hernia	First trimester	More studies needed	
	Maternal fatty liver may result in stillbirth		Established	
Ticarcillin disodium	Known to be a teratogenic in mice			B
Tobramycin sulfate (Nebcin)	No increased evidence of malformation; possibly ototoxic		More studies needed	C
Trimethoprim-sulfamethoxazole (Bactrim, Septra)	Teratogenic in animals—primarily cleft palate; may cause fetal resorption. No documented teratogenesis in humans	First trimester	More studies needed	C
Zidovudine (AZT) (Retrovir)	No documented fetal effects		Few human studies	C
Antineoplastic agents				
Aminopterin	Abortifacient and teratogenic; ocular teratogen; cranial anomalies	First trimester	Well documented	X
Azathioprine (Imuran)	By itself, not teratogenic; may cause neonatal immunosuppression	Near term	Studies needed when combined with other drugs	D

Table 25-5. (continued)

Agent	Significance or effect	Stage of pregnancy during which effects occur	Documentation	Category
Busulfan (Myleran)	Questionable cleft palate; minor effects such as low birth weight, neutropenia	Cleft palate—first trimester; neutropenia—near term	More studies needed	D
Chlorambucil (Leukeran)	Questionable cleft palate	First trimester	More studies needed	D
Cisplatinum	No documented fetal effects			D
Cyclophosphamide (Cytoxan)	Severe stunting; fetal death; extremity defects; also normal infants born	First trimester	More studies needed	D
Cytosine arabinoside (Cytosar-U)	Possible intrauterine growth retardation and fetal death	Throughout	More studies needed	
Dactinomycin	Ocular abnormalities in animals	First trimester	More studies needed	D
Ethyl carbamate	No documented problems		More studies needed	
Mercaptopurine	Isolated reports of malformations	First trimester	More studies needed	D
Methotrexate	Abortifacient; any live-born infant likely to be severely malformed	First trimester	Fairly well documented	D
Procarbazine hydrochloride	Possible renal abnormalities	First trimester	More studies needed	D
Triethylenemelamine	No known abnormalities		More studies needed	
Vinblastine sulfate	Normal infants after intrauterine exposure		More studies needed	D
Vincristine sulfate	Possible renal anomalies	First trimester	More studies needed	D
Antithyroid agents				
Methimazole	Goiter; mental retardation (risk is slight, however—probably 30%)	From wk 14 on	Fairly well documented	D
Potassium iodide	Goiter; mental retardation	From wk 14 on	Fairly well documented	X

Propylthiouracil	Goiter; mental retardation (risk is slight, however—probably 30%)	From wk 14 on	Fairly well documented	D
Radioiodine	Congenital hypothyroidism; cretinism	From wk 14 on	Fairly well documented	X
Asthma drugs				
Albuterol (Metaproterenol)	Does not cause birth defects; adverse effects related to cardiovascular and metabolic effects of drug	Near term	Fairly well documented	C
Aminophylline	No increase in abnormalities; tachycardia, vomiting, jitteriness in fetus after medication given to mother	Near term	Fairly well documented	C
Cromolyn	No increase in fetal anomalies reported; high doses cause fetal growth retardation and stillbirth in animals	Throughout	More studies needed	C
Terbutaline	Does not cause birth defects; adverse effects as for albuterol	Near term	Fairly well documented	B
Theophylline	No documented birth defects; transient tachycardia, irritability, and vomiting may occur in newborns	Near term	Fairly well documented	C
Autonomic drugs				
Atropine	Sympathomimetic effects	Near term	Documented: When used to treat bradycardia, safety uncertain	C
Decamethonium bromide	Does not cross placenta in usual dose			

Table 25-5. (continued)

Agent	Significance or effect	Stage of pregnancy during which effects occur	Documentation	Category
Epinephrine	May decrease strength of uterine contractions	Labor		C
	May be associated with an increase in major and minor malformations			
Gallamine triethiodide	Does not cross placenta in usual dose	First trimester	More studies needed	
Scopolamine	May decrease duration of labor; anticholinergic effects, including tachycardia and heart rate variability	Labor		C
Succinylcholine chloride	Crosses placenta slowly; may result in temporary ileus	Labor		
Tubocurarine chloride	Crosses placenta 6–10 min after injection	Labor		
Cardiovascular drugs				
Angiotensin I–converting inhibitors, including captopril	Decreased uterine blood flow with increased fetal morbidity and mortality; may cause oligohydramnios	Second and third trimesters	More studies needed. Use with extreme caution if at all in pregnancy	C (according to manufacturer)
Aldomet	Decrease of intracranial volume after first trimester exposure	After first trimester	Probably the preferred antihypertensive in pregnancy	C
Beta-adrenergic blocking agents including propranolol, atenolol, metaprolol, and labetalol	Possible association with teratogenesis	First trimester	More studies needed	C
	Neonatal hypoglycemia; IUGR; neonatal bradycardia and respiratory depression	Near term		

Captopril	Embryocidal in animals; one reported case of fetal malformation	First trimester	More studies needed	C
Diazoxide	Teratogenic in animals	First trimester	More studies needed	D
	May produce severely depressed infants	Labor and delivery	More studies needed	
Digitoxin	One report of fetal death from maternal overdose	Uncertain	More studies needed	B
Digoxin	Equilibration between mother and fetus after one wk of treatment; lack of documented effects on fetus	Uncertain	More studies needed	B
Heparin	Probably little fetal effect as does not cross placenta; maternal osteoporosis and thrombocytopenia	Throughout	Maternal effects well established	C
Hydralazine	Questionable skeletal defects	First trimester	More studies needed	C
	Thrombocytopenia, tachycardia	Throughout		
Nifedipine	Possible fetal hypoxemia and acidosis	Throughout	More studies needed	C (according to manufacturer)
Quinidine	May cause neonatal thrombocytopenia	Throughout	More studies needed; probably a relatively safe drug in pregnancy	C
Reserpine	Teratogenic in animals	First trimester	More human data needed	D
	SGA	Throughout	More studies needed	
	Nasal blockage; bradycardia; possible interference with temperature regulation	Near term	More studies needed	
Spironolactone	Possible antiandrogenic effects	Throughout	More studies needed	D

Table 25-5. (continued)

Agent	Significance or effect	Stage of pregnancy during which effects occur	Documentation	Category
Verapamil	May cause decrease in uterine blood flow and cause fetal hypoxia and bradycardia	Throughout	Well documented but of questionable significance	C (according to manufacturer)
Central nervous system drugs				
Amphetamines	Possible association with congenital heart defects and biliary atresia; cleft palate	Fourth through twelfth wk	More studies needed	D
	Withdrawal syndrome in neonate	Near term	Fairly well documented	
Barbiturates	All cross the placenta	Near term		B
	Also stored in fetal liver, brain, and placenta; fetal concentration greater than maternal concentration; fetus may be addicted; neonatal bleeding, coagulation defects, thrombocytopenia; possible congenital malformation, enzyme induction	First and second trimesters	Coagulation problems need to be studied further; enzyme induction well documented; more studies needed in which other antiepileptic drugs are not given also	
Bromides	May be associated with growth retardation, dermatitis, lethargy, dilated pupils	Throughout	More studies needed	D
Carbamazepine (Tegretol)	May cause anomalies including craniofacial defects, fingernail hypoplasia, and developmental delay	First trimester	More studies needed	D
Chloral hydrate (Noctec)	May cause withdrawal	Near term	Fairly well established	C

Chlordiazepoxide hydrochloride (Librium)	Possible increased incidence of congenital anomalies if taken during first 42 d of pregnancy	First 42 d	More studies needed	D
	Neonatal depression, hypotonia, and hypothermia; neonatal withdrawal syndrome	Near term	Fairly well documented	
Chlorpromazine	Thrombocytopenia	Near term	More studies needed	C
	Chromosomal anomalies	Early	More studies needed	
	Possible goiter	From wk 14 on	More studies needed	
	Extrapyramidal effects; jaundice; may cause pigmentary retinal opacity in fetus; urinary retention	Near term	More studies needed	
Diazepam (Valium)	Possible increased incidence of congenital anomalies, including cleft palate	First 42 d	More studies needed	D
	Cord blood level approximately equal to maternal blood level; hypotonia, hypothermia, impaired cold response; possible withdrawal symptoms, decreasd beat-to-beat variability in neonatal heart rate; thrombocytopenia; withdrawal syndrome may last up to 10 d	Near term	More studies needed	
Ethchlorvynol (Placidyl)	Withdrawal symptoms	Near term	Fairly well documented	D
Ethosuximide (Zarontin)	Congenital malformations	First trimester	More studies needed	C
Ethyl alcohol	SGA; fetal alcohol syndrome; microcephaly; acute alcohol withdrawal	Throughout	Fairly well documented	D
	Failure to thrive; possible liver abnormalities and hepatoblastoma		More studies needed	
Fluoxetine hydrochloride (Prozac)	No documented adverse fetal effects		Few human studies	B

Table 25-5. (continued)

Agent	Significance or effect	Stage of pregnancy during which effects occur	Documentation	Category
Imipramine hydrochloride (Presamine, Tofranil)	Possible craniofacial and CNS lesions; questionable association with limb reduction defects	Throughout	Probably of low teratogenic potential when used in therapeutic dose	D
Lithium carbonate	Possible alteration in cardiac rhythm; altered thyroid function tests in fetus; possible goiter; jaundice; electrolyte imbalance; neonatal hypotonia; CNS depression	Near term	More studies needed	D
	Ebstein's anomaly and other cardiac anomalies	First trimester	Fairly well documented	
Lysergic acid diethylamide (LSD)	Chromosomal damage; limb and skeleton anomalies	First trimester	Of limited teratogenic potential	
Meprobamate (Equanil, Miltown)	Questionable increase of anomalies, including hypospadias, when taken in the first 42 d of pregnancy	First trimester	More studies needed	D
	Newborn flaccidity; thrombocytopenia	Neonatal period	More studies needed	
Nortriptyline hydrochloride (Aventyl)	Bladder distention; depression	Near term	More studies needed	D
Phenmetrazine hydrochloride (Preludin)	Unconfirmed studies suggest skeletal and visceral anomalies	First trimester	More studies needed	C
Phenothiazine derivatives	Retinopathy; urinary retention; extrapyramidal reactions; hyperbilirubinemia	Near term	More studies needed	C

Phensuximide (Milontin)	Congenital malformations	First trimester	More studies needed	C
Phenytoin sodium (Dilantin)	High incidence of anomalies (abnormal genitalia, cleft lip and palate, hypoplasia of distal phalanges, diaphragmatic hernia, fetal hydantoin syndrome)	First and second trimesters	Fairly well documented; 10–15% incidence of anomalies when used in first trimester	D
	Hemorrhagic disease	Near term	Fairly well documented	
Primidone (Mysoline)	Reported to have a high association with congenital anomalies	First trimester	More studies needed	D
	Neonatal hemorrhagic effects	Near term	Fairly well documented	
Prochlorperazine (Compazine)	No definite effect on fetus substantiated; extrapyramidal effects and jaundice reported; possibility of permanent neurologic damage cannot be excluded	Near term for jaundice; throughout pregnancy for extrapyramidal effects and neurologic damage	More studies needed	C
Promethazine hydrochloride (Phenergan)	Possible association with congenital hip dislocation	Uncertain	More studies needed	C
	May interfere with platelet aggregation	Near term	Fairly well documented	
Thalidomide	Severely teratogenic, but teratogenicity not dose-related; phocomelia, hearing defects, abnormalities of gut musculature, cerebrovascular system, and ophthalmic defects also reported	First trimester	Well documented	
Trimethadione (Tridione)	Possible congenital heart disease; mental retardation; cleft lip and palate; neural and skeletal disease; possibly embryotoxic	Throughout	More studies needed; prior studies involved patients using more than one antiepileptic agent	X

Table 25-5. (continued)

Agent	Significance or effect	Stage of pregnancy during which effects occur	Documentation	Category
Valproic acid	Possible association with microcephaly; possible fetal hydantoin syndrome; hepatotoxic at high levels	Throughout	More studies needed	D
Contrast agents				
Diatrizoate meglumine (Hypaque)	Increased neonatal PBI for 3–8 d		Fairly well documented	
Iodopyracet (Diodrast)	May cause fetal goiter; increased neonatal PBI for 3–8 d		Fairly well documented	
Iophendylate (Pantopaque)	Prolonged elevation of neonatal PBI		Fairly well documented	
Diuretics				
Acetazolamide	Limb defects	First trimester	More studies needed	C
Ammonium chloride	Fetal acidosis	Near term	More studies needed	B
Furosemide (Lasix)	Increased fetal urine output without circulatory imbalance; possible electrolyte imbalance	Near term	More studies needed	C
Thiazides	Bone marrow depression; thrombocytopenia; neonatal death; ascites; possible chronic hypokalemia, hypoglycemia	Near term	More studies needed	D
	Possible teratogenic effects	First trimester	More studies needed	
Hematologic drugs				
Bishydroxycoumarin (dicumarol)	Possible fetal hemorrhage; death	Throughout	Fairly well documented	D
	Fetal anomalies	First trimester	More studies needed	
Phenindione	Hypoplasia of nasal bones and skeletal deformities	First trimester	More studies needed	D

Warfarin sodium (Coumadin)	Hemorrhage death in utero; numerous fetal deformities reported, including hypoplastic nasal bridge, stippled epiphyses, broad-based phalanges, ophthalmic abnormalities; fetal warfarin syndrome; CNS defects	Throughout	Fairly well documented	D
Hormone substances				
Androgens	Masculinization of female fetus; possibly embryotoxic	Throughout	Well documented; the risk of incidental brief exposure is probably minimal	D
Bromocriptine	No evidence of teratogenicity exists; should be stopped with pregnancy; patients with adenomas should be observed carefully for growth			C (X after conception)
Chlomiphene citrate	Possibly teratogenic if taken early in pregnancy	First trimester	More studies needed	X (according to manufacturer)
Corticosteroids	Cleft palate	Early	More studies needed	B
	Newborn adrenal failure	Late	More studies needed	
	Placental insufficiency	Late	More studies needed	
	Possible acceleration of fetal lung maturity	Late	More studies needed; variable from one compound to another	
Diethylstilbestrol (DES)	Anomalies of female reproductive tract, including adenosis; increased incidence of clear cell adenocarcinoma of vagina	Early	Fairly well documented	X
Estrogens (synthetic)	Possible masculinization of female fetus; may be embryotoxic	Throughout	More studies needed	D

Table 25-5. (continued)

Agent	Significance or effect	Stage of pregnancy during which effects occur	Documentation	Category
Oral contraceptives	Possible limb reduction defects; possible cardiac anomalies; questionable Pierre Robin syndrome	Early	More studies needed	D
Progestational agents (synthetic)	Possible masculinization of female fetus; may be embryotoxic; also as above for oral contraceptives	Throughout	Fairly well documented	D
Testosterone	Masculinization of female fetus; advanced bone age	Throughout	Fairly well documented	
Vaccines				
BCG vaccine	Questionable direct fetal effects; febrile response may interrupt pregnancy	Throughout	Vaccination not recommended	
Cholera	Questionable direct fetal effects; febrile response may interrupt pregnancy	Throughout	Vaccination not recommended	
Diphtheria toxoid	Frequent febrile maternal response; no direct adverse fetal effects	Throughout		
Influenza virus	May result in abortion; no malformations confirmed		Vaccination may be indicated during pregnancy	
Measles virus	Infected fetus; may increase abortion rate	Throughout	More studies needed	
Mumps	Infected fetus with uncertain effects on fetal development	Throughout	More studies needed	
Pertussis	Maternal febrile response may lead	Early		

	to abortion; no fetal anomalies reported		
Poliomyelitis	Probably safe for the pregnant woman		
Rabies	Serious maternal allergic and neurologic side effects; give only when clearly indicated	Throughout	
Rubella vaccine	Rubella syndrome	Throughout	More studies needed
Smallpox	Fetal vaccinia	Throughout	Fairly well documented
Tetanus toxoid	Probably safe during pregnancy		
Typhoid	No harmful effects documented; typhoid-paratyphoid causes more severe side effects and should be used only in case of an epidemic		
Yellow fever	Vaccination should be postponed to second trimester because of paucity of data; give only if exposure to disease is unavoidable		
Vitamins			
Ascorbic acid (C)	MDR has no adverse side effects; deficiency may lead to abortion and premature delivery	Throughout	More studies needed
Cyanocobalamin	MDR dosage has no known adverse fetal effects		
Folic acid	Deficiency has severe effects on developing embryo, with resorption and congenital malformations in a wide variety of species; possibly related to neural tube defects	Early pregnancy	More studies needed for humans
Niacinamide	MDR dosage has no adverse fetal effects; pellagra does not appear to disturb human gestation		

Table 25-5. (continued)

Agent	Significance or effect	Stage of pregnancy during which effects occur	Documentation	Category
Pantothenate, calcium	MDR dosage has no adverse fetal effects; dysmorphogenetic effects in animals with deficiency; questionable whether human deficiency can occur			
Pyridoxine hydrochloride (B_6)	MDR dosage has no known adverse fetal effects; deficiency has a questionable association with nausea and vomiting of pregnancy; possible maternal neurologic problems at high doses	Throughout	Established for high dose only; more studies needed	
Riboflavin (B_2)	MDR has no adverse fetal effects; deficiency may be related to prematurity and abortion	Early	More studies needed	
Thiamine (B_1)	MDR has no adverse effects on infant; deficiency may lead to abortion	Early	More studies needed	
Vitamin A	Intracranial hypertension; growth retardation	Throughout	Established for large dose only	
Vitamin D	Mental retardation; hypercalcemia	Throughout	Established for large dose only	
	Possibly related to aortic stenosis	First trimester	More studies needed	
Vitamin K	Excess may lead to hyperbilirubinemia; deficiency may cause fetal hemorrhage	Near term	Fairly well documented	

Miscellaneous				
Agent Orange	Possible increased abortion, stillbirths, and malformations	Throughout	More studies needed	
Brompheniramine	Possible increased incidence of syndactyly	First trimester	More studies needed	
Cadmium	Teratogenic in rodents; may be embryotoxic	First trimester	More studies needed	
Caffeine	Possible intrauterine growth retardation, skeletal abnormalities, shortening of pregnancy	Throughout	More studies needed	
Carbon monoxide	Increased carboxyhemoglobin concentration resulting in cellular hypoxia; in animals exposed to carbon monoxide, decreased fetal weight and increased perinatal mortality are noted; at high doses, if mother and fetus survive, fetus may exhibit somatic and neurologic anomalies	Throughout	More studies needed	
Cholinesterase	Transient muscular weakness	Throughout	Fairly well documented	
Cimetidine (Ranitidine)	Possible transient liver impairment in newborn	Near term	More studies needed	B
Cocaine	Possible congenital anomalies including prune-belly syndrome, hydronephrosis, renal and ureteral agenesis, ambiguous genitalia, hypospadias	First trimester	Fairly well documented	
	Incidence of abruptio placenta, spontaneous abortion, prematurity, impaired fetal growth, and neurobehavioral deficits	Throughout	Fairly well documented	

Table 25-5. (continued)

Agent	Significance or effect	Stage of pregnancy during which effects occur	Documentation	Category
Danocrine	Genital tract ambiguity, including urogenital sinus formation	First trimester	Fairly well documented	X (?)
Dioxane	Extremely teratogenic in experimental animals; increased abortion, cleft palate, and kidney abnormalities	First trimester	More studies needed	
Diphenhydramine hydrochloride (Benadryl)	Thrombocytopenia	Near term	More studies needed	C
	Possible association with cleft palate	First trimester	More studies needed	
Doxylamine succinate and pyridoxine hydrochloride (Bendectin)[b]	Possible relation to limb reduction defects, cardiovascular abnormality, esophageal atresia; potentially teratogenic (limited, if teratogenic at all)	First trimester		
Etretinate	Multiple anomalies documented including facial dysmorphosis, syndactylia, absence of terminal phalanges, neural tube closure defects, hip malformations, low-set ears, and high palate	First trimester	Well documented. May be present at teratogenic levels for some years after discontinuing drug	X
Guaifenesin	Thrombocytopenia; possible increase in inguinal hernias	Near term	More studies needed	C
Hexamethonium compounds	Paralytic ileus in fetus; hypotension	Throughout	More studies needed	C
Hyperthermia-inducing agents	Mental retardation; facial dysmorphosis; microphthalmus; microcephaly; cleft lip and palate; neural tube defects	First trimester	More studies needed	

Indomethacin	Thrombocytopenia; possible premature closure of ductus arteriosus	Near term	More studies needed	D
	Oligohydramnios	Throughout	Fairly well documented	
Isotretinoin (Accutane)	Central nervous system malformation; cardiac, ear, and thymus malformations; cleft palate, facial dysmorphosis; risk of spontaneous abortion	First trimester	Well documented	X
Lead	Possibly teratogenic	Early	More studies needed	
	Possible neurologic birth defects; SGA	Throughout	More studies needed	
Meclizine hydrochloride (Antivert)	Documented teratogen in animals; no clear evidence of human teratogenesis	Early	More studies needed	B
Metoclopramide (Reglan)	No documented fetal effects		Few human studies	B
Organic mercury	Brain damage, cerebral palsy, and blindness	Throughout	Fairly well documented	
Nicotine	SGA; increased incidence of prematurity, stillbirths, and abortions; neonatal irritability	Throughout	Evidence suggestive but not conclusive	
Oxytocin	Fetal electrolyte abnormalities	Near term	Fairly well documented	
Penicillamine	Skin hyperelastosis	Throughout	Fairly well established	D
Phenacetin	Questionable hemoglobinemia	Throughout	More studies needed	B
Phenylpropanolamine	Possible increase in minor malformations, including hypospadias and eye and ear malformations	First trimester	More studies needed	C
Podophyllum resin	Absorption may result in fetal peripheral neuropathy and death in utero	Throughout	More studies needed	

Table 25-5. (continued)

Agent	Significance or effect	Stage of pregnancy during which effects occur	Documentation	Category
Polychlorinated biphenyls (PCBs)	SGA; eye defects; abnormal skin coloration	Throughout	Fairly well established	
Quinine	Many defects reported, including CNS anomalies	First trimester	More studies needed	D
	Maternal and neonatal thrombocytopenia; hemolysis in G-6-PD–deficient newborns	Near term	Fairly well established	
Serotonin	Multiple anomalies of skeleton and organs	First trimester	More studies needed	
Spermicides	Increased abortion; limb reduction defects; neoplasms, hypospadias, and chromosomal abnormalities	First trimester	More studies needed; risk, if it exists at all, must be slight	
X-ray therapy	Microcephaly; mental retardation	Throughout	Fairly well established; medical diagnostic radiation (< 10 rad) has little or no teratogenic effect	

SGA = small for gestational age; PPHN = persistent pulmonary hypertension of the newborn; PCB = paracervical block; CNS = central nervous system; G-6-PD = glucose 6-phosphate dehydrogenase; IGUR = intrauterine growth retardation; RDS = respiratory distress syndrome; PBI = protein-bound iodine; MDR = minimum daily requirement.

[a]*Near term* implies the time period near labor and delivery as well as the neonatal period.

[b]No longer commercially available.

Selected Readings

ACOG Technical Bulletin, No. 64, *Immunization During Pregnancy,* May 1982.

ACOG Technical Bulletin, No. 84, *Teratology,* Feb. 1985.

Barber, R. K. B. Symposium on drugs in pregnancy. *Obstet. Gynecol.* 58(5) (Suppl.):1s, 1981.

Berkowitz, R. L. *Handbook for Prescribing Medications During Pregnancy.* Boston: Little, Brown, 1981.

Briggs, G. B., et al. *Drugs in Pregnancy and Lactation* (3rd ed.). Baltimore: Williams & Wilkins, 1989.

Council on Scientific Affairs. Effects of toxic chemicals on the reproductive system. *J.A.M.A.* 253:3431, 1985.

Guze, B., and Guze, P. Psychotropic medication use during pregnancy. *West. J. Med.* 151:296–298, 1989.

Heinonen, O., et al. *Birth Defects and Drugs in Pregnancy.* Littleton, MA: Publishing Sciences Group, 1977.

Jones, K. L., et al. Pattern of malformation in the children of women treated with carbamazepine during pregnancy. *N. Engl. J. Med.* 320:1661, 1989.

Knoben, J. E., and Anderson, P. O. *Handbook of Clinical Drug Data* (6th ed.). Hamilton, IL: Drug Intelligence Publications, 1988.

Longo, L. D. Environmental pollution and pregnancy: Risks and uncertainties for the fetus and infant. *Am. J. Obstet. Gynecol.* 137:162, 1980.

Mattison, D. R., et al. Effects of drugs and chemicals on the fetus. Parts 1–3. *Contemp. Obstet. Gynecol.* 34:163–176, 97–110, 131–145, 1989.

Niebil, J. R. *Drug Use in Pregnancy* (2nd ed.). Philadelphia: Lea & Febiger, 1988.

Rayburn, W. F., and Zuspan, F. P. *Drug Therapy in Obstetrics and Gynecology* (2nd ed.). New York: Appleton-Century-Crofts, 1986.

Shepard, T. H. *Catalog of Teratogenic Agents* (3rd ed.). Baltimore: Johns Hopkins Press, 1980.

Shepherd, T. H. Human teratology. *Adv. Pediatr.* 33:225, 1986.

Werler, M. W., et al. The relation of aspirin use during the first trimester of pregnancy to congenital cardiac defects. *N. Engl. J. Med.* 321:1639–1642, 1989.

26 Perinatal Ultrasound

Mark C. Williams

Since its introduction into clinical obstetrics, fetal ultrasound imaging has become an essential component in obstetric management.

I. **Applications.** The three general applications for obstetric ultrasound imaging (OUI) are

A. **Biometry.** Direct ultrasonic measurements of the fetus provide information that can be used to estimate gestational age. When combined with appropriate clinical information, they can be used to document normal or altered growth patterns of fetal organ systems, making the detection of many disorders possible.

B. **Structural assessment.** High-resolution ultrasonic images, sometimes in combination with ultrasonic Doppler investigations, can detect relatively minute structural abnormalities of the fetal gastrointestinal, genitourinary, cardiac, and central nervous systems. Additionally, multiple gestations can be diagnosed and abnormalities of placentation detected.

C. **Assessment of fetal well-being.** Real-time ultrasound is used to perform biophysical profiles (BPPs) and amniotic fluid volume assessments in the antepartum interval. These tests provide invaluable information on the fetal status and have helped lessen perinatal mortality.

In addition, ultrasound is helpful for determining the presence (or absence) of intrauterine gestations when bleeding or pain is present in early pregnancy.

II. **General principles**

A. **Safety concerns.** Ultrasound imaging uses focused, high-frequency sound waves in order to generate images. These sound waves transmit energy and can theoretically cause damage to the fetus. Ultrasound at much higher intensities has been shown to disrupt biologic systems. The two principal mechanisms of damage are **heat** and **cavitation.** The relative susceptibility of a given organ system is related to the intensity and duration of ultrasound exposure, its distance from the sound source, and the thermal dissipation characteristics of the organ system (related to blood flow through the organ).

In a recent review of the safety of ultrasound in obstetrics, the Food and Drug Administration (FDA) stated that although no definite effects could as yet be documented for current exposure levels, the possibility of long-term side effects could not be excluded. Further, the report warned that such effects might be subtle in nature and not easily detected.

Apparently the potential for fetal damage with exposure to the energy levels of clinical OUI is small. Nevertheless, studies should **only** be performed for specific clinical indications.

B. **Imaging modalities**

1. **Traditional ultrasound imaging.** Ultrasound images are generated by a combination of a sound source/receiver (transducer) and electronic processor, which send out timed high-frequency pulses of sound (usually in the range 2–8 MHz) and then calculate the time delay between signal generation and return. Because the average speed of sound waves in human tissues is known (1540 m/second), this delay in signal return can be displayed as depth on a display device. A tracing of this information from one point over time is used to generate an "M-mode" image of moving structures. By simultaneously obtaining images from adjacent points, real-time cross-sectional imaging of underlying structures is possible. This image can be oriented in a linear, curvilinear, or radial manner, depending on the shape of the transducer ap-

paratus. Both transabdominal and transvaginal transducers are commonly employed in obstetric and gynecologic ultrasound.

a. **Imaging frequency.** The exact frequency employed for imaging depends on the clinical setting. Transducers of 5 or 6 MHz are used when possible because they provide superior resolution. Unfortunately, such high-frequency sound waves are easily attenuated by bodily tissues and do not adequately image fetuses located more than 6–8 cm from the transducer. When this is a problem, lower-frequency transducers of 3–4 MHz are used.

b. **Tissue interfaces.** Highly dense structures such as bones reflect a large portion of an incident sound signal, sometimes resulting in a shadowing of structures lying behind them. Fluid-filled structures generate few return images (are hypoechoic) and appear empty on the display. Interfaces between areas of differing tissue densities (e.g., fluid-tissue, tissue-bone) are the most easily visualized; fetal imaging is more difficult if little difference exists between the structure of interest and surrounding tissues (e.g., distinguishing fetal abdominal circumference [AC] from uterus if oligohydramnios is present, distinguishing renal parenchyma from surrounding retroperitoneal structures if calyceal structures are not well developed).

2. **Doppler ultrasound.** Ultrasound technology is also used to measure the direction (and velocity) of fluid flow by means of Doppler ultrasound. The Doppler effect, as used in obstetrics, finds that predictable changes in the frequency of a sound wave occur when it is reflected by moving red blood cells. Cells moving toward a sound wave source will reflect sound waves back at a higher frequency; cells traveling away from a source will reflect sound at a diminished frequency. The magnitude of this change is proportional to the velocity of the cells. By comparing initial and returning sound frequencies, a "Doppler shift" is calculated. This information can then be combined ("duplexed") with simultaneous standard ultrasound images to provide information regarding blood flow in a given area. Such information is usually color coded and superimposed on a standard sonographic image. Color flow Doppler ultrasound has proved extremely valuable for evaluating fetal cardiac defects and identifying loops of umbilical cord (preferably avoided during amniocentesis). Fetal cardiac Doppler ultrasound evaluations use a relatively high amount of sound energy to generate their images but have recently been approved by the FDA.

a. **Blood flow velocity.** Doppler ultrasound can also be used to calculate blood flow velocity, either in direct terms (i.e., cm/second) or expressed as various modified ratios of systolic to diastolic flow velocity (e.g., the S/D ratio, Pourcelot index, pulsatility index). These measurements have been performed for various fetal vessels, including the umbilical artery, the aorta, the carotids, and the middle cerebral artery, in attempts to facilitate diagnosis of fetal disease states.

Although Doppler velocimetry shows promise as a means of fetal assessment, it has not yet been incorporated into most antepartum fetal assessment programs. Currently, the most significant use for Doppler velocimetry is assessment of fetal umbilical artery blood flow after 24–26 weeks of pregnancy. Routine Doppler velocimetric assessment is not currently recommended.

C. **Types of ultrasonographic studies**

1. **Level I scan.** The level I scan is the basic minimum ultrasound evaluation. Except in special circumstances, this information should be obtained whenever OUI is performed. A level I scan should include

a. A **general description** of the intrauterine contents, including the number and orientation of fetuses, the placement of the placenta with relation to the uterine cavity and the cervix, and some estimation of the amniotic fluid volume (individual estimations for all fetuses in multiple gestations).

b. The following **fetal features should be measured:**

(1) Biparietal diameter (BPD)

(2) Head circumference (HC)

(3) Abdominal circumference (AC)
(4) Femur length (FL)

c. For all fetuses beyond 22 weeks' gestation, an **estimated fetal weight** (EFW) should be calculated from proved regression equations, or by using suitable fetal weight nomograms. This estimated weight should then be interpreted as a percentile for gestational age (e.g., "The EFW based on a BPD/AC table was 1720 grams, placing the fetus at the 25% for gestational age").

d. A **survey of the fetal anatomy,** including the intracranial anatomy and ventricular structures, a "four-chamber" cardiac image, the kidneys and bladder, the stomach, and the umbilical cord insertion. If possible, the presence of a three-vessel umbilical cord should be documented.

e. Some comment as to the **fetal heart rate and rhythm.**

f. A **cursory evaluation for other problems,** such as an abnormally thickened (hydropic) placenta, an overly distended fetal bladder, or cystic dilatation of a renal pelvis, evidence of fetal ascites or other effusions, or uterine abnormalities (such as leiomyomata).

g. In multifetal gestations, the **presence of a dividing membrane should always be sought** (as this effectively excludes the possibility of a monochorionic, monoamniotic pregnancy). Fetuses beyond 24 weeks' gestation should be evaluated for growth retardation and discordance. **Discordance** in twins has been defined as either a difference in EFWs of more than 25% or differences in fetal BPDs of more than 4 mm.

2. Level II scan. A level II scan is a more extensive exam of the entire fetus, often with special attention focused to a specific fetal organ system. The level II study is best performed under the direct supervision of an experienced sonographer as a "live," real-time exam. Static images may be used to document salient findings, but videotaped images often prove far more useful, as they more easily capture dynamic features of some anomalies and help convey the three-dimensional nature of others.

If questions remain after an initial level II exam, further studies should be considered at a regional obstetric referral center.

3. Biophysical profile. As originally described by Manning and colleagues [2], the BPP is a scoring system that has proved to be a valuable method of fetal antepartum assessment. Its principal advantage over other methods of fetal evaluation is that it retains sensitivity (i.e., the ability to diagnose impending fetal compromise) but offers improved specificity (fewer falsely "positive" or abnormal exams).

a. Sonographic criteria. Four sonographic criteria (**fetal breathing movements, gross body/limb movements, general body tone,** and **amniotic fluid volume)** and a **nonstress fetal cardiotocogram** are scored as either normal or abnormal, with 2 points assigned for normal findings, and none if a category is judged abnormal. These scores are then totaled, with scores of 8 or 10 normal, 4 or less very abnormal, and scores of 6 equivocal. Clinical use of the BPP is discussed in Chap. 22.

Remember that the BPP and other similar tests are clinical applications of available technology. They must be interpreted in light of all relevant data pertaining to a given patient, and caution should be used in inferring a particular prognosis from test results viewed outside the actual clinical context.

4. "Limited study." In certain circumstances, it is acceptable to perform a **limited ultrasonic evaluation.** In such cases, a specific ultrasonic finding is usually being surveyed serially, such as the BPP or amniotic fluid volume. If a limited study is elected, a previous complete level I scan should have been performed, and the determination made that a repeat complete study is not warranted.

III. Overview of technique for various fetal measurements. Four fetal measurements are essential to every fetal ultrasound examination.

A. Biparietal diameter. The fetal BPD is measured in a plane transverse to the long axis of the head, which allows visualization of the midline falx cerebri, the cavum septum pellucidum, and the thalamus (which can be seen straddling the midline centrally) (Fig. 26-1). It is often possible to see small portions of the anterior and

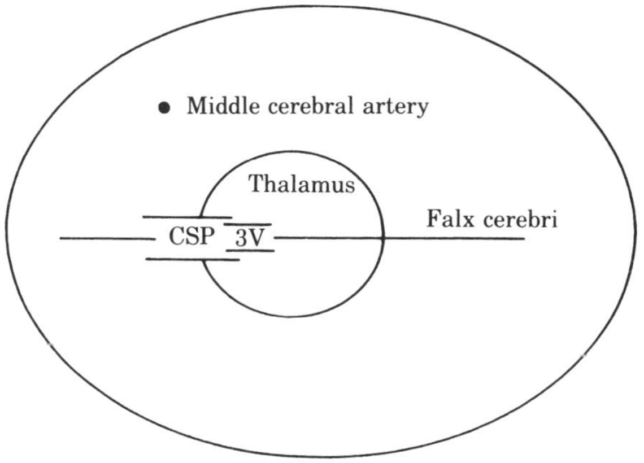

Fig. 26-1. Intracranial anatomy for the biparietal diameter. (CSP = cavum septum pellucidum; 3V = third ventricle.)

posterior lateral ventricles, slightly lateral to the falx, and third ventricle (in the midline slightly anterior to the thalamus). On occasion, high-resolution equipment allows visualization of the middle cerebral artery near the Sylvian fissure. If structures such as the cerebellum, orbits, or basal skull (the petrous ridges and wings of the sphenoid give an X-shaped appearance) are seen, a more accurate plane should be sought prior to obtaining measurements of the head.

1. **Technically difficult studies.** Due to fetal positioning, occasionally it will be impossible to obtain an accurate BPD. In such circumstances, it is usually best to report that the measure was "not technically possible," rather than reporting and according clinical significance to a suspect measurement that may later be erroneous.
2. **Imaging landmarks.** The BPD is traditionally measured from the external surface of the cranium anteriorly to the internal surface of the cranium posteriorly. The cranium is most often found to be slightly elliptic in shape. Some fetuses will present with cranial shapes that are either overly rounded (brachycephalic) or an exaggerated narrowed, longitudinally lengthened elliptic shape (dolichocephaly).

   In order to assess the degree of alteration in fetal head shape, the cephalic index has been developed. It is obtained by dividing the transverse cranial diameter by the occipito-frontal diameter. Cephalic indices of 0.74–0.83 are within one standard deviation of the mean.

   Brachycephaly and dolichocephaly are not intrinsically abnormal, but can result in false estimates of gestational age (EGA) or EFW. Infants with brachycephaly will tend to have overestimated EFW and EGA determinations, due to the exaggerated width of the BPD measurement relative to the overall fetal size. The converse is true for dolichocephalic infants. This problem can be overcome by using other parameters to assess gestational age (such as FL and HC), and by using EFW nomograms based on HC or FL, or both, in combination with AC.

B. Head circumference. The HC is measured in the same plane as the BPD. It can be measured directly with computer planimeters, or its length accurately estimated by measuring the diameters of the head in the occipito-frontal dimension (OFD) and transverse dimension (TD). All measures can be obtained from the external surface of the relevant portions of the cranium, or at a midpoint within the cranial bones. If the OFD and TD are used to estimate the HC, the following formula can be used:

$$HD = \tfrac{1}{2} \times (OFD + TD) \times 3.1416$$

This formula is modeled for a circle but closely approximates the results obtained if formulas for elliptic circumference are used.

The HC has the advantage of being unaffected by alterations in the shape of the fetal head. As such, it is an ideal parameter for estimating fetal weight. Unfortunately, HC offers a much wider range of possible values than BPD, and nomograms relating HC to EFW are less often employed clinically. If computers or hand calculators are used to directly compute EFW, regression equations using HC are good options.

C. Abdominal circumference. The fetal AC is measured in a plane perpendicular to the long axis of the torso (Fig. 26-2). It should contain the stomach bubble and the midportion (not umbilical insertion) of the hepatic vein. The superior poles of the kidneys usually lie slightly caudad to this plane.

In order to obtain this cross section, it is usually best to orient the transducer parallel to the spine slightly caudad to the heart. The transducer should then be rotated 90 degrees, with care taken to avoid oblique transabdominal planes. The AC should then be measured several times, until two or three consistent values have been obtained. As with the HC, if computed planimetry is unavailable, two diameters can be obtained and an estimated AC calculated with the following formula:

$$AC = \tfrac{1}{2} \times (D1 + D2) \times 3.1416$$

The AC measurement is very sensitive to intrauterine growth retardation (IUGR), as evidenced by the use of FL/AC and HC/AC ratios in screening for IUGR. The AC is best not used to assist in the determination of gestational age.

D. Femur length. The femur portion measured in OUI is the ossified portion of the diaphysis. The epiphyseal cartilages are hypoechoic (not easily visualized by OUI) because they are not well calcified in utero. The femur itself is somewhat bowed, but the proper FL should be the linear distance between the proximal and distal diaphyses (Fig. 26-3).

Embryologically, the distal femoral epiphysis becomes ossified at 28–35 weeks gestation. At times, this observation can be used to help assess fetal gestational age or to predict fetal lung maturity [1, 3].

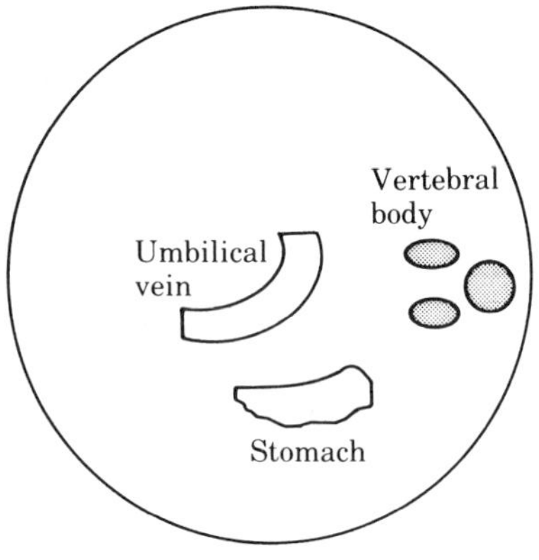

Fig. 26-2. Cross-sectional anatomy for the fetal abdominal circumference.

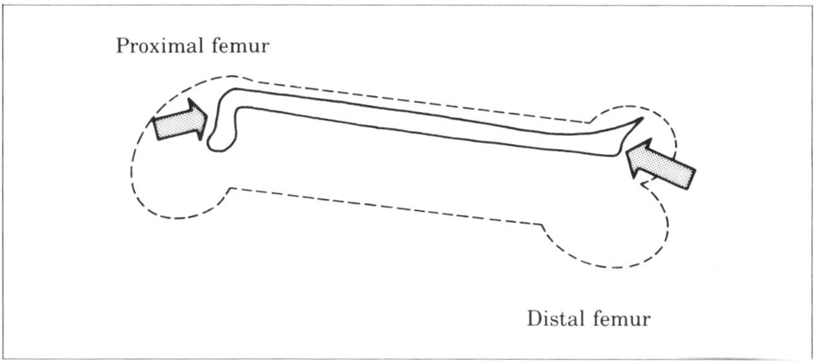

Fig. 26-3. The femur length is measured at the locations marked with arrows.

E. Other fetal measures. For a more complete discussion of fetal biometry, the reader is referred to a list of excellent references at the end of this chapter. These texts also provide appropriate nomograms for estimation of fetal weight and gestational age–specific tables of fetal measurements.

IV. Indications for OUI evaluation. As experience with OUI has accumulated, the indications for such imaging have broadly expanded. Routine OUI is not considered standard care in the United States and should be reserved for specific medical indications. Although no long-term adverse effects from OUI, as currently employed, have been documented in humans, subtle long-term effects may still become evident.

A. The National Institutes of Health's 1984 *Consensus Report on Safety of Ultrasound* reported a number of indications for OUI:

1. **Estimation of gestational age** for confirmation of clinical dating among patients who are to undergo elective repeat cesarean delivery, induction of labor, or elective pregnancy termination.
2. **Evaluation of fetal growth** among patients with suspected or known medical complications associated with either IUGR or macrosomia. These conditions include severe preeclampsia, chronic hypertension, chronic renal disease, and severe diabetes mellitus.
3. **Vaginal bleeding of undetermined etiology** in pregnancy.
4. **Determination of fetal presentation** when the fetal presentation cannot be adequately assessed in labor, or the fetal presentation is variable in late pregnancy.
5. **Suspected multiple gestation** if multiple fetal heart rate patterns are present, the fundal height is larger than expected for gestational age, or fertility-enhancing medications have been taken.
6. **As an adjunct to amniocentesis,** OUI facilitates avoidance of the fetus and placenta and decreases the risk to the fetus.
7. **Uterine size/dates discrepancy.** OUI facilitates accurate assessment of gestational age and detection of conditions such as oligohydramnios and polyhydramnios.
8. **Pelvic mass** noted on clinical exam.
9. **Suspected hydatidiform mole** based on symptoms such as hypertension, proteinuria, or ovarian cysts, or a combination, or the absence of fetal heart tones by Doppler ultrasound after 12 weeks of gestation.
10. **For cervical cerclage,** as an adjunct to timing of the procedure and placement of the cerclage suture.
11. **Suspected ectopic pregnancy** or when pregnancy occurs in a patient at high risk of ectopic pregnancy.
12. **Suspected intrauterine fetal demise.**
13. **As an adjunct to special procedures** such as fetoscopy, intrauterine trans-

fusion, percutaneous fetal blood sampling, shunt catheter placement, or chorionic villus sampling.

14. **Suspected uterine anomaly,** such as clinically significant leiomyomata, uterus didelphys, or bicornuate uterus.
15. **Localization of intrauterine contraceptive device.**
16. **Surveillance of ovarian follicle development.**
17. **Biophysical profile** for fetal well-being after 28 weeks of gestation.
18. **Observation of intrapartum events** such as the version or extraction of the second twin.
19. **Suspected polyhydramnios or oligohydramnios.**
20. **Suspected abruptio placentae.**
21. **As an adjunct to external breech version.**
22. **Estimation of fetal weight and presentation** in premature rupture of membranes and preterm labor.
23. **Abnormal maternal serum alpha fetoprotein** (MS-AFP) value for clinical gestational age when drawn. OUI provides an accurate assessment of gestational age and detects several conditions that may cause elevations of MS-AFP, such as multiple gestations, anencephaly, and the "vanishing twin" syndrome.
24. **Serial evaluation of identified fetal anomaly.**
25. **History of previous congenital anomaly.**
26. **Serial evaluation of fetal growth in multiple gestation.**
27. **Estimation of gestational age** in patients presenting late for prenatal care.

V. Application of OUI to several common clinical problems

A. Discordant uterine size for gestational age

1. **Uterine fundal height less than expected for dates.** If gestational age is well established, a pubic symphysis–uterine fundus ("fundal height") measurement 3 cm or more smaller than expected for gestational age is considered abnormal (in general after 28 weeks' gestation, the fundal height approximately equals the gestational age in weeks).
   a. **Uncertain pregnancy dating.** In poorly dated pregnancies (see sec. **D),** a size/dates discrepancy often merely reflects incorrect pregnancy dating (i.e., overestimation of gestational age by menstrual history). Fetal measures of BPD, HC, and FL can be used to estimate gestational age, and in combination with the fetal AC can be used to estimate fetal weight and serially evaluate fetal growth.
   b. **Good pregnancy dating.** If the gestational age is known with some certainty, the EFW can be compared to the expected EFW for gestational age. Fetuses falling below the tenth percentile for gestational age are considered growth retarded. Ratios of HC/AC and FL/AC can also be used to assess for possible IUGR. Interpretation of the HC/AC ratio somewhat depends on fetal gestational age (1.12—24.0 weeks, 1.05—32 weeks, and 0.98—40 weeks); the FL/AC ratio (normally approximately 0.20–0.22) does not vary during pregnancy. Both ratios are helpful in assessing for asymmetric IUGR. Together, these various measures and ratios provide a relatively sensitive and specific means of assessing gestational age and fetal growth. The two general categories of IUGR are **asymmetric growth retardation** and **symmetric growth retardation.** Asymmetric growth retardation is thought to be caused by preferential fetal shunting of blood to the cerebral circulation under conditions of nutritional deprivation, resulting in a relative decrease in the splanchnic blood flow and reduced abdominal growth. As the condition persists and compensatory mechanisms are overwhelmed, fetal growth parameters become symmetrically retarded, resulting in abnormally decreased EFW with paradoxically normal FL/AC and HC/AC ratios. Symmetric IUGR can also be falsely diagnosed in infants who are growing at rates normal for themselves but below the tenth percentile for the general population.
2. **Uterine fundal height more than expected for date.** The finding of a fundal height 3 cm or more greater than expected for gestational age is considered large for dates.

a. Potential causes of fundal height being more than expected for age include
  (1) Incorrect pregnancy dating
  (2) Large-for-gestational-age fetus
  (3) Multiple gestation
  (4) Polyhydramnios

If no prior ultrasonic evaluations have been performed to establish pregnancy dating, the possibility of incorrect pregnancy should be considered. **Repeat evaluation should be considered near term** to assess interval growth and evaluate for possible fetal macrosomia.

B. High-risk pregnancy

1. Complications. OUI facilitates the management of pregnancies at risk for complications. Firmly established pregnancy dating allows more precise evaluation of fetal growth. Precise knowledge of obstetric dating also may affect decisions regarding certain therapeutic interventions (choice of tocolytic agents, use of fetal lung–maturing agents) or timing of delivery in complicated pregnancies. The following pregnancy complications are best managed by an ultrasound evaluation obtained at 14–16 weeks to confirm pregnancy dating, followed by serial sonographic evaluation of fetal growth and EFW:
  (a) Chronic renal disease
  (b) Collagen vascular disease
  (c) Diabetes or prior gestational diabetes
  (d) Hypertension or prior preeclampsia
  (e) Isoimmunization (Rhesus or other)
  (f) Lupus anticoagulant present
  (g) Maternal malignancy
  (h) Multiple gestations

2. Evaluation. Serial evaluations of fetal growth in most cases are best initiated at 24–26 weeks' gestation and then repeated at monthly intervals. Fetuses not progressing normally for gestational age (using population-specific percentile growth tables) should be followed with other methods of antepartum assessment (such as contraction stress tests, nonstress tests, or BPPs).

In multifetal gestations, normal growth tables are not well established, as a population of "normal" twin gestations has not been easily defined. In general, twin gestations at term yield fetuses weighing approximately 10% less than matched singleton fetuses. Serial evaluations of EFW should be evaluated for discordant growth. Fetuses with differences of more than 25% in EFW or BPDs varying by more than 4 mm exhibit abnormal discordance and should be placed into an antepartum assessment protocol as described before.

Patients thought to be at risk of preterm labor may benefit from early ultrasonic confirmation of pregnancy dating, as accurate pregnancy dating often facilitates the management of preterm labor. They do not require serial sonographic evaluation unless other indications of IUGR are noted.

C. Suspected fetal anomaly. OUI has been found to be an effective method of diagnosing major fetal anomalies, with a sensitivity of approximately 85% and close to 100% specificity for major anomalies.

1. History. Patients with family or obstetric histories suggestive of fetal anomalies should undergo a thorough ultrasonic evaluation to screen for fetal anomalies. This evaluation should initially survey all fetal organ systems and then focus on the index organ system (i.e., that system with a history of prior anomaly). The timing of this study is sometimes difficult, as major CNS abnormalities (such as anencephaly) are often detectable by 16–18 weeks of gestation, whereas cardiac structure is much more easily assessed at 22 weeks of gestation.

2. Maternal serum alpha fetoprotein abnormalities. MS-AFP determinations between 15 and 20 weeks of gestation have been used to assess pregnancies for the possibility of CNS abnormalities. OUI is a valuable adjunct for evaluating fetal anatomy and potential viability when abnormal MS-AFP values are present.
  (a) Elevated MS-AFP values are often associated with open neural tube defects. They are also associated with ventral abdominal wall de-

fects, multiple gestations, fetal demise (in multifetal gestations), and other less common conditions.

With an elevated MS-AFP, an ultrasound evaluation should always be performed to establish the correct EGA. If the corrected EGA places the MS-AFP in the normal range, no further evaluation is necessary. Otherwise, a thorough fetal ultrasonic evaluation is required, with special care taken to visualize intracranial structures and the entire neural tube. A negative ultrasonic evaluation does not negate the significance of an elevated MS-AFP. Small neural tube defects are not always detected by even the most thorough ultrasound evaluation. The risk of an open neural tube defect after a normal ultrasonic evaluation is 5–10%.

If the cause for an elevated MS-AFP is not obvious, an ultrasound-guided amniocentesis should be performed to directly measure the amniotic fluid alpha fetoprotein (AF-AFP) and the amniotic fluid acetylcholinesterase and to perform a fetal karyotype. Acetylcholinesterase is found in high concentrations within the CNS and is present in the amniotic fluid very early in pregnancy. If found after 14 weeks' gestation, amniotic fluid acetylcholinesterase is considered direct evidence of an open neural tube defect. Contamination of amniotic fluid with fetal blood can raise the level of AF-AFP but does not affect the level of amniotic fluid acetylcholinesterase.

(b) Decreased MS-AFP levels. Patients with decreased MS-AFP levels are at increased risk for having infants with chromosomal abnormalities such as trisomies 21 and 18. Such syndromes cannot be reliably excluded by ultrasound evaluation. Thus, amniocentesis for fetal karyotype should be offered too in these circumstances.

3. Abnormalities of amniotic fluid volume. Abnormalities of amniotic fluid volume may be indicators of functional abnormalities within the renal, gastrointestinal, or CNS systems. Oligohydramnios may also reflect ruptured amniotic membranes.

a. Polyhydramnios. No exact definition for polyhydramnios exists, but two suggested definitions are

(1) Subjectively increased amniotic fluid volume and a largest pocket diameter in excess of 7 cm

(2) Amniotic fluid index (the sum of largest vertical amniotic fluid pocket depths from the four uterine quadrants) of 20 or greater [6, 7]

Polyhydramnios is often seen in association with diabetic pregnancies, isoimmunization syndromes, open neural tube defects, and fetal anomalies affecting the fetal swallowing mechanism (esophageal atresia, tracheoesophageal fistula), or the gastrointestinal tract (duodenal atresia, others). If polyhydramnios is judged severe, fetal chromosomal evaluation should be considered, as these features are at increased risk of chromosomal abnormalities.

b. Oligohydramnios. Oligohydramnios is defined as an amniotic fluid volume less than expected for gestational age. It is of great clinical significance, as severe reductions in amniotic fluid volume may alter fetal mobility and predispose to abnormal facies, limb contractures, and pulmonary hypoplasia. In the term pregnancy, oligohydramnios (with intact membranes) is highly associated with adverse fetal outcomes and requires careful management.

(1) Etiology. Oligohydramnios can be caused by rupture of membranes or decreased production of amniotic fluid. After 18 weeks of gestation, the fetal kidneys produce most amniotic fluid. Renal agenesis, dysplasia, or obstruction of the urinary system may cause oligohydramnios.

(2) Quantitation. Two commonly used methods of quantitating oligohydramnios are the amniotic fluid index [6, 7] and the largest pocket-size method.

(a) The **amniotic fluid index** [6, 7] has been described. Indices of 5 or less are defined as oligohydramnios.

(b) The **largest pocket method** defines oligohydramnios as a largest amniotic fluid pocket of less than 1 × 1 cm. Additionally, pockets of 1 × 1 cm to 2 × 2 cm are considered to be borderline oligohydramnios. Patients with diminished amniotic fluid volumes should be carefully followed for the onset of oligohydramnios with serial sonographic evaluation.

4. **Single umbilical artery.** The presence of three umbilical blood vessels (two arteries and one vein) should be confirmed. Two-vessel umbilical cords (single umbilical artery) occur in up to 1% of pregnancies, are associated with fetal anomalies in 20–50% of liveborn infants, and are found disproportionately among cases of intrauterine fetal demise. Fetuses with two-vessel cords should be carefully evaluated for other coexisting anomalies.

   If definite fetal anomalies are identified by OUI, consideration should be given to fetal karyotypic analysis after amniocentesis or percutaneous fetal blood sampling. The incidence of karyotypic abnormalities increases slightly if one anomaly is present. The presence of two or more anomalies is much more strongly associated with fetal karyotypic abnormalities.

D. **Uncertain dating of pregnancy.** Patients who do not have well-established menstrual dating (i.e., history confirmed by early physical examination) should have an ultrasound evaluation to confirm (or establish) the EGA and estimated date of confinement (EDC).

Patients should be questioned as to prior ultrasound evaluations at other facilities, and every effort should be made to obtain this information. If such studies have been performed by suitably experienced practitioners, the earliest available sonographic study is generally used to establish obstetric dates.

1. **Estimated gestational age.** The margin of error associated with ultrasonic determination of EGA is approximately 10% of the determined gestational age (± 1-week margin of error prior to 12 weeks' gestation, ± 1–2 weeks' error from 12–20 weeks' gestation, and ± 2–3 weeks' error after 20 weeks of gestation).

   If a scan is performed between 7 and 10 weeks of gestation, the fetal crown-rump length should be used to determine the EGA. For scans obtained later in pregnancy, the EGAs associated with the fetal BPD, HC, and FL should be obtained and (as available) averaged.

   If a scan is attempted prior to 6 weeks of gestation and no fetal pole is clearly visible, the gestational sac measure should not be used to establish the EGA. A repeat scan should be scheduled several weeks later to document fetal cardiac activity within the uterus (essentially excluding the possibility of ectopic gestation), and the pregnancy dated using the later scan.

   If the ultrasound estimates an EGA that (within the procedural error limits) agrees with the menstrual dates, the menstrual dates are considered confirmed. For pregnancies that are less than 24 weeks' gestation by ultrasound with "dates/sono" discrepancies of more than two to three weeks, it is usually safe to accept the ultrasound EGA as the correct obstetric EGA.

2. **Growth retardation.** In pregnancies of more than 24 weeks' gestation by ultrasound with reported menstrual EGAs three or more weeks more advanced, the possibility of growth retardation should be considered. If the abdominal circumference is decreased in size for ultrasound gestational age, asymmetric IUGR may be present. If FL/AC and HC/AC ratios are within normal limits (i.e., if all fetal measures are symmetric), the possibility of symmetric IUGR should be considered. If underlying maternal disease is present, this diagnosis is made more likely. When growth retardation is felt to be a reasonable possibility, the fetus should be monitored in an antepartum assessment program and a repeat sonogram obtained in approximately three weeks. If the repeat exam shows normal growth for assigned ultrasonic gestational age, the obstetric EGA should be accepted and antepartum assessment discontinued. If little or no growth occurs, the fetus should be managed as a high-risk pregnancy, followed with careful antepartum testing, and consideration should be given to early delivery.

3. **Changing the EDC.** Once properly established, the EDC should be strictly

adhered to. If better information becomes available and it is judged necessary to change the EDC, this information should be carefully documented in the patient's chart.

4. **Serial scans.** OUI allows accurate interval assessment of fetal growth throughout pregnancy. Pregnancies at risk for IUGR (maternal disease states, multiple gestations) should be scanned initially early in pregnancy, and then at intervals throughout pregnancy. A commonly used scheme uses a 16-week scan to confirm gestational age followed by scans at four-week intervals starting at 24 or 26 weeks of gestation.

   The fetus can also be surveyed at intervals if anomalies such as hydrocephalus or hydronephrosis are noted, or if the fetus is at risk of hydrops or cardiac compromise. Changing fetal findings may necessitate therapeutic intervention or early delivery.

E. Unexplained abdominal pain or vaginal bleeding

1. **Ectopic pregnancy.** The management of unexplained abdominal pain and vaginal bleeding in pregnancy has been greatly aided by the increasing availability of abdominal (and vaginal) ultrasound. If an ectopic pregnancy is suspected, ultrasonic evaluation of the uterine cavity should be performed and a serum beta-human chorionic gonadotropin (β-HCG) titer performed. If the β-HCG titer is in excess of 6500, an intrauterine gestation should be seen by transabdominal ultrasonic evaluation, and if not, an ectopic gestation is likely. Recently, it has also been reported that if vaginal ultrasound evaluation is performed, a β-HCG titer in excess of 1800 without evidence of intrauterine pregnancy is strongly suggestive of an ectopic gestation [4, 5].
2. **Abnormalities of placentation.** Abnormal placentation is strongly associated with bleeding complications in all stages of pregnancy. Ultrasonic studies allow relatively precise delineation of the site of placentation. It is important to remember that prior to 20 weeks' gestation, the placenta is frequently seen to be "low lying." In 60–90% of second-trimester marginal placenta previas, normal placentation will be noted at term. Placentas found to be implanted both anteriorly and posteriorly (e.g., central placenta previa) most commonly do not resolve.

References

1. Mahony, B. S., et al. Epiphyseal ossification centers in the assessment of fetal lung maturity: Sonographic correlations with the amniocentesis lung profile. *Radiology* 159:521–524, 1986.
2. Manning, F. A., et al. Fetal biophysical profile scoring: A prospective study of 1,184 high risk patients. *Am. J. Obstet. Gynecol.* 140:289, 1981.
3. McLeary, R. D., and Kuhns, L. R. Sonographic evaluation of the distal femoral epiphyseal ossification center. *J. Ultrasound Med.* 2:437–438, 1983.
4. Nyberg, D. A., et al. Abnormal pregnancy: Early diagnosis by ultrasound and serum chorionic gonadotropin levels. *Radiology* 158:393–396, 1986.
5. Nyberg, D. A., et al. Ectopic pregnancy: Diagnosis by sonography correlated with quantitative HCG levels. *J. Ultrasound Med.* 6:145–150, 1987.
6. Phelan, J. P., et al. Amniotic fluid volume assessment with the four-quadrant technique at 36–42 weeks' gestation. *J. Reprod. Med.* 32:540–542, 1987.
7. Phelan, J. P., et al. Amniotic fluid index measurements during pregnancy. *J. Reprod. Med.* 32:601–604, 1987.

Selected Readings

Callen, P.. W. (ed.). *Ultrasonography in Obstetrics and Gynecology* (2nd ed.). Philadelphia: Saunders, 1988.

Mahony, B. S., Callen,, P. W., and Filly, R. A. The distal femoral epiphyseal ossification center in the assessment of third trimester age: Sonographic identification and measurement. *Radiology* 155:201–204, 1985.

Nyberg, D. A., Mahony, B. S., and Pretorius, D. H. (eds.). *Diagnostic Ultrasound of Fetal Anomalies: Text and Atlas*. Chicago: Year Book, 1990.

Reed, K. L., Anderson, C. F., and Shenker, L. (eds.). *Fetal Echocardiography: An Atlas*. New York: Liss, 1988.

Romero, R., et al. *Prenatal Diagnosis of Congenital Anomalies*. East Norwalk, CT: Appleton & Lange, 1988.

Sabbagha, R. E. (ed.). *Diagnostic Ultrasound Applied to Obstetrics and Gynecology* (2nd ed.). Philadelphia: Lippincott, 1987.

Labor and Delivery

27 Normal Labor

Jeanne Ann Conry

Labor is the process by which contractions of the gravid uterus expel the fetus. A **term pregnancy** occurs between 37 and 42 weeks from the last menstrual period (LMP). **Preterm labor** is that occurring prior to 37 weeks' gestational age. Termination of pregnancy prior to 20 weeks' gestation is defined as either spontaneous or therapeutic **abortion.** The distinction between spontaneous abortion and preterm labor in the 20–24 week gestational-age group is imprecise. **Post-dates pregnancy** occurs after 42 weeks and requires careful monitoring.

I. **Evaluation of the laboring patient.** Evaluation of the patient presenting with the complaint of labor includes history, physical examination, selected laboratory tests, and fetal monitoring. A clinical impression and management plan are formulated from the information obtained.

A. **History**

1. **History of the present labor**

a. **Contractions.** The frequency, duration, onset, and intensity of uterine contractions should be determined. Contractions that effect progressive cervical effacement and dilatation are usually regular and intense (the patient can no longer walk or talk during them). They may be accompanied by a "bloody show," the passage of blood-tinged mucus from the dilating cervical os. Braxton Hicks contractions are felt by many patients during the last weeks of pregnancy. These are usually irregular, mild, and do not effect cervical change. Table 27-1 lists factors that differentiate true labor from false labor.

a. **Rupture of membranes.** The patient may present with the complaint of leaking fluid alone or in conjunction with uterine contractions. The time of occurrence is important because prolonged rupture increases the risk of chorioamnionitis. If it is not offered as a complaint, the question of leakage of fluid must be raised to determine the status of fetal membranes. The patient may report a large gush of fluid with continued leakage, leaving little doubt as to its source. She may, however, report merely increased moisture on her underclothes and be uncertain whether it represents urine, vaginal secretions, cervical mucus, or amniotic fluid. Physical examination and microscopic evaluation are necessary. The patient should be questioned regarding the color of the liquid to determine the presence of blood or meconium in it.

(1) **The extent, if any, of vaginal bleeding** should be ascertained. Spotting or blood-tinged mucus is common in normal labor. Heavy vaginal bleeding merits complete investigation because it may be abnormal and reflect a significant disorder. The topic of third-trimester bleeding is covered in Chap. 20.

c. **Fetal movement.** Most patients are aware of their fetus's baseline level of activity. If the patient reports significant or progressive decrease in fetal movement from this baseline, fetal well-being must be confirmed. Such evaluations can involve continuous fetal monitoring with a nonstress test, a contraction stress test, or biophysical profile (see Chap. 22).

2. **History of present pregnancy.** The history of the present pregnancy may be obtained by interviewing the patient in labor or by reviewing a prenatal record. The prenatal record may be from your own institution or from an outside source. The patient, of course, may have had no prenatal care or have no record of

Table 27-1. Differentiating true labor and false labor

Factors	True labor	False labor
Contractions	Regular intervals	Irregular intervals
Interval between contractions	Gradually shortens	Remains long
Intensity of contractions	Gradually increases	Remains same
Location of pain	In back and abdomen	Mostly in lower abdomen
Effect of analgesia	Not terminated by sedation	Frequently abolished by sedation
Cervical change	Progressive effacement and dilation	No change

it. If a prenatal record is available, important items should be verified with the patient.

a. **Gestational age** is best determined by data in the prenatal record. The later the patient presents for initial prenatal care, the more difficult it becomes to determine accurately the **estimated gestational age** (EGA). Important landmarks for determining gestational age include (1) the first day of the LMP—the **estimated date of confinement** (EDC) is calculated as 40 weeks from this date; (2) the date of the last ovulation (as determined by a basal body temperature chart) or the date of conception—EDC is calculated as 38 weeks from this date; (3) fetal heart tones first heard with a Doppler instrument 10–12 weeks from the LMP or with a fetoscope 18–20 weeks from the LMP; (4) quickening (maternally perceived fetal movement), which occurs approximately 17 weeks from the LMP; (5) uterine size before 16 weeks' EGA as determined by an experienced physician; and (6) ultrasound measurement of fetal size prior to 24 weeks of gestation.

   (1) **Accurate dating** requires evaluation during the first half of pregnancy. The patient presenting in labor with an uncertain LMP and no prenatal care may be difficult to date with accuracy. Uncertain gestational age presents a significant problem because of different management strategies for term, preterm, and postterm pregnancies. In these situations the only alternative is to use bedside ultrasound in the labor and delivery suite. Confirmatory amniocentesis to assess fetal lung maturity may be necessary in difficult cases.

b. **Medical problems arising during the gestation.** The patient should be questioned specifically regarding any medical problems arising during the pregnancy. Hospitalizations should be noted, as well as any new medications prescribed. A history of recurrent urinary tract infections and pyelonephritis or any infectious diseases requiring treatment should be elicited. History of glucose intolerance and treatment with diet or insulin should be noted. If any blood pressure elevation has been recorded during the pregnancy, the time of onset, severity, and treatment should be determined. Seizure history, noting frequency and medications, is pertinent for obstetric care.

c. **Review of systems.** An obstetrically oriented review of symptoms should be carried out. Severe headaches, scotomatas, hand and facial edema, or epigastric pain may suggest preeclampsia. Generalized pruritus may be secondary to cholestasis of pregnancy or hepatitis. Dysuria, urinary frequency, or flank pain may indicate cystitis or pyelonephritis.

3. **Past pregnancies.** Each past pregnancy, its duration and outcome, should be reviewed. Particular attention should be paid to preterm deliveries, operative deliveries, prolonged or difficult labors, dystocias, malpresentation, eclampsia or preeclampsia, placental abruption or placenta previa, and blood loss re-

quiring transfusion. Other medical facilities may need to be contacted for records to verify or clarify certain points.

4. **Medical history.** Any and all active medical problems should be evaluated and the extent of the disease determined. The stress of labor can aggravate many medical problems and jeopardize both maternal and fetal well-being.

B. **Physical examination.** Although active labor is not the optimal setting for physical examination, a general physical examination with emphasis on the abdomen and pelvis can be performed between painful contractions. Any signs of intercurrent medical illness or abnormalities of major organ systems should be elicited and carefully noted. Special note should be taken of those parts of the physical examination that may be potentially positive because of that individual patient's history.

1. **General examination**

a. **Vital signs.** A complete set of vital signs should be taken immediately on admission. Blood pressure should be taken **between** contractions, and if the woman is extensively obese, a large cuff should be used. Abnormal readings should be rechecked. An elevated body temperature, especially if associated with ruptured membranes, may indicate chorioamnionitis. An elevated pulse or respiratory rate in the absence of any other abnormality is observed commonly in the normal patient in active labor.

b. **Head.** Examination of the head should include fundoscopy to rule out vascular abnormalities, hemorrhages, or exudates that may suggest such diseases as diabetes or hypertension. Pale conjunctivae (or nail beds) may suggest anemia. Facial as well as hand and ankle edema are common in toxemia. The thyroid gland should be palpated to rule out goiter or other masses.

c. **Chest.** Examination of the chest may reveal the presence of a pneumonic process or significant cardiac murmurs (other than the physiologic systolic ejection murmur so common in pregnancy), and provides a baseline in case complications such as pulmonary edema or pneumonia develop. Distended neck veins suggest cardiopulmonary congestion, which, although rare, is a serious complication of labor and should be recognized early so that proper therapy may be instituted. Auscultation of the lungs for wheezes and crackles is especially important in those with asthma or hypertension.

d. **Abdomen.** An attempt should be made to palpate major abdominal viscera for pain or masses, although this is difficult with a term-sized uterus. Epigastric tenderness may suggest toxemia.

e. **Extremities.** Examination of extremities should include an assessment of peripheral edema. Although mild ankle edema commonly is found near term in normal pregnancies, severe lower extremity or hand edema may suggest preeclampsia. A brief neurologic examination should be performed, because the presence of deep-tendon hyperreflexia and clonus may suggest impending seizure activity.

2. **Obstetric abdominal examination**

a. **Uterine size.** Until the middle of the third trimester, the distance (cm) from the pubic symphysis to the uterine fundus approximates the gestational age in weeks. Toward term, the measurement becomes progressively less reliable because individual variation in fetal size becomes greater and fundal height varies with the degree of engagement of the presenting part. **Estimation of fetal weight** should be attempted by careful palpation of the gravid uterus, mentally adjusting for amniotic fluid volume, thickness of the maternal abdomen, and the proportion of the fetus engaged in the pelvis. Fundal size larger than expected by the gestational age suggests incorrect dates, fetal or maternal anomalies, or multiple gestation. It may be possible to determine **multiple gestation** by abdominal palpation, but a sonogram is required for confirmation.

b. **Leopold's maneuvers.** It is essential to determine the position of the fetus within the uterus for labor management. This may be accomplished with the four maneuvers described by Leopold for examination of the abdomen (Fig. 27-1). A bedside ultrasound can confirm the position.

(1) The **first maneuver** determines which fetal pole occupies the uterine fundus (e.g., the breech with a vertex presentation). The breech moves with the fetal body. The vertex is rounder, harder, and feels more globular than the breech and can be maneuvered separately from the fetal body.

(2) With the **second maneuver,** the lateral aspects of the uterus are palpated to determine on which side the fetal back or fetal extremities (the so-called small parts) are located. The small parts are less firm than the back, and often movement is apparent.

(3) The **third maneuver** is performed with the examiner facing caudally, and the presenting part is made to move from side to side. If this is not done easily, engagement of the presenting part probably has occurred.

(4) The **fourth maneuver** reveals the presentation. With the fetus presenting by vertex, the cephalic prominence may be palpable on the side of the fetal small parts, confirming flexion of the fetal head (occiput presentation). Extension of the head (face presentation) is suspected when the cephalic prominence is on the side of the fetus opposite the small parts.

c. **The lie of the fetus** is a description of the relationship of the long axis of the fetus to the long axis of the mother. The lie is longitudinal with a vertex or breech presentation, or otherwise transverse or oblique as with a shoulder presentation.

d. **Presentation** describes that part of the fetus that is lowest in the pelvis—the vertex, the breech, or the shoulder. Most commonly seen is a **vertex** presentation, in which the **occiput** is lowest. With deflexion of the fetal head, however, the **brow** or **face** may be the lowest part. In a **breech** presentation, the fetal buttocks (the breech) are the presenting part. The breech presentation has several variations. When the fetal legs are extended above the pelvis, the presentation is termed **frank breech.** The feet and buttocks presenting together is a **complete breech,** whereas one foot alone is a **single-footling breech,** and both feet presenting is a **double-footling breech.** Although all abnormal presentations have an increased incidence of cord prolapse, footling breeches are especially at risk. A **shoulder** presentation requires a transverse lie. **Compound** presentations (e.g., vertex and an extremity together rarely are seen with term pregnancies.

e. **Position** of the presenting part is best determined by vaginal examination (see sec. **3.c.[3]**).

f. **Auscultation** of the fetal heart tones should be performed. We routinely perform continuous monitoring, carefully noting baseline heart rate, variability, accelerations, and decelerations.

3. **Pelvic examination.** Inspection and palpation of the perineum and the pelvis are of primary importance in the evaluation of the laboring patient. Information elicited includes the presence or absence of perineal, vaginal, and cervical lesions, including herpes; the adequacy of the bony pelvis; the integrity of the fetal membranes; the degree of cervical dilatation and effacement; and the station of the presenting part. In most instances, undiagnosed third-trimester vaginal bleeding and preterm premature rupture of the membranes preclude digital examination of the cervix until further evaluation is performed.

a. **Inspection.** Inspection of the perineum for **herpetic lesions,** large vulvar varicosities, large condylomas, and evidence of poorly repaired or broken-down perineal lacerations should be carried out. If any question of active genital herpes exists, the vagina and cervix should be inspected with the use of a speculum.

(1) **Diagnosis of ruptured membranes** may sometimes be visually confirmed from across the room. Often, however, it is necessary to perform a sterile speculum examination to determine the status of the fetal movements. The sterile speculum is inserted into the vagina and a light source positioned so the cervix and posterior vagina can be visualized.

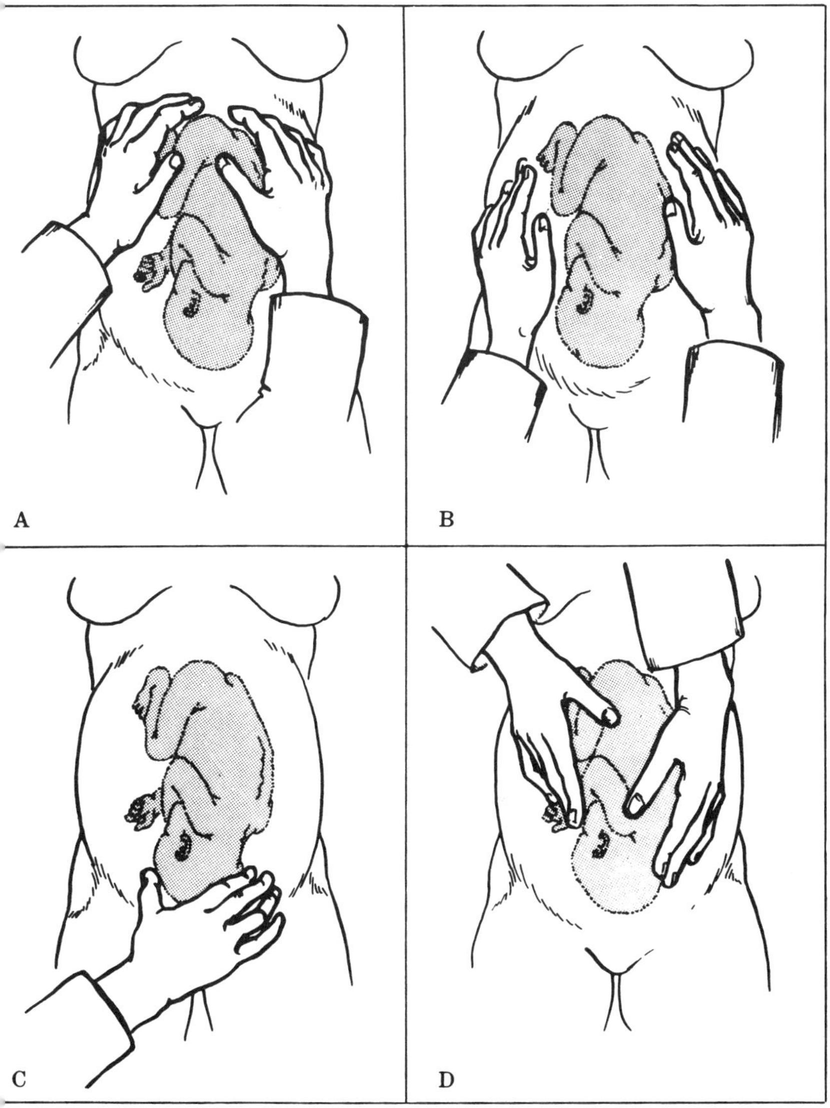

Fig. 27-1. Leopold's maneuvers to diagnose fetal presentation and position of the fetus. **A.** Palpation of the upper pole. **B.** Determining the side of the small parts. **C.** Palpation of the lower pole. The vertex is freely movable, and the breech moves with the body. **D.** Is the prominence of the presenting part on the side opposite the small parts, as with the face presentation, or is it on the same side, as with vertex presentation? (From K. Niswander, *Obstetric and Gynecologic Disorders: A Practitioner's Guide*. Flushing, N.Y.: Medical Examination, 1975.)

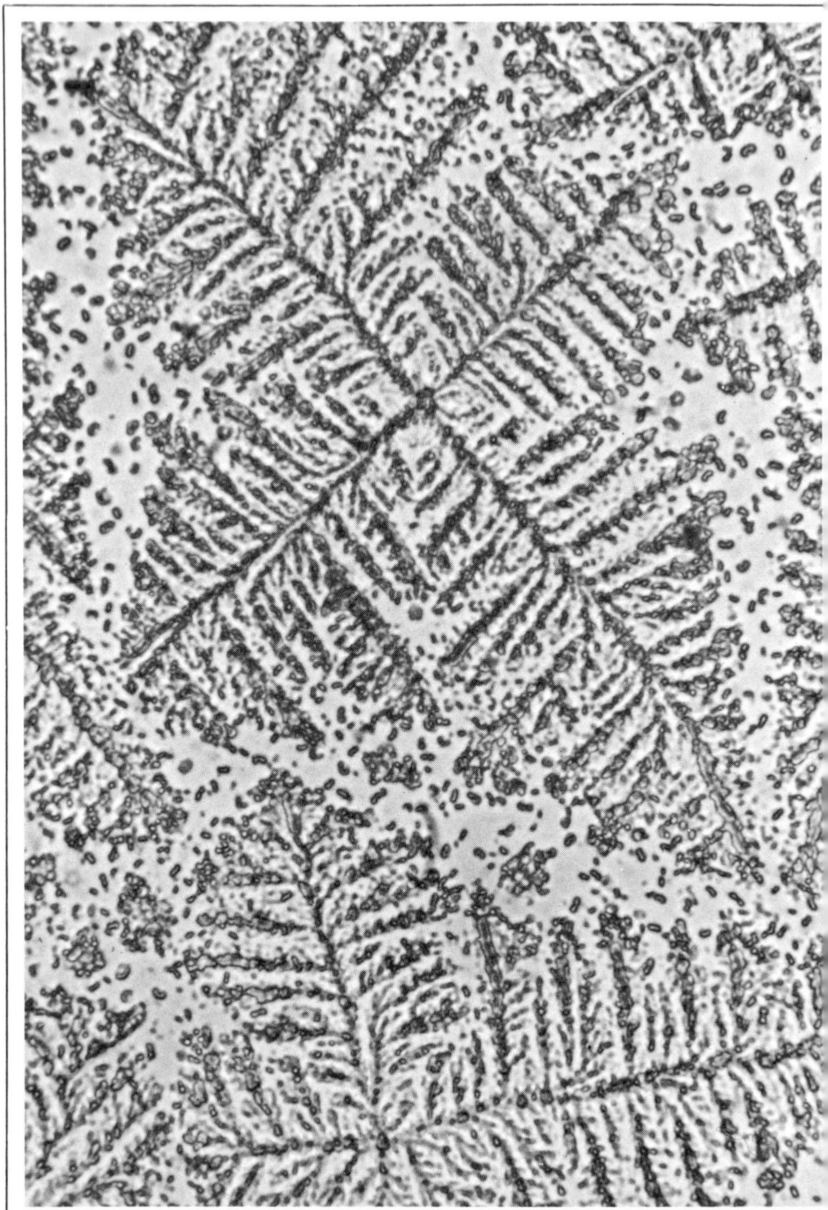

Fig. 27-2. "Ferning" in smear from the vagina suggests that amniotic fluid is present in the vagina.

(2) **Cultures are obtained then for anyone suspected of preterm labor or chorioamnionitis.** With preterm rupture of membranes, a sample of amniotic fluid from the vaginal pool should be obtained at this time to evaluate fetal lung maturity. Direct transcervical visualization of fetal scalp, feet, umbilical cord, or other fetal parts confirms ruptured membranes. Otherwise, any fluid pooled in the posterior vaginal fornix is sampled with a sterile cotton swab, smeared on a glass slide, and applied to nitrazine paper. **Ferning** of the air-dried fluid under the microscope suggests amniotic fluid (Fig. 27-2). The alkaline pH of amniotic fluid causes nitrazine paper to turn a deep blue, a positive test. Unfortunately, blood and sometimes urine may cause false-positive results. If bloody amniotic fluid is noted (port-wine fluid), further investigation to rule out abruptio placentae should be undertaken. The absence or presence of meconium in the amniotic fluid should be noted. Meconium is fetal stool. Its presence in and release from the fetal gastrointestinal tract increase with advancing gestational age. Although it may be released into the amniotic fluid during hypoxic stress, this is not a pathognomonic finding since it also can be present under normal conditions.

b. Palpation of the cervix

(1) **Dilatation** of the cervix describes the degree of opening of the cervical os. The cervix can be described as undilated or closed (0 cm), fully dilated (10 cm), or any point between these two extremes (0–10 cm).

(2) **Effacement** of the cervix describes the process of thinning that the cervix undergoes before or during labor (Fig. 27-3). The thick, prelabor cervix is approximately 3 cm long and is said to be uneffaced or to have 0% effacement. With complete or 100% effacement, the cervix is paper-thin. As a general rule, primiparas begin to efface the cervix before dilatation begins, whereas multiparas begin to dilate before significant effacement has been reached.

c. Palpation of the fetal presenting part

(1) **Identification** of the presentation should be confirmed by digital palpation of the fetal presenting part. The novice often assumes it to be a vertex, but identification must be positively made on every occasion. Vertex presentation can be confirmed by palpation of the suture lines of the fetal skull. Palpation of the fetal buttocks, feet, face, or arm confirms other presentations. Inability to identify the presenting part with certainty demands an ultrasound examination.

(2) **Station** refers to the relationship between the fetal presenting part and pelvic landmarks. When the presenting part is at **zero station,** it is at the level of the ischial spines, which are the landmarks for the midpelvis. This is important in the vertex presentation because it implies that the largest part of the fetal head, the biparietal diameter, has entered the pelvis. If the presenting part is 1 cm above the spines, it is described as −1 station. If it is 2 cm below the spines, the station is +2. The presenting part is described as **floating** when it is palpated at above −3 station. At +3 station, the presenting part is on the perineum, and it may distend the vulva with a contraction and be visible to an observer (Fig. 27-4).

(3) **Position** of the presenting part is described as the relationship between a certain pole of the presenting part and the surrounding pelvis, as follows: anterior = closest to the symphysis; posterior = closest to the coccyx; and transverse = closest to the left or right vaginal sidewalls. The index landmark in a vertex presentation is the occiput, which is identified by palpating the lambdoid sutures forming a Y with the sagittal suture; it is the sacrum in a breech presentation; and the mentum (or chin) in a face presentation. Figures 27-5 and 27-6 demonstrate the various vertex positions. **Occiput anterior** implies the occiput is closest to the maternal pubis. **Right occiput transverse** implies it is directed toward the right side of the maternal pelvis. Breech and face presentations

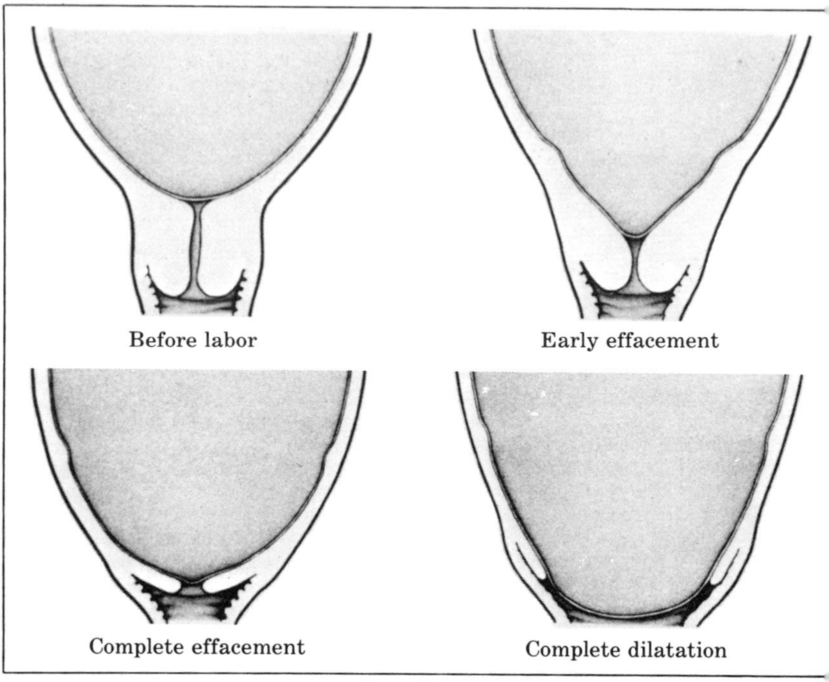

Fig. 27-3. Cervical effacement and dilatation in the primigravida. (From *Mechanism of Normal Labor,* Ross Clinical Education Aid, No. 13. Columbus, OH: Ross Laboratories, 1975.)

are described in a similar fashion (e.g., right sacrum transverse, right mentum transverse).

d. **Evaluation of pelvic adequacy.** The shape of the maternal pelvis may be visualized as a cylinder with a gentle anterior curve toward the outlet. The curve forms because the posterior border of the pelvis (the sacrum and the coccyx) is longer than the anterior border (the symphysis pubis). The lateral borders (the innominate bones) are more or less parallel in the gynecoid pelvis. Dystocia may be encountered when abnormalities of these bony elements are present. Pelvic adequacy can be judged clinically by measuring pelvic diameters at certain levels.

Even in the most experienced hands, clinical pelvic measurements are merely **estimations.** Unless the maternal pelvis is grossly contracted, adequacy is proved only by a trial of labor. The maternal pelvis is one of three factors that determines the success of labor. A large fetus or inadequate uterine contractions, even with an adequate pelvis, may prevent vaginal delivery.

(1) The **inlet** of the true pelvis is limited by the symphysis pubis anteriorly, sacral promontory posteriorly, and the iliopectineal line laterally. The **anteroposterior** (AP) diameter of the inlet may be estimated by determining the diagonal conjugate measurement. The diameter (the distance from the sacral promontory to the inner inferior surface of the symphysis pubis) is measured clinically by attempting to touch the sacral promontory with the vaginal examining finger while simultaneously noting where the inferior border of the symphysis touches the examining finger (Fig. 27-7). A measurement greater than 12 cm suggests adequacy.

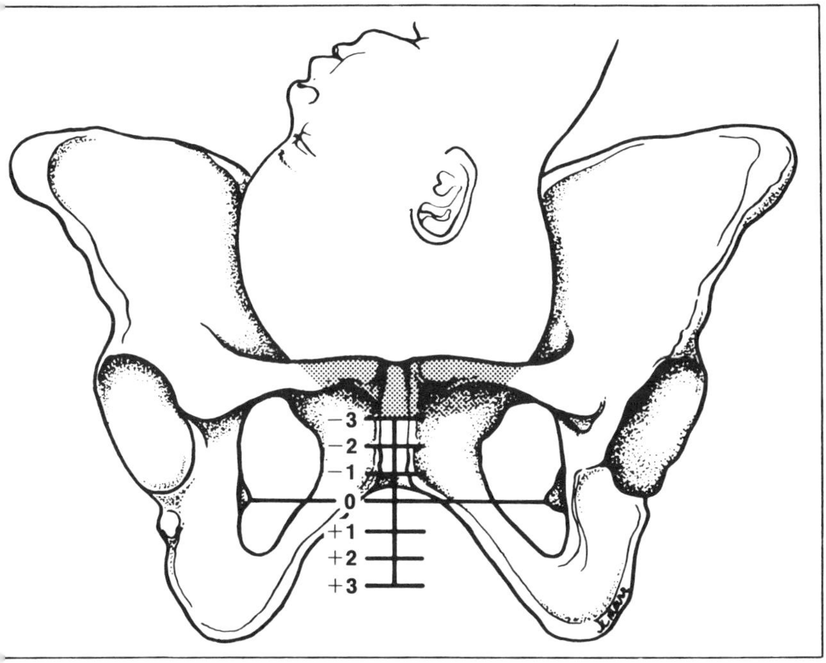

Fig. 27-4. Estimation of descent of fetal head into the pelvis. Zero station is diagnosed when the fetal vertex has reached the level of the ischial spines. (From K. Niswander, *Obstetrics: Essentials of Clinical Practice* [2nd ed.]. Boston: Little, Brown, 1981.)

(2) The **midpelvis** is bordered anteriorly by the symphysis pubis, posteriorly by the sacrum, and laterally by the ischial spines. A gently curved concave sacrum adds adequacy to the midpelvis. The interspinous diameter is estimated by palpating the ischial spines (Fig. 27-8). An estimated distance of less than 9 cm suggests midpelvis contraction. Experience is required to estimate this diameter with accuracy.

(3) The **outlet** is limited anteriorly by the arch of the symphysis pubis, posteriorly by the tip of the coccyx, and laterally by the ischial tuberosities. This transverse diameter of the outlet can be estimated by placing a clenched fist between the two ischial tuberosities. A measurement of 8 cm or more suggests an adequate diameter. The AP measurement is estimated by judging the prominence of the tip of the sacrum and by noting the angle made by the pubic rami. A narrow pelvic arch decreases the effective AP diameter. Dystocia as a result of an abnormal outlet alone is unusual, although with midpelvic inadequacy, the outlet is also usually inadequate.

C. Laboratory tests. Routine laboratory tests at the initial prenatal visit should include a complete blood cell count (CBC); blood type; Rh determination; antibody screen; serologic test for syphilis; rubella antibody titer; urinalysis and urine culture; Pap smear; cervical cultures for gonorrhea and *Chlamydia;* **hepatitis B surface antigen** (HBsAg) determination if the patient population is at risk for hepatitis B. During labor, the CBC, urinalysis, and serologic test for syphilis should be repeated. Thc HBsAg is repeated for high-risk patients. Patients with a history of glucose intolerance should have a timed (fasting or postprandial)

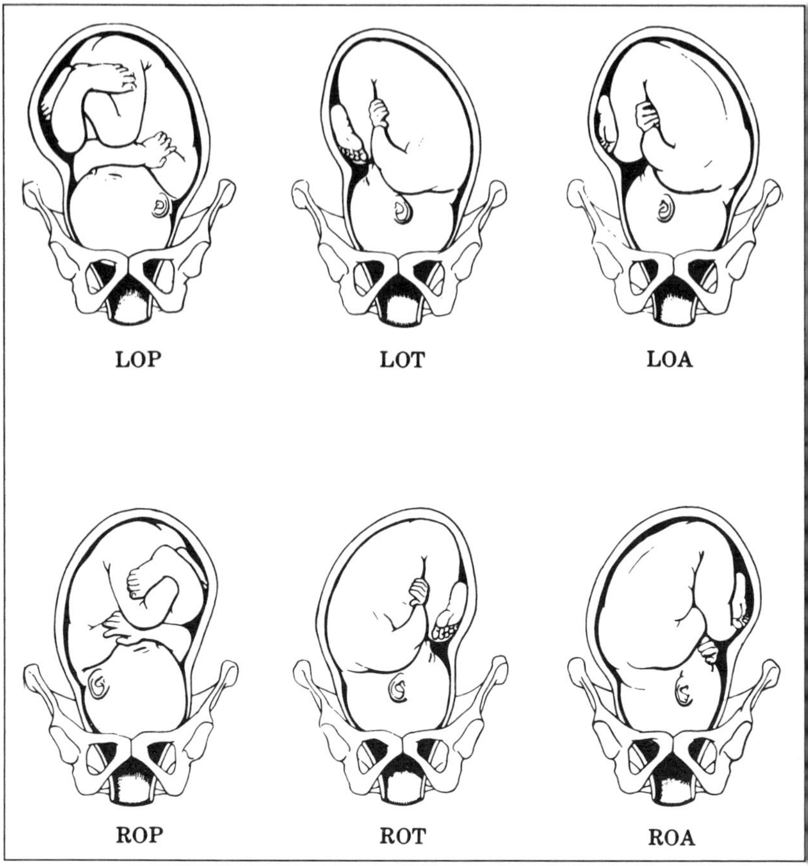

Fig. 27-5. Various vertex presentations. (LOP = left occiput posterior; LOT = left occiput transverse; LOA = left occiput anterior; ROP = right occiput posterior; ROT = right occiput transverse; ROA = right occiput anterior.) (From *Obstetrical Presentation and Position,* Columbus, OH: Ross Laboratories, 1975.)

blood glucose determination. If preeclampsia is a possibility, a CBC including a platelet count, renal function tests, liver function tests, and a uric acid value should be ordered. Fibrinogen and clotting parameters should be evaluated if the diagnosis of abruptio placentae is being considered. If the patient has a history of postpartum hemorrhage, is a grandmultipara, or is likely to have a cesarean section, a blood type is ordered to facilitate rapid cross-matching of blood. Specific laboratory tests should be ordered as required for specific physical findings, diseases, or complications.

D. Formulation of impression and plan. With the pertinent information from the history, examination, and laboratory testing taken into account, a clinical impression is made, and the patient is placed either objectively (using a system for awarding points to certain risk factors) or subjectively into a risk category. The process of deciding which patients require invasive procedures such as amniotomy, placement of internal fetal monitors, fetal scalp pH sampling, or intensive care–level monitoring of maternal vital functions begins with the initial clinical impression. The assessment and plan necessarily interface with the desires, plans,

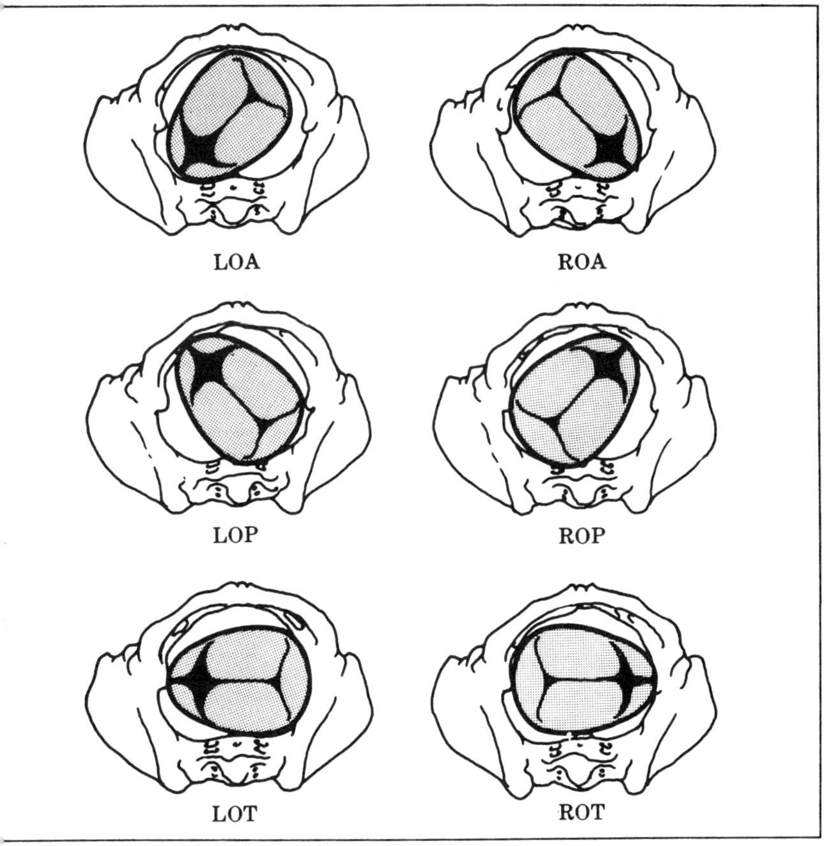

Fig. 27-6. Vaginal palpation of the large and small fontanelles and the frontal, sagittal, and lambdoidal sutures determines the position of the vertex. (LOA = left occiput anterior; ROA = right occiput anterior; LOP = left occiput posterior; ROP = right occiput posterior; LOT = left occiput transverse; ROT = right occiput transverse.) (From K. Niswander, *Obstetric and Gynecologic Disorders: A Practitioner's Guide.* Flushing, N.Y.: Medical Examination, 1975.)

and goals that the patient has expressed regarding her labor. The practitioner must be cognizant of and respect the patient's desires regarding her birthing process, while not compromising the level of care given to the mother and fetus. The high-risk patient presenting in labor needs detailed counseling regarding the nature of her problems, the rationale for tests and procedures, and any options that are available for her medical management.

II. Management of normal labor. Labor is a normal physiologic function of pregnancy. Despite this, complications occur such as intrapartum fetal death and fetal distress, dysfunctional labor, uterine rupture, chorioamnionitis, maternal and fetal hemorrhage, and even maternal death. The purpose for management of labor is to achieve progress toward delivery in a reasonable period of time, while providing maternal support and avoiding any significant compromise to the mother or fetus.

A. Distinguishing normal from abnormal progress in labor

1. Labor is divided in three stages. The **first stage** of labor encompasses the

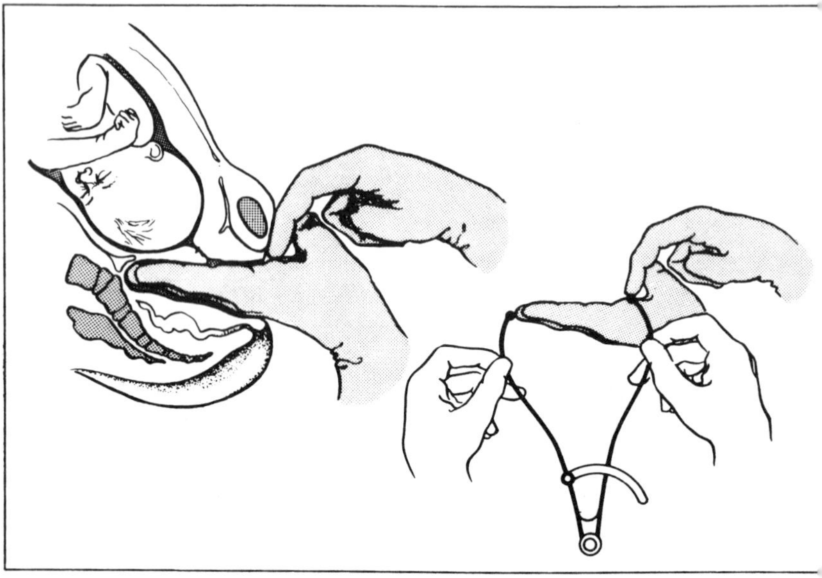

Fig. 27-7. Estimation of diagonal conjugate measurement. Vaginal fingers reach for the promontory of the sacrum, with note taken of the point at which the symphysis pubis touches the metacarpal bone *(left)*. The distance is measured with the calipers *(right)*. (From K. Niswander, *Obstetrics: Essentials of Clinical Practice* [2nd ed.]. Boston: Little, Brown, 1981.)

interval of time from the onset of labor until the cervix has become fully dilated (10 cm). This stage is further subdivided into a latent and an active phase. The **latent phase** is characterized by slow dilatation of the cervix to approximately 4 cm, or a point at which the rate of change in cervical dilatation is noted. The **active phase** ensues and is characterized by more rapid dilatation until 10 cm is achieved. The **second stage** of labor begins with complete dilatation of the cervix and ends with delivery of the infant. It is characterized by voluntary and involuntary pushing during uterine contractions to enhance descent of the presenting part and achieve delivery of the infant. The **third stage** of labor denotes the interval from delivery of the infant to delivery of the placenta (afterbirth). It is further discussed in sec. **III.**

2. **Assessment of progress in labor** requires periodic digital examination of the cervix to assess change in effacement, cervical dilatation, and descent of the presenting part. Vaginal examinations should be timely enough to adequately determine the progress of labor while still being limited for the sake of patient comfort and to minimize the risk of infection when the membranes are no longer intact. In Fig. 27-9, the average nulliparous labor has been represented cervicographically. The latent phase of labor is variable in length, and distinguishing between the normal and abnormal latent phase may be difficult. In the active phase of labor, the average rate of cervical dilatation is 1.5 cm/hour in the multipara and 1.2 cm/hour in the nullipara. However, acceptable standard deviations from these values are uncertain. Except in the case of complete arrest of dilatation, effacement, and descent, diagnosing abnormality of the active phase may be difficult. The average second stage of labor is one-half hour in a multipara and one hour in the primipara. Chapter 30 is devoted to the controversial topic of diagnosis and management of abnormal labor.
3. **Amniotomy** (artificial rupture of the membranes) is usually accomplished by

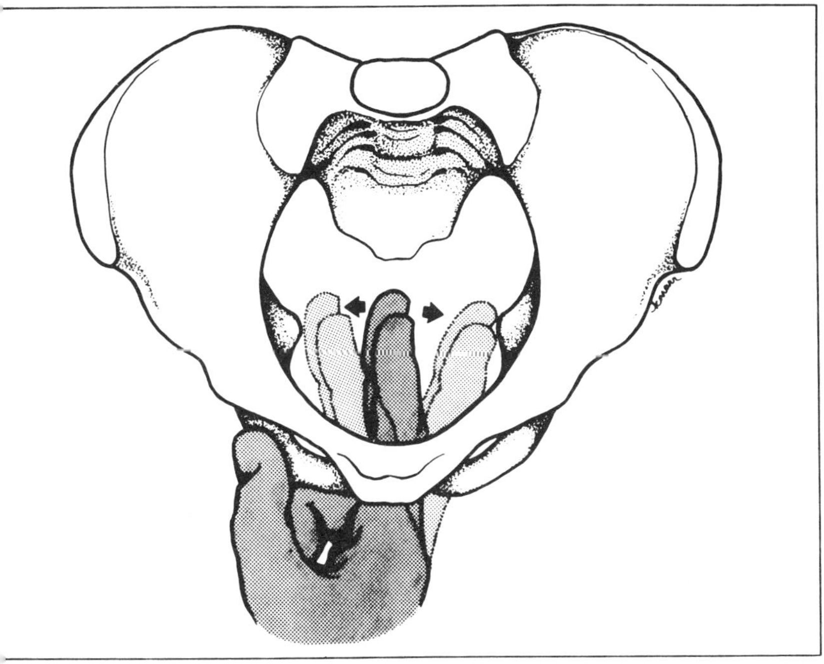

Fig. 27-8. Palpation of ischial spines to estimate interspinous diameter. (From K. Niswander, *Obstetrics: Essentials of Clinical Practice* [2nd ed.]. Boston: Little, Brown, 1981.)

puncturing the membranes with a sterile plastic instrument that is guided between two gloved fingers.

a. **Indications** for amniotomy include (1) visualizing the amniotic fluid for quantity and evidence of meconium or blood, (2) gaining direct access to the fetus for placement of internal fetal monitors, and (3) attempting to induce or accelerate labor.

   There is little debate that amniotomy is the only definitive way to visualize the amniotic fluid and to gain direct access to the fetal scalp. The effect of amniotomy on the speed of labor, however, is more controversial. Studies of the effect of amniotomy on duration of labor predominantly suggest that amniotomy performed in the active phase of labor significantly shortens labor [19, 29]. Performed during or before the latent phase of labor, however, amniotomy has been shown not to be beneficial to the course of labor.

b. **Risks** of amniotomy include several serious complications. Rupture of a fetal vessel traversing the fetal membranes (vasa praevia) at the site of amniotomy is rare but can cause fetal exsanguination. Prolapse of the umbilical cord between the presenting part and the cervix can occur at amniotomy and cause severe fetal compromise unless operative delivery is performed rapidly. Cord prolapse can be avoided by not performing amniotomy until the head is engaged in the pelvis and well applied against the cervix. Cord prolapse, of course, can also occur with spontaneous rupture of membranes.

c. Several studies have suggested **side effects** from amniotomy, including temporary fetal acidosis, increased incidence of variable fetal heart rate decelerations, and increased incidence of caput succedaneum and molding of the fetal skull [19]. The overall neonatal outcome in early amniotomy versus late spontaneous rupture has been similar in the majority of studies. In

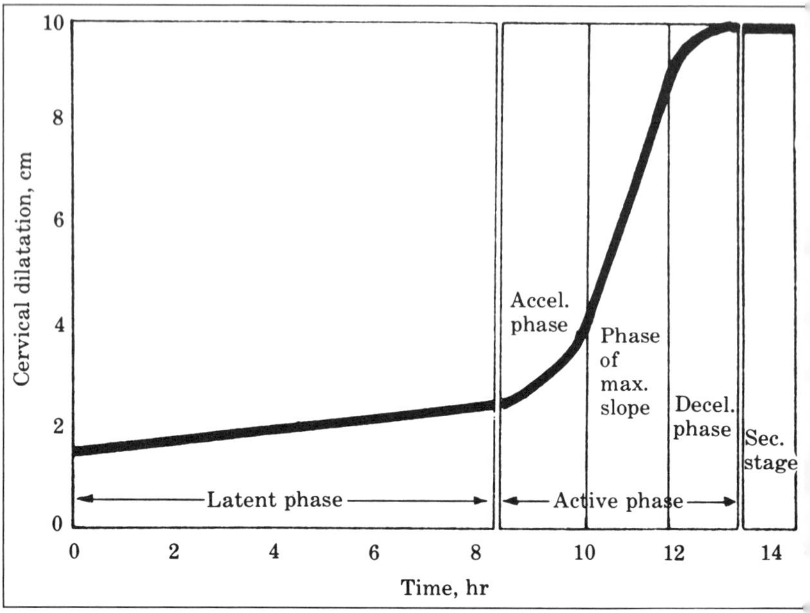

Fig. 27-9. Composite of the average dilatation curve for nulliparous labor. (From E. A. Friedman, *Labor: Clinical Evaluation and Management* [2nd ed.]. New York: Appleton-Century-Crofts, 1978.)

summary, the **various indications for amniotomy have rendered it integral** to the practice of modern obstetrics and it is used frequently at most institutions. The procedure has a few risks, and these must be weighed against the expected benefits each time artificial rupture of membranes is contemplated. Moreover, it should be understood when performing amniotomy to hasten labor that no controlled study has proved that a more rapid labor is superior for the mother or fetus compared to a slower, spontaneous labor.

B. Mechanisms of labor in the vertex presentation. The process of labor and delivery is marked by characteristic changes in fetal position or **cardinal movements** in relation to the maternal pelvis. These spontaneous adjustments of attitude are made to effect efficient passage through the pelvis as progressive descent of the fetus is accomplished.

1. **Engagement** is the descent of the largest transverse diameter, the biparietal diameter, to a level below the pelvic inlet. An occiput below the ischial spines is engaged.
2. **Descent** of the head is a discontinuous process occurring throughout labor. Because the transverse diameter of the inlet is wider than the AP diameter, and because the longest diameter of the fetal head is the AP diameter, in most instances the fetus enters the pelvis in an occiput transverse alignment.
3. **Flexion.** To decrease this AP diameter of the fetal head, flexion occurs as the head encounters the levator muscle sling, thereby decreasing the diameter by approximately 2.0 cm (occipitomental, 12.0 cm, to occipitofrontal, 10.5 cm). Later, further flexion occurs, reducing the diameter to 9.5 cm (suboccipitobregmatic) (Fig. 27-10).

   In the midpelvis, the architecture of the passageway changes so that now the AP diameter of the maternal pelvis is longer than the transverse diameter.
4. **Internal rotation.** The fetus accommodates to this change by rotation of the head from the transverse orientation (occiput transverse) to an AP alignment

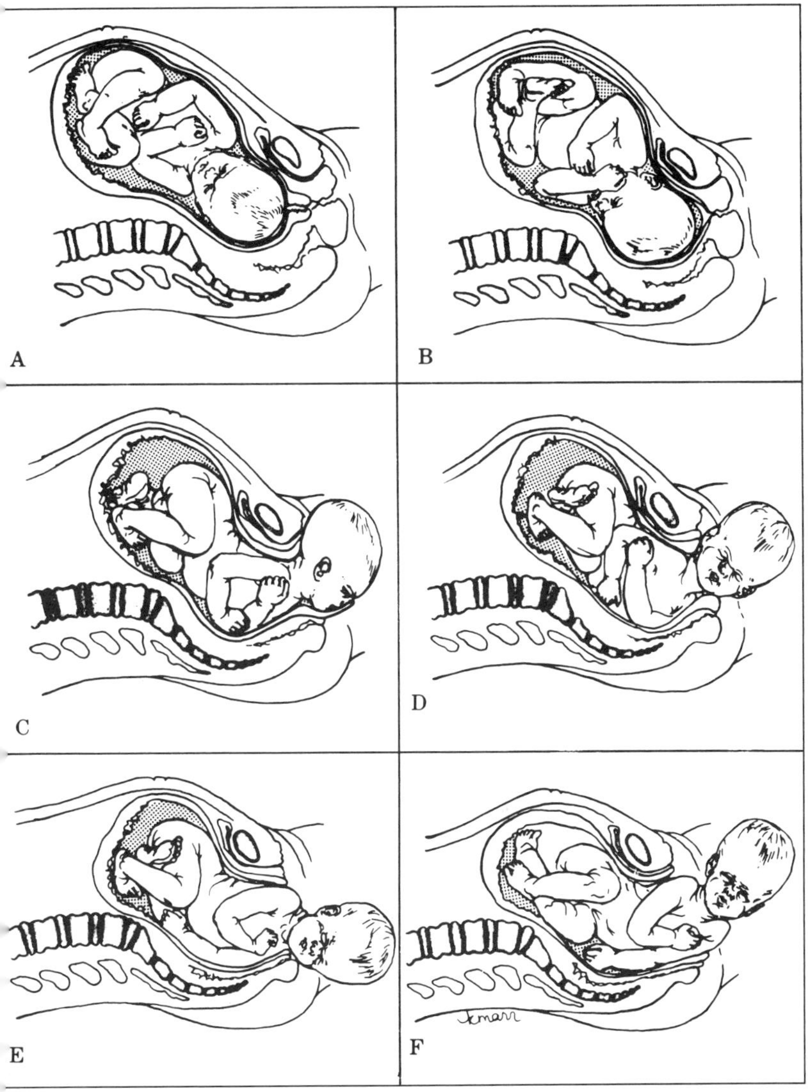

Fig. 27-10. Mechanism of labor in the left occiput anterior position. **A.** Engagement and flexion of the head. **B.** Internal rotation. **C.** Delivery by extension of the head. **D.** External rotation. **E.** Delivery of the anterior shoulder. **F.** Delivery of the posterior shoulder. (From K. Niswander, *Obstetric and Gynecologic Disorders: A Practitioner's Guide*. Flushing, N.Y.: Medical Examination, 1975.)

(usually occiput anterior), thus accomplishing internal rotation. Further descent to the level of the introitus occurs with the head in the AP plane.

5. **Extension.** Delivery of the head from the usual occiput anterior position through the introitus is accomplished by extension of the head. Little actual descent occurs with extrusion of the head because the head is delivered by a reversal

of the flexion that occurred as it entered the pelvis. The face appears over the perineal body, while the symphysis pubis acts as a fulcrum where it impinges on the occiput.

6. **External rotation.** Following delivery of the head, the fetal head rotates back toward the original transverse orientation (external rotation or restitution) when the fetal shoulders assume the AP diameter as they enter the midpelvis. The remainder of the delivery proceeds with presentation of the anterior shoulder beneath the symphysis pubis and the posterior shoulder across the posterior fourchette (Fig. 27-10).

C. **Intrapartum fetal assessment.** Some form of evaluation of fetal well-being during labor is necessary to improve on the natural rate of intrapartum fetal demise and intrapartum fetal asphyxia. The clinical decision involves the use of **intermittent** auscultation of the fetal heart versus **continuous** electronic fetal monitoring (external or internal), with fetal scalp pH sampling performed as necessary.

1. **Intermittent auscultation of the fetal heart rate** is performed every 15 minutes throughout the active phase of labor and at least every 5 minutes or after each push during the second stage. Electronic fetal heart rate monitoring and its interpretation are discussed in some detail in Chap. 22.

2. No prospective, controlled studies clearly demonstrate the value of **continuous electronic fetal monitoring** [14, 33]. Two retrospective studies published in the early 1980s compared the outcome of monitored patients with that of premonitoring era patients in the same institution. These studies showed the incidence of intrapartum stillbirth, severe birth asphyxia, low Apgar scores, and long-term neurologic damage to be significantly improved in the monitored group [15, 23], findings not confirmed in prospective investigations.

3. **Risks and complications.** Intermittent auscultation imparts no direct risk to the fetus except that evidence of a fetus in distress may be missed. Significant variable decelerations and evidence of uteroplacental insufficiency could escape diagnosis by this modality, however, and subject a compromised fetus to continued labor [14]. External electronic fetal heart rate monitoring, likewise, has no direct ill effect on the mother or fetus, but the tendency to keep the patient supine to obtain optimal fetal heart rate recordings sometimes causes aortocaval compression. The main risk of electronic fetal heart rate monitoring is inaccurate pattern interpretation, thereby allowing fetal distress to go unrecognized or, conversely, supporting unnecessary intervention to "save" a healthy fetus.

   To most accurately assess the fetal heart rate pattern and the amplitude, duration, and frequency of uterine contractions, internal fetal scalp electrodes and intramniotic pressure catheters are used. The most common complication of the scalp electrode is fetal scalp septic dermatitis or cellulitis, with an incidence of less than 1% in most series [32]. Rarer and more serious complications include cranial osteomyelitis, generalized gonococcal sepsis, and cerebrospinal fluid leakage with associated meningitis [25, 26, 31]. Again, the benefits must be carefully weighed against the risks. At the University of California, Davis (UCD), virtually all patients are monitored electronically. This approach is particularly beneficial in the high-risk obstetric population. Internal fetal monitors are used liberally where indicated: in patients too obese or uncooperative to be monitored externally; during oxytocin augmentation of labor; in the patient whose external tracing is not reassuring; and in the patient attempting vaginal delivery after a prior cesarean section.

D. **Maternal preparation, position, anesthesia, and analgesia**

1. **Physical preparation.** Physical preparation of the laboring patient is straightforward. Those patients who are physically unclean and in whom delivery is not imminent are encouraged to shower. The constipated patient or one who has hard stool palpable in the rectum may have a Fleet enema. Shaving of the perineum may sometimes facilitate episiotomy repair but has no effect on the rate of infection and is not routinely performed at UCD. The routine insertion of an indwelling intravenous catheter is recommended for fluid administration during labor and venous access for administration of drugs, anesthetic agents,

or blood. Intravenous fluids are administered to replace the large insensible fluid losses that occur during labor because oral intake usually is limited to ice chips or sips of water. Gastric emptying is minimal during labor, and keeping the stomach empty for the possibility of emergency anesthesia is warranted. The infused fluid is usually Ringer's lactate or 0.45% normal saline with or without 5% dextrose. Intravenous fluid infused rapidly or given as a bolus should **not** contain dextrose because the maternal blood glucose can rise rapidly, which may further compromise an already acidotic fetus [21]. Dextrose administration throughout labor helps prevent starvation ketosis.

2. **Maternal position.** Maternal position in labor has consequences for both maternal comfort and fetal well-being. The dorsal supine position with the gravid uterus resting on the aorta and inferior vena cava can cause maternal hypotension and placental hypoperfusion.

   Patients in the latent phase of labor frequently are most comfortable if they are allowed to walk. No risk of fetal compromise exists as long as an initial monitoring strip is reassuring and the membranes are intact. Studies comparing patients who were ambulatory during the active phase of labor versus those who were confined to bed have found some acceleration of the first stage of labor and decreased numbers of operative deliveries in the ambulatory group, with equal fetal outcome [5]. In the late active phase, it was difficult to keep the ambulatory group walking [13]. In the active phase, bed rest on the patient's side is a good position and allows intermittent or continuous fetal monitoring to be performed. One study [12] showed that continuous fetal monitoring may be carried out in the ambulatory patient by telemetry with no difference in fetal outcome but significantly less subjective pain than in control.

3. **Analgesia and anesthesia.** The goal of pain control in labor is to provide the patient the comfort to experience her birth process as fully as she desires while avoiding significant fetal compromise. The modalities that meet these needs include psychoprophylaxis, narcotic and analgesic drugs, and regional anesthesia.

   a. **Psychoprophylaxis.** Over the past several decades, various psychoprophylactic methods have been devised and popularized to reduce the amount of analgesia required for labor and delivery. The central theme in such methods is that preparation for childbirth through the use of antenatal instruction will ease anxiety for the parturient and her partner. An informed patient can prepare herself to control her reactions at the time of labor. Emphasis is placed on simplified methods of establishing **self-control,** for example, by concentrating on something innocuous, such as a given breathing pattern, instead of the pain of the contraction. This allows labor to be better tolerated. The **Lamaze method** probably is the most popular example of psychoprophylaxis for labor.

   b. **Narcotic and analgesic drugs.**

      (1) **Timing.** An analgesic appropriate during one phase of labor may be entirely inappropriate at another time. Common analgesic regimens are provided in Table 27-2. In a prolonged early latent phase of labor, mild sedation with a short-acting barbiturate or ataractic such as hydroxyzine (Vistaril), secobarbital (Seconal), or sodium pentobarbital (Nembutal) may be sufficient. In addition, these medications frequently will relieve the discomfort experienced by the patient in false labor, thus, in effect, confirming the diagnosis. These drugs should have little effect on the progress of the patient in true labor. Barbiturates have lost some popularity because of their prolonged depressant effect on the newborn. Hydroxyzine is rapidly transmitted across the placenta, but no effect on Apgars or neurologic function has been found [2]. Narcotics are best avoided until the active phase of labor is reached (i.e., 3–4 cm of dilatation in the primigravida and 5 cm in the multipara) [9]. Once the active phase of labor has begun, any of the following methods of pain relief may be instituted.

      (2) **Commonly used drugs.** The most common form of analgesia during labor

Table 27-2. Common analgesic regimens during labor

Drug	Dose (mg)	Route	Peak effect in fetus	Duration	Effect	Problems
For early or latent-phase labor, or with suspected false labor						
Secobarbital (Seconal)	100–300	PO[a], rectal	2–4 hr	3–6 hr	Sedation, sleep	Respiratory depression; fetal depression if fetus delivered during peak effect
Pentobarbital (Nembutal)	30–100	PO[a], rectal, IM	2–4 hr	3–6 hr		
Promethazine hydrochloride (Phenergan)	25–50	PO[a], rectal, IM	1–3 hr	4–6 hr	Sedation, antiemetic, antianxiety agent; augments narcotic effects	Anticholinergic effects; other rare serious effects (see *PDR*)
Hydroxyzine (Vistaril)	50–100	PO[a], IM	30–150 min	4–6 hr	Sedation, tranquilization, narcotic and barbiturate augmentation; antiemetic	Drowsiness, drying of mouth

For active-phase labor[b]						
Meperidine hydrochloride (Demerol)[c]	50–100	IV IM	10–60 min 30–150 min	30–120 min 2–4 hr	IM slower onset, longer lasting; analgesia, sedation	Respiratory depression, dizziness, sweating, nausea, vomiting
Nalbuphine hydrochloride (Nubain)	5–10	IV SC	15–30 min 30–45 min	1–2 hr 2 hr	Analgesic, agonist/ antagonist; sedation	Respiratory depression, confusion, nausea
Butorphanol tartrate (Stadol)	1–2 0.5–1	IM IV	30–60 min 15–45 min	3–4 hr 1½–3 hr	Rapid onset, short duration; analgesia, greater sedative effects	Respiratory depression, dizziness, nausea, vomiting

[a]Oral medications should be avoided in labor, except for an antacid when inhalation anesthesia is planned.
[b]If delivery is imminent within 3 hours of administering meperidine or within 1½ hours of giving alphaprodine, naloxone hydrochloride (Narcan), 0.4 mg IV, may be given 5 minutes prior to delivery.
[c]Promethazine or hydroxyzine may be used to augment the analgesia.
Source: From L. S. Goodman and A. Gilman, *The Pharmacologic Basis of Therapeutics* (5th ed.). New York: Macmillan, 1975; *Physicians' Desk Reference (PDR)* (40th ed.), Oradell, N.J.: Medical Economics, 1986.

is a **parenterally administered narcotic.** "Twilight sleep," using morphine and scopolamine, is only of historic interest and has been replaced by the use of meperidine hydrochloride (Demerol), nalbuphine (Nubain), or butorphanol tartrate (Stadol). The narcotics may also be used intravenously, in which case their effect is more rapid and their duration of action shorter. Narcotic dosages should be reduced when they are used concomitantly with a sedative.

(3) Dosages. Meperidine usually is given in a dose of 50–100 mg IM q3–4h or 10–25 mg IV q1.5–3.0h. Butorphanol is used in dosages of 2 mg IM q3–4h or 0.5–1.0 mg IV q1.5–2.0h. Many have noted that butorphanol provides an added quality of sedation that often is useful in anxious patients. Nalbuphine is used in dosages of 5–10 mg SC or IV q2–3h, depending on the patient's response.

(4) Precautions. It should be emphasized that parenteral narcotics cross the placenta and may depress the fetus. This effect is manifested most commonly by a loss of either reactivity (acceleration above baseline) or beat-to-beat variability in the fetal heart rate tracing. It should be remembered that the fetal metabolism of these drugs is several times slower than in the mother. Parenteral narcotics should be avoided if it is anticipated that their peak action will not have been dissipated by the time delivery is accomplished. This determination is not always easy to make; therefore, a narcotic antagonist, preferably naloxone hydrochloride (Narcan), in both the adult (0.4 mg IV or IM) and neonatal (0.01 mg/kg) dilutions, should be readily available. The primary undesirable effect of narcotics is on the respiratory center. If the newborn is provided with good air exchange, little harm is likely to result. Patient-controlled analgesia has been used successfully at other institutions [6, 27], but recent studies have shown no benefit to the mother and an increased need for naloxone [28].

c. Regional anesthesia. Aside from psychoprophylaxis, many experts consider regional anesthesia the preferred method for vaginal delivery. Certainly, if there is any concern in interpreting the fetal monitoring, a regional anesthetic is preferred over parenteral. The various methods include epidural, spinal, caudal, paracervical, and pudendal block.

The pain of labor and delivery originates primarily in three areas: the **uterus, cervix,** and **perineum.** Somatic sensory nerves supplying the perineum run in a direct manner along the sacral roots S2, S3, and S4. The pain of uterine contractions is transmitted on sympathetic nerves following a circuitous course through the pelvis and entering the spinal cord at segments T11 and T12.

(1) Epidural anesthesia is the most elegant of the regional blocks. The indication is relief of pain during labor.

(a) Contraindications include patient refusal, infection in the lumbar area, clotting defect, active neurologic disease, sensitivity to the local anesthetic, hypovolemia, and septicemia.

(b) Risks include hypotension, respiratory arrest, toxic drug reaction, and rare neurologic complications. The physician administering the block should have the experience and equipment at hand to deal with all complications.

(c) Effects. Epidural anesthesia has no significant effect on the progress of labor. It has not been demonstrated to directly affect the uterus, but contractions may decrease in intensity or frequency following initial catheter placement. Conversely, maternal relaxation following cessation of pain may result in rapid dilatation [8, 9].

Adverse effect on the fetus is minimal if maternal hypotension and resultant placental hypoperfusion are avoided. Given cautious hydration and dosing in preeclamptics, epidural anesthesia is the preferred form of analgesia for operative deliveries. It is the technique of choice in patients with cardiac disease, except with severe aortic or pulmonary stenosis, where hypotension should be avoided [8].

(d) Procedure. The procedure is begun by adequately hydrating the patient with a preload of 500–1000 ml of intravenous fluid. A lumbar epidural block is performed by entering the epidural space between L2 and S1 (usually L3–L4), and threading a plastic catheter into the space (Fig. 27-11). The catheter is aspirated to ascertain that the tip is not in the cerebrospinal fluid blood vessel. A 2-ml test dose of local anesthetic is given to confirm proper catheter placement (Table 27-3). The full dose then is given: 12–16 ml for a standard epidural block (T10–S5), 6 ml for segmental anesthesia (T10–T12), or 16–20 ml for surgical anesthesia (T5–T6). The dose may be repeated as necessary to serve as anesthesia and analgesia throughout labor or given as continuous dosing [8].

(2) Spinal anesthesia. Spinal anesthesia, usually in the form of a **low saddle block**—so designated because the area anesthetized would occupy a saddle—is commonly used for delivery. Unlike the epidural block, it is used after full dilatation has been reached or after the presenting part is at a level where vaginal delivery can be accomplished. At UCD, epidural anesthesia is preferred for labor and delivery.

(a) Procedure

(i) An **intravenous line** should be in place and the patient should

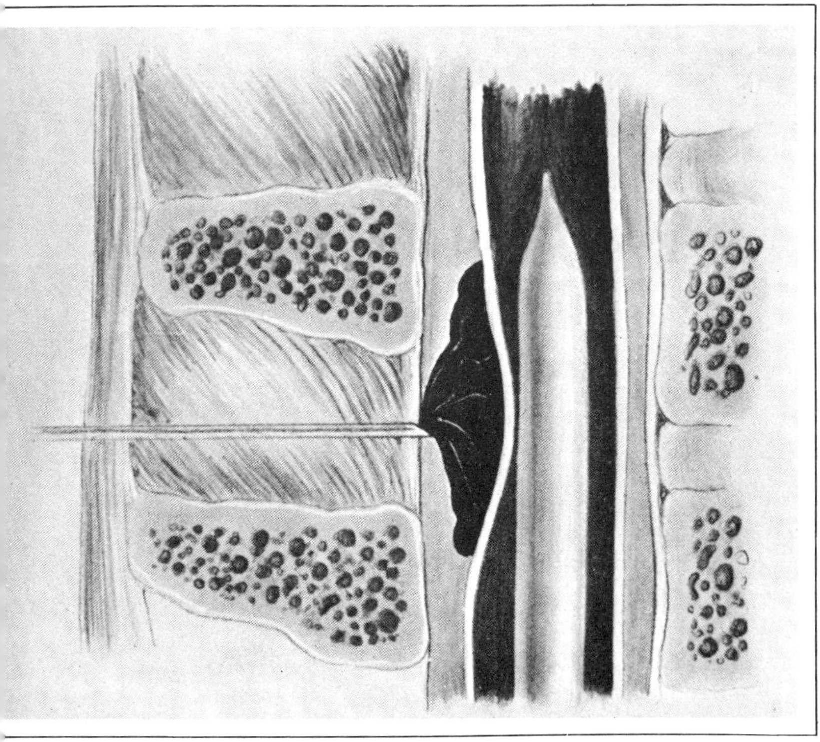

ig. 27-11. Epidural anesthesia. The anesthetic agent has been introduced into the pidural space. (From D. Moore, *Regional Block* [4th ed.]. Springfield, IL: Thomas, 967.)

Table 27-3. Commonly used local anesthetics for peripheral or regional blocks

Drug	Concentration (%)	Maximum dose (mg)	Onset of action (min)	Duration of action	Most common use	Remarks
Lidocaine (xylocaine without epinephrine)[a]	0.5–2 (usually 1)	300	5–15	1–3 hr	Paracervical, pudendal, local for episiotomy, epidural, saddle block	Allergic response, fetal bradycardia without paracervical block, hypotension
Chloroprocaine hydrochloride (Nesacaine)[b]	2–3	1000	5–15	30–90 min	Epidural, local, paracervical block	Safest for obstetrics; local irritation, short-acting
Tetracaine hydrochloride (Pontocaine)[b]	0.5[c]	100	6–15	75–150 min	Spinal, saddle block	Potent in small volume
Mepivacaine hydrochloride (Carbocaine)[a]	0.5–1	500	10–15	1–3 hr	Paracervical, epidural, caudal block	
Bupivacaine hydrochloride (Marcaine)[a]	0.25–0.75	225	10–20	100–300 min	Epidural, caudal, lumbar sympathetic block	Long-acting, good motor blockade at higher concentrations; do not use as paracervical block

[a] Amide compounds—less readily metabolized, greater liability for adverse reaction, some antiarrhythmic effect on heart.
[b] Ester compounds—fewer systemic effects, less chance of allergic response.
[c] 1% diluted with 10% dextrose produces approximately a 0.5% solution.

have received a fluid load of 300–500 ml before the administration of the anesthetic, to prevent a hypotensive response to the sympathetic blockade created by the anesthetic.

(ii) With a **small-gauge needle** (22- to 26-gauge), the subarachnoid space is entered most commonly in the L4–L5 or L5–S1 interspace, and the anesthetic is administered when a free flow of cerebrospinal fluid is evident. (See Table 27-3 for drugs.)

(iii) The patient, if sitting, is brought to the **upright position** and kept there for a period of 30–90 seconds to allow the hyperbaric anesthetic solution to settle. This creates the **saddle effect.**

(iv) The patient then is placed in the **lithotomy position** and the delivery is completed, usually **(though not always)** with forceps.

(b) Contraindications include those listed for epidural anesthesia as well as placenta previa, abruptio placentae, and fetal distress.

(i) Relative contraindications include chronic backache, history of spinal headache, and chronic headache.

(c) Complications include hypotension, respiratory arrest, headache, and neurologic complications.

(3) Paracervical block has been a popular form of analgesia because it is simple, reliable, and seemed very safe for the patient. It has fallen out of use because of its frequent association with fetal bradycardias following placement of the block.

(a) The **cause** may be fetal toxicity from the local anesthetic, uterine artery vasoconstriction, or hypercontractility of the uterus. Bradycardia has been associated with virtually all local anesthetic agents [22, 24].

(b) The **technique** for paracervical block is presented both for historic perspective and because it may be useful in cases in which other anesthetics are contraindicated or pose a greater risk to the fetus. The block is performed by single or continuous injection of the anesthetic agent on each side of the cervix to block Frankenhäuser's ganglion. The shallow injection technique described by Bloom and colleagues [1] was associated with no fetal bradycardia.

(4) Pudendal block usually is reserved for the actual delivery and provides anesthesia in the distribution of the pudendal nerve.

(a) Procedure. With the patient in the lithotomy position and with the operator using a spinal needle and an Iowa trumpet, lidocaine, carbocaine, or Nesacaine is infiltrated through the sacrospinous ligament on both sides just medial and inferior to its insertion into the ischial spine (Fig. 27-12). This often is adequate anesthesia for outlet forceps delivery and episiotomy repair, although failure is common (10–15%). Aspiration of blood prior to infiltration of the anesthetic demands repositioning of the needle.

E. Vaginal labor and delivery after cesarean section. At the UCD Medical Center, patients with a one or two prior low transverse cesarean sections are offered a trial of labor and vaginal delivery. Management of this situation is included in this chapter because the literature supports the premise that a properly conducted **vaginal birth after cesarean** (VBAC) carries no added maternal or fetal morbidity [4].

1. The complication of concern with VBAC is rupture of the previous uterine incision with resultant maternal and fetal morbidity. In 1978, more than 89% of patients with previous cesarean sections were delivered by repeat cesarean, largely because of the fear of uterine rupture. However, in an extensive review of the literature from 1950–1980, Lavin and colleagues [16] reported a 0.7% rate of uterine rupture and a 0.93% perinatal death rate. Twelve of the fourteen deaths resulted from rupture of vertical uterine scars, and the two deaths from transverse scar rupture were unmonitored patients. More recent series suggest a very low rate of uterine rupture and a high success rate in patients with a single previous low transverse uterine incision [4, 17, 20]. The safety and

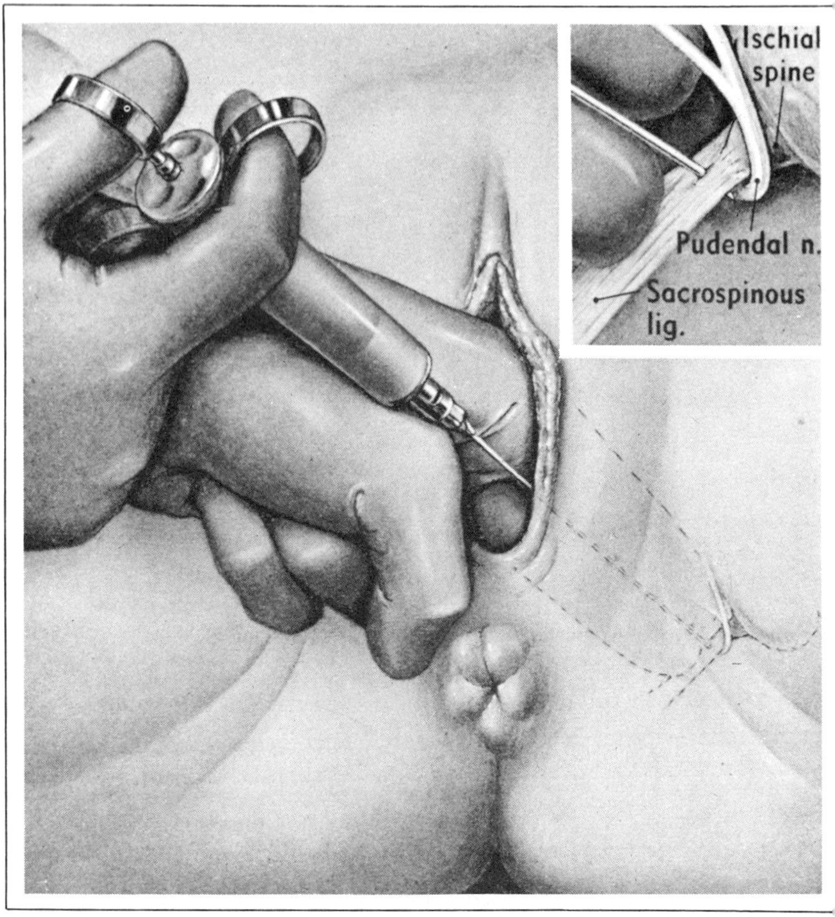

Fig. 27-12. Technique of pudendal block. (From J. Bonica, *Principles and Practice of Obstetric Analgesia and Anesthesia*. Philadelphia: Davis, 1967.)

efficacy of continuous epidural anesthesia and oxytocin augmentation during VBAC have been described [3, 4, 10].

2. **Procedure.** At UCD, an operating room and staff, anesthesiologists, and blood bank are available around the clock, and obstetricians are in-house to respond appropriately to uterine rupture or any other more common obstetric emergency. Patients attempting VBAC are admitted to the labor floor, an intravenous line is started, and blood is submitted for typing and a screen. **Membranes are ruptured as soon as accessible,** and a fetal scalp electrode and intrauterine pressure catheter are inserted to monitor the fetus and quality of labor. **Oxytocin** and **epidural anesthesia** are used for the usual obstetric indications. After the third stage of labor, the uterine incision is not examined. Results have been favorable, and the patients frequently appreciate the chance to participate in a normal labor and delivery.

III. Normal delivery

A. Management of spontaneous delivery of the infant

1. **Preparation.** As the multiparous patient approaches complete dilatation or the

nulliparous patient begins to crown the fetal scalp with a push, preparations are made for delivery. If delivery is to take place in a combined labor and delivery room, equipment is opened and materials readied to receive the neonate.

2. **Maternal position.** The mother's position on the delivery room table is usually restricted to the dorsal lithotomy position with left lateral tilt (to displace the uterus from the great vessels). This position has been encouraged to allow the obstetrician adequate access to the perineum. In a labor room setting, patients may naturally tend to push and deliver on their sides, sitting, or in the knee-chest position.
   a. Relatively few **controlled comparisons** of the benefits of various delivery positions have been published. One study [18] advocated the "half-sitting" position that can be used in a delivery room setting with stirrups. Patients found this position more comfortable, required fewer operative deliveries, and had equivalent fetal outcome to controls.
   b. **Procedure.** The perineum is prepped with iodine solution and an attempt is made to avoid maternal fecal contamination of the perineum. Delivery anesthesia is chosen at this time. Many deliveries may be performed without anesthesia if that is the patient's and physician's preference. If episiotomy is contemplated, the midline perineum is infiltrated with local anesthetic or a pudendal block is placed.
3. **Maneuvers of delivery from an occiput anterior position**
   a. **Delivery of the head.** The fetal head is delivered by extension. As the flexed head passes through the vaginal introitus, the smallest diameter (occipitobregmatic) is presented if the vertex is maintained in a state of flexion. **Maintaining flexion** and **pushing the perineum back over the face and under the chin before the head is allowed to extend appears to be the least traumatic method** [11]. Extending the fetal head by lifting the fetal chin with a towel-covered hand on the perineum (Ritgen maneuver) can accelerate the delivery process but may be more traumatic to the perineum. Once the fetal head has been delivered, external rotation and restitution to the occiput transverse position occurs. The nose and oropharynx of the fetus should be suctioned with the bulb syringe. If **meconium staining** is present, the nasopharynx, oropharynx, and fetal stomach should be suctioned thoroughly with a DeLee device attached to wall suction prior to delivery of the shoulders to minimize meconium aspiration. **Care should be taken not to stimulate the posterior pharyngeal mucosa too vigorously,** because a vagal response so stimulated could cause a fetal bradycardia. A finger should be slipped into the vagina along the fetal neck to see if a nuchal cord is present. If one is present, it can usually be reduced over the vertex or over the body and loosened. If this cannot be accomplished easily, the cord should be doubly clamped and divided between the clamps and the remainder of the delivery carried out.
   b. **Delivery of the shoulders.** Delivery of the anterior shoulder is accomplished by gentle but firm downward traction on the fetal head toward the floor. Direct suprapubic pressure from an assistant to effect this maneuver may be required. With the anterior shoulder delivered, the posterior shoulder now is delivered with vertical traction directed upward on the vertex (see Fig. 27-9). The perineal body should be watched to avoid extensions of the episiotomy or the occurrence of lacerations. When both shoulders have passed through the introitus, the remainder of the delivery requires little assistance in most cases.
   c. **Final steps.** Grasping the infant around the back of the neck with one hand and gliding the other hand toward the vagina to the baby's buttocks, the operator delivers the infant. **Care should be taken to keep the baby's head downward** to facilitate drainage of nasopharyngeal secretions. The infant can usually be cradled in one arm and tucked against the operator's abdomen, leaving the other hand free to perform the steps that follow. The secretions from the nose and oropharynx should again be suctioned, and the umbilical cord doubly clamped and divided, leaving 2–3 cm of cord. A brief

examination of the proximal end of the cord may prevent clamping part of an omphalocele or umbilical hernia. The baby is transferred to the mother's abdomen for initial bonding or to the crib, where necessary resuscitation or other procedures can be performed.

4. **Episiotomy.** This incision of the perineum enlarges the vaginal orifice at the time of delivery. The incision may be made with scissors or a knife and may be made in the midline (**medial** episiotomy) or begun in the midline and extended laterally (**mediolateral** episiotomy). Episiotomy is one of the most frequently performed obstetric procedures and one of the more controversial.

   a. **Major indications**

      (1) Prevention of more extensive lacerations [7].

      (2) Prevention of postpartum pelvic relaxation from stretching of the endopelvic fascia.

      (3) Prevention of trauma to the fetal head.

   b. **Risks versus benefits.** An episiotomy has never been shown unequivocally to accomplish these goals in any prospective clinical trial [30]. However, an episiotomy is simpler to repair than a laceration. As with any other surgical procedure, the risks of episiotomy must be compared with the benefits. Pain and edema are the most frequent associated postepisiotomy findings, usually resolving within a few days. Dyspareunia, however, may be a complaint of a significant number of women several weeks post partum. Infection can be one of the most serious complications of episiotomy, leading to significant morbidity and rarely maternal mortality [30].

   c. **Timing.** If indicated, an episiotomy should be performed when 3–4 cm diameter of fetal scalp is visible during a contraction. Excessive blood loss can occur if performed earlier. If performed too late, excessive stretching of the perineum and vagina may have already occurred.

   d. **Method.** With adequate local, pudendal, or spinal anesthetic in place, the perineum is elevated from the fetal head and medial episiotomy is performed by incising the triangularly shaped perineum toward the anus and into the vagina. An adequate incision should be made for the episiotomy to be of value. Care must be taken to avoid cutting into the anal sphincter or the rectum unless this degree of exposure is deemed necessary. If a short perineum is encountered, a mediolateral episiotomy should be considered [7]. Delivery is performed with care taken by the obstetrician to prevent extension of the episiotomy by applying pressure at the perineal apex with a towel-covered hand. **Note: It must be remembered that most deliveries can be performed without episiotomy and the proposed benefits have never been proved.**

B. **Delivery of the placenta**

1. **Spontaneous delivery.**

   a. **Timing.** Usually, the placenta separates spontaneously from the uterine wall within approximately five minutes of delivery. No attempt should be made to extract the placenta prior to its separation.

   b. **Separation** is indicated when

      (1) The fundus changes to a globular shape.

      (2) The fundus changes to a firm consistency.

      (3) A gush of blood appears vaginally.

      (4) The umbilical cord appears to lengthen.

   When separation has occurred, gentle fundal massage and firm but gentle traction on the cord sometimes will effect delivery of the placenta rapidly. We use the Brandt-Andrews maneuver, a cephalad shearing motion exerted with the abdominal hand on the uterus while traction on the cord is simultaneously exerted (Fig. 27-13). The abdominal hand should prevent uterine inversion.

2. **Manual extraction.** If the placenta has not separated after 30 minutes and the patient is anesthetized adequately, manual removal may be performed to reduce potential excess blood loss. Intrauterine bacterial contamination is a theoretic risk but is not a common complication.

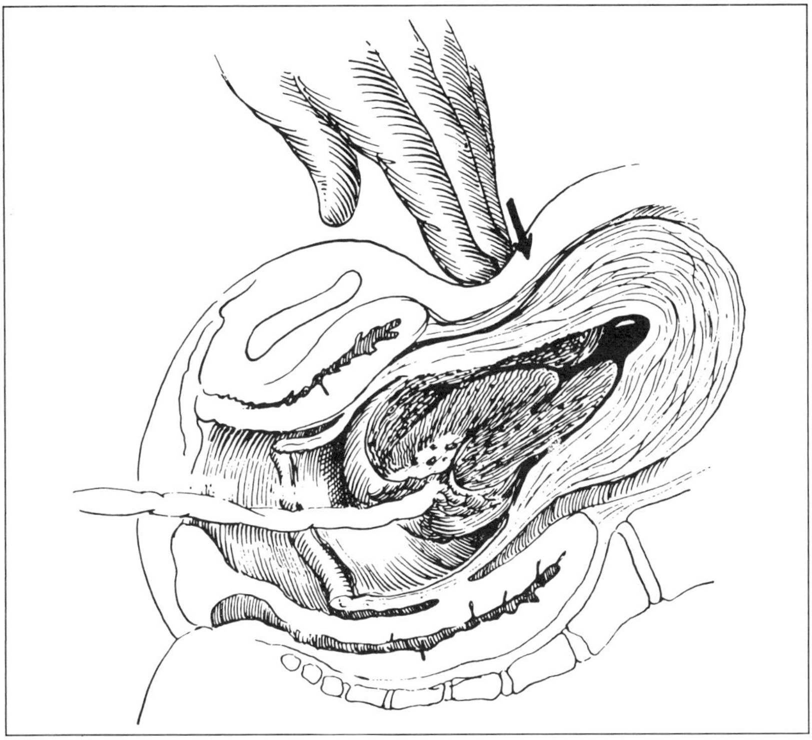

Fig. 27-13. Brandt-Andrews delivery of the placenta. After the fundus is firm, moderate tension is exerted on the umbilical cord while the other hand "shears off" the placenta from the uterine wall by upward kneading pressure on the anterior uterine wall. (From J. R. Wilson, *Atlas of Obstetric Technic* [2nd ed.]. St. Louis: Mosby, 1969. Daisy Stilwell, medical illustrator.)

a. **Procedure.** One hand should grasp the fundus and hold it downward firmly. Care should be taken by physicians to adequately protect themselves with an extra glove and arm cover. With the other hand, reach into the uterine cavity and gently peel off the placenta in a circumferential fashion until separation is complete. The placenta can now be removed. Vigorous fundal massage will minimize subsequent bleeding.

3. **Examination of the placenta.** The placenta should be examined for missing cotyledons or other evidence of undelivered remnants. The membranes should be inspected for vessels that run blindly to an edge, suggesting a succenturiate lobe that may not have been removed. The cut end of the cord should be examined for the presence of two arteries and a vein. The absence of one umbilical artery may suggest a congenital anomaly in the newborn. When abnormalities of the placenta are suspected, pathologic evaluation is warranted.

C. **Active prophylaxis against postpartum atony.** Although the fundus usually contracts well after delivery, this is not always the case. A poorly contracted uterus can lead to rapid and severe blood loss. Therefore, it is wise to take active measures to avoid excessive blood loss caused by postpartum uterine atony. **Gentle but firm external fundal massage should always be part of postpartum management.** It usually is wise to give an oxytocic agent either intramuscularly with the delivery of the anterior shoulder (10 units oxytocin) or in an intravenous drip following the delivery of the placenta (20 units in 1000 ml of 5% dextrose in water at 100 drops/minute). The latter is preferable because it allows for a more controlled third stage. Oxytocin can cause marked hypotension if administered as an intravenous bolus. Occasionally, oxytocin is insufficient. Methylergonovine maleate (Methergine), 0.2 mg IM, often produces sufficient uterine contractility to correct atony. However, methylergonovine is contraindicated in patients who are hypertensive (hypertension may be aggravated) and should be avoided as well in patients who are hypotensive (further peripheral vasoconstriction in a patient in hypovolemic shock may result in digit loss secondary to vascular insufficiency). If bleeding persists despite such active prophylaxis, 250 μg of 15-methyl prostaglandin is indicated, and appropriate treatment must be continued as discussed in Chap. 20.

D. Repair of lacerations and episiotomy

1. **Lacerations of the birth canal.** After delivery of the placenta, the physician should inspect the birth canal for lacerations. The vaginal sidewalls and fornices should be palpated and inspected. Lacerations involving the periurethral tissues can be missed unless the labia minora are separated. Lacerations usually are linear and cephalad and may be repaired in an interrupted or continuous fashion. By placing the palm of one hand into the vagina as a retractor, the cervix can be exposed. The anterior lip of the cervix should be examined and elevated to allow visualization of the entire cervix.
2. **The episiotomy.** The episiotomy is repaired with 2-0 or 3-0 absorbable suture material. Interrupted sutures are required to approximate the deep tissues of the perineal body. Running interlocking sutures are used to repair the vaginal mucosa, with care being taken to include its apex. The perineum is reapproximated with subcutaneous and subcuticular running sutures.
3. **A laceration extending through the anal sphincter** (third-degree) should be repaired with interrupted sutures, incorporating the fascia of the muscle for strength. When the rectal mucosa is involved (fourth-degree), this structure should be reapproximated in two layers with intestinal suture, and care should be taken to avoid including suture material in the luminal surface of the intact mucosa. The remainder of the repair is routine.

IV. Assisted delivery. When it is not possible to achieve spontaneous vaginal delivery, then operative delivery is required. This may be either by cesarean section or an instrumented vaginal delivery. The latter entails the use of either forceps or a vacuum extractor. This is discussed in detail in Chap. 30.

References

1. Bloom, S. L., et al. Effects of paracervical blocks on the fetus during labor: A prospective study with the use of direct fetal monitoring. *Am. J. Obstet. Gynecol.* 114:218, 1972.
2. Chautigan, R. C., and Osthemer, G. W. Effect of maternally administered drugs on the fetus and newborn. *Adv. Perinat. Med.* 5:181–242, 1986.
3. Clark, R. B. Regional anesthesia. *Obstet. Gynecol. Annu.* 13:131, 1984.
4. Clark, S. Rupture of the scarred uterus. *Obstet. Gynecol. Clin. North Am.* 15:737–744, 1988.
5. Diaz, A. G., et al. Vertical position during the first stage of the course of labor and neonatal outcome. *Eur. J. Obstet. Gynecol. Reprod. Biol.* 11:1, 1980.
6. Evans, J. M., Rosen, J., and Hoffman, M. Apparatus for patient-controlled administration of IV narcotics during labour. *Lancet* 1:17–18, 1976.
7. Green, J. S. Factors associated with rectal injury in spontaneous deliveries. *Obstet. Gynecol.* 73(1):732–733, 1989.
8. Fishburne, J. I. Current concepts concerning the use of analgesia and anesthesia during labor and delivery. *Adv. Clin. Obstet. Gynecol.* 23:68–88, 1984.
9. Fishburne, J. I. Systematic analgesia during labor: Symposium on obstetric anesthesia and analgesia. *Clin. Perinatol.* 9:29–53, 1982.
10. Flam, B. L., et al. Vaginal delivery following cesarean section: Use of oxytocin

augmentation and epidural anesthesia with internal tocodynamic and internal fetal monitors. *Am. J. Obstet. Gynecol.* 148:759, 1984.
11. Goodlin, R. C. On protection of the maternal perineum during birth. *Obstet. Gynecol.* 62:393, 1983.
12. Haukkamaa, M., et al. The monitoring of labor by telemetry. *J. Perinat. Med.* 10:17, 1982.
13. Hemmink, E., and Saarikoski, S. Ambulation and delayed amniotomy in the first stage of labor. *Eur. J. Obstet. Gynecol. Reprod. Biol.* 15:129, 1983.
14. Hon, E. H., and Petrie, R. H. Clinical value of FHR monitoring. *Clin. Obstet. Gynecol.* 18:21, 1975.
15. Ingemarsson, E., Ingemarsson, I., and Svenningson, H. W. Impact of routine fetal monitoring during labor and fetal outcome with long-term follow-up. *Am. J. Obstet. Gynecol.* 141:29, 1981.
16. Lavin, J. P., et al. Vaginal delivery in patients with a prior cesarean section. *Obstet. Gynecol.* 59:135, 1982.
17. Martin, J., Morrison, J., and Wiser, W. Vaginal birth after cesarean section. The demise of routine repeat abdominal delivery. *Obstet. Gynecol. Clin.* 15:719–736, 1988.
18. Marttila, M., et al. Maternal half-sitting position in the second stage of labor. *J. Perinat. Med.* 11:286, 1983.
19. McKay, S., and Mahan, C. S. How worthwhile are membrane stripping and amniotomy? *Contemp. Obstet. Gynecol.* 26:173, 1983.
20. Meier, P. R., and Porreco, R. P. Trial of labor following cesarean section: A two-year experience. *Am. J. Obstet. Gynecol.* 144:671, 1982.
21. Milner, R. D. G. Fetal Fat and Glucose Metabolism in Fetal Physiology and Medicine. In R. W. Beard and P. W. Nathaniels (eds.), *The Basis of Perinatology.* New York: Dekker, 1984. P. 153.
22. Morishima, H. O., Covino, B. G., and Yell, M. Bradicardia in the fetal baboon following paracervical block anaesthesia. *Am. J. Obstet. Gynecol.* 140:775, 1981.
23. Mueller-Heubach, E., et al. Effects of electronic fetal heart rate monitoring on perinatal outcome and obstetric practices. *Am. J. Obstet. Gynecol.* 137:758, 1980.
24. Nesheim, B. L. Which local anesthetic is best suited for paracervical blocks. *Acta Obstet. Gynecol. Scand.* 12:261, 1983.
25. Nieburg, P., and Gross, S. J. Cerebrospinal fluid leak in a neonate associated with fetal scalp electrode monitoring. *Am. J. Obstet. Gynecol.* 147:839, 1983.
26. Overturf, G. D., and Balfour, G. Osteomyelitis and sepsis: Severe complications of fetal monitoring. *Pediatrics* 155:244, 1975.
27. Rayburn, W. R., et al. IV meperidine during labor: A randomized comparison between nursing and patient-controlled administration. *Obstet. Gynecol.* 74:702–706, 1974.
28. Scott, J. Obstetric analgesia. *Am. J. Obstet. Gynecol.* 106:959–978, 1970.
29. Stewart, P., et al. Spontaneous labour: When should the membranes be ruptured? *Br. J. Obstet. Gynaecol.* 89:39, 1982.
30. Thacker, S. B., and Banta, H. D. Benefits and risks of episiotomy: An interpretive review of the English language literature, 1860–1980. *Obstet. Gynecol. Surv.* 38:322, 1983.
31. Thadepalli, H., et al. Gonococcal sepsis secondary to fetal monitoring. *Am. J. Obstet. Gynecol.* 126:510, 1976.
32. Wagener, M. M., et al. Septic dermatitis of the neonatal scalp and maternal endomyometritis with internal fetal monitoring. *Pediatrics* 74:81, 1984.
33. Wood, C., et al. A controlled trial of fetal heart rate monitoring in a low-risk obstetric population. *Am. J. Obstet. Gynecol.* 141:527, 1981.

28 Preterm Labor

Mark C. Williams

Preterm labor (PTL) is an obstetric complication with a high associated neonatal morbidity rate, especially if not promptly diagnosed and treated. To reduce the impact of PTL, many interventions and strategies have been attempted. These include improved methods of **identifying patients at risk** for PTL, **tocolytic therapy** (medications to stop uterine contractions), and therapy directed toward **reducing subsequent neonatal morbidity** if tocolytic therapy proves ineffective.

I. **Natural history. Preterm labor** is currently defined as labor occurring prior to the completion of 37 gestational weeks from the first day of the last menses. Previously, **preterm birth** had been used to describe any delivery of an infant weighing less than 2500 gm. The latter definition is no longer used, as it falsely includes growth-retarded infants of more than 37 weeks' gestation.

PTL continues to be a significant obstetric problem both in the United States and worldwide. In the United States, the frequency of delivery prior to 37 weeks among whites is approximately 7%; that of American blacks is 15%. Although the preterm birth rate among blacks has decreased by 15–20% over the past 25 years, the mean gestational age of preterm birth has not. Despite advances in neonatal care and in the medical treatment of PTL, premature birth due to PTL still accounts for 20–30% of neonatal mortality. Most of these deaths occur in infants born prior to 32 weeks' gestation, as survival currently approaches 100% in infants born at later gestations.

A. **Factors associated with PTL**

1. Maternal in utero exposure to diethylstilbestrol
2. Increased uterine volume, as in multiple gestation and polyhydramnios
3. Infection
4. Low pre-pregnancy maternal weight
5. Maternal age of less than 18 or more than 40 years
6. Number of second-trimester pregnancy terminations
7. Previous preterm delivery
8. Sociocultural factors such as low socioeconomic status
9. Smoking
10. Uterine anomalies

The essential problem with PTL is that despite multiple approaches, little progress has been made toward significantly reducing its occurrence, much less eliminating it.

B. **Attempts have been made to develop scoring systems to identify women at risk of PTL** [6]. These systems are able to predict PTL in some, but not all, populations.

C. Although **tocolytic medications** have proved effective at stopping **active** preterm labor, they have not succeeded in prolonging pregnancies sufficiently to lower the rate of preterm birth. Recent attempts to decrease PTL by **home monitoring** of uterine contractile patterns in patients thought to be at high risk for PTL have been promising but remain controversial.

D. It is important to realize that PTL is not actually a disease entity, but rather the final common diagnosis arrived at by one of many pathways. It would be simplistic to believe that any single diagnostic or therapeutic approach would be sufficient to prevent or minimize PTL.

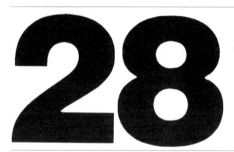

II. **Physiology.** The precise mechanism of labor initiation in humans is uncertain, but smooth muscle contractile physiology has been found applicable to PTL. This knowledge has provided a scientific basis for investigating tocolysis of labor.

A wide variety of hormones and compounds influence **myometrial contractility** including oxytocin, prostaglandins, and steroid hormones (such as estrogen and progesterone), magnesium sulfate ($MgSO_4$), and medications such as calcium channel blockers and beta-sympathomimetics. Myometrial contractions can be caused by alterations in cell membrane electrical potential, or by alterations in intracellular Ca^{+2} concentration, usually by intracellular adenylcyclase activation. At Ca^{+2} concentrations greater than 10^{-7}M, cellular contractions are possible. The principal mechanisms are discussed here.

A. Adenylcyclase activation. Myometrial cellular contraction results from the union of actin and phosphorylated myosin. It requires intracellular Ca^{+2} concentrations of greater than 10^{-7}M. Several cellular subsystems affect the activation (phosphorylation) of myosin. Figure 28-1 demonstrates the binding of compounds to specific cell membrane receptors that lead to activation of the cell membrane enzyme complex.

Within the myocyte, cyclic-AMP (cAMP) activates protein kinase A (Fig. 28-2). Protein kinase A then phosphorylates certain membrane proteins (ultimately causing decreased intracellular Ca^{+2}), and phosphorylates myosin light-chain kinase (MLCK). After phosphorylation, MLCK-P has decreased affinity for calmodulin. As the calmodulin-MLCK interaction is necessary for myometrial contraction, uterine contractility is decreased.

B. Cellular ionic alterations. Intracellular concentrations of ions such as Na^+, K^+, and Ca^{+2} also affect myometrial contractility. Cellular contraction involves influx of Na^+ and the exit of K^+. Inflow of Ca^{+2} into the cell can be influenced by alterations in cell membrane electrical potential (voltage-dependent channels), as well as by systems not influenced by electrical potential (voltage-independent channels). As previously noted, decreased intracellular Ca^{+2} below a certain level will diminish uterine contractility. Medications such as $MgSO_4$ may alter membrane potential and favor the exit of Ca^{+2} from the cell; calcium channel blockers may decrease the conductivity of Ca^{+2} into the cell.

C. Oxytocin. The precise relation between oxytocin and labor is unclear. Oxytocin is thought to bind with a specific cell membrane receptor, which then activates processes mediated by prostaglandins, which go on to produce cellular contractions.

D. Prostaglandins. Prostaglandins are ubiquitous, biologically active compounds that have significant effects on uterine contractility. Certain prostaglandins (such as $PGF_{2\alpha}$ and PGE_2 stimulate uterine contractions, whereas others (such as PGI_2)

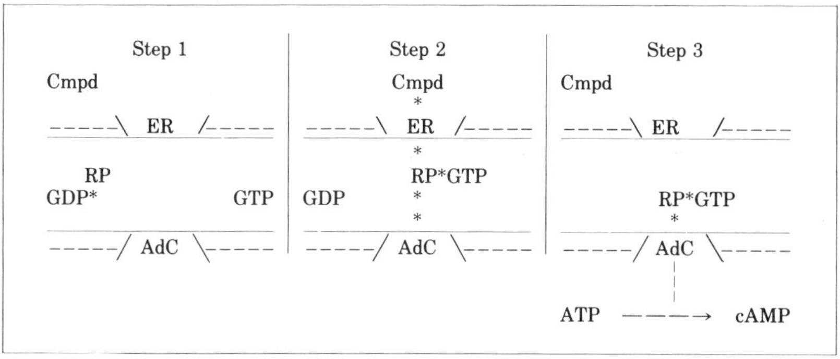

Fig. 28-1. Adenylcyclase activation in the myocyte. (AdC = membrane-bound adenylcyclase; ER = external cellular receptor for Cmpd; GDP = guanosine diphosphate; GTP = guanosine triphosphate; Cmpd = hormone [e.g., beta-sympathomimetic]; RP = regulatory protein; * = complex.)

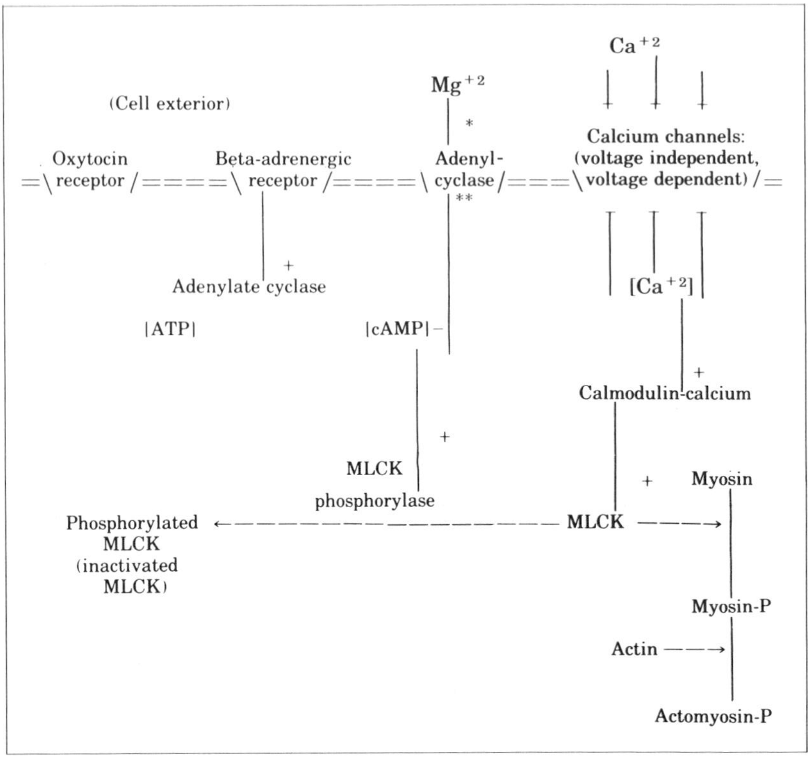

Fig. 28-2. Mediators of uterine contraction. (* = extracellular Mg^{+2} may either stimulate membrane-bound adenylcyclase to increase intracellular [cAMP], or activate membrane Ca^{+2}-dependent adenylcyclase to promote egress of intracellular Ca^{+2} ions; ** = stimulation of Na-K ATPase by elevated intracellular [cAMP] causes exchange of intracellular Na^{+} for extracellular K^{+}, and causes electrical changes favoring exit of Ca^{+2} from the cell; MLCK = myosin light-chain kinase.)

promote uterine relaxation. Activation of certain extracellular membrane receptors may lead to activation of processes resulting in intracellular prostaglandin release.

1. **Prostaglandin synthetase inhibitors** are known to be potent inhibitors of uterine contractility, both in vitro and in vivo. By inhibiting cyclooxygenase, which is necessary for conversion of arachidonic acid into prostaglandin derivatives, they block intracellular contractile processes.

III. Diagnosis. The diagnosis of PTL is often difficult. Studies on PTL frequently document 40–60% efficacy for placebo therapy. Many of these "placebo successes" may represent falsely diagnosed PTL. In its early stages, PTL is not easily differentiated from gastroenteritis, Braxton Hicks ("false labor") contractions, or other conditions causing mild abdominal discomfort. If patients are properly educated or monitored for abnormal uterine activity, it is possible to document increased uterine contractions and initiate tocolytic therapy or treat the underlying condition (such as a urinary tract infection) causing the increase in uterine contractions.

It is important to note that uterine contractions are suggestive, but **not diagnostic,** for PTL. The diagnosis is made from the combined findings of uterine contractions

and cervical change. The exact predictive significance of contractions without cervical changes is unclear.

A. **Symptoms** suggestive of PTL include persistent lower abdominal cramping or discomfort occurring with some regularity, possibly every 15 minutes or less. In many cases, the patients may note a subjective increase in the intensity of lower abdominal cramps, which calls their attention to the condition.

   Patients noting such symptoms after 19–20 weeks of gestation should be observed for labor. They should be monitored for uterine contractions with an external uterine contraction monitor. Prior to 25 weeks' gestation, it is often difficult to monitor the fetal heart rate reliably. As delivery at this age is almost uniformly fatal, such heart rate monitoring is not necessary.

B. **History and examination**

   1. **The patient's history** should be reviewed and the patient thoroughly evaluated for other causes of lower abdominal pain.
   2. A **sterile speculum exam** of the vagina should then be performed. During this exam, cervical cultures for group B streptococcus, *Chlamydia,* and *Neisseria gonorrhoeae* can be collected. The vagina should also be assessed for evidence of leakage of amniotic fluid. If **premature rupture of membranes** is suspected, no pelvic exam should be performed until that diagnosis has been established or excluded (see Chap. 29). Further, if the history is suggestive of **placenta previa,** this diagnosis should be excluded by ultrasound evaluation of the uterus prior to manual vaginal examination.
   3. In patients not thought to have premature rupture of membranes or placenta previa, a **manual pelvic exam** should be performed. This exam should include a careful digital evaluation of the **internal** cervical os. Factors to be assessed include cervical dilation; effacement; consistency; fetal position within the vagina (i.e., anterior versus posterior); and fetal station within the pelvis. The findings of this exam should be carefully documented. This exam should then be repeated in 30–60 minutes. If PTL appears likely, it is advisable to place an intravenous line and begin hydration with normal saline or Ringer's lactate. If changes are noted to have occurred between two exams conducted within 12–24 hours of each other, the diagnosis of PTL is confirmed and therapy should be initiated.
   4. **A presumptive diagnosis of PTL** can be made in certain circumstances without documenting cervical change. Patients presenting with evidence of uterine contractions and advanced cervical dilation (i.e., dilation of the internal os greater than 2 cm or cervical effacement of > 80%), especially at less than 32 weeks' gestation, should be considered for immediate tocolytic therapy. In such cases, the fetal risks of preterm birth outweigh those of tocolytic therapy.

IV. Management

A. **General considerations.** After the diagnosis of PTL has been confirmed, appropriate therapy should be instituted. Management considerations include the choice of an appropriate tocolytic agent, whether to initiate fetal pulmonary maturation therapy, and the possible use of vitamin K to lessen the possibility of intraventricular hemorrhage (IVH). Additionally, Morales and colleagues [27] have recently reported that empiric antibiotic therapy may improve the efficacy of tocolytic therapy.

B. **Tocolytic therapy.** A number of medications are used to inhibit the contractions of PTL. These include beta-sympathomimetic agents, $MgSO_4$, prostaglandin synthetase inhibitors, and calcium channel blockers. Of all the medications available, only the beta-sympathomimetic agent **ritodrine** (Yutopar) currently has FDA approval for labor tocolysis. Nevertheless, there is extensive favorable clinical experience with **$MgSO_4$** and **terbutaline.** Both are frequently used in the treatment of PTL in the United States. Other agents such as indomethacin (Indocin) and nifedipine (Procardia) have also occasionally been used, but experience with them is limited, and they are not as yet widely used in obstetrics.

   Tocolysis is best accomplished by the use of a single tocolytic agent at doses adequate to either halt or significantly reduce uterine contractility. The most commonly used agents for initial, single-drug treatment are beta-sympathomimetics such as ritodrine (Yutopar) or terbutaline, and $MgSO_4$ [2, 9, 19, 39]. If the initial agent is unable to provide adequate tocolysis at maximum dose, it is generally advisable to attempt therapy with another agent, preferably one that acts by a different mechanism. In 10–20% of cases, the second agent will prove effective.

1. **Beta-sympathomimetics.** The beta-sympathomimetic agents ritodrine (Yutopar), terbutaline (Brethine), hexoprenaline, isoxsuprine, and salbutamol have been used for tocolysis. In the United States, although ritodrine is the only medication with an FDA-approved indication for tocolysis of labor, terbutaline is also frequently used. These agents stimulate uterine cell membranes beta-adrenergic receptors, resulting in increased intracellular concentrations of cAMP. cAMP then causes a decrease in intracellular Ca^{+2} concentration and decreases the uterine contractility.
   a. **Common side effects** of beta-sympathomimetic therapy (due to stimulation of cardiac beta-2-receptors) include tachycardia, shortness of breath, chest pain, and altered glucose and potassium homeostasis (hyperglycemia and hypokalemia). As a relatively selective beta-2-agonist, ritodrine offers some theoretic advantage, but its use is still often associated with these side effects.
   b. **Contraindications.** Beta-sympathomimetic therapy is contraindicated in those with significant history of ischemic cardiac disease, or with a cardiac condition likely to be aggravated by tachycardia. Patients with hyperthyroidism or hypertension should not receive beta-sympathomimetic agents. Blood glucose levels may be elevated by beta-sympathomimetics. Diabetes may be aggravated by beta-sympathomimetic therapy, with subsequent hyperglycemia. If used in diabetes, blood sugars should be followed closely, and insulin doses may need to be increased.
   c. **Dosage and route of administration.** Tocolysis with beta-sympathomimetic agents has been associated with adult respiratory distress syndrome (ARDS) [3, 35]. This association may be more closely related to maternal infection than tocolysis [18]. Nevertheless, it is recommended that fluid intake be carefully restricted to approximately 100 ml/hour (total fluids). Hankins [16] has also suggested that infusions of fluids with a low salt content may help prevent ARDS.
      (1) **Ritodrine** is available in oral and intravenous forms. For treatment of acute PTL the intravenous infusion is recommended.
         (a) **Intravenous.** The initial infusion rate should be 50–100 μg/minute of ritodrine in 5% dextrose in water, with incremental increases of 50 μg/minute q15–30min until adequate tocolysis is achieved. The maximum dose is 350 μg/minute. The infusion rate may need to be decreased if the patient experiences side effects. If **chest pain** develops, the medication should be temporarily discontinued and a 12-lead electrocardiogram tracing obtained. If the patient's pulse exceeds 130, the dose should be decreased. Continue the medication for 12–24 hours of uterine quiescence.
         (b) **Oral.** The usual dose of ritodrine is 10 mg PO q2h for the initial 24 hours of oral therapy, followed by 10–20 mg PO q4–6h.
      (2) **Terbutaline** has been found effective as a tocolytic in acute preterm labor by Stubblefield and Heyl [39]. It is also commonly used as prophylactic tocolysis to prevent recurrent PTL, usually given as an oral medication. (**Note:** Although intravenous administration of terbutaline has also been used to treat PTL, intravenous ritodrine is the preferred intravenous beta-sympathomimetic tocolytic at this time.) Recently, Lam and colleagues [21] have advocated its administration by subcutaneous pump. Administration information for subcutaneous (injection) and oral routes are provided below.
         (a) **Subcutaneous.** SC injection of 0.25 mg initially, and hourly until adequate tocolysis is achieved, followed by transfer to oral terbutaline therapy.
         (b) **Oral.** A dose of 2.5–5.0 mg PO q4–6h, with doses deferred if maternal

pulse is greater than 130. Some experts recommend titrating the oral dose to a maternal pulse 20–25% greater than the nontreated maternal resting pulse. It is not known whether this method is more efficacious than regular scheduled dosing.

2. Magnesium sulfate

a. Mechanism. The precise physiologic mechanism for the tocolytic effect of $MgSO_4$ is not known with certainty. It is known to affect excitation, excitation-contraction propagation, and contraction of the muscle cell. The final pathway for all these processes is a decrease in intracellular Ca^{+2} ion concentration, which decreases the ability of the cell to phosphorylate myosin light chains during cellular contractions.

b. Dosage and administration

(1) Contraindications and cautions. $MgSO_4$ therapy is contraindicated in patients with heart block, myasthenia gravis, or significant myocardial disease. It should be used with care in patients with decreased renal function, as it is primarily cleared by renal excretion. $MgSO_4$ therapy sometimes is associated with respiratory depression. The patient's respiratory status should be carefully monitored when receiving other medications with similar effects, such as narcotic analgesics or other sedative-hypnotic agents.

(2) For **tocolysis** of acute PTL, $MgSO_4$ is usually administered by an IV bolus of 4–6 gm in 100 ml of normal saline, given over 30–45 minutes. The loading dose is followed by IV infusions of 2–4 gm/hour, titrated as necessary to eradicate (or significantly diminish) uterine contractions. Mild contractions may persist after cervical change has been halted. In such cases, it is often best to examine the patient regularly and document progression of cervical change before increasing the dose or changing to another agent.

(3) Therapeutic serum levels. Serum levels of 5.5–7.5 mg/dl are usually necessary to inhibit labor [19]. These levels are most often achieved by initial infusion rates of 3 or 4 gm/hour. It is also possible to monitor the patient for inadvertent overdosage by evaluating deep tendon reflexes, as these are usually diminished at serum magnesium levels of 7–10 mg/dl. Ultimately, respiratory depression occurs with serum levels greater than 12 mg/dl.

(4) Contractions refractory to therapy. If uterine contractions are refractory to therapy, or if high doses of $MgSO_4$ are necessary, it is important to evaluate serum Mg^{+2} levels. Patients with rapid clearance of Mg^{+2} may benefit from larger doses of $MgSO_4$, whereas patients with therapeutic levels may require alternate therapy or the addition of a second agent (see sec. **IV.B.3,4** and sec. **V**).

(5) Decreased renal function. Patients with decreased renal function require significantly lower doses and should have serum Mg^{+2} levels carefully monitored.

c. Complications. In comparison with the other major therapeutic alternative currently available for the tocolysis of preterm labor (beta-sympathomimetic agents), $MgSO_4$ therapy is generally well tolerated. Common side effects include a warm or flushed feeling as therapy is initiated, palpitations, headache, and oral dryness. Diplopia and difficulty focusing the eyes also sometimes occur.

(1) Inadvertent overdosage of $MgSO_4$ is observed fairly often. This can lead to severe depression of voluntary musculature and the respiratory system. Initial loading doses should be carefully checked. If excessive magnesium is administered, intravenous administration (slow push) of calcium gluconate is helpful. The patient's respirations should then be supported until respiratory depression has resolved.

3. Prostaglandin synthetase inhibitors. Prostaglandin synthetase inhibitors have been shown to be effective tocolytics [28, 32]. Their use in pregnancy sometimes causes decreased amniotic fluid volume, which usually resolves within one to two days of discontinuation of the medication. A small number of infants may also develop narrowing of the ductus arteriosus in utero [26]. This effect was found to appear at gestational ages prior to 32 weeks' gestation and resolved within 24 hours of discontinuation of indomethacin therapy.

a. **Selection.** At this time, prostaglandin synthetase inhibitors are best held as alternate tocolytic agents. Their use is best reserved for occasions when more commonly used agents are either contraindicated or have failed. They should not be used for tocolysis of labor after 32 weeks of gestation. Prior to starting therapy, the patient should be informed of the small possibility of premature closure of the fetal ductus arteriosus and alternate therapy discussed.

b. **Contraindications.** Prostaglandin synthetase inhibitors are contraindicated in patients with a history of salicylate allergy, drug-associated asthma, coagulation abnormalities, or significantly impaired hepatic or renal function. They are relatively contraindicated with a prior history of peptic ulcer disease.

c. **Indomethacin** is well absorbed after oral or rectal administration and is strongly protein bound. Rectal administration is preferred in PTL, as gastric emptying may be delayed. An initial dose of 100 mg should be given per rectum, followed by 25 mg q6h for a maximum of 48 hours of therapy. Continuous electronic fetal monitoring is advised, as it is extremely difficult to visualize the fetal ductus. Amniotic fluid volumes should be evaluated daily and therapy discontinued if oligohydramnios appears to be developing.

d. **Complications.** Prostaglandin synthetase inhibitors are generally well tolerated. Although their inhibition of cyclooxygenase appears to be rapidly reversible in vivo, they have occasionally been associated with postpartum hemorrhage [38].

4. **Calcium channel blockers** affect smooth muscle contractility by altering the passage of the Ca^{+2} ion into the cell. Their physiologic properties have allowed their use in such disparate conditions as malignant hypertension, migraine headache disorder, and certain cardiac dysrhythmias. These generally beneficial properties would seem to allow calcium channel blockers to be used in many patients where traditional agents such as beta-sympathomimetics are contraindicated. Offsetting these favorable properties are the findings of fetal acidosis and intrauterine demise noted when they have been used in sheep and Rhesus monkeys. Research now indicates that animal experimentation may not correlate directly with human experience. Some studies of calcium channel blockers in human pregnancies affected by hypertension [40] and PTL [37] have been more favorable. A prospectively randomized study comparing nifedipine (Procardia) with ritodrine found comparable tocolytic efficacy [9] and no detrimental effects in human fetuses exposed to nifedipine [10, 11, 12]. If their use is elected, an initial dose of 10 mg should be administered. The sublingual route is preferred. Up to three more initial doses of 10 mg should be given at 15- to 20-minute intervals, until contractions are resolved. The medication should then be continued at 10 mg q6h for several days.

V. **Additional therapeutic considerations: It is important to understand that the preterm delivery rate in Western countries has not been reduced despite the widespread use of multiple tocolytic agents.** The reasons remain unclear but are likely to be related to the difficulty of predicting and diagnosing preterm labor and preterm delivery risk factors.

A. **Alternate single-agent tocolysis.** Beta-sympathomimetics and $MgSO_4$ are most commonly used for initial therapy. If both have been tried individually, and significant uterine contractions remain, alternate therapy may be considered. Both prostaglandin synthetase inhibitors [8, 15, 20, 28, 32] and calcium channel blocking agents [9, 10, 37, 40] have been reported as potentially efficacious, although neither group has been evaluated sufficiently to consider them "first line" therapy. Neither medicine has been approved for this use by the FDA.

B. **Multiple-agent tocolysis.** Although the concurrent use of multiple tocolytic medications is generally ill-advised, under certain circumstances it may be considered [13, 15, 17, 20, 34]. It should be understood that such treatment is of a "heroic" nature and is **only justified under the most extreme conditions.** Such circumstances might include PTL prior to 28–30 weeks' gestation with cervical dilatation greater than 2–3 cm that is not responsive to initial single-agent therapy. In such circumstances, even two days of successful tocolysis may allow sufficient time for fetal lung–maturing therapy to have an effect. If multiple-agent tocolysis is attempted, the patient should be informed of the circumstances requiring this therapy, as well as other options available to her. Meticulous fluid restriction should be used to reduce the risk of pulmonary edema and ARDS.

In cases of PTL refractory to tocolysis, underlying infection is often present. **If chorioamnionitis appears likely, tocolysis is contraindicated.** Other infections, such as pyelonephritis, do not preclude tocolysis, but may predispose the patient to ARDS [7]. Scrupulous fluid restriction (total oral and intravenous < approximately 100 ml/hour) is mandatory. If corticosteroids are administered, a leukocytosis to approximately 30,000 cells/μL with increased immature cells may be present for 24–36 hours. White blood cell count elevations in excess of this often precede overt infection and suggest careful clinical evaluation of the patient.

1. **The optimal combination of medications for dual tocolytic therapy is not known.** The addition of indomethacin to either $MgSO_4$ or ritodrine [15, 20] may be the most efficacious combination. Combination therapy with ritodrine and $MgSO_4$ has also been reported [17, 34] but may not add significantly to therapeutic efficacy [13]. In view of current concerns regarding calcium channel blockers and their use in pregnancy, they should not be used in combination with other agents. As experience with calcium channel blockers becomes more widely available, this recommendation may be subject to change.
2. It is unlikely that addition of a third therapeutic agent to a tocolytic regimen would contribute significantly to its efficacy. **"Triple" tocolysis is not recommended.**

C. Adult respiratory distress syndrome. Tocolysis of PTL is frequently associated with maternal ARDS. Although it was first thought to be a complication of corticosteroid therapy for fetal pulmonary maturation, subsequent research indicates that latent infection may be the actual cause [7, 18]. In order to avoid ARDS, patients should be carefully fluid restricted [3]. Total (intravenous and oral) fluid intake should be restricted to 100–125 ml/hour and 2.0–2.5 liters/day. Intravenous infusions of 5% dextrose are less likely to result in fluid retention during tocolysis [18]. For tocolysis, solutions of 5% dextrose or 0.25 normal saline are strongly recommended [16].

D. Accelerating fetal lung maturity

1. **Corticosteroid therapy.** During experimentation with corticosteroid medications in sheep, Liggins [22] found that fetal lambs receiving this medication had accelerated maturation of the pulmonary tissues. Subsequent experimentation has documented this effect in humans.

   The mechanism for reduced respiratory distress syndrome in neonates receiving in utero corticosteroid therapy is unclear. It is possible that corticosteroids cause induction in enzyme systems responsible for pulmonary surfactant, or that this therapy causes the release of surfactant stored in type II pneumatocytes.

   Liggins [22] and the Perinatal Collaborative Group [4] provided convincing evidence that corticosteroid therapy was of significant benefit for fetuses delivered between 30 and 34 weeks of gestation. Since then, numerous other investigators have evaluated other gestational-age-range groups and derived similar conclusions. Black female infants have shown the largest decrease in neonatal respiratory distress syndrome, whereas white male infants have shown much less improvement. Subsequent research has expanded the use of corticosteroids to fetuses of 25–26 weeks' gestation. No effect has ever been documented for gestations of more than 34 weeks.

   Both **betamethasone** (24-mg total dose, given as 12 mg twice at 12- or 24-hour intervals) and **dexamethasone** (20-mg total dose, given as 5-mg doses at 6-hour intervals) are commonly employed. Therapy must be initiated 24–48 hours before delivery for the desired effect.
2. **Alternate therapies.** The process of fetal pulmonary development is undoubt-

edly quite complex. Hormones such as thyroxine and prolactin have been shown to have important effects on the development of other physiologic systems, and animal studies indicate that thyroxine may play an important role in pulmonary development. Morales and colleagues [30] found that administration of thyroxine-releasing hormone and betamethasone to patients at risk of preterm delivery decreased neonatal pulmonary complications. The value of thyroxine-releasing hormone in promoting fetal lung maturity is currently being assessed by a multicenter, national collaborative group.

Although such alternate therapies are considered experimental now, they may eventually become accepted therapy in cases at high risk of preterm delivery.

E. **Antibiotic therapy. Infection** is thought to play a significant role in many cases of PTL. The use of antibiotics to prevent PTL has been evaluated but not found to be of clinical relevance, due to costs of screening and disease prevalence. Alternately, the use of antibiotics as adjuncts to the treatment of PTL has been assessed. McGregor and colleagues [25] and Morales and colleagues [27] have reported that antibiotics favorably influence the efficacy of tocolysis among patients without obvious cause for PTL. Newton and colleagues [31], however, found that combined ampicillin and erythromycin did not improve efficacy of tocolysis. If confirmed by other studies, prophylactic antibiotic therapy may offer a potentially significant advance in the therapy of PTL. If antibiotic prophylactic therapy is elected, ampicillin (2 gm IV q6h) should be initiated after cervical cultures have been obtained. It should be continued until cultures are negative at 48 hours, and then discontinued. Patients with penicillin allergy should receive an equivalent cephalosporin with adequate coverage for group B streptococcus.

F. **Neonatal intraventricular hemorrhage.** Infants born prior to 32–34 weeks' gestation are at increased risk of IVH. Pomerance and colleagues [36] and Morales and colleagues [29] have reported that maternal administration of large doses of vitamin K prior to delivery may decrease neonatal IVH. Their observations are considered somewhat controversial but may eventually be accepted. If high rates of IVH are found at a given institution, prophylactic maternal vitamin K therapy (10 mg IM) should be considered.

VI. **Maintenance tocolytic therapy.** Tocolysis should be continued at the minimum dosage necessary to adequately minimize uterine contractility for a minimum of 12–24 hours. After this, maintenance tocolytic therapy should be considered. The evidence supporting such treatment is based on work by Creasy and colleagues [5] and others. Creasy found that patients with prior PTL who subsequently received prophylactic oral tocolysis were less frequently readmitted with recurrences of PTL, but **no significant difference in gestational age achieved was noted between the two study groups** (placebo, 36 days prolongation; oral ritodrine, 34 days prolongation). Later investigators have found some prophylactic agents to be superior to others, but they have rarely been compared to placebo. Although prophylactic tocolysis is commonly used, its efficacy or necessity is not universally agreed on.

A. **Prophylactics**

1. **Beta-sympathomimetics** are widely used prophylactic agents. If prophylaxis against recurrent PTL is elected, either ritodrine (at doses of 10–20 mg PO q4–6h) or terbutaline (2.5–5.0 mg PO q4–6h) may be considered. These agents occasionally cause significant maternal tachycardia. The patient should be instructed to obtain her pulse prior to taking the medicine, and to defer administration when it is greater than 115. Terbutaline has been found to induce glucose intolerance when used in pregnancy [1, 23]. Patients maintained on terbutaline for any significant time should be evaluated with a one-hour 50-gm glucose tolerance test.

   If oral beta-sympathomimetics are not well tolerated, other therapeutic options include oral magnesium gluconate and the subcutaneous terbutaline pump.

2. **Oral magnesium prophylaxis** was compared against oral ritodrine by Martin and colleagues [24]. Magnesium gluconate (at dosages of 1 gm q2–4h) was found of equivalent efficacy to oral ritodrine and had marginally fewer maternal side effects. Long-term magnesium therapy has been found to have potential effects on maternal bone calcium levels. The significance of this observation to prophylactic PTL prophylaxis has not yet been assessed.

3. **Subcutaneous terbutaline pump.** Lam and colleagues [21] have advocated the use of the terbutaline pump for prophylactic tocolysis. Its efficacy is currently under study.

References

1. Angel, J. L., et al. Carbohydrate intolerance in patients receiving oral tocolytics. *Am. J. Obstet. Gynecol.* 159(3):762–766, 1988.
2. Beall, M. H., et al. A comparison of ritodrine, terbutaline, and magnesium sulfate for the suppression of preterm labor. *Am. J. Obstet. Gynecol.* 153:854, 1985.
3. Bloss, J. D., et al. Pulmonary edema as a delayed complication of ritodrine therapy: A case report. *J. Reprod. Med.* 32(6):469–471, 1987.
4. Collaborative Group on Antenatal Steroid Therapy. Effect of antenatal dexamethasone administration on the prevention of respiratory distress syndrome. *Am. J. Obstet. Gynecol.* 141:276, 1981.
5. Creasy, R. K., et al. Oral ritodrine maintenance in the treatment of preterm labor. *Am. J. Obstet. Gynecol.* 137:212, 1980.
6. Creasy, R., Gummer, B., and Liggins, G. System for predicting spontaneous preterm birth. *Obstet. Gynecol.* 55:692, 1980.
7. Cunningham, F. G., et al. Pulmonary injury complicating antepartum pyelonephritis. *Am. J. Obstet. Gynecol.* 156(4):797–807, 1987.
8. Dudley, D. K. L., and Hardie, M. J. Fetal and neonatal effects of indomethacin used as a tocolytic agent. *Am. J. Obstet. Gynecol.* 151:181, 1985.
9. Ferguson, J. E., et al. A comparison of tocolysis with nifedipine or ritodrine: Analysis of efficacy and maternal, fetal, and neonatal outcome. *Am. J. Obstet. Gynecol.* 163(1 Pt. 1):105–111, 1990.
10. Ferguson, J. E., et al. Cardiovascular and metabolic effects associated with nifedipine and ritodrine tocolysis. *Am. J. Obstet. Gynecol.* 161(3):788–795, 1989.
11. Ferguson, J. E., et al. Neonatal bilirubin production after preterm labor tocolysis with nifedipine. *Dev. Pharmacol. Ther.* 12(3):113–117, 1989.
12. Ferguson, J. E., et al. Nifedipine pharmacokinetics during preterm labor tocolysis. *Am. J. Obstet. Gynecol.* 161(6 Pt. 1):1485–1490, 1989.
13. Ferguson, J. E., Hensleigh, P. A., and Kredenster, D. Adjunctive use of magnesium sulfate with ritodrine for preterm labor tocolysis. *Am. J. Obstet. Gynecol.* 148(2):166, 1984.
14. Forman, A., Anderson, K.-E., and Ulmsten, U. Inhibition of myometrial activity by calcium antagonists. *Semin. Perinatol.* 5(3):288–294, 1981.
15. Gamissans, O., et al. A study of indomethacin combined with ritodrine in threatened preterm labor. *Eur. J. Obstet. Gynecol. Reprod. Biol.* 8(3):123–128, 1978.
16. Hankins, G. D. V. Complications of Beta-sympathomimetic Tocolytic Agents. In Clark, S. L., Phelan, J. P., and Cotton, D. B. (eds.), *Critical Care Obstetrics.* Oradell, NJ: Medical Economics Books, 1987. Pp. 192–207.
17. Hatjis, C. G., et al. Efficacy of combined administration of magnesium sulfate and ritodrine in the treatment of preterm labor. *Obstet. Gynecol.* 69:317, 1987.
18. Hatjis, C. G., and Swain, M. Systemic tocolysis for premature labor is associated with an increased incidence of pulmonary edema in the presence of maternal infection. *Am. J. Obstet. Gynecol.* 159(3):723–728, 1988.
19. Hollander, D. I., Nagey, D. A., and Pupkin, M. J. Magnesium sulfate and ritodrine hydrochloride: A randomized comparison. *Am. J. Obstet. Gynecol.* 156:433, 1987.
20. Katz, Z., et al. Treatment of premature labor contractions with combined ritodrine and indomethacine. *Int. J. Gynecol. Obstet.* 21:337–342, 1983.
21. Lam, F., et al. Use of subcutaneous terbutaline pump for long-term tocolysis. *Obstet. Gynecol.* 72:810, 1988.
22. Liggins, G. C. The Prevention of RDS by Maternal Betamethasone Administration. In *Lung Maturation and the Prevention of Hyaline Membrane Disease.*

Report of the 70th Ross Conference on Pediatric Research. Columbus, OH: Ross Laboratories, 1976. P. 97.

23. Main, E. K., Main, D. M., and Gabbe, S. G. Chronic oral terbutaline therapy is associated with maternal glucose intolerance. *Am. J. Obstet. Gynecol.* 157:644, 1987.
24. Martin, R. W., et al. Comparison of oral ritodrine and magnesium gluconate for ambulatory tocolysis. *Am. J. Obstet. Gynecol.* 158:1440–1445, 1988.
25. McGregor, J. A., et al. Adjunctive erythromycin for idiopathic preterm labor: Results of a randomized, double-blinded, placebo-controlled trial. *Am. J. Obstet. Gynecol.* 154(1):98–103, 1986.
26. Moise, F. J., et al. Indomethacin in the treatment of premature labor: Effects on the fetal ductus arteriosus. *N. Engl. J. Med.* 319:327–331, 1988.
27. Morales, W. J., et al. A randomized study of antibiotic therapy in idiopathic preterm labor. *Obstet. Gynecol.* 72(6):829–833, 1988.
28. Morales, W. J., et al. Efficacy and safety of indomethacin versus ritodrine in the management of preterm labor: A randomized study. *Obstet. Gynecol.* 74(4):567–572, 1989.
29. Morales, W. J., et al. The use of antenatal vitamin K in the prevention of early neonatal intraventricular hemorrhage. *Am. J. Obstet. Gynecol.* 159(3):774–779, 1988.
30. Morales, W. J., et al. Fetal lung maturation: The combined use of corticosteroids and thyrotropin-releasing hormone. *Obstet. Gynecol.* 73(1):111–116, 1989.
31. Newton, E. R., Dinsmoor, M. R., and Gibbs, R. S. A randomized, blinded, placebo-controlled trial of antibiotics in idiopathic preterm labor. *Obstet. Gynecol.* 74(4):562–566, 1989.
32. Niebyl, J. R., et al. The inhibition of premature labor with indomethacin. *Am. J. Obstet. Gynecol.* 136:1014, 1980.
33. Niebyl, J. R., and Witter, F. R. Neonatal outcome after indomethacin treatment for preterm labor. *Am. J. Obstet. Gynecol.* 155:747, 1986.
34. Ogburn, P. L., et al. Magnesium sulfate and β-mimetic dual-agent tocolysis in preterm labor after single-agent failure. *J. Reprod. Med.* 30(8):583, 1985.
35. Philipsen, T., et al. Pulmonary edema following ritodrine-saline infusion in preterm labor. *Obstet. Gynecol.* 53:304, 1981.
36. Pomerance, J. J., et al. Maternally administered antenatal vitamin K: Effect on neonatal prothrombin activity, partial thromboplastin time, and intraventricular hemorrhage. *Obstet. Gynecol.* 70:235, 1987.
37. Read, M. D., and Wellby, D. E. The use of calcium antagonist (nifedipine) to suppress preterm labour. *Br. J. Obstet. Gynaecol.* 93:933–937, 1986.
38. Reiss, U., et al. The effect of indomethacin in labour at term. *Int. J. Obstet. Gynaecol.* 14:369, 1976.
39. Stubblefield, P. G., and Heyl, P. S. Treatment of premature labor with subcutaneous terbutaline. *Obstet. Gynecol.* 59(4):457, 1982.
40. Ulmsten, U. Treatment of normotensive and hypertensive patients with preterm labor using oral nifedipine, a calcium antagonist. *Arch. Gynecol.* 236(2):69–72, 1984.

Selected Readings

Ballard, P. Combined hormonal and lung maturation. *Semin. Perinatol.* 8:123, 1981.

Creasy, R. K., and Resnik, R. (eds.). *Maternal-Fetal Medicine: Principles and Practice* (2nd ed.). Philadelphia: Saunders, 1989.

Iams, J. D. (ed.). Preterm labor. *Clin. Obstet. Gynecol.* 31:3, 1988.

Iams, J. D., et al. Does extra-amniotic infection cause preterm labor? Gas-liquid chromatography studies of amniotic fluid in amnionitis, preterm labor, and normal controls. *Obstet. Gynecol.* 70(3 Pt. 1):365–368, 1987.

Joshi, A. K., Chen, C. I., and Turnell, R. W. Prevalence and significance of group B streptococcus in a large obstetric population. *Can. Med. Assoc. J.* 137(3):209–211, 1987.

McDonald, H., Vigneswaran, R., and O'Loughlin, J. A. Group B streptococcal colonization and preterm labour. *Aust. N. Z. J. Obstet. Gynaecol.* 29(3 Pt. 2):291–293, 1989.

Ulmsten, U., Andersson, K. E., and Wingerup, L. Treatment of premature labor with the calcium channel antagonist nifedipine. *Arch. Gynecol.* 229:1–5, 1980.

29 Premature Rupture of Membranes

Mark C. Williams

I. General principles. Premature rupture of membranes (PROM) is defined as rupture of the amniotic membranes prior to the onset of labor, regardless of gestational age. When PROM is noted in a pregnancy prior to 37 completed weeks of gestation, the term **preterm premature rupture of membranes** (PPROM) is usually applied. The time interval between rupture of membranes and the onset of labor is termed the **latency period;** the time interval between rupture and delivery is termed the **interval period.** Depending on precise definitions, PROM has been reported to occur in 3–19% of pregnancies and has been associated with up to 35% of preterm deliveries.

A. Etiology. Various factors have been thought to be associated with PROM:

1. **Infectious etiologies** (amnionitis, cervicitis, and vaginal colonization with group B streptococci and other vaginoses)
2. Conditions associated with **increased uterine volume** (polyhydramnios and multiple gestations)
3. **Coitus**
4. **Fetal anomalies**
5. **Lower socioeconomic status**
6. **Biochemical structural abnormalities** (Ehlers-Danlos syndrome)
7. **Structural alterations** possibly related to dietary deficiencies of ascorbic acid or copper.

Because these factors often coexist, the demonstration of exact causality has proved difficult.

From a patient management standpoint, it is best to consider the condition of PROM prior to term as clinically distinct from PROM after 37 completed weeks of gestation. Term patients with PROM seem to have a distinctly lower rate of infectious complications, and a plausible biochemical mechanism for PROM at term has been identified. As pregnancies approach 38–40 weeks' gestation, a gradual decrement in membrane tensile strength occurs. A similar defect is also likely to explain the increased incidence of PROM noted with the Ehlers-Danlos syndrome. The membrane tensile strength hypothesis has been tested in PPROM, and no generalized changes in membrane strength have been noted. Bacteria have been shown in multiple studies as being capable of enzymatically altering the tensile strength of the amniotic membrane. Much research has been directed at investigating an infectious mechanism for PPROM, and many pieces of evidence indicate infection may have a central role in PPROM.

B. Natural history. The expected latency interval in PROM is inversely correlated with gestational age. The earlier in gestation that PROM occurs, the longer the latency period can be expected to extend. Taken as a whole, patients experiencing PROM at term will undergo onset of labor within 24 hours in 80–90% of cases, with less than 10% having latency periods in excess of 48 hours. Among preterm gestations with PPROM, 60–80% will undergo onset of labor within 24 hours, but 20–40% may have latency periods in excess of 7 days.

1. **Complications.** Pregnancies affected by PROM are at increased risk for such obstetric complications as umbilical cord prolapse, chorioamnionitis, and postpartum endometritis. Patients with PPROM are at increased risk of abruptio placentae, with a reported incidence of 4.0–6.3%. This is 2–3 times greater than the frequency noted among control patient groups with intact amniotic membranes. The risk of abruptio placentae appears especially increased among PPROM patients with a history of recent vaginal bleeding.

When the amniotic fluid volume in PPROM remains significantly reduced for any length of time, the fetus is at risk of developing a fetal compression syndrome. Findings associated with fetal compression include abnormal (Potter) facies, contractures of the extremities, and most significantly, pulmonary hypoplasia. The incidence of these abnormalities is related to gestational age at the time of PROM, the degree of amniotic fluid reduction, and the duration of these conditions.

2. **Morbidity and mortality.** Accurate statistics regarding maternal and fetal morbidity and mortality of PPROM in the second trimester have only recently become available. This lack of objective information owes to previously held perceptions of uniformly poor outcomes and the common practice of recommending induction of labor and delivery in all such cases. More recently, some clinicians have opted for a course of expectant management. The available published studies of PPROM are limited to relatively small numbers of patients but have generally reported consistent findings. Several of these are summarized here.
   a. In a retrospective study of PPROM prior to 34 weeks' gestation, van Dongen [13] found a neonatal mortality of 29% (14 in 48 infants). Four of these deaths could be directly attributed to pulmonary hypoplasia, with three cases of pulmonary hypoplasia with PPROM prior to 20 weeks' gestation and a fourth case with PPROM at 26 weeks' gestation. It was stated that "[PPROM] before 20 weeks' gestation will certainly lead to lung hypoplasia."
   b. Blott and Greenough [3] found a neonatal mortality of 36% among 30 patients with PPROM occurring in the second trimester. Compressive limb abnormalities were seen in 27% of the infants.
   c. Thibeault and colleagues [12] found positional joint abnormalities in 21 in 76 (28%) infants with PPROM of greater than five days. In this series, the abnormalities usually responded to physical therapy and did not require other intervention.
   d. Taylor and Garite [11] evaluated 53 cases of PROM between 16 and 25 weeks of gestation and found that gestational age at time of PPROM had less effect on neonatal survival than did gestational age at birth and birth weight. Thirteen of 18 infants born after 26 weeks' gestation survived.
3. **Prognosis.** As is evidence from these studies, the prognosis with PPROM is often guarded, but need not preclude expectant management or attempts to improve fetal survival and decrease associated morbidities. A review of current literature does, however, indicate that PPROM prior to 20 weeks' gestation with associated nonresolving oligohydramnios has little chance of attaining a viable infant.

   Finally, it should be noted that spontaneous leakage of fluid will resolve and amniotic fluid volume (AFV) reaccumulate in up to 5% of cases. This is especially true if leakage of fluid is noted subsequent to genetic amniocentesis.

C. **Diagnosis.** Because PROM significantly affects pregnancy outcome and management decisions, care must be taken to establish the diagnosis when it is suggested either by a history of leaking fluid per vagina or by an ultrasound finding of decreased AFV.

When PROM is suspected, direct digital examination of the cervix or vagina should be avoided until a decision to deliver has been made. Leakage of fluid can usually be documented by a sterile speculum examination of the vagina performed after the patient has been allowed to rest in a supine position for 20–30 minutes. The posterior fornix should be examined for evidence of pooling of fluid. If gross pooling is not evident, direct observation of the cervix during a Valsalva maneuver or with coughing may show evidence of free flow of fluid from the cervical os.

1. **Vaginal fluids** obtained either from the posterior fornix or the cervical os may be directly examined for evidence of amniotic fluid. The most commonly used techniques are the "fern" test and the nitrazine test. Other methods of analyzing pooled vaginal fluids for evidence of PROM have been evaluated. Pooled vaginal fluid can be cytologically stained for fetal squamous cells and fat

globules. Although cytologic staining methods are quite specific, they are of limited clinical utility. They are often falsely negative in preterm gestations and require special dyes and techniques not readily performed in labor areas. Amniotic fluid can be chemically analyzed for compounds known to be present in large concentrations in amniotic fluid and either absent or in low concentration in the normal vaginal fluids of pregnancy, such as prolactin, alpha fetoprotein, and human placental lactogen. Assays for these compounds have shown some promise as markers for PROM. Evaluation for "ferning" and alteration of vaginal pH continue to provide the best, most easily accessible methods of primary evaluation for PROM.

a. **The fern test** is performed by obtaining a sample of fluid on a sterile cotton-tipped applicator from the posterior vaginal fornix during the sterile speculum exam. If a pool of fluid is not in evidence, fluid may be obtained from the external portion of the cervical os. The sample is then smeared thinly on a clean glass slide, allowed to air dry, and examined with a microscope at × 5–10 magnification for evidence of an arborized (fernlike) pattern. To prevent false-negative results, care should be taken to allow adequate time for complete drying of the slide, and the entire slide should be inspected. Any evidence of arborization should be read as a positive test. Both fingerprint-stained slides and dried saline irrigating solution samples have been reported to cause falsely positive arborization patterns.

b. **The nitrazine test** relies on the fact that amniotic fluid (pH 7.0–7.5) is significantly more alkaline than normal vaginal secretions (pH 4.5–5.5). A sample of vaginal fluid obtained on a sterile cotton-tipped applicator should be smeared on a piece of nitrazine pH paper. A color change to blue-green (pH 6.5) or blue (pH 7.0) is strong evidence for the presence of amniotic fluid. False-positive results may result if specimens are contaminated by blood, urine, semen, or antiseptic cleansing agents.

4. **Amniotic fluid volume.** When evaluations for arborization and pH change do not provide evidence of amniotic fluid leakage in spite of a suggestive clinical history, the patient should undergo ultrasound evaluation to assess the AFV. PROM will usually be associated with a decreased AFV, but fluid pockets measuring larger than 3 × 3 cm are often present. **If the AFV is noted to be significantly reduced, whether or not PROM is ultimately confirmed, the fetus should be carefully evaluated for the presence of normal-appearing kidneys and bladder.** Renal agenesis with subsequent oligohydramnios will occasionally present in a manner similar to PROM, but the optimal management often differs significantly.

5. **Amniocentesis.** If vaginal fluid analysis is inconclusive and ultrasound findings are suggestive of PROM, it is possible to confirm the diagnosis by instilling 1–2 ml of **sterile dye** within the amniotic cavity by amniocentesis and then placing a sterile cotton gauze within the vagina. The patient would be maintained in a supine position and the gauze removed after 30–40 minutes. If PROM is present, the cephalad portion of the gauze will be stained. Regardless of the state of the amniotic membranes, the urine will eventually be noted to pass the dye.

a. **Procedure.** Amniocentesis is best performed under continuous ultrasound needle guidance. In cases of PROM, it should be performed only by a physician experienced in amniocentesis, and only if an adequate fluid pocket can be visualized. (When AFV is extremely reduced, loops of umbilical cord may falsely appear to be fluid pockets. Attempts to perform amniocentesis under such conditions may inadvertently cause damage to the umbilical cord.) It is advisable to **monitor fetal heart rate** for a short time after amniocentesis if any difficulty is encountered with the procedure.

b. **Dyes.** Various dyes have been used for instillation, including Evans blue (Food and Drug Administration class C); indigo carmine (class C), the preferred agent; and methylene blue (class D if intraamniotic). Care should be taken to ensure exclusive intraamniotic instillation, as intravenous administration of indigo carmine can (rarely) have adverse effects. Evans blue T

1824 is a good alternative. Methylene blue can no longer be recommended for general use in intraamniotic instillation, as in large doses it has been associated with fetal hemolytic anemia, hyperbilirubinemia, methemoglobinemia, and a higher likelihood of fetal staining. Methylene blue has been reported to have weak (but not statistically significant) associations with congenital malformations in humans.

II. Management considerations

A. Initial Management

1. Evaluation. The evaluation of suspected PROM is described in sec. **I.C.** To minimize the risk of infection, manual examination of the vagina and cervix should be avoided. During the initial evaluation, cultures of the cervix for group B streptococci should be obtained. Additional cultures for *Neisseria gonorrhoeae* and *Chlamydia* should also be performed if these organisms have a high prevalence in the existing clinical environment.

a. Pooled vaginal fluid can be collected using a DeLee suction trap or with a sterile catheter/syringe system. Free-flowing fluid obtained in this manner may be accurately analyzed for **evidence of fetal lung maturity,** with the usual criteria of lecithin-sphingomyelin ratio greater than 2 or the presence of phosphatidylglycerol providing strong evidence for fetal lung maturity. If the fluid obtained is contaminated by blood or meconium, only the presence of phosphatidylglycerol will accurately predict fetal lung maturity.

b. Amniocentesis is usually not required in PROM but may be indicated in certain clinical situations. **Amniotic fluid cultures** in PROM show infection in approximately 10% of cases, and amniocentesis affords an accurate way to document infection prior to overt chorioamnionitis. It may be necessary to confirm the diagnosis by dye instillation if the previously described clinical methods do not **prove** amniotic fluid leakage. The erroneous diagnosis of PROM may result in unnecessary hospitalization and intervention. Falsely negative studies for PROM may not allow an optimal management plan to be developed. If amniocentesis is performed to confirm PROM, samples of fluid may also be obtained for bacterial culture and fetal lung maturity analysis.

(1) Risks. Amniocentesis is not without risk to the fetus, and the relative benefits and risks to patient and fetus should be assessed before attempting the procedure. Factors such as fluid pocket size, placental location, and proximity of the prospective pocket to umbilical cord and vital fetal structures should be taken into account.

B. Long-term management. After the diagnosis has been confirmed, the exact management strategy will depend on a variety of factors including gestational age, apparent well-being of the fetus, fetal lung maturity, fetal presentation, evidence of maternal or fetal infection, signs of labor, and, at times, cervical "ripeness" for induction. In general terms, three categories of pharmacologic intervention may be considered: **fetal lung maturation therapy, antibiotic prophylaxis,** and **tocolysis of labor.** In the case of PROM at term, **induction of labor** is also a consideration. Before addressing management concerns specific to various gestational-age ranges, the broader issues of fetal lung maturation therapy and antibiotic therapy will be discussed.

III. Therapeutic interventions

A. Fetal lung maturation therapy

1. Corticosteroids such as betamethasone and dexamethasone have been used to promote fetal lung maturation in PPROM.

a. Controversial therapy. In spite of extensive investigation, the use of corticosteroid (CCS) medications to promote fetal lung maturation continues to be very controversial. When more general considerations regarding the possibility of unrecognized side effects are set aside, **three predominant issues remain:**

1. What is the contribution of the condition of PROM itself as a maturing influence on the fetal pulmonary structures?

2. To what extent do various pharmacologic interventions influence the neonate's pulmonary function and decrease the incidence of neonatal respiratory distress syndrome?
3. Should CCS or other therapy directed toward pulmonary maturity be attempted?

2. **PROM itself has been shown in many studies to promote fetal lung maturation.** This maturing effect may help explain the great disparity in the literature regarding CCS fetal lung maturation therapy. Some investigators [2, 9] have found CCS therapy to enhance fetal lung maturity; other excellent studies, including a national collaborative study [5], have failed to document this finding. A possible explanation for these differing results was offered by Spinnato [10], a participant in the national collaborative study. He found that in the indigent population studied, the incidence of immature fetal lung studies obtained from consecutive patients admitted with PROM prior to 34 weeks' gestation was quite low (8 in 73 patients, 11%). Since most prior studies had not controlled for possibly preexisting fetal lung maturity prior to randomization of treatment, he felt that they may not have been able to detect improvement in a relatively small proportion of their subjects.

3. Another consideration regarding CCS therapy in PROM is that **CCS use may increase the infectious morbidity** of this condition. Although not uniformly observed, several studies have documented an increase in maternal postpartum endomyometritis after CCS administration. This effect appears limited to the maternal infectious morbidity, as most studies have not found an attendant rise in neonatal infectious morbidity. Finally, it has been reported that prophylactic antibiotic therapy may correct the tendency to chorioamnionitis in PROM [1, 9]. After administration of CCS type medications, a leukocytosis to 20,000–30,0000/ml for approximately 48 hours is commonly noted. This effect is related to demargination of peripheral white blood cell counts and does not in and of itself signify infection. It may unfortunately mask a rising white blood cell count due to infection.
   a. **Indications.** No unanimity of opinion exists regarding CCS fetal lung maturation therapy in PROM. Most authors feel CCS use should be either avoided or restricted to experimental protocols. This is certainly the case for situations where pulmonary maturity either has been documented or is relatively likely, based on gestational age. Nevertheless, CCS therapy may be a consideration for fetuses at 25–28 weeks' gestation, or for fetuses of less than 34 weeks' gestation with documented immature lung indexes. CCS therapy should only given if an index period of 48 hours is anticipated, as this appears to be the minimum effective time interval for this therapy. Finally, it is conceivable that current investigations involving multiagent regimens, such as the recent work by Morales and colleagues [8] using combinations of CCS and thyroid-releasing hormone, may eventually provide a more effective means of promoting fetal lung maturity in PROM.

B. Antibiotic usage

1. **Empiric therapy.** Although PROM appears to have a significant association with underlying infection, the exact role for antibiotic therapy has yet to be defined.
   a. **Therapeutic options**
      (1) Initiation of empiric antibiotic therapy after collection of initial cultures from the amniotic sac (by amniocentesis) or from the cervical os, or both has been accomplished, but prior to positive culture results.
      (2) Withholding antibiotic therapy until positive evidence of infection (i.e., the presence of bacteria or leukocytosis in amniotic fluid obtained by amniocentesis or positive cervical or amniotic fluid culture), or cervical Gram's smear showing frequent white blood cells.
      (3) Observation for clinical evidence of chorioamnionitis and initiation of antibiotic therapy after the diagnosis of chorioamnionitis and the decision to deliver the fetus have been made.
   b. **Patient evaluation.** As no single strategy has been shown superior to others

the decision to initiate antibiotic therapy in PROM will depend on an appraisal of the individual patient's likelihood of underlying infection, as well as the potential risks to the fetus and mother should underlying infection be either inadequately treated or initially left untreated. Both Amon and colleagues [1] and Morales and colleagues [9] have found evidence that initial therapy with antibiotics, such as ampicillin, started on presentation but prior to positive culture results, may decrease the infectious morbidity associated with PROM among patients with group B streptococcal colonization. If empiric antibiotic therapy is elected, ampicillin given 1–2 gm IV q6h is recommended in nonallergic patients. In cases of penicillin allergy, depending on the individual allergic history, alternate medications such as cephalothin or oral erythromycin may be considered. Antibiotic therapy should be discontinued at 48 hours if cultures are negative. Patients found to culture positive for such organisms as group B streptococcus or *N. gonorrhoeae* require suitable antibiotic therapy for at least seven days. The need to treat such infections as mycoplasma, *Ureaplasma,* and nonspecific vaginosis is less well established but may reasonably be considered. All patients with positive cultures should have repeat cultures after therapy is finished to verify that the identified organism is no longer present.

2. **Surgical prophylaxis.** Patients with PROM are at high risk for postoperative infection. Patients with no clinical evidence of infection should receive perioperative antibiotic prophylaxis after the umbilical cord has been clamped. A wide variety of single- and multiple-dose antibiotic regimens have been shown effective, and the clinician should choose the regimen most appropriate for a given institution based on clinical experience and prevailing sensitivity patterns. Patients who have evidence of infection should receive a full course of broad-spectrum parenteral antibiotic therapy, as described next.
3. **Overt infection**
   a. **Chorioamnionitis.** In PROM, the diagnosis of chorioamnionitis is best made on clinical grounds. Finding such as maternal or fetal tachycardia, increasing uterine tenderness to palpation, maternal fever, and rising white blood cell count (in the absence of recent CCS therapy) all suggest this diagnosis. Although rising C-reactive protein titers are relatively sensitive indicators of early infection, they have generally been found to have poor specificity (approximately 50% false-positives) and therefore add little to the diagnosis of infection.
      (1) **Therapy.** When chorioamnionitis complicating PROM has been diagnosed, appropriate antibiotic therapy should be promptly initiated and delivery expedited. If delivery is imminent, some clinicians advocate withholding treatment until after delivery has occurred (in order to avoid masking a fetal infection); others believe that immediate initiation of therapy will best minimize infectious morbidity in mother and child. The difficulty in accurately estimating the time interval to vaginal delivery strengthens the argument for immediate therapy. It may be helpful to develop an antibiotic prophylaxis policy in consultation with the pediatric physicians who will be caring for the infant after delivery.
      (2) **Cesarean section.** The diagnosis of chorioamnionitis with PROM is not a sufficient reason to perform a cesarean section, as such intervention has not been shown to improve neonatal outcome. Moreover, it will greatly increase the infectious risk to the mother. Usual obstetric indications for cesarean section apply in PROM.
      (3) **Microbes** frequently associated with chorioamnionitis include *Bacteroides* species (25%), *Escherichia coli* (10%), group B streptococci (12%), and other aerobic streptococci (13%). A polymicrobial infection is often present. Adequate therapy for this infection requires a regimen with sufficient antimicrobial spectrum to treat this diverse group of pathogens. A commonly employed regimen is ampicillin (2 gm IV q6h) in combination with gentamicin (loading dose of 1.5–2.0 mg/kg followed with a dose of approximately 1 mg/kg q8h). Certain extended-spectrum peni-

cillins and cephalosporin antibiotics may offer a comparable antimicrobial spectrum without the potential ototoxicity and nephrotoxicity of regimens employing aminoglycosides. Patients with evidence of chorioamnionitis who ultimately require cesarean section should also receive clindamycin or another antimicrobial regimen with good activity against anaerobic bacteria.

C. **Tocolysis.** As with other topics in PROM, the use of tocolytic agents, such as beta-sympathomimetics and magnesium sulfate, is still debated. Pregnancies in the range of 25–34 weeks' gestation have been considered as potential candidates for tocolysis by various investigators.

1. **Indications.** Tocolysis in PROM can generally be categorized as either an attempt to

a. **Prolong the latency interval for several days in order to allow fetal lung maturation** to occur, or

b. **Achieve extended latency intervals sufficient to significantly lessen the common neonatal complications** associated with preterm birth.

Most studies regarding tocolysis in PPROM have been of a retrospective design; however, two prospectively randomized studies have recently been published—with conflicting results [4, 6]. Since obvious benefit has not been demonstrated in the limited number of prospectively randomized studies available, and because tocolytic therapy in combination with underlying maternal infection may predispose to maternal pulmonary edema, it seems most prudent at this time to avoid the use of tocolytic agents in PPROM unless they are part of a study protocol.

IV. Management recommendations

Using the following considerations as a guide, it is possible to offer some recommendations for groups of **patients classed by gestational age.** These are meant to provide a starting point for an individualized care plan. Future medical developments and specific circumstances may cause significant alterations in these generalized care strategies.

A. Gestational age less than 35 weeks

1. **Consideration of risks.** Appropriate management of PPROM requires a careful assessment of the various risks to mother and fetus of the available expectant management and therapeutic options. Clinical features of PPROM that make this condition both challenging and controversial include the significant potential for maternal and fetal morbidity and mortality, as described. A decision to expedite delivery may place the mother at risk of cesarean section due to either a failed induction of labor or because of electronic fetal heart rate monitoring suggestive of fetal distress.

2. **Patient participation.** In PROM and PPROM, an optimal management plan will be obtained after a careful discussion of the relevant maternal and fetal aspects with the patient and her family. **It is of the utmost importance that the patient be actively involved in planning a strategy.** In cases of extreme prematurity, it may be helpful to involve a neonatologist in the discussion.

a. **Issues** that should be addressed include the following:

(1) **The likelihood of neonatal survival** based on the institution's statistical experience with infants at each gestational age or birth weight. The prematurely delivered infant is at risk of such common dangers of prematurity as neonatal respiratory distress syndrome, intracranial hemorrhage, and necrotizing enterocolitis.

(2) **The potential risks to the fetus while remaining in utero,** including abruptio placentae, cord accidents, pulmonary hypoplasia, infection, fetal compression syndrome.

(3) The **potential risks to and benefit for the mother and fetus if therapeutic interventions such as antibiotic therapy or fetal lung maturation therapy are attempted,** and how much time will be required for therapy to be effective. Both tocolysis and CCS therapy may predispose to maternal adult respiratory distress syndrome.

(4) **Whether the latency interval and fetal outcome likely to be achieved justify potential risk to future maternal fertility** should infection or other complications develop over time (e.g., PPROM with anhydramnios and fetal chest constriction at 22 weeks will probably not result in a satisfactory fetal outcome, whereas PPROM at 22 weeks with decreased but present amniotic fluid and no evidence of chest compression may in some circumstances result in a viable infant). The risk to the patient of developing intrauterine infection in the latter case may be judged as acceptable (or not) after adequate discussion with the patient.

(5) **The appropriate site for care.** Some institutions allow selected patients to remain at home with PPROM after an appropriate observation interval; others advise hospitalized bed rest until delivery. (At this time, only patients with a fetus in vertex presentation who show no evidence of recent vaginal bleeding should be considered for outpatient management.)

3. **Gestational age less than 22 weeks.** The patient should be evaluated for PPROM and the diagnosis confirmed. Amniotic fluid may not present an arborization pattern at this gestational age. A thorough ultrasound examination should be performed to detect correctable anomalies (e.g., posterior urethral valves) and exclude other causes of oligohydramnios (renal agenesis). If severe oligohydramnios is present and persists over several days, strong consideration should be given to induction of labor. In spite of generally poor outcomes, expectant management in this group of patients is occasionally successful. If fluid leakage resolves or some AFV is maintained, a more favorable fetal prognosis may be present and observation may be placed in a more favorable light. Leakage noted within several weeks of amniocentesis should be initially observed, as it may resolve. Neither tocolytics nor CCS fetal lung maturation therapy is likely to benefit the patient. Prophylactic initial antibiotic therapy while awaiting culture results should be considered.

4. **Gestational age 23–25 weeks.** Considerations are similar to those of estimated gestational ages less than 22 weeks. However, as fetal weight increases, a more favorable prognosis may be present. Ultrasound evaluation is urged to confirm pregnancy dating and assess for possible anomalies. Stronger consideration toward expectant management is probably warranted, especially if estimated fetal weight is greater than 500–600 gm. As fetal weight approaches 500 gm and gestational age approaches 25 weeks, transfer of the patient to a high-risk obstetric center with complete neonatal services is recommended. Prophylactic antibiotics should be considered, but neither tocolytics nor CCS therapy is likely to benefit the fetus, as lung formation is only in its early stages at this time.

5. **Gestational age 25–35 weeks**

a. **Tests.** Ultrasound is recommended to evaluate for possible anomalies, fetal presentation, and AFV. Attempts to diagnose fetal pulmonary hypoplasia in utero have not yet provided sufficient precision to be adopted into clinical practice.

b. **Optimal management.** Significant disagreement exists among major institutions regarding optimal management. Management options range from immediate induction of labor to tocolysis of labor. Expectant management offers many advantages, but other management options may be preferable in varying clinical situations.

(1) **Expectant management.** Patients managed expectantly should be regularly evaluated for onset of chorioamnionitis, and a regular schedule of electronic fetal heart rate monitoring should be established. Special emphasis should be placed on new-onset variable decelerations, as they may indicate umbilical cord compromise. AFV should be assessed at least weekly. Prophylactic antibiotic administration during the initial 48 hours after PPROM, but prior to culture results, should be considered. If CCS fetal lung maturation therapy is attempted, antibiotics should be concomitantly administered. The use of tocolytics is very controversial but

in certain circumstances may be considered in an attempt to lengthen the latency interval and allow fetal maturation. Tocolytics in PPROM may best be restricted to experimental protocols until their efficacy is better established.

(2) Latency interval. As the latency interval increases, and for fetuses greater than 28–30 weeks' gestation, it is best to constantly evaluate the patient and fetus for indications for delivery. PPROM predisposes to placental abruption, and precipitous deliveries often occur, even among carefully observed patients. The fetal presentation and planned route of delivery should always be carefully documented in the medical record. Cesarean section is generally recommended for nonvertex presentations among fetuses in this gestational-age range. Selected fetuses of greater than 34 weeks' gestation with documented abdominal circumferences greater than head circumference (e.g., head–abdominal circumference < 1.0) meeting published criteria may be considered for vaginal breech delivery. Careful discussion of delivery options with the parturient is recommended if breech delivery is contemplated.

B. Gestational age greater than 35 weeks

1. Tests. Patients thought to have experienced rupture of membranes at gestation

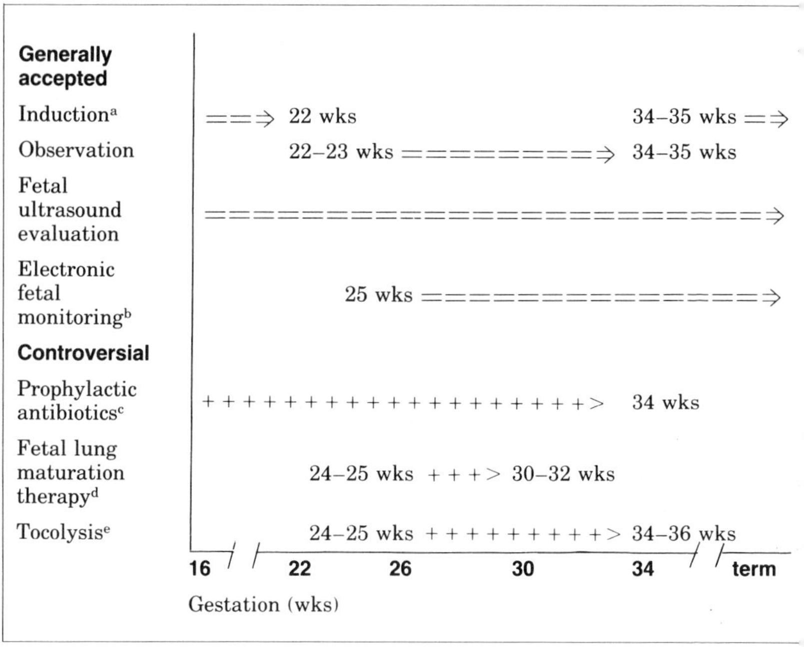

Fig. 29-1. Timetable for generally accepted and controversial management considerations in PPROM.

[a]Evaluate the amniotic fluid volume. If severe oligohydramnios persists prior to 22 weeks, consider induction; if gestation is past 34–35 weeks, evaluate for fetal lung maturity and induce when mature.

[b]External monitoring should be done on a regular basis to evaluate for abnormal decelerations and the usual criteria of fetal well-being.

[c]Initiate until cultures are negative at 48 hours.

[d]Obtain amniotic fluid for lung maturity profile. If immature, consider fetal lung maturation therapy *and* antibiotics.

[e]In rare circumstances, tocolysis may offer some therapeutic benefit.

ages of more than 35 weeks should be carefully evaluated to confirm amniotic fluid leakage. If there is any question about **pregnancy dating,** an ultrasound evaluation should be obtained. If the gestational age is uncertain, it may also be advisable to obtain a sample of amniotic fluid for fetal lung maturity studies. If institutional epidemiologic studies show a high prevalence of specific infections, such as group B streptococci, cultures for these organisms should be obtained.

2. **Pharmacologic intervention.** Little support is given in the literature for any pharmacologic intervention in this group of patients. Neither tocolysis, antibiotics, nor CCS therapy has been shown of benefit.
3. **Optimal management.** Patients may be managed by either expectant management or aggressive induction of labor. If any question of pregnancy dating or fetal lung maturity exists (as in delayed fetal lung maturation associated with gestational diabetes), it is best to opt for expectant management.
   a. **Labor.** In most cases, these patients will begin spontaneous labor within 24–48 hours. A small proportion of patients will not enter labor, and it will be necessary to consider induction of labor. The prevailing practice in such situations is to induce labor by oxytocin infusion if labor does not spontaneously ensue after 6–12 hours. In most cases, labor proceeds normally and vaginal delivery is attained. Nevertheless, in cases of poor cervical "inducеability" (low Bishop score), it may be reasonable to defer active induction of labor for several days. Kappy [7] evaluated the conservative management of PROM in term patients and found a significantly lower cesarean section rate among patients treated in this manner (39% and 12% cesarean rates, respectively, among patients with induced versus spontaneous labor).
   b. If **expectant management** of PROM at term is a consideration, cervical exams per vagina should be avoided. A initial sterile speculum exam of the cervix is recommended to ascertain which patients will be candidates for this treatment option.

   Figure 29-1 depicts one possible scheme for the management of PPROM and PROM.

V. **Summary.** PPROM and PROM are extremely complex areas of obstetrics. Proper management requires an up-to-date knowledge of recent research, as well as careful attention to clinical details.

References

1. Amon, E., et al. Ampicillin prophylaxis in preterm premature rupture of the membranes: A prospective randomized study. *Am. J. Obstet. Gynecol.* 159(3):539–543, 1988.
2. Arias, F., Knight, A. B., and Tomich, P. B. A retrospective study on the effects of steroid administration and prolongation of the latent phase in patients with preterm premature rupture of the membranes. *Am. J. Obstet. Gynecol.* 154(5):1059–1063, 1986.
3. Blott, M., and Greenough, A. Neonatal outcome after prolonged rupture of the membranes starting in the second trimester. *Arch. Dis. Child.* 63(10):1146–1150, 1988.
4. Bourgeois, F. J., et al. Early versus late tocolytic treatment for preterm premature membrane rupture. *Am. J. Obstet. Gynecol.* 159(3):742–748, 1988.
5. Collaborative Group on Antenatal Steroid Therapy. Effect of antenatal dexamethasone administration on the prevention of respiratory distress syndrome. *Am. J. Obstet. Gynecol.* 155:2, 1986.
6. Garite, T. J., et al. A randomized trial of ritodrine tocolysis versus expectant management in patients with premature rupture of membranes at 25 to 30 weeks of gestation. *Am. J. Obstet. Gynecol.* 157(2):388–393, 1987.
7. Kappy, K. A., et al. Premature rupture of membranes at term: A comparison of induced and spontaneous labors. *J. Reprod. Med.* 27(1):29, 1982.
8. Morales, W. J., et al. Fetal lung maturation: The combined use of corticosteroids and TRH. *Obstet. Gynecol.* 73(1):111–116, 1989.

9. Morales, W. J., et al. Use of ampicillin and corticosteroids in premature rupture of membranes: A randomized study. *Obstet. Gynecol.* 73(5 Pt. 1):721–726, 1989.
10. Spinnato, J. A. Infrequency of pulmonary immaturity in an indigent population with preterm premature rupture of the membranes. *Obstet. Gynecol.* 69(6):942, 1987.
11. Taylor, J., and Garite, T. J. Premature rupture of membranes before fetal viability. *Obstet. Gynecol.* 64(5):615–620, 1984.
12. Thibeault, D. W., et al. Neonatal pulmonary hypoplasia with premature rupture of fetal membranes and oligohydramnios. *J. Pediatr.* 107(2):273–277, 1985.
13. van Dongen, P. W., et al. Lethal lung hypoplasia in infants after prolonged rupture of membranes. *Eur. J. Obstet. Gynecol. Reprod. Biol.* 25(4):287–292, 1987.

Selected Readings

Alger, L. S., and Pupkin, M. J. Etiology of preterm premature rupture of the membranes. *Clin. Obstet. Gynecol.* 29(4):758–770, 1986.

Crenshaw, C., Jr. (guest ed.). Preterm premature rupture of the membranes. *Clin. Obstet. Gynecol.* 29(4):735–860, 1986.

Fisk, N. M. Modifications to selective conservative management in preterm premature rupture of the membranes. *Obstet. Gynecol. Surv.* 43(6):328–334, 1988.

Graham, J. M., Jr. Causes of limb reduction defects: The contribution of fetal constraint and/or vascular disruption. *Clin. Perinatol.* 13(3):575–591, 1986.

Miller, J. M., Jr., and Pastorek, J. G., II. The microbiology of premature rupture of the membranes. *Clin. Obstet. Gynecol.* 29(4):739–757, 1986.

Monif, G. R., Hume, R., Jr., and Goodlin, R. C. Neonatal considerations in the management of premature rupture of the fetal membranes. *Obstet. Gynecol. Surv.* 41(9):531–537, 1986.

Nagey, D. A., and Saller, D. N., Jr. An analysis of the decisions in the management of premature rupture of the membranes. *Clin. Obstet. Gynecol.* 29(4):826–834, 1986.

Romero, R., et al. Infection in the pathogenesis of preterm labor. *Semin. Perinatol.* 12(4):262–279, 1988.

Rudd, E. G. Premature rupture of the membranes: A review. *J. Reprod. Med.* 30(11):841–848, 1985.

Schwartz, M. F. Genetic aspects of premature rupture of the membranes. *Clin. Obstet. Gynecol.* 29(4):771–778, 1986.

Veille, J. C. Management of preterm premature rupture of membranes. *Clin. Perinatol.* 15(4):851–862, 1988.

Diagnosis of PROM

Fisk, N. M., et al. Is C-reactive protein really useful in preterm premature rupture of the membranes? *Br. J. Obstet. Gynaecol.* 94(12):1159–1164, 1987.

Fribourg, S. Safety of intraamniotic injection of indigo carmine. *Am. J. Obstet. Gynecol.* 140:350–351, 1981.

McEnery, J. K., and McEnery, L. N. Unfavorable neonatal outcome after intraamniotic administration of methylene blue. *Obstet. Gynecol.* 48:74s–75s, 1976.

Morrison, L., and Wiseman, H. J. Intra-amniotic injection of Evans blue dye. *Am. J. Obstet. Gynecol.* 113:1147, 1972.

Phocas, I., et al. Vaginal fluid prolactin: a reliable marker for the diagnosis of prematurely ruptured membranes. Comparison with vaginal fluid alpha-fetoprotein and placental lactogen. *Eur. J. Obstet. Gynecol. Reprod. Biol.* 31(2):133, 1989.

Rochelson, B. L., et al. A rapid colorimetric AFP monoclonal antibody test for the diagnosis of preterm rupture of the membranes. *Obstet. Gynecol.* 69(2):163, 1987.

Infection/Antibiotics

Alger, L. S., et al. The association of *Chlamydia trachomatis, Neisseria gonorrhoeae,* and group B streptococci with preterm rupture of the membranes and pregnancy outcome. *Am. J. Obstet. Gynecol.* 159(2):397–404, 1988.

Bobitt, J. R., Damato, J. D., and Sakakini, J. Jr. Perinatal complications in group B streptococcal carriers: a longitudinal study of prenatal patients. *Am. J. Obstet. Gynecol.* 151(6):711–717, 1985.

Fortunato, S. J. et al. Steady-state cord and amniotic fluid ceftizoxime levels continuously surpass maternal levels. *Am. J. Obstet. Gynecol.* 159(3):570–573, 1988.

Gravett, M. G., et al. Independent associations of bacterial vaginosis and *Chlamydia trachomatis* infection with adverse pregnancy outcome. *J.A.M.A.* 256(14):1899–1903, 1986.

Gravett, M. G., and Eschenbach, D. A. Possible role of *Ureaplasma urealyticum* in preterm premature rupture of the fetal membranes. *Pediatr. Infect. Dis.* 5(6 Suppl.):S253–S257, 1986.

Matorras, R., et al. Group B streptococcus and premature rupture of membranes and preterm delivery. *Gynecol. Obstet. Invest.* 27(1):14–18, 1989.

McGregor, J. A., et al. Bacterial protease-induced reduction of chorioamniotic membrane strength and elasticity. *Obstet. Gynecol.* 69(2):167–174, 1987.

Morales, W. J., and Lim, D. Reduction of group B streptococcal maternal and neonatal infections in preterm pregnancies with premature rupture of membranes through a rapid identification test. *Am. J. Obstet. Gynecol.* 157(1):13–16, 1987.

Morales, W. J., Washington, S. R., and Lazar, A. J. The effect of chorioamnionitis on perinatal outcome in preterm gestation. *J. Perinatol.* 7(2):105–110, 1987.

Muller, M., et al. Rupture of fetal membranes and premature delivery associated with group B streptococci in urine of pregnant women. *Lancet* 2(8394):69–70, 1984.

Ray, D. A., et al. Maternal herpes infection complicated by prolonged premature rupture of membranes. *Am. J. Perinatol.* 2(2):96–100, 1985.

Romero, R., et al. Prostaglandin concentrations in amniotic fluid of women with intra-amniotic infection and preterm labor. *Am. J. Obstet. Gynecol.* 157(6):1461–1467, 1987.

Romero, R., et al. Intraamniotic infection and the onset of labor in preterm premature rupture of the membranes. *Am. J. Obstet. Gynecol* 159(3):661–666, 1988.

Sbarra, A. J., et al. Effect of bacterial growth on the bursting pressure of fetal membranes in vitro. *Obstet. Gynecol.* 70(1):107–110, 1987.

Simon, C., et al. Bacteriological findings after premature rupture of the membranes. *Arch. Gynecol. Obstet.* 244(2):69–74, 1989.

CORTICOSTEROIDS

Avery, M. E., et al. Update on prenatal steroid for prevention of respiratory distress. Report of a conference—September 26–28, 1985. *Am. J. Obstet. Gynecol.* 155(1):2–5, 1986.

MacKenna, J., and Brame, R. G. Fetal lung maturity and phospholipids. *Obstet. Gynecol. Annu.* 14:222, 1985.

Ohlsson, A. Treatments of preterm premature rupture of the membranes: A meta-analysis. *Am. J. Obstet. Gynecol.* 160(4):890–906, 1989.

ABRUPTIO PLACENTAE

Gonen, R., Hannah, M. E., and Milligan, J. E. Does prolonged preterm premature rupture of the membranes predispose to abruptio placentae? *Obstet. Gynecol.* 74(3 Pt. 1):347–350, 1989.

Nelson, D. M., Stempel, L. E., and Zuspan, F. B. Association of prolonged, preterm premature rupture of the membranes and abruptio placentae. *J. Reprod. Med.* 31(4):249–253, 1986.

Vintzileos, A. M., et al. Preterm premature rupture of the membranes: A risk factor for the development of abruptio placentae. *Am. J. Obstet. Gynecol.* 156(5):1235–1238, 1987.

MANAGEMENT STRATEGIES

Douvas, S. G., et al. Treatment of premature rupture of the membranes. *J. Reprod. Med.* 29(10):741–744, 1984.

Garite, T. J. Premature rupture of the membranes: the enigma of the obstetrician. *Am. J. Obstet. Gynecol.* 151(8):1001–1005, 1985.

Gazaway, P., and Mullins, C. L. Prevention of preterm labor and premature rupture of the membranes. *Clin. Obstet. Gynecol.* 29(4):835–849, 1986.

Hauth, J. C., et al. Term maternal and neonatal complications of acute chorioamnionitis. *Obstet. Gynecol.* 66(1):59–62, 1985.

Morales, W. J., and Lazar, A. J. Expectant management of rupture of membranes at term. *South. Med. J.* 79(8):955–958, 1986.

Olofsson, P., Rydhstrom, H., and Sjoberg, N. O. How Swedish obstetricians manage premature rupture of the membranes in preterm gestations. *Am. J. Obstet. Gynecol.* 159(5):1028–1034, 1988.

NONINFECTIOUS NEONATAL MORBIDITY IN PPROM

Blackmon, L. R., Alger, L. S., and Crenshaw, C. Jr. Fetal and neonatal outcomes associated with premature rupture of the membranes. *Clin. Obstet. Gynecol.* 29(4):779–815, 1986.

Hewitt, B. G., and Newnham, J. P. A review of the obstetric and medical complications leading to the delivery of infants of very low birthweight. *Med. J. Aust.* 149(5):234, 1988.

Johnson, A., et al. Ultrasonic ratio of fetal thoracic to abdominal circumference: An association with fetal pulmonary hypoplasia. *Am. J. Obstet. Gynecol.* 157(3):764–769, 1987.

Moretti, M., and Sibai, B. M. Maternal and perinatal outcome of expectant management of premature rupture of membranes in the midtrimester. *Am. J. Obstet. Gynecol.* 159(2):390–396, 1988.

30 Abnormal Labor and Delivery

Katherine M. Gillogley

With the rising cesarean section rate in the United States, abnormal labor and its management have been increasingly focused on by physicians, the lay public, third-party payers, and legislative bodies. Failure to progress in labor is one of the major factors contributing to the rise in the cesarean section rate [16].

Dystocia (difficult labor) can theoretically be attributed to one or more of three etiologies: uterine dysfunction, fetal malpresentation or abnormality, or pelvic abnormality. Other abnormalities of labor include precipitous labor, umbilical cord prolapse, abruption, uterine rupture, retained placenta, uterine inversion, and postpartum hemorrhage. Fetal distress is discussed in Chap. 22.

I. Uterine dysfunction

A. Diagnosis. The diagnosis of abnormal progress of labor is made by graphing cervical dilatation and descent against time (Friedman curve, see Fig. 27-10). The average and upper limits of normal times for lengths of latent phase, active phase, and second stage as well as rate of cervical dilatation in the active phase are found in Table 30-1.

1. Definitions

a. Prolonged latent phase is diagnosed when the latent phase exceeds 20 hours in nulliparas or 14 hours in multiparas. The latent phase must be distinguished from false labor, although this is often done retrospectively.

b. Protraction disorder of the active phase is diagnosed when the rate of cervical dilatation is less than 1.2 cm/hour in the nullipara or 1.5 cm/hour in the multipara.

c. Diagnosis of **secondary arrest of labor** in the active phase is made when no cervical change occurs over two hours. **Arrest of descent** is diagnosed when no descent of the presenting part occurs over one hour after complete cervical dilatation is reached.

d. Prolonged second stage is reached after two hours in the nullipara without a regional anesthetic and after three hours with regional anesthesia. In the multipara, prolonged second stage is recognized after one hour without anesthesia and two hours with a regional anesthetic.

e. Precipitous labor is recognized when delivery occurs within one hour of the onset of labor.

2. Uterine contraction monitoring. The frequency of uterine contractions can be determined by palpation and external or internal uterine contraction monitoring. The intensity of contractions cannot be determined by an external uterine contraction monitor. With an internal uterine pressure catheter, baseline uterine pressure as well as intensity of contractions is noted in mm Hg. Montevideo units are calculated by multiplying the mean change from the baseline at the peak of the contractions by frequency of contractions in 10 minutes. In women with normal spontaneous labor, 95% will exhibit uterine contraction patterns of greater than 100 Montevideo units [22].

B. Etiology. Uterine dysfunction may occur primarily as an inadequate contraction or uncoordinated contraction pattern, or as secondary to malpresentation, cephalopelvic disproportion, or other factor that in retrospect would make vaginal delivery impossible.

Factors that may contribute to uterine dysfunction include sedation, anxiety,

Table 30-1. Labor duration

	Nulliparas	Multiparas
Latent phase		
Mean (hr)	6.4	4.8
Upper limit (hr)	20.1	13.6
Active phase		
Mean (hr)	4.6	2.4
Upper limit (hr)	11.7	5.2
Dilatation rate		
Lower limit (cm/hr)	1.2	1.5
Second stage		
Upper limit (hr)	2.9	1.1

Source: E. A. Friedman, *Labor: Clinical Evaluation and Management* (2nd ed.). New York: Appleton-Century-Crofts, 1978.

anesthesia, supine position, unripe cervix, chorioamniotis, overdistention of the uterus, or uterine fibroids.

C. Management

1. **Prolonged latent phase** (Fig. 30-1). Friedman [8] reports an 85% response rate with administration of sedation to patients with this disorder. Ten percent of patients are retrospectively diagnosed with false labor and five percent require oxytocin. Amniotomy is not recommended unless other indications are present (e.g., fetal heart rate abnormalities). Morphine or nalbuphine hydrochloride (Nubain) 10–15 mg IM or SC may be administered if false labor is suspected. Hydroxyzine (Vistaril), 100 mg PO, may be used alternatively. O'Driscoll and colleagues [18] recommend an active approach to the management of prolonged latent phase using amniotomy and oxytocin, provided the diagnosis of labor is made.
2. **Protraction and arrest disorders** (Figs. 30-2, 30-3). Before consideration of the use of oxytocin, malpresentation and obvious cephalopelvic disproportion must be ruled out. If the presenting part is engaged, amniotomy and placement of an internal pressure catheter are performed. Position of the vertex is ascertained. Several treatment methods have been recommended with variations of the active management model currently the most popular.
3. **Active management of labor.** In this model of labor management by O'Driscoll

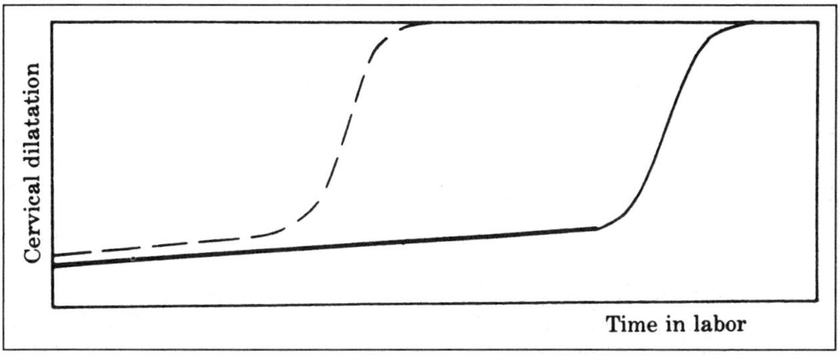

Fig. 30-1. Prolonged latent phase pattern *(solid line)*. Broken line illustrates average dilatation curve for nulliparas. (From E. A. Friedman, *Labor: Clinical Evaluation and Management* [2nd ed.]. New York: Appleton-Century-Crofts, 1978.)

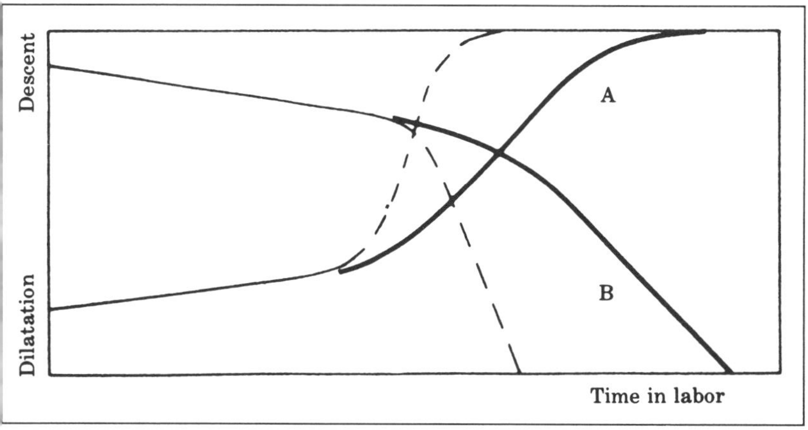

Fig. 30-2. Protraction disorders of labor. **A.** Protracted active phase. **B.** Protracted descent pattern. Broken lines illustrate average normal dilatation and descent patterns. (From E. A. Friedman, *Labor: Clinical Evaluation and Management* [2nd ed.]. New York: Appleton-Century-Crofts, 1978.)

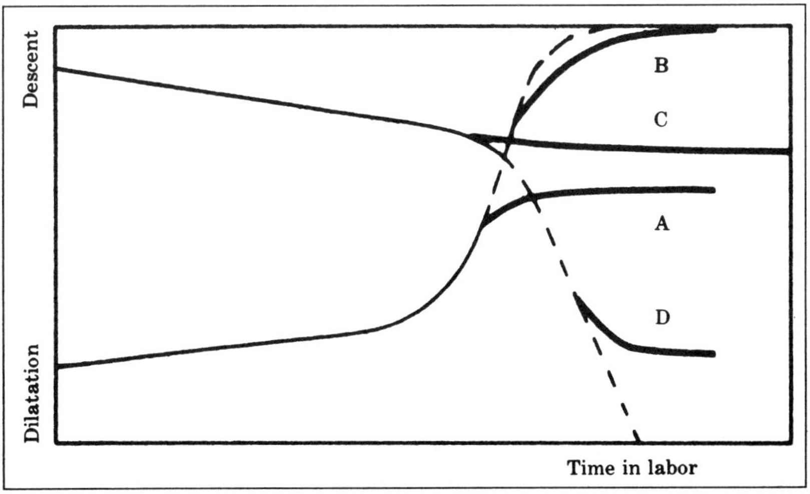

Fig. 30-3. Arrest disorders of labor. **A.** Secondary arrest of dilatation. **B.** Prolonged deceleration. **C.** Failure of descent. **D.** Arrest of descent. Broken lines illustrate normal dilatation and descent curves. (From E. A. Friedman, *Labor: Clinical Evaluation and Management* [2nd ed.]. New York: Appleton-Century-Crofts, 1978.)

and colleagues [18], once the diagnosis of labor is made, progress of labor is closely followed and graphed with hourly cervical examinations. Artificial rupture of membranes is performed as long as the presenting part is engaged. If the rate of cervical dilatation is less than 1 cm/hour, oxytocin infusion is started. Cesarean section is performed if the patient has not delivered within 12 hours after the diagnosis of labor unless delivery is anticipated within an hour. At Dublin Maternity Hospital in Ireland, where the model originated, the cesarean section rate is 4.8%.

a. **Variations** of this model have developed because of controversy concerning the timing of artificial rupture of membranes, management of latent phase, absolute labor time limits, and the manner in which oxytocin is administered.

4. **Ambulation.** Ambulation and an upright sitting position have been found in a small randomized study to be as effective as oxytocin in labors with failure of progression in the active phase [20]. Several other randomized studies in normal labor patients showed an increase in uterine activity and shorter labor lengths with the ambulation group compared to the supine group [15]. As this approach to management of protraction and arrest disorders has not been studied extensively, its use should be reserved for selected cases and used more widely to prevent uterine dysfunction in the normal laboring patient. If there is a concern about the need for continuous fetal monitoring, telemetry may be useful.
5. **Amniotomy.** Significant controversy exists about the benefit of amniotomy on the progress of normal labor. However, in clinical practice, amniotomy is generally performed when a protraction or arrest disorder is diagnosed in the active phase.
6. **Maternal position change or manual rotation, or both.** When the vertex position is not occiput anterior, the knee-chest or upright sitting position is useful. If spontaneous rotation does not occur, manual rotation to occiput anterior can be attempted.
7. **Operative delivery.** Cesarean section for failure to progress can be considered when the arrest of labor in the active phase persists despite adequate uterine contractions for more than two hours. Labor is frequently augmented with oxytocin before cesarean section, even if there appear to be adequate uterine contractions, provided the fetal heart rate is normal and no contraindications exist. With arrest of descent in the second stage, forceps or vacuum extraction may be considered after the exclusion of potential macrosomia and criteria for station and position have been met.
8. **Guidelines for use of oxytocin.** Significant controversy exists concerning the correct way to administer oxytocin. O'Driscoll and colleagues [18] recommend starting at 6 mU/minute and increasing by 6 mU/minute q15min to a maximum of 40 mU/minute, not exceeding seven contractions q15min. Seitchik and colleagues [22, 23] have demonstrated that nearly 40 minutes are required for the plasma level of oxytocin to reach its maximum level after an increase in dose. They state that with 40-minute dosage-increment intervals, 70–75% of patients requiring oxytocin augmentation that deliver vaginally require doses less than 5 mU/minute. The American College of Obstetricians and Gynecologists (ACOG) currently recommends an initial dose of 0.5 mU/minute for augmentation, which is increased q30–60min by 1–2 mU/minute until adequate contractions are achieved [12]. The advantage of the lower starting dose and longer interval to dosage increase is the overall decrease in oxytocin dose required and less hyperstimulation. The disadvantage of this regimen is the longer time to achieve adequate contractions in the occasional patient who requires higher doses of oxytocin.

   The standard dilution for oxytocin is 10 units/1000 ml IV fluid, administered by IV pump. In the United States electronic fetal monitoring is used for patients requiring oxytocin treatment. Close monitoring of uterine contraction frequency is required to avoid hyperstimulation.

   a. **Risks.** The risks of oxytocin augmentation include hyperstimulation, fetal distress, uterine rupture, water intoxication, cardiac arrhythmia, hypersensitivity reaction, and postpartum hemorrhage. Water intoxication is exceedingly rare with the current methods of administration.
   b. **Contraindications.** Absolute contraindications to administration of oxytocin are those that are contraindications to labor. Oxytocin use is acceptable in the patient attempting a trial of labor after a previous low transverse cesarean section.

II. Fetal malpresentation and abnormalities

A. Occiput malpresentations

1. **Diagnosis.** The diagnosis of occiput posterior, occiput transverse, and asynclitism is made primarily by vaginal exam, although Leopold's maneuvers and ultrasound may be helpful in the diagnosis. On vaginal examination, the occiput (located by palpating the posterior fontanelle, which is triangular in shape) is in the posterior part of the pelvis for occiput posterior. With occiput transverse, the sagittal suture is in the transverse diameter of the pelvis (see Fig. 27-6). **Asynclitism** is diagnosed when the biparietal diameter is not parallel to the diameters of the pelvis (e.g., one of the parietal bones is presenting).
2. **Treatment.** As **occiput anterior with flexion is the ideal presentation,** any other occiput presentation descends through the pelvis with greater (less optimal) diameters. If the pelvis is ample or the fetal head is small, delivery may occur without rotation with occiput posterior positions or with late spontaneous rotation with occiput transverse positions. It is desirable to diagnose persistent occiput posterior or transverse positions before the second stage so that maneuvers such as maternal position change and manual rotation are more likely to be successful. In the second stage, a skilled operator with forceps may rotate the fetal head to occiput anterior. However, these procedures are becoming less common today, with the relative safety of cesarean section and the potential for higher fetal morbidity with difficult midforceps procedures.

B. Brow presentation

1. **Diagnosis.** Brow presentation is diagnosed when the fetal head is partially extended and the fetal brow is palpable on vaginal examination (Fig. 30-4).
2. **Incidence.** 0.2% of deliveries.
3. **Treatment.** Before delivery can occur, flexion to a vertex position or deflexion to a face presentation must occur. This will occur in approximately two-thirds of cases. If cephalopelvic disproportion is suspected, the conversion has not taken place, and labor is arrested, cesarean section is appropriate.

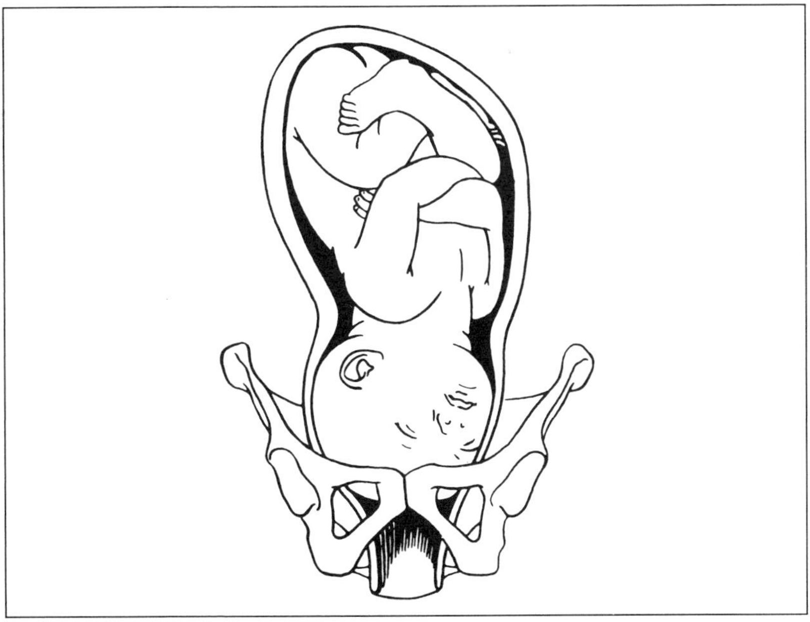

Fig. 30-4. Brow presentation. (From *Obstetrical Presentation and Position,* Ross Clinical Education Aid, No. 18. Columbus, OH: Ross Laboratories, 1975.)

C. **Face presentation**
   1. **Diagnosis.** Face presentation occurs when the fetal head is completely extended. The diagnosis is made when facial features of the fetus are palpated on vaginal examination. The reference point for describing the position is the chin (mentum) (Fig. 30-5).
   2. **Incidence.** 0.2% of deliveries.
   3. **Treatment.** With an ample pelvis, a mentum anterior presentation can deliver without rotation. A mentum posterior must rotate before vaginal delivery. If the mentum posterior position persists, cesarean section must be performed.

D. **Breech presentation**
   1. **Diagnosis.** Breech presentation may be diagnosed by Leopold's maneuvers, vaginal examination, or ultrasound. The point of reference in describing the position of the breech is the sacrum. Breech presentations are classified as frank, complete, or footling (Fig. 30-6). Breech presentations at term or preterm in labor have a higher incidence of congenital anomalies (6.3% versus 2.4%) [3]. Thus ultrasound evaluation of fetal anatomy should be performed if time and resources permit.
   2. **Incidence.** 3–4% of deliveries.
   3. **Etiology.** Breech presentation is found more commonly with preterm gestations, congenital anomalies, and uterine anomalies.
   4. **External breech version.** If the diagnosis of breech is made before labor and at or after 37 weeks of gestation, external breech version may be attempted if no contraindications exist. The procedure must be performed on a labor and delivery unit and preparations should be made in order to perform an emergency cesarean section if necessary. After a reactive nonstress test is obtained, a tocolytic agent is administered. The breech is then elevated out of the pelvis, and the fetal head directed into the pelvis with a forward or backward roll under ultrasound guidance. The success rate is 60–70% [25]. Complications include fetal distress secondary to abruption or cord accident.
   5. **Delivery of the breech.** Recognized complications of vaginal breech delivery include entrapment of the fetal head, spinal cord injury secondary to hyperextension of the fetal head, brachial plexus injury, lower Apgar scores, prolapse of the umbilical cord, asphyxia, intracranial hemorrhage, and trauma to in-

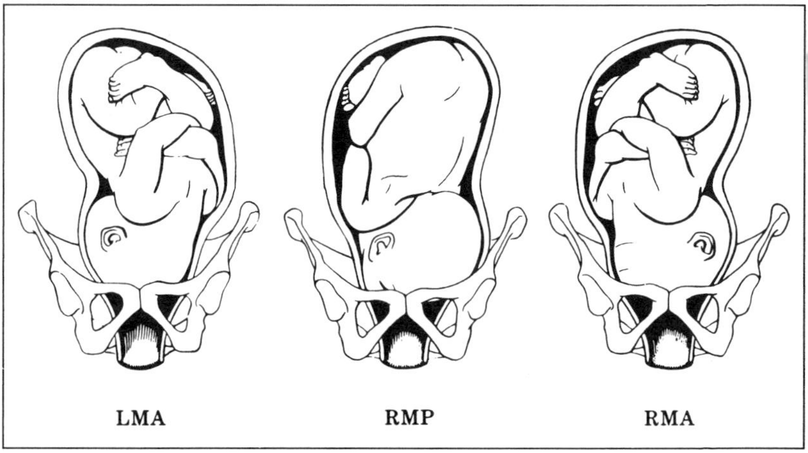

Fig. 30-5. Types of face presentation. (LMA = left mentum anterior; RMP = right mentum posterior; RMA = right mentum anterior.) (From *Obstetrical Presentation and Position,* Ross Clinical Education Aid, No. 18. Columbus, OH: Ross Laboratories, 1975.)

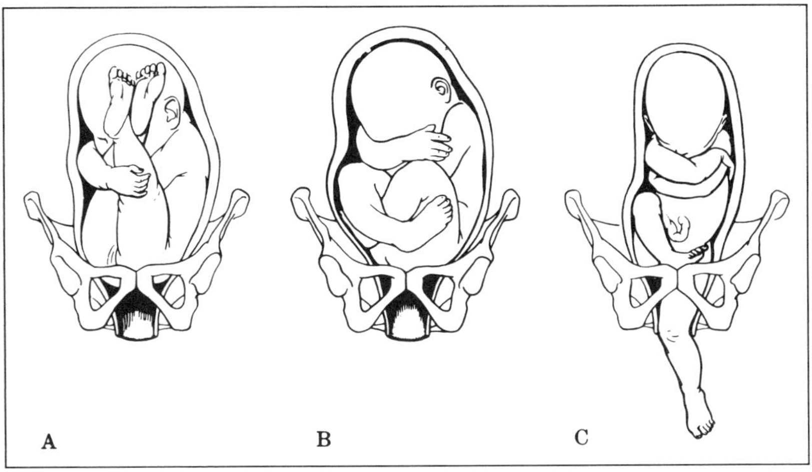

Fig. 30-6. Types of breech presentation. **A.** Frank breech. **B.** Complete breech. **C.** Footling breech. (From *Obstetrical Presentation and Position,* Ross Clinical Education Aid, No. 18. Columbus, OH: Ross Laboratories, 1975.)

ternal organs. With the demonstration of higher fetal morbidity rates, many centers began to deliver most breeches by cesarean section. However, Collea and colleagues [6] in a series of 208 term frank breech presentations, which were randomized to vaginal delivery or cesarean section, showed that when specific criteria are followed, fetal morbidity attributed to birth trauma for vaginal breech delivery declines to 3.3%. These criteria include frank breech presentation, estimated fetal weight between 2500 and 3800 gm, adequate pelvis by pelvimetry, and no hyperextension of the fetal head.

6. **Pelvimetry.** Pelvimetry may be performed by conventional x-ray pelvimetry or computed tomography (CT) pelvimetry. CT pelvimetry delivers one-third of the radiation dose to the fetus, compared to conventional x-ray pelvimetry and has been used successfully in breech management protocols [13]. The same pelvic measurements are used as in conventional x-ray pelvimetry (Table 30-2).

Assisted breech delivery is accomplished by allowing the buttocks and trunk to deliver spontaneously to the level of the umbilicus. An assistant should be present. The back is kept facing up, and when the level of the scapulae is

Table 30-2. Minimal measurements for x-ray pelvimetry

Pelvic plane	cm
Inlet	
Transverse	11.5
Anterior-posterior	10.5
Midpelvis	
Transverse	10.0
Anterior-posterior	11.5

Source: J. V. Collea et al. The randomized management of term frank breech presentation: Vaginal delivery vs. cesarean section. *Am. J. Obstet. Gynecol.* 131:186, 1978.

reached, the arms are delivered by sweeping each across the chest, after rotation of each shoulder anteriorly. The fetal body is held in the horizontal plane by the assistant. The head is flexed using the Mauriceau-Smelli-Veit maneuver (finger over each maxilla) or suprapubic pressure, or both. Episiotomy is recommended in most circumstances. Piper forceps may be used at this point to deliver the aftercoming head.

E. Transverse lie

1. **Diagnosis.** Transverse lie is diagnosed by Leopold's maneuvers with confirmation by sonography (Fig. 30-7).
2. **Incidence.** 0.3% at term.
3. **Etiology.** Transverse lie is more common in multiparous women, preterm and multiple gestations, and patients with placenta previa and uterine leiomyomata.
4. **Management.** If diagnosed before labor and at or after 37 weeks, the external version may be performed if no contraindications exist. Guidelines similar to external breech version apply. If diagnosed in labor, cesarean section must be performed. A vertical uterine incision is frequently necessary for atraumatic delivery. The transverse lie is at high risk for prolapse of the umbilical cord if rupture of the membranes occurs.

F. Compound presentation is diagnosed by vaginal examination when more than one presenting part is palpated (e.g., fetal head and hand). Ultrasound should be performed to confirm the presentation. As long as the vertex precedes the extremity as labor progresses, vaginal delivery can be expected. If on ultrasound, the presentation is breech or the lie transverse, the aforementioned guidelines apply.

G. Multiple pregnancy

1. **Diagnosis.** Multiple pregnancy is suspected when size is greater than dates, with the diagnosis made by ultrasound. An attempt to locate an amniotic membrane should be made, as there are greater risks in the monoamniotic twin pregnancy, such as cord entanglement.
2. **Incidence.** The incidence of twins varies between countries and racial groups, with the incidence of monozygotic twins staying constant. The rate in the United States is approximately 1 in 90. The incidence of triplets is approximately 1 in 8000.
3. **Management.** The multiple pregnancy prenatally requires close surveillance. Preterm labor, preeclampsia, polyhydramnios, congenital anomalies, intrauterine growth retardation, and intrauterine fetal demise have a higher in-

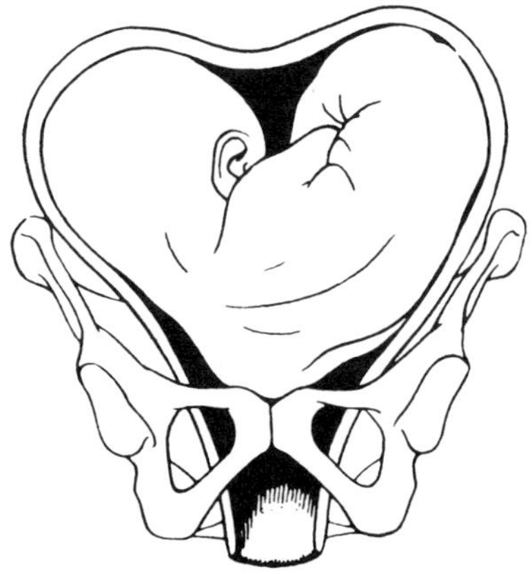

Fig. 30-7. Shoulder presentation. (From *Obstetrical Presentation and Position,* Ross Clinical Education Aid, No. 18. Columbus, OH: Ross Laboratories, 1975.)

cidence in multiple gestation. Twin-twin transfusion may occur, leading to anemia and intrauterine growth retardation in one twin with hydramnios and heart failure in the other. Frequent prenatal visits and serial ultrasound examinations are used to monitor the development of complications.

a. **Intrapartum management** depends on the presentation and gestational age of the twins, as well as other obstetric factors that are present. Vertex-vertex presentation is most common, followed by vertex-breech presentation. Vaginal delivery of the vertex-vertex presentation is performed unless other complications exist. The delivery of other types of presentations of twins is controversial. If breech delivery is to be attempted vaginally, the same criteria should be used as in singleton gestations.

b. **During labor,** electronic fetal heart rate monitoring is performed on both fetuses. The progress of labor is followed as in singletons. Oxytocin may be used if a protraction or arrest disorder occurs. Delivery is performed in a delivery/operating room with anesthesia personnel and pediatric team in attendance. After delivery of the first infant, ultrasound and vaginal examination are performed to ascertain the position of the second fetus. For vertex presentations, the membranes are ruptured when the head is engaged to facilitate monitoring. Oxytocin is used if regular contractions fail to resume. After delivery of the second infant and placentas, the patient is closely observed for hemorrhage.

H. **Fetal malformations.** Hydrocephalus and fetal tumors, such as cystic hygroma, abdominal tumors, and sacrococcygeal teratomas may be the cause of dystocia. Dystocia may occur before descent of the head, as in hydrocephalus, or may occur later as an abdominal dystocia. Today, with the liberal use of ultrasound, many congenital anomalies are being detected prior to labor. Hydrocephalus may be suspected in labor when large fontanelles and widespread suture lines are present or an indentable cranium is palpated on vaginal examination. Cesarean section is the treatment of choice when dystocia is caused by one of these.

III. Pelvis abnormalities

A. **Dystocia** may also be caused by

1. **Pelvic tumors** occupying the pelvis such as uterine leiomyomata and ovarian tumors.
2. **Abnormal bony pelvis** secondary to malnutrition, heredity, kyphosis, scoliosis, or trauma.
3. **Vaginal abnormalities** such as a longitudinal or transverse vaginal septum.
4. **Cervical abnormalities** secondary to scar tissue from previous cone biopsy or cerclage.

B. **Diagnosis.** Clinical pelvimetry prenatally and in labor can be used to assess the adequacy of the bony pelvis, although unless grossly abnormal, most will advocate augmentation with oxytocin when dystocia occurs. X-ray and CT pelvimetry are reserved in most cases for decisions about breech vaginal delivery. Causes of soft tissue dystocia are diagnosed by vaginal examination or ultrasound.

IV. Other abnormalities of labor

A. **Cord prolapse.** Umbilical cord prolapse occurs more commonly with breech presentations, transverse lie, and polyhydramnios. It may occur with artificial rupture of the membranes if the head is not well applied to the cervix. While a hand holds up the presenting part and the patient is placed in Trendelenburg's position, preparations are made for emergency cesarean section. If cord prolapse occurs with a malpresentation and the fetal heart rate is normal, no manipulation of the fetus should be made before emergent cesarean section is performed.

B. **Uterine rupture** may occur in a previously surgically scarred uterus, with trauma, or spontaneously. It may be asymptomatic (uterine window) and be noted at time of repeat cesarean section or cause fetal distress, hemorrhage, or fetal death, or a combination. **Risk factors** for uterine rupture in labor are previous uterine operation, overdistended uterus, and injudicious use of oxytocin.

1. **Incidence.** 1 in 1500 deliveries.
2. **Diagnosis.** In labor, uterine rupture is often diagnosed by the onset of fetal distress, vaginal bleeding, and abdominal pain. A change in abdominal contour

may be noted. A loss of uterine pressure may be noted if an internal pressure catheter is present. Rupture of the lower segment of the uterus may remain asymptomatic until vaginal delivery has occurred and postpartum hemorrhage ensues. With trauma, as in a motor vehicle accident, fetal distress or fetal death may be a sign that uterine rupture or abruption has occurred.

3. **Management.** With diagnosis of uterine rupture, immediate emergency cesarean section should be performed. In most cases, the uterine defect can be repaired and hysterectomy avoided. The integrity of the bladder should be checked intraoperatively.

C. **Abruption.** See Chap. 20.

D. **Shoulder dystocia**

1. **Incidence.** 1 in 300 deliveries.
2. **Risk factors.** Diabetes, suspected macrosomic infant, obesity, prolonged second stage, midpelvic delivery by forceps or vacuum, previous shoulder dystocia.
3. **Morbidity.** Fractured clavicle or humerus, brachial plexus injury, asphyxia, fetal or neonatal death.
4. **Management.** The impeding factor of most shoulder dystocias is the impaction of the anterior shoulder beneath the symphysis pubis. Many shoulder dystocias will resolve with the McRoberts maneuver, which consists of flexing the thighs at the hips and pulling them to the maternal abdomen [10]. Suprapubic pressure by an assistant may be used concomitantly. A generous episiotomy should be cut. If this is not successful, Wood's corkscrew maneuver may be used. The shoulders are rotated 180 degrees or to an oblique diameter, disengaging the impacted shoulder. Delivery of the posterior arm is also sometimes used but associated with a greater incidence of humerus and clavicle fractures. A method of last resort, the Zavanelli maneuver, has been described in which the head is replaced back into the vagina and cesarean section performed [21].

V. **Third-stage abnormalities**

A. **Retained placenta.**

1. **Diagnosis.** Retained placenta is diagnosed when the placenta has not delivered spontaneously within 30 minutes of delivery.
2. **Etiology.** Most cases of retained placenta are idiopathic; however, rarely **placenta accreta** is the cause, which is abnormal penetration of the placenta to the deciduomyometrial junction. **Placenta increta** is penetration into the myometrium, and **placenta percreta** is penetration through to the serosal surface of the uterus.
3. **Management.** If the placenta remains undelivered after gentle traction on the umbilical cord while performing the Brandt-Andrews maneuver (see Fig. 27-13), and 30 minutes have passed since delivery of the infant, the vagina and cervix should be examined manually. If the placenta has not passed through the cervix into the vagina, manual extraction is necessary. Anesthesia personnel should be summoned. The perineum and vagina are prepared with Betadine. After establishment of adequate general or regional anesthesia, the entire hand is placed inside the uterus. After location of the placenta, the fingers shear the placenta off the uterine wall, starting at the edges of the placenta, developing a plane of separation. After the entire placenta is manually separated from the uterine wall, the hand grasps the placenta and removes it from the uterus. The uterine cavity is then checked for retained fragments. A gauze sponge wrapped around two fingers is useful for this purpose. Occasionally curettage with a Hunter's curet may be necessary for adherent fragments. Oxytocin is administered. Methylergonovine maleate (Methergine), 0.2 mg, or 15-methylprostaglandin 0.25 mg (1 ampule) IM, may be necessary if uterine atony is present.

B. **Uterine inversion**

1. **Incidence.** 1 in 15,000 deliveries.
2. **Diagnosis.** Uterine inversion can be **complete** or **partial.** Complete uterine inversion usually presents as a mass attached to the placenta as it delivers. Partial uterine inversion may be noted with uterine exploration for postpartum hemorrhage.

3. **Management.** Anesthesia personnel should be summoned emergently. Immediately after discovery, the placenta is removed and attempts are made to replace the uterus back into the pelvis with firm, steady pressure on the fundus. Tocolytic agents such as terbutaline or magnesium sulfate may be used to relax the uterus [5]. General anesthesia using halothane will also permit uterine relaxation sufficient to replace the uterus in cases where initial attempts have failed. Laparotomy rarely may be necessary to reinvert the uterus. After the uterus is successfully replaced, oxytocin is administered. Methylergonovin maleate (Methergine), 0.2 mg IM, or 15-methylprostaglandin, 1 ampule (250 μg) IM, or both, may also be administered to prevent or treat atony.

C. **Postpartum hemorrhage.** See Chap. 32.

VI. **Operative delivery**

A. **Forceps**

1. **Definitions** are from ACOG [2].
   a. **Outlet forceps.** The requirements include that "the scalp is visible at the introitus without separating the labia, the fetal skull has reached the pelvic floor, the sagittal suture is in the anterioposterior diameter or in the right or left occiput anterior or posterior position, and the fetal head is at or on the perineum" [2]. This excludes rotations of greater than 45 degrees.
   b. **Low forceps.** "The application of forceps when the leading point of the skull is at station +2 or more" [2]. This category also includes rotations of greater than 45 degrees.
   c. **Midforceps.** "The application of forceps when the head is engaged but the leading point of the skull is above station +2" [2].
2. **Types.** Variations between forceps include differences in shanks, locking mechanisms, fenestration of blades, and modifications for special uses (Fig. 30-8).
   a. **Parallel shank** (Simpson's, DeLee, Hawks-Dennen). This type is particularly useful for the molded, long fetal head.
   b. **Overlapping shank** (Elliot, Tucker-McLane, Luikart, Laufe). This type is useful for the round, unmolded head.
   c. **Piper.** This type of forceps is used with breech presentation for the delivery of the aftercoming head.
   d. **Barton and Kielland's forceps** are used for rotations of 90 degrees or more.
3. **Principles.** Indications for the use of forceps include prolonged second stage, fetal distress, or maternal conditions such as cardiac disease. Before the decision is made to perform a forceps operation, fetal position, station, and size should be carefully evaluated. Preparations for forceps delivery include establishing adequate anesthesia by pudendal, spinal, or epidural block and emptying the bladder with a catheter. Electronic fetal monitoring is performed throughout the procedure. For direct occiput anterior or occiput posterior positions, the left blade, held by the left thumb and forefinger, is inserted on the maternal left side, guided by the right hand into the vagina. The opposite is repeated for the right blade. Each blade is inserted into the posterior vagina and gently guided into place on its respective side, with the handle starting almost perpendicular to the floor and sweeping in an arc to the horizontal in the midline. If the forceps application is correct, the shanks should lock without difficulty. Before traction is applied, the application is checked. The sagittal suture should be equidistant from the blades. The posterior fontanelle should be one finger-breadth above the level of the shanks for the occiput anterior position. Traction is applied downward during contractions, with the patient pushing. Episiotomy is performed when the fetal head distends the perineum.
4. **Outcome.** Fetal complications of forceps deliveries include facial palsies, cephalohematomas, skull fractures, brachial plexus palsies, asphyxia, hyperbilirubinemia, death, and intracranial hemorrhage. Maternal complications of forceps deliveries include vaginal, cervical, rectal, and bladder lacerations; pelvic hematomas; and hemorrhage. Most authorities agree that properly performed outlet forceps operations should have morbidity rates similar to spontaneous vaginal deliveries. Most would also agree that "difficult" midforceps operations have little place in modern obstetrics. Controversy exists whether

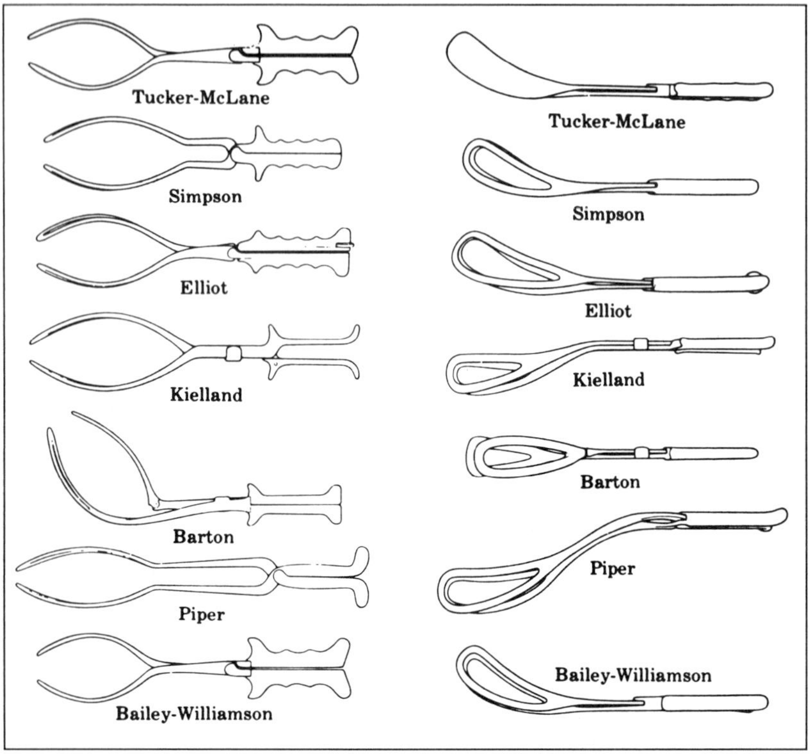

Fig. 30-8. Commonly used forceps. (From R. Douglas and W. Stromme, *Operative Obstetrics* [3rd ed.]. New York: Appleton-Century-Crofts, 1976.)

any midforceps procedures should be performed today. Hayasi [11] and Friedman [9] have addressed opposite points of view in two interesting reviews of the literature on the safety of midforceps.

B. Vacuum extraction

1. Types

a. Malmström. Metal cup, first vacuum extractor.

b. Silastic cup. Pliable, electric pump.

c. Mityvac. Plastic, hand pump.

2. Principles. Indications and preparations for the use of a vacuum extractor are similar to that for forceps. The vacuum extractor is applied to the fetal head, checking that no vaginal tissue is underneath the suction cup. Vacuum is applied only during contractions. The woman is encouraged to push.

3. Outcome. Reported fetal complications include cephalohematomas, brachial plexus palsies, hyperbilirubinemia, asphyxia, and retinal and intracranial hemorrhage. Vaginal and rectal lacerations are the more common maternal complications. Vacuum extraction and forceps deliveries have been compared and vacuum extraction found to be associated with less maternal trauma and more shoulder dystocia, fetal cosmetic injuries, and neonatal jaundice than forceps deliveries. No significant difference was found in the incidence of cephalohematomas [4].

C. Cesarean section

1. Types

a. The **low transverse (Kehr's) uterine incision** is the most commonly performed, as this is least likely to rupture with subsequent pregnancies. If separation of the scar occurs, it is more likely to be incomplete (**uterine window**) and less likely to be catastrophic.

b. The **vertical or classic uterine incision** extends into the thicker portion of the myometrium and is used when the lower uterine segment is undeveloped, such as a preterm footling breech or transverse lie. The risk of rupture during labor is several times greater and more likely to be complete, thus a trial of labor is contraindicated. Elective repeat cesarean section should be scheduled at 38 weeks, provided fetal lung maturity is documented.

c. The **low vertical incision** theoretically is contained within the lower uterine segment, thus reducing the risk of subsequent rupture. However, in most instances where this incision is chosen, the lower uterine segment is not well developed and the incision extends into the main body of the uterus.

2. Indications. Failure to progress, fetal distress, malpresentation, active herpes, placenta previa, prior cesarean section.

3. Morbidity. Endometritis; wound infection; anesthetic accident; bladder, ureter, vascular, or bowel injury; cervical lacerations; thromboembolic events; hemorrhage; pulmonary and urinary infections; ileus; iatrogenic prematurity; transient tachypnea of the newborn; fetal scalp laceration. The infectious morbidity can be reduced by using prophylactic antibiotics in cases with rupture of membranes or labor.

4. Vaginal delivery after cesarean section is an option that should be offered to women with prior low transverse cesarean sections and with no recurrent obstetric reason for cesarean section. The overall success rate is approximately 79% [7]. The risk of rupture in labor with a prior low transverse cesarean section is approximately 0.7% [14, 17]. The risk of dehiscence (uterine window) is 4% in both trials of labor or elective repeat cesarean section [17]. Vaginal delivery after prior cesarean section for cephalopelvic disproportion or failure to progress has a success rate of 61%. Half of the women in one trial delivered infants larger than those delivered at the cesarean section for failure to progress [24]. Recently more reports of trials of labor following multiple cesarean sections have emerged. The success and morbidity rates appear to be similar to vaginal delivery after one previous section [19].

5. Elective repeat cesarean section. The most significant preventable complication of elective repeat cesarean section is **iatrogenic prematurity.** If performed at 38 weeks' completed gestational age, fetal lung maturity should be demonstrated by an lecithin-sphingomyelin ratio of at least 2 : 1 or if **phosphtidylglycerol** is present. At 39 weeks, it may be performed without amniocentesis, if dates were confirmed with pelvic examination prior to 16 weeks' gestation, heart tones auscultated 30 weeks prior by Doppler or 20 weeks prior by fetoscope, and either a positive pregnancy test 36 weeks prior or ultrasound prior to 24 weeks [1]. An additional option for patients with a prior low transverse uterine scar is to wait for the onset of labor. This is especially useful in the patient with uncertain dates or late care, thus obviating the need for amniocentesis.

References

1. ACOG. Assessment of Fetal Maturity Prior to Repeat Cesarean Delivery or Elective Induction of Labor. ACOG Committee Opinion No. 72, August 1989.
2. ACOG. Obstetric Forceps. ACOG Committee Opinion No. 71, August 1989.
3. Brenner, W. E., Bruce, R. D., and Hendricks, C. H. The characteristics and perils of breech presentation. *Am. J. Obstet. Gynecol.* 118:700, 1974.
4. Broekhuizen, F. F., et al. Vacuum extraction versus forceps delivery: Indications and complications, 1979–1984. *Obstet. Gynecol.* 69:338, 1987.
5. Catanzarite, V. A., et al. New approaches to the management of acute puerperal uterine inversion. *Obstet. Gynecol.* 68:7S, 1986.
6. Collea, J. V., Chein, C., and Quilligan, E. J. The randomized management of

term frank breech presentation: A study of 208 cases. *Am. J. Obstet. Gynecol.* 137:235, 1980.
7. Flamm, B. L. Vaginal birth after cesarean section: Controversies old and new. *Clin. Obstet. Gynecol.* 28:735, 1985.
8. Friedman, E. A. Dysfunctional Labor (Vol. 2). In J. J. Sciaar (ed.), *Gynecology and Obstetrics*. New York: Lippincott, 1988. Pp. 7–8.
9. Friedman, E. A. Midforceps delivery: No? *Clin. Obstet. Gynecol.* 30:93, 1987.
10. Gonik, B., Stringer, C. A., and Held, B. An alternate maneuver for management of shoulder dystocia. *Am. J. Obstet. Gynecol.* 145:882, 1983.
11. Hayashi, R. H. Midforceps delivery: Yes? *Clin. Obstet. Gynecol.* 30:90, 1987.
12. Induction and augmentation of labor. *ACOG Tech. Bull.* 110, November, 1987.
13. Kopelman, J. N., et al. Computed tomographic pelvimetry in the evaluation of breech presentation. *Obstet. Gynecol.* 68:455, 1986.
14. Lavin, J. P., et al. Vaginal delivery in patients with a prior cesarean section. *Obstet. Gynecol.* 59:135, 1982.
15. Lupe, P. J., and Gross, T. L. Maternal upright posture and mobility in labor—A review. *Obstet. Gynecol.* 67:727, 1986.
16. National Institutes of Health Consensus Development Task Force. Statement on cesarean childbirth. *Am. J. Obstet. Gynecol.* 139:902, 1981.
17. Nielsen, T. F., Ljungblad, U., and Hagberg, H. Rupture and dehiscence of cesarean section scar during pregnancy and delivery. *Am. J. Obstet. Gynecol.* 160:569, 1989.
18. O'Driscoll, K., Foley, M., and MacDonald, D. Active management of labor as an alternative to cesarean section for dystocia. *Obstet. Gynecol.* 63:485, 1984.
19. Phelan, J. P., et al. Vaginal birth after cesarean. *Am. J. Obstet. Gynecol.* 157:150, 1987.
20. Read, J. A., Miller, F. C., and Paul, R. C. Randomized trial of ambulation versus oxytocin for labor enhancement: A preliminary report. *Am. J. Obstet. Gynecol.* 139:669, 1981.
21. Sandberg, E. C. The Zavanelli maneuver: A potentially revolutionary method for the resolution of shoulder dystocia. *Am. J. Obstet. Gynecol.* 1551:479, 1985.
22. Seitchik, J. The management of functional dystocia in the first stage of labor. *Clin. Obstet. Gynecol.* 30(1):42, 1987.
23. Seitchik, J., et al. Oxytocin augmentation of dysfunctional labor. IV. Oxytocin pharmacokinetics. *Am. J. Obstet. Gynecol.* 150:225–228, 1984.
24. Seitchik, J., and Rao, V. Cesarean delivery in nulliparous women for failed oxytocin-augmented labor: Route of delivery in subsequent pregnancy. *Am. J. Obstet. Gynecol.* 143:393, 1982.
25. Van Dorsten, J. P., Schifrin, B. S., and Wallace, R. L. Randomized control trial of external cephalic version with tocolysis in late pregnancy. *Am. J. Obstet. Gynecol.* 141:417, 1981.

31 Diseases of the Placenta

Richard H. Oi

The placenta is a fetal organ, the development and function of which are directly related to the growth and well-being of the fetus. Many indirect ways of assessing antepartum placental function that contribute to the intrauterine evaluation of the fetus are being and have been developed. Direct examination and assessment of the placenta, while possible only during the postnatal period, still can contribute to the assessment of the neonate, help to explain certain antenatal events, and aid in the management of the puerpera. The placenta should be briefly examined immediately on its delivery, specifically to anticipate retained fragments or cotyledons, and should be reexamined more thoroughly after completion of the postdelivery evaluation. Cord blood is conveniently obtained after delivery of the infant and prior to placental delivery. The subsequent placental examination should be conducted in a systematic fashion and a schema consistently used.

Placental Examination

I. Size and weight

A. The normal weight ratio of placenta to fetus at term is 1 : 6 to 1 : 7. The placenta usually is discoid and measures 15–20 cm in its greater diameter and 2–3 cm in its thickest portion. It weighs between 400 and 600 gm.

B. Large placentas with weight ratios of 1 : 3 and 1 : 2 are seen with severe erythroblastosis, congenital syphilis, and some class A–C diabetic pregnancies. A less prominent alteration of the placental-fetal ratio is seen in pregnancies of chronic cigarette smokers, who have a slight increase in placental versus fetal weight.

C. Small placentas may be seen in patients with chronic hypertension, as well as with pregnancy-induced hypertension. This change in placental weight is associated with intrauterine growth retardation or small-for-gestational-age infants.

II. The umbilical cord averages 50–70 cm long and should be examined for knots, the pattern of insertion into the fetal surface of the placenta or membranes, and the number of vessels present in the cord. A cord length of at least 40 cm seems necessary in order not to complicate normal vaginal delivery.

A. True knots occur in approximately 1% of deliveries and lead to a perinatal loss of approximately 6%. They probably occur as a result of fetal tumbling movements and a cord of excessive length and may contribute to signs of fetal bradycardia in labor. **False knots** are focal dilatations or varices of the umbilical vessels and are of no clinical significance.

B. Nuchal cord (loops of cord around the fetal neck) occurs in approximately 20–24% of deliveries and usually is associated with a cord length of greater than 70 cm. It does not usually cause any fetal morbidity or mortality but may be the cause of fetal heart rate decelerations during labor.

C. The cord insertion into the fetal surface is generally in the central portion but slightly eccentric.

1. In a **battledore placenta,** the cord insertion is at the placental margin, and except for occasional inadvertent separation on traction during delivery, it is of no clinical significance (Fig. 31-1).

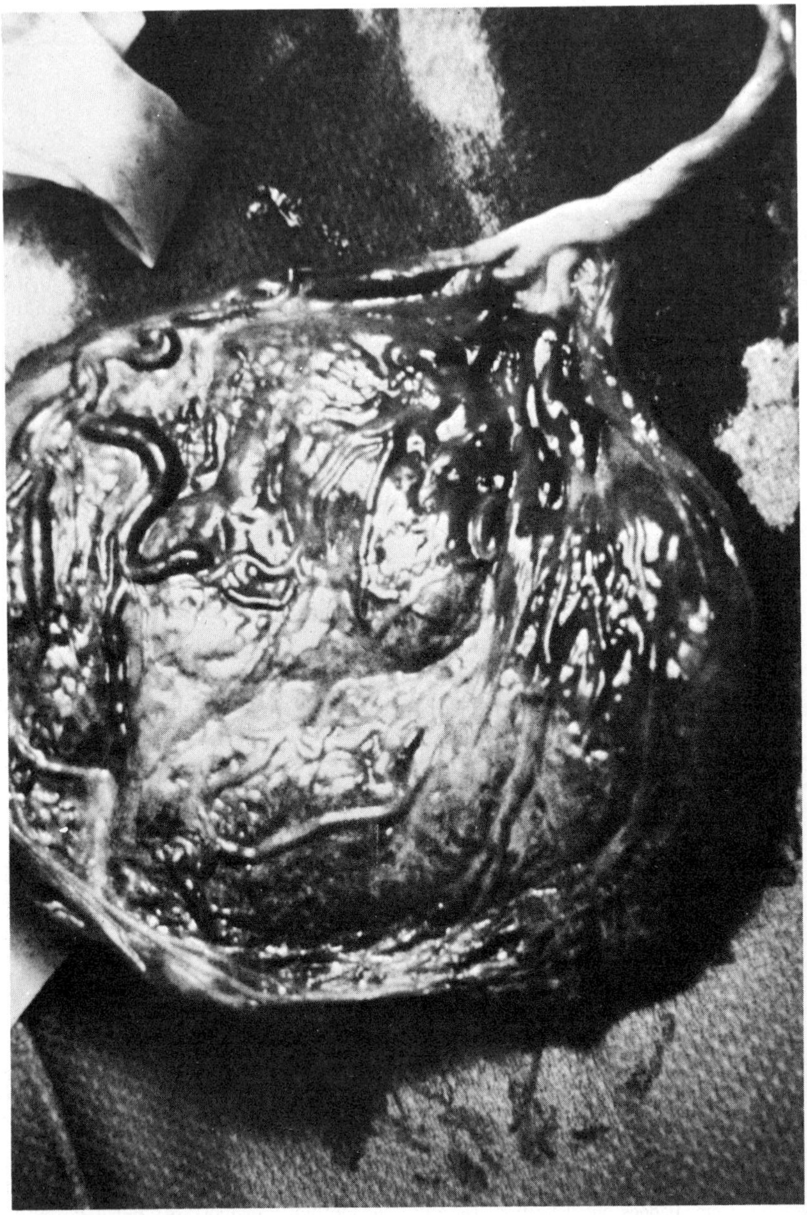

Fig. 31-1. Battledore placenta.

2. **Velamentous (membranous) insertions**

a. In these insertions, the umbilical cord inserts on the placental membranes and traverses the membranes before being distributed onto the fetal surface of the placenta (Fig. 31-2). That portion of membranes containing the fetal vessels may present over the cervical os and in front of the fetal presenting part; this constitutes **vasa praevia.** Vasa praevia should be suspected when rupture of the membranes during labor is attended by a bloody discharge. Prompt intervention is indicated to avoid fetal exsanguination. Rarely, an anemic, distressed, flaccid fetus will be delivered and should be transfused immediately if a velamentous insertion with torn fetal vessels is noted. Velamentous vessels are encountered with greater frequency in twin placentas, and fetal hemorrhage with exsanguination of one or both fetuses may occur.

b. Velamentous insertions occur in approximately 1% of singleton placentas, and up to 25% of infants may have defects unrelated to chromosomal abnormalities.

D. Absence of one umbilical artery

1. Of singleton pregnancies, 0.2–1.1% will demonstrate a single umbilical artery in the cord, which may indicate that anomalies are present in the infant. The malformations are not specific to any organ system, are frequently multiple, and are often lethal. The anomalies include those of the genitourinary and cardiovascular systems, cleft palates, and musculoskeletal abnormalities. Low birth weight is seen more frequently when only a single artery is found in the cord, and the finding of only one artery is more prevalent in diabetic mothers as well as with autosomal trisomies. The incidence of anomalies associated

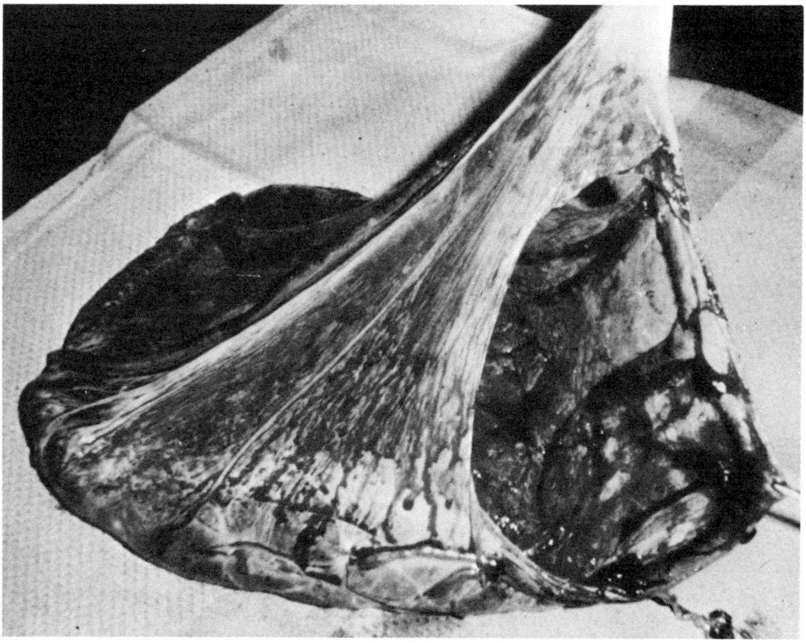

Fig. 31-2. Velamentous insertion with fetal vessels coursing through the membranes. Note vessel paralleling the margin of ruptured membranes.

with a single umbilical artery ranges from 25–50%; this finding, therefore, necessitates careful evaluation of the neonate.

2. Twin pregnancies have a higher incidence of a single umbilical artery (7%) in one of the twins, but this usually is not associated with the same degree of risk of congenital anomalies as in singleton pregnancies.

III. Maternal surface

A. Postpartum hemorrhage

1. Retention of placental cotyledons

a. Etiology. Fragments of placental cotyledons may be retained in the uterus after delivery of the placenta, and serious hemorrhage may result.

b. Evaluation and treatment. The retention of the cotyledons can be suspected by noting areas of disruption on the maternal surface. Immediate, careful, and thorough exploration of the uterine cavity should be performed to remove any remaining fragments. Occasionally, general anesthesia may be required to relax the uterus and to alleviate the discomfort of the procedure.

2. Another cause of serious hemorrhage in the postpartum period is a **retained succenturiate** (accessory) **lobe** of the placenta (see sec. **IV.F**).

B. Retroplacental clots or hematomas

1. The presence of clots on the maternal surface may be associated with

a. Marginal sinus or lake rupture. Clots noted at the margin of the placenta found in pregnancies that are delivered after what appears clinically to be a minor degree of abruption are designated as marginal sinus or marginal lake rupture. This is often the only finding in cases of third-trimester bleeding in which placenta previa and abruptio placentae are ruled out.

b. Abruptio placentae. Retroplacental hematomas are seen with abruptio placentae and may present as a fresh, adherent clot or as an older hematoma that has caused a depression in the maternal surface and become firm and laminated. They may also be seen in placentas complicated by toxemia of pregnancy without clinical evidence of abruption. The surface area occupied by the clot correlates, in general, but not consistently, with the clinical severity of the abruption.

2. **Evaluation and confirmation** occur after the fact, the therapy for abruption having been accomplished by delivery of the fetus and placenta.

C. Intervillous fibrin deposition can be identified as innumerable, irregular, speckled areas of whitish fibrinous material that on light palpation of the maternal surface gives a granular sensation. This is accentuated when **calcifications** also are present. These changes are seen most frequently in mature placentas and do not appear to have any clinical significance.

D. Infarctions of the placenta can occasionally be suspected when a relatively focal, firm, organized area is noted on the maternal surface (Fig. 31-3). More often, however, infarctions are identified only by taking multiple sections through the placenta and identifying either acute hemorrhage infarctions or older, more organized infarctions.

1. Infarctions frequently are seen at the placental margin and represent physiologic changes of degeneration and atrophy. They may be seen throughout the placenta in normal pregnancies but more often are associated with pathologic pregnancies, especially with toxemia or maternal chronic vascular disease.

2. Fresh infarctions appear as dark purplish areas contiguous with the decidual surface. As infarctions become older, they appear yellow and pale to gray-white, and they become firm.

3. True infarctions occur when the spiral arterioles leading into the intervillous space are compromised. Prolonged vascular spasm such as with toxemia or thrombosis in vessels narrowed by atheromatous lesions secondary to hypertensive disorders of pregnancy may lead to placental infarctions. Fetal compromise may occur, resulting in growth retardation. Placental abruptions and infarctions often are seen together as they are both the result of vascular compromise.

IV. Fetal surface

A. Fetal membranes over the placenta are thin and translucent, beneath which a steel-blue hue is noted on the fetal surface.

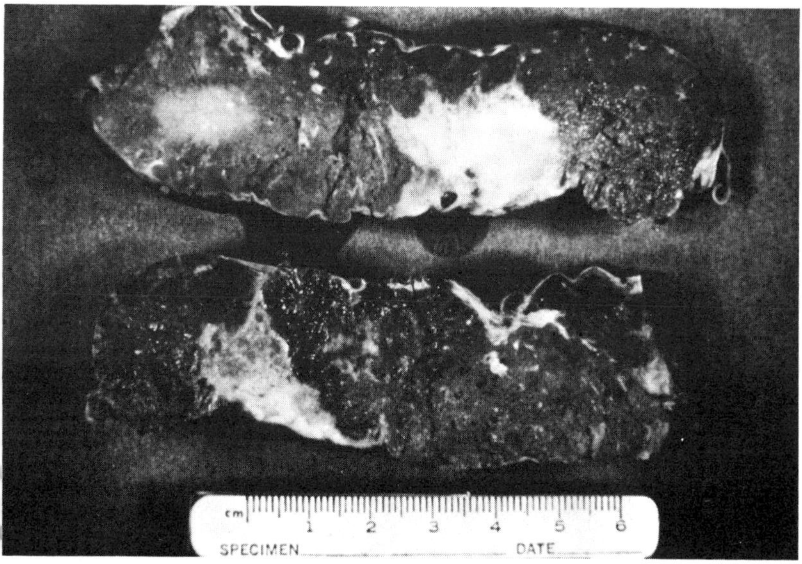

Fig. 31-3. Infarctions of the placenta with the base of the infarction at the decidual margin of the placenta.

1. **Meconium staining** can be identified as a brown-green stain that can be removed easily if the staining is recent.
2. **Chorioamnionitis** is associated with an opaque, whitish, thickened membrane over the fetal surface in a placenta that, in addition, may have a foul odor.

B. Subchorionic fibrin deposition appears as either small nodules or larger collections of gray-white fibrinlike material beneath the chorionic plate. This usually is seen in mature placentas and does not have any known clinical significance.

C. Chorionic cysts up to 4–5 cm in diameter may occur on the fetal surface of the placenta; they appear as thin-walled cystic structures containing clear serous or gelatinous material. Hemorrhage may occur into these cysts. They seem not to have any clinical significance.

D. Amnion nodosum

1. **Description.** This appears as multiple 2- to 3-mm gray-white plaquelike deposits on the fetal surface, especially near the insertion of the umbilical cord (Fig. 31-4). These are surface deposits of fetal squamous cells (vernix) and are dislodged easily.
2. **Evaluation.** These deposits are seen in instances of oligohydramnios and therefore are consistently associated with some anomaly or abnormality of the urinary system (e.g., renal agenesis [Potter's disease], cystic kidneys, or obstruction of the urinary system). This finding should be reported immediately to the neonatologist attending the infant.

E. Squamous metaplasia also appears as small gray-white granules on the fetal membranes but, unlike amnion nodosum, is not removed easily. It is seen in mature placentas but only infrequently in immature placentas. It has no clinical significance other than suggesting a mature gestation.

F. Succenturiate lobes

1. **Description.** These are accessory lobes of the placenta that may be located at various distances from the placental margin and may be another cause of serious hemorrhage in the postpartum period. They probably represent persistent areas of the chorionic tissue that did not undergo atrophy (the chorion

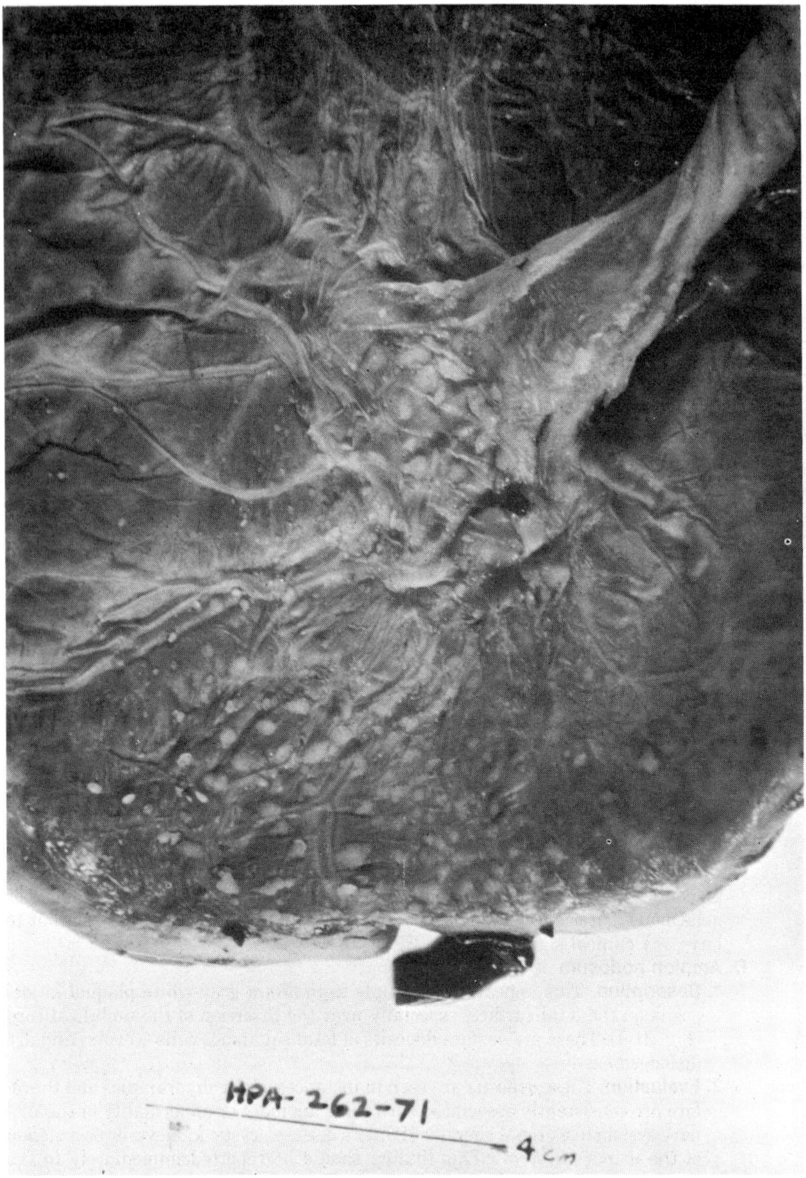

Fig. 31-4. Amnion nodosum.

laeve). Fetal arterial and venous vessels, instead of eventually penetrating into the chorionic plate before reaching the placental margin, will be seen to continue over the membranes to the accessory lobe (Fig. 31-5).

2. **Evaluation and treatment.** The presence of disrupted vessels **at the placental margin** is diagnostic of a succenturiate lobe, and prompt exploration of the uterine cavity is indicated to remove the accessory lobe. As with retained cotyledons, exploration and removal can be accomplished without additional analgesia or anesthesia, but on occasion general anesthesia may be necessary.

G. **Circumvallate placenta.** The presence of chorionic villi beyond the chorionic plate, which is outlined by a fold of chorion laeve, characterizes a circumvallate placenta (Fig. 31-6). If the fold occurs at the placental margin, **placenta marginata** is the designation.

1. **Significance.** Clinically, hemorrhage and premature labor and, in some instances, hydrorrhea have been noted with circumvallate placentas. More often, however, a circumvallate placenta is an incidental finding at delivery.
2. **Evaluation and treatment.** A circumvallate placenta should be considered when uterine contractions, hydrorrhea, and intermittent bleeding occur in the late second and early third trimesters of pregnancy. There is no specific therapy other than expectant management. In most instances, premature labor and delivery occur.

Twin Placentas

I. **Classification of fetal membranes**

A. **Dichorionic, diamniotic twin placenta.** Each twin has developed within its own amniotic as well as chorionic membrane. Thus what separates the twins can be shown to consist of two thin, translucent amniotic membranes that are separated

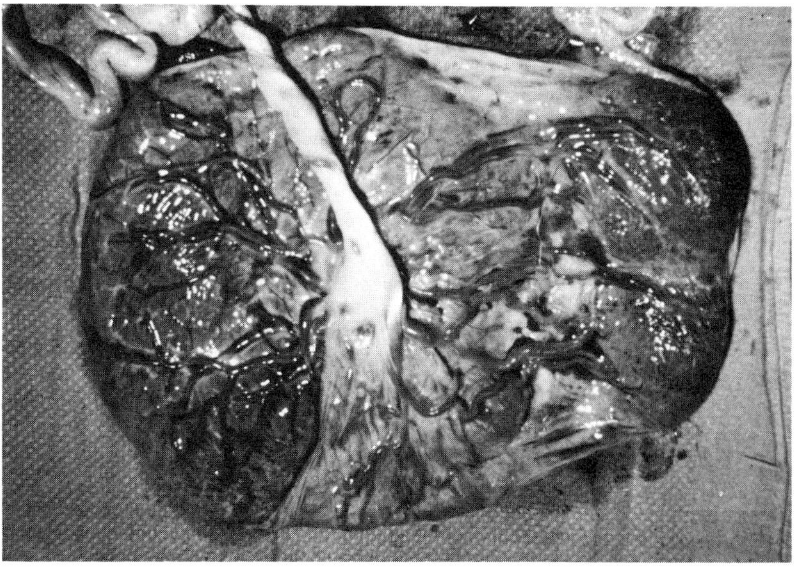

Fig. 31-5. Succenturiate lobe. Note fetal vessels reaching the edge of the placenta and extending for a short distance over the membranes to an accessory lobe (*to the right*).

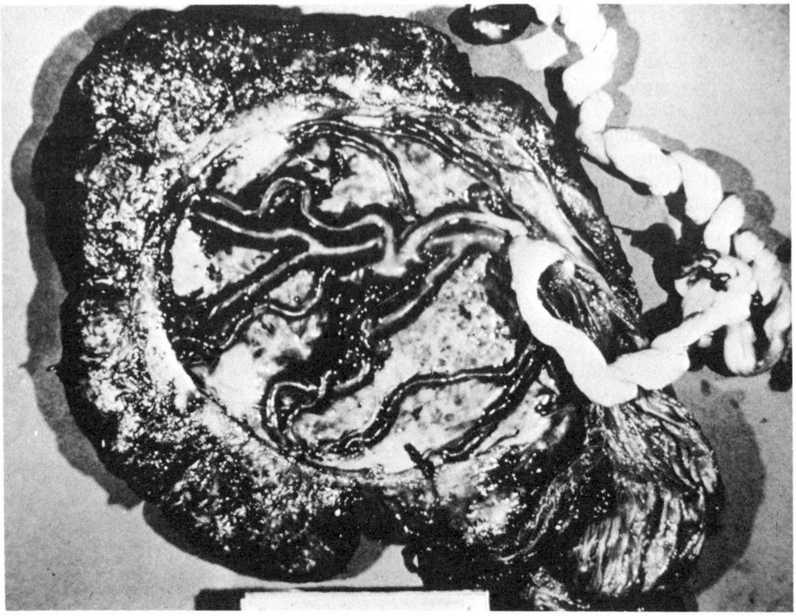

Fig. 31-6. Circumvallate placenta. The chorionic plate appears to be limited by a circumferential fibrous band beyond which there is further placental development.

easily and "peeled" from the intervening fused chorionic membranes of each twin. This can, however, be misleading, and confirmation is best obtained by histologic section of the membranes occurring between the fetal compartments.

B. Monochorionic, diamniotic twin placenta. Each twin has developed its own amniotic membrane and both are surrounded by a single chorionic membrane. The fused amniotic membranes separating the twins can be peeled from each other without any intervening chorion, since the chorionic membrane encircles both amniotic cavities and arises from the placental margins only. Histologic sections will confirm the presence of two amnions without an intervening chorionic membrane.

C. Monoamniotic, monochorionic placentas will not have any membranous structures separating the twins. Instead, the fetal surface will show the two umbilical cords closely approximated in their insertions. Cord entanglements with obstruction of the fetal circulation may occur and cause fetal death.

D. Monochorionic twins experience a greater perinatal loss than with dichorionic placentation, especially as related to vascular anastomoses. **Vascular anastomoses** only occur in monochorionic twin placentas and are the rule, rather than the exception, in these instances. Depending on what vessels are involved in the anastomoses (arterial-to-arterial, arterial-to-venous, venous-to-venous) and what caliber of vessel is involved (large vessels on the chorionic plate or vessels at the level of the cotyledons), various effects may be noted:

1. Completely normal infants
2. Twin transfusion syndrome—severe hydramnios and unequal development of the twins
3. Normal twin with an acardiac monster or fetus papyraceous

II. Monozygotic versus dizygotic twins

A. Monozygotic. Single-ovum twins can be associated with all of the three types of placentation, depending on when the twinning occurred relative to placental formation. Most demonstrate monochorionic placentation, but approximately 30% have dichorionic placentas.

B. Dizygotic. Twins from two fertilized ova always have dichorionic placentas, and the placentas are fused in most instances.

III. Umbilical cord

A. Velamentous insertions are more common in twin placentas.

B. Cords with a single umbilical artery also are more common (7%).

Neoplasms of the Placenta

Only two significant neoplastic processes occur in the placenta: chorioangioma and trophoblastic proliferations.

I. Chorioangioma is a benign proliferation of fetal capillaries usually associated with the chorionic plate. It varies in size from a few millimeters to a large tumor of 7–8 cm. Chorioangioma may be associated with hydramnios, congestive heart failures, and fetal malformations, especially with the larger tumors. Maternal complications such as toxemia and possibly abruptio placentae may also be associated with chorioangiomas. However they are more commonly found incidentally at the delivery of a normal infant.

II. Trophoblastic proliferations of the placenta histologically occur as hydatidiform mole, invasive mole (chorioadenoma destruens), and choriocarcinoma.

A. Hydatidiform mole (molar pregnancy)

1. Definition. Hydatidiform moles are abnormal placentas, the villi of which are swollen, edematous, and vesicular, resembling a bunch of grapes (Fig. 31-7). Histologically, edematous villi are noted with absent or, at least, diminished numbers of fetal capillaries; most characteristic is a marked trophoblastic

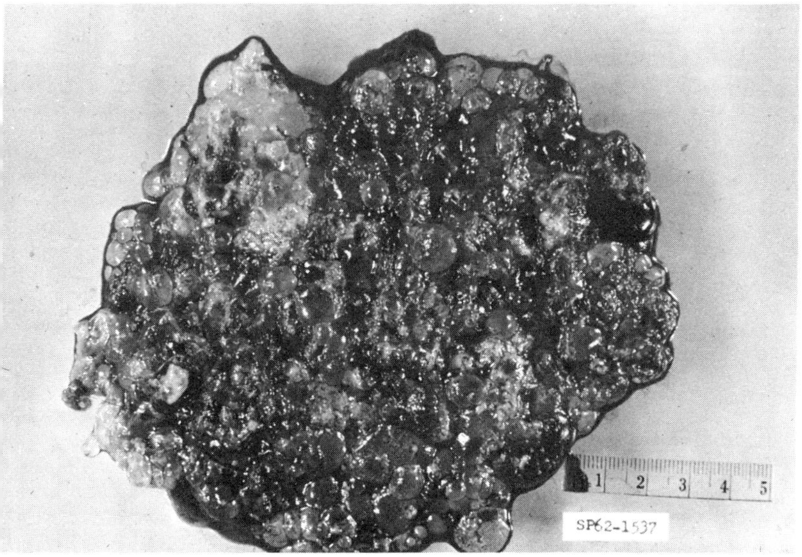

Fig. 31-7. Hydatidiform mole with swollen, edematous, and vesicular villi, resembling a bunch of grapes.

hyperplasia with and without atypia. An occasional hydatidiform mole may be associated with a fetus or fetal tissues and is described as a **partial hydatidiform mole.** Partial moles are predominantly associated with polyploid chromosomal abnormalities, especially triploidy, and are perhaps less often associated with malignant sequelae. **Complete or classic hydatidiform moles** reveal an exclusively female karyotype (XX), but the chromosomal complement is made up of two identical male haplotypes. These moles may originate from a duplication of the male genome without genetic contribution from the female. The reported incidence ranges from 1 in 1000 to 1 in 1700 pregnancies in the United States, and 1 in 125 to 1 in 200 in Taiwan, in other Asian countries, and in Mexico. In the United States, an incidence of 1 in 600 therapeutic abortions has been noted.

2. **Clinical profile**
   a. **Age.** Hydatidiform moles occur more frequently in older women, especially those older than 40 years. They also are reported to occur more frequently in women younger than 20 years. Parity is of no significance.
   b. **Symptoms** (usually occur before the eighteenth week of amenorrhea)
      (1) **Vaginal bleeding** occurs in almost all patients, and substantial quantities of blood may fill the endometrial cavity, causing **uterine enlargement** and **anemia.**
      (2) **Hyperemesis gravidarum** occurs in 20–30% of patients and may require parenteral fluid and electrolyte and antiemetic therapy.
      (3) **Toxemia of pregnancy** occurs in 10–30% of patients. Preeclampsia or eclampsia occurring early in gestation suggests a molar pregnancy.
      (4) Clinical evidence of **hyperthyroidism** with warm skin, tachycardia, tremor and thyroid enlargement occurs in a small percentage of patients. Thyroid storm may occur, precipitated by toxemia or surgical manipulation.
      (5) **Trophoblastic embolization** occurs in 2–3% of patients and is characterized by acute respiratory symptoms of cough, tachypnea, and cyanosis.
      (6) **Disseminated intravascular coagulation** may occur with the onset of symptoms or during therapy, as thromboplastic substances may be released into the maternal circulations.
   c. **Signs**
      (1) In 50% of cases, the **uterus is large for the date of gestation** as a result of the molar tissue proliferation and also because of intrauterine bleeding that distends and enlarges the uterine cavity.
      (2) **Theca lutein cysts** resulting in bilateral ovarian enlargement, 8 cm or larger, occur in 20–40% of cases. They may undergo torsion and become infarcted.
3. **Diagnosis.** The diagnosis should be suspected in an amenorrheic gravida with hyperemesis gravidarum or toxemia before the twenty-fourth week of pregnancy. Thyrotoxicosis and trophoblastic embolization may occur occasionally. The diagnosis should especially be suspected if the uterus is larger than expected for the length of gestation (seen in one-half of cases) or if bilateral ovarian enlargement consistent with theca lutein cysts is noted. Expulsion of hydropic vesicles is prima facie evidence of molar pregnancy, and management may proceed from this finding. Otherwise, the necessary diagnostic procedures include
   a. **Ultrasonography.** Precise diagnosis can be readily made by the characteristic snowstorm pattern of multiple intrauterine echoes.
   b. **Quantitative urinary human chorionic gonadotropin (HCG) excretion.** After 12 weeks of pregnancy, values over 500,000 IU/24 hours usually are associated with moles, and values of greater than 1 million IU/24 hours are almost always associated with hydatidiform moles. Multiple gestations may have levels greater than 500,000 IU and must be considered when titers are disproportionately elevated. Low to normal values, however, have been noted with molar pregnancies. The individual value, therefore, is not diagnostic but helps to confirm the diagnosis and is important as a baseline "tumor marker."

c. **Arteriography** is the ultimate in invasive techniques and rarely is necessary, since confirmation usually can be obtained by ultrasonography.

4. **Management.** Once the diagnosis has been established, prompt **evacuation** of the uterus is indicated, as patients with molar pregnancies are at risk for serious complications, such as blood loss, hypervolemia, toxemia, and thyrotoxicosis. A complete blood cell count (CBC), electrolyte panel, quantitative beta-HCG determination, and chest roentgenogram are obtained. Liver and renal function tests are also useful before evacuation.
   a. **Suction curettage** is the method of choice in evacuating the uterus, especially if the patient is interested in maintaining her reproductive function. Laminaria tents are useful in aiding cervical dilatation, and suction curettage under general anesthesia is performed using the largest vacuum curet available. Blood should be matched and available, and oxytocin, 10–20 units in 1000 ml fluid, should be running during the procedure. Sharp curettage should follow, to remove all molar tissues. These curettings are sent for histologic examination as a separate specimen and are not combined with the initially suctioned material.
   b. **Abdominal hysterectomy** with the molar pregnancy in situ may be performed in patients who are no longer interested in childbearing. Ovarian enlargements caused by theca lutein cysts should not be removed, since they regress spontaneously after removal of the molar tissues and the reduction of the HCG level.
   c. Rh-negative women who are unsensitized, especially those with partial hydatidiform moles in whom fetal tissues are identified, should receive Rh_0 (D) immunoglobulin.

5. **Follow-up**
   a. **Spontaneous remission** occurs in 80% of patients after evaluation, but in 20% malignant sequelae will occur. Careful follow-up evacuation or removal of the molar pregnancy is therefore very important.
   b. **Evaluation**
      (1) **Chest roentgenograms** should be obtained at the time of evacuation and at 4 and 8 weeks postoperatively if the HCG titers are decreasing as expected.
      (2) **Pelvic examination** is performed 2–4 weeks after evaluation and monthly thereafter to detect clinical evidence of recurrence.
      (3) **Quantitative HCG.** Assay for specific HCG beta subunit should be performed every week until three consecutive negative values have been obtained, then every month for six months, and then every two months for six months.
   c. **Effective contraception** must be used during this period, since pregnancy will elevate the HCG titer and confuse the early detection of malignant sequelae. Oral contraception is acceptable.
   d. Three consecutive negative HCG values are considered to be evidence of remission. Subsequent negative titers, as described in sec. **5.b.(3)**, are required before the patient should be allowed to consider pregnancy.
   e. **Recurrent molar pregnancy**
      (1) Recurrent hydatidiform mole incidence ranges from 1 in 150 to 1 in 50.
      (2) There appears to be increased risk of developing malignant sequelae with repetitive moles.

6. **Malignant sequelae** (gestational trophoblastic disease)
   a. **Diagnosis** is based on the following findings:
      (1) There is a twofold or greater increase in titer over any two-week period.
      (2) The level of HCG plateaus with no decline in titer over any three-week interval.
         (a) A postevacuation beta-HCG regression curve can be used to follow the expected decrease in serum HCG levels (Fig. 31-8).
         (b) Use of the curve allows interpretation of limited numbers of titers, especially in the noncompliant patient, avoids overinterpretation of the values, and minimizes the possibility of overtreatment.

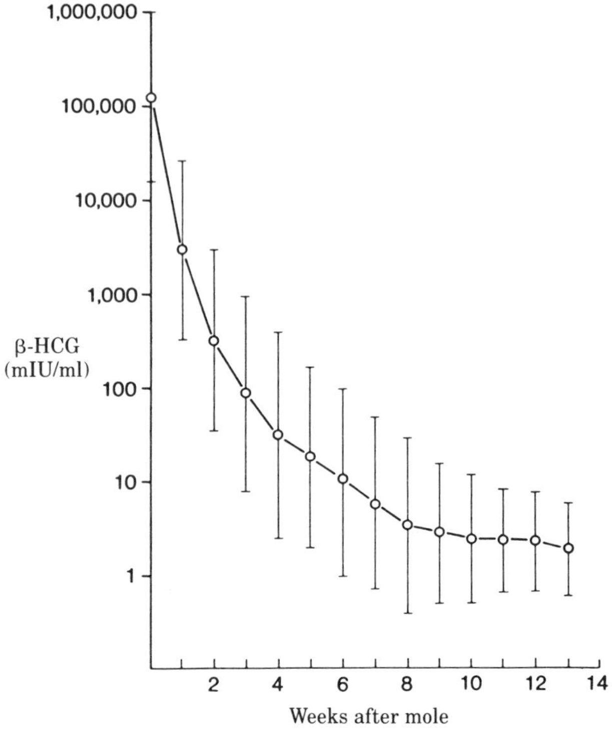

Fig. 31-8. The mean value and 95% confidence limits describing the normal postmolar beta–human chorionic gonadotropin (β-HCG) regression curve. (From J. B. Schlaerth et al., Prognostic characteristics of serum human chorionic gonadotropin titer regression following molar pregnancy. *Obstet. Gynecol.* 58:478, 1981.)

- **(3)** The HCG titer continues to be greater than 500 units 60 days after evacuation.
- **(4)** There is clinical evidence of metastases:
  - **(a)** The chest roentgenogram shows a lesion.
  - **(b)** The uterus is enlarged and there is vaginal bleeding.
  - **(c)** Persistent theca lutein cysts are present.
  - **(d)** Cervical or vaginal metastatic lesions are identified.
  - **(e)** Bizarre neurologic symptoms occur, indicating central nervous system metastasis.

b. Evaluation

- **(1)** Clinical examination to detect evidence of subinvolution, theca lutein cysts, or vaginal lesions
- **(2)** Chest roentgenograms to identify metastases
- **(3)** Blood studies
  - **(a)** CBC, differential cell count, platelet count
  - **(b)** Prothrombin time, partial thromboplastin time
  - **(c)** Electrolytes, blood urea nitrogen (BUN), creatinine
  - **(d)** Liver function studies

(e) Thyroid panel
(f) Blood and Rh typing
(4) Liver and brain scan (computed tomography)
(5) Intravenous pyelogram
(6) Pelvic ultrasonic scan to rule out pregnancy and, if possible, to identify invasion into the myometrium
(7) Beta-HCG titer

c. Determine by this evaluation whether the sequelae represent nonmetastatic trophoblastic disease (NMTD) confined to the uterus or metastatic trophoblastic disease (MTD).

B. Nonmetastatic trophoblastic disease

1. **Definition.** If, after the evaluation just outlined in sec. **A.6.b,** no evidence of disease presents outside the uterus, the diagnosis is NMTD.
   a. NMTD is preceded by molar pregnancy in 75% of cases, with the remainder following term pregnancy, abortion, and ectopic pregnancy (rare).
   b. Histologically, most are **invasive moles** (chorioadenoma destruens).
      (1) Hydropic villi with absent fetal vessels and with marked trophoblastic proliferation are seen invading the myometrium. The tumor may penetrate the full thickness of the myometrium to cause severe intraperitoneal bleeding.
      (2) NMTD is usually locally invasive only and rarely metastatic to lung, vagina, or vulva.
2. **Therapy**
   a. Single-agent chemotherapy with either methotrexate, 0.3–0.4 mg/kg/day IM or IV for 5 days; **or** dactinomycin, 10–12 μg/kg/day IV for 5 days.
      (1) Repeat the course after toxic symptoms subside and the leukocyte count and platelet count return to normal (leukocyte count > 1500, platelet count > 100,000). This usually occurs within 5–10 days, and repeat courses are delivered every two weeks.
      (2) Repeat the liver panel, BUN, serum creatinine, CBC, and pelvic examination before each course.
      (3) Therapy should be continued for one or two courses after the first normal HCG titer is obtained. Titers are then obtained monthly for 12 months, after which the disease is considered in remission.
   b. **Intermittent high-dose methotrexate with folinic acid (citrovorum factor)** appears to be preferred to single-agent chemotherapy as it is less toxic, achieves remission earlier, and requires minimal numbers of courses of therapy.
      (1) Methotrexate, 1 mg/kg IM, is given on days 1, 3, 5, and 7 at 4 P.M., and CBC, platelet count, and liver function studies are obtained at 8 A.M.; citrovorum factor, 0.1 mg/kg IM, is given on days 2, 4, 6, and 8 at 4 P.M.
      (2) Complete blood cell count, platelet count, and liver function tests (especially serum glutamic-oxaloacetic transaminase) are obtained 3 times/week for two weeks and then as often as the situation dictates.
      (3) Subsequent courses
         (a) If weekly HCG titers continue to fall, withhold therapy.
         (b) Administer a second course if (1) the HCG plateaus for two or more weeks or rises; or (2) metastases or new lesions appear.
         (c) Retreat with the second course at the same dose if the response is adequate (i.e., if the HCG has decreased). If the initial response was inadequate, doses of both methotrexate and citrovorum factor are increased by increments of 0.5 mg/kg and 0.05 mg/kg, respectively.
         (d) Failure of response to two consecutive schedules of methotrexate and citrovorum factor is considered drug resistance, and alternative agents should be used.
      (4) Methotrexate and citrovorum factor may be used as an adjuvant to hysterectomy; remove the uterus midway during therapy.
   c. **Toxic symptoms** may occur abruptly and patients are best treated in the hospital.

- **(1)** Bone marrow suppression—leukopenia, thrombocytopenia. Discontinue therapy or do not initiate a new course if
  - **(a)** The white blood cell count is less than 3000/ml and neutrophils number fewer than 1500
  - **(b)** The platelet count is less than 100,000/ml
  - **(c)** The BUN or liver enzymes are elevated significantly
- **(2)** Hepatotoxicity—liver necrosis.
- **(3)** Gastrointestinal toxicity—stomatitis, diarrhea, ulceration, perforation.
- **(4)** Skin reactions—rash, alopecia.

d. If resistance to single-agent therapy occurs—that is, (1) titer is rising, (2) titer plateaus after two courses, (3) titer is not normal after four courses of treatment, or (4) new metastases have appeared—switch to another single agent (methotrexate versus dactinomycin) or consider hysterectomy if childbearing is not a factor.

e. If childbearing is not a consideration and NMTD is suspected, abdominal hysterectomy may be performed on the third day of a five-day course of either methotrexate or dactinomycin. The specimen should be carefully examined for the presence of residual disease and the patient followed with titers and, if necessary, with chemotherapy as described in **a.**

f. After remission, the patient should continue to be followed with HCG titers, chest roentgenography, and pelvic examination, as was noted in sec. **A.5** for hydatidiform mole.

g. Pregnancy outcome after treatment for hydatidiform mole is not associated with any increase in fetal wastage or congenital anomalies.

C. Metastatic trophoblastic disease

1. Definition. MTD is present when the evaluation indicates malignant sequelae and the disease has been found to extend beyond the uterus and is metastatic to the lung, vagina, brain, or liver.

a. Ninety-five percent of MTD is histologically **choriocarcinoma** and shows sheets of atypical cytotrophoblastic and syncytiotrophoblastic cell proliferation invading and causing necrosis and hemorrhage.

b. Antecedent molar pregnancy is noted in 50% of cases. The remainder occur after abortion or term gestation.

c. Extremely vascular lesions are common, and they may cause substantial hemorrhage.

d. This disease usually occurs within several months of the antecedent gestational event, although later occurrences have been reported.

2. Evaluation. Staging studies in detecting MTD are outlined in secs. **A.6.a** and **A.6.b.** In addition

a. Abdominal computed tomography scans and ultrasonography may aid in identifying other visceral involvement.

b. Lumbar puncture and assay of both cerebral spinal fluid and serum HCG may have potential use in detecting central nervous system metastases and assessing the efficacy of therapy with central nervous system involvement.

3. Patients with MTD are subclassified as high-risk for failure of single-agent chemotherapy or poor-prognosis patients, and low-risk for failure of therapy or good-prognosis patients on the basis of the following criteria:

a. Good prognosis, low risk

- **(1)** Initial urinary HCG titer less than 100,000 IU/24 hours or serum HCG titer less than 40,000 mIU/ml
- **(2)** Duration of symptoms less than four months
- **(3)** No liver or brain metastases; metastases confined to lungs or pelvis
- **(4)** No prior chemotherapy

b. Poor prognosis, high risk

- **(1)** Urinary HCG titer greater than 100,000 IU/24 hours or serum HCG titer greater than 40,000 mIU/ml.
- **(2)** MTD identified more than four months after antecedent molar pregnancy or gestational event or from onset of symptoms

(3) Liver or brain metastases
(4) MTD following term pregnancy instead of molar pregnancy

4. Therapy for a low-risk patient with good prognosis

a. Patients are treated as for NMTD (see sec. **B.2**), including high-dose methotrexate with citrovorum factor.

b. Patients are followed as for NMTD (see sec. **B.2.f**).

c. Failure of therapy (i.e., new metastatic lesions appear, or titers do not decrease progressively) is an indication for multiagent treatment (see sec. **5**). Hysterectomy may also be reconsidered with treatment failure of MTD.

5. Therapy for a high-risk patient with poor prognosis. Aggressive combination chemotherapy with adjuvant radiotherapy or surgical therapy is critical for gaining disease remission.

a. Intensive, almost continual therapy and monitoring, long-term additional maintenance therapy, and prompt intervention with radiotherapy or surgery would justify managing these patients in major oncology centers, if not trophoblastic disease centers.

b. In general terms, combination chemotherapy is employed, using either MAC (methotrexate, dactinomycin, and chlorambucil or cyclophosphamide) or the modified Bagshawe protocol, which consists sequentially of hydroxyurea, vincristine, and then a modification of doxorubicin hydrochloride and melphalan. Both treatment protocols are well described and the treatment complications outlined [1, 2].

(1) Severe complications should be anticipated with either regimen, including severe leukopenia and thrombocytopenia with secondary sepsis, and bleeding (intraperitoneal, intrapleural, hepatic, and intracerebral or spinal cord hemorrhage).

(2) Cerebral or hepatic metastases should be treated with irradiation in conjunction with chemotherapy to decrease the risk of hemorrhage.

(3) Surgical intervention may be required to remove isolated metastases, especially lung lesions.

c. Chemotherapy is continued until three consecutive negative HCG titers are obtained, and then two additional courses are delivered.

d. Titer determinations are continued after remission every two weeks for three months, then every two months for six months, and finally every six months indefinitely.

6. Central nervous system metastases require that management be modified to avoid intracranial hemorrhage. Radiation directed toward preventing hemorrhage should precede the combination chemotherapy.

D. Survival statistics

1. There is an excellent chance for cure (approaching 100%) of NMTD and low-risk MTD patients.

2. High-risk MTD patients or those with a poor prognosis have a 50–80% chance of being cured.

a. Prognosis (approximately 90%) is excellent if only lung metastases are present.

b. Central nervous system metastases reduce survival to approximately 50%, and patients with liver disease have even poorer prognoses.

Hydramnios and Oligohydramnios

I. Hydramnios

A. Description. Hydramnios (also called **polyhydramnios**), an excess of amniotic fluid, occurs in 0.5–1.5% of gravidas. Volumes in excess of 2000 ml at term are considered pathologic, and 1700 ml is considered the upper limit of normal at between 30 and 37 weeks' gestation. The disease usually is clinically evident when the volume of fluid reaches approximately 3000 ml.

1. In **chronic hydramnios,** the fluid accumulates over a relatively long period of time and is associated with the following:
   a. **Fetal anomalies**
      (1) Central nervous system defects such as anencephaly, hydrocephalus, and meningocele
      (2) Gastrointestinal anomalies such as esophageal and duodenal atresia
   b. **Maternal conditions** such as diabetes, erythroblastosis, and twin gestation
   c. **Placental and umbilical cord vascular conditions** (those related to monovular multiple gestations, and chorioangiomas)
2. In **acute hydramnios,** which is much less common than chronic hydramnios, the collection of excessive fluid may occur within a few hours or days and requires a much more active management program. Perinatal loss secondary to preterm delivery is the usual outcome.

B. Diagnosis. The diagnosis is suspected when the following signs and symptoms are present:
1. Excessive uterine enlargement, noted either by the patient or physician, becomes apparent, usually between 21 and 37 weeks' gestation.
2. In rare instances, abdominal distention with pain, respiratory symptoms with dyspnea, and severe edema may herald the onset of the disease. In some cases, maternal symptoms are so severe as to require immediate therapeutic relief.
3. Confirmation of the diagnosis is best made with **ultrasonography,** which will identify large, echoless areas within the uterine cavity and which also may identify fetal anomalies.
4. Amniotic fluid analysis for **alpha fetoprotein** may be useful because of the many instances of fetal central nervous system anomalies.
5. Amniotic fluid **prolactin levels** may be determined and found to be lower than expected for the gestational age.

C. Treatment
1. **Expectant management** may be indicated in patients without severe symptoms after a thorough investigation has failed to reveal any evident fetal anomaly.
2. More severe symptoms will require **hospitalization with bed rest.** Diuretics and salt restriction have been unsuccessful therapeutic tools.
3. If respiratory symptoms are severe or abdominal pain demands relief, **transabdominal amniocentesis** with slow drainage of fluid may be used (500 ml/hour). Too rapid withdrawal may result in premature separation of the placenta or premature labor. Other complications include preterm labor and intrauterine infection.
4. Amniotic fluid reaccumulates rapidly. **Repeated amniocentesis** may give patients some relief and diminish the risk of premature labor. However, premature labor is to be expected in the majority of cases.

D. Complications of labor
1. Malpresentations, especially breech presentations
2. Umbilical cord prolapse
3. Hemorrhage during and after delivery

E. Fetal risk
1. The disease carries a poor fetal prognosis, with an expected fetal death rate of nearly 50%. Death usually is a result of anomalies incompatible with extrauterine existence or a result of the effects of immaturity.
2. Major fetal anomalies occur in 20–30% of cases.
3. A normal-appearing fetus should be investigated immediately for the possibility of gastrointestinal anomalies, especially esophageal and duodenal atresia.
4. It should be reassuring that in at least 60% of cases, there is no fetal or maternal disease.

F. Maternal effects. Uterine dysfunction and prolonged labor are reported as frequent concomitants to hydramnios because of uterine overdistention. Most patients, however, experience normal patterns of uterine activity. Postpartum uterine atony and subsequent hemorrhage should be anticipated, and a dilute solution of IV oxytocin (10–20 units/1000 ml fluid) should be administered promptly with delivery of the infant.

II. Oligohydramnios

A. Description. Oligohydramnios is recognized when there is a markedly decreased quantity of amniotic fluid—volumes of only a few milliliters to 60 ml. It may occur at any time during pregnancy and often is unrecognized. It frequently is a lethal syndrome, resulting in very early pregnancy losses, and in late pregnancy it is associated with fetal anomalies, especially intrauterine growth retardation.

B. Fetal effects. The condition is associated most often with fetal anomalies that diminish or restrict the flow of fetal urine into the amniotic cavity. The classic example is renal agenesis (Potter's disease). Polycystic kidneys and obstructive lesions of the urinary outflow tract, such as urethral stenosis, are other examples. **Amnion nodosum,** gray-white nodules on the fetal surface of the placenta, occurs with oligohydramnios, and its identification should prompt a search for fetal urinary tract abnormalities (see sec. **IV.D** under Placental Examination).

As previously noted, it also is associated with intrauterine growth retardation and frequently is seen with the postmaturity syndrome. It should be considered a potentially grave sign of increasing fetal compromise and distress.

C. Treatment. Oligohydramnios rarely causes any maternal symptoms, and so treatment is directed to those fetal conditions that may be corrected or reversed.

References

1. Hammond, C. B., et al. Treatment of metastatic trophoblastic disease: Good and poor prognosis. *Am. J. Obstet. Gynecol.* 115:451, 1973.
2. Surwit, E. A., et al. A new combination chemotherapy for resistant trophoblastic disease. *Gynecol. Oncol.* 8(1):110, 1979.

Selected Readings

Benirschke, K. A review of the pathologic anatomy of the human placenta. *Am. J. Obstet. Gynecol.* 84:1595, 1962.

Benirschke, K., and Driscoll, S. G. *The Pathology of the Human Placenta.* New York: Springer, 1967.

Fox, H. *Pathology of the Placenta.* Philadelphia: Saunders, 1978.

Goldstein, P. P., and Berkowitz, R. S. (eds.). Gestational trophoblastic neoplasms: An invitational symposium. *J. Reprod. Med.* 26:179, 1981.

Morrow, C. P. (ed.). Trophoblastic disease. *Clin. Obstet. Gynecol.* 27:151, 1984.

Philipson, E. H., Sokol, R. J., and Williams, T. W. Oligohydramnios: Clinical associations and predictive value for intrauterine growth retardation. *Am. J. Obstet. Gynecol.* 146:271, 1983.

Queenan, J. T., and Gadow, E. L. Polyhydramnios: Chronic vs acute. *Am. J. Obstet. Gynecol.* 108:349, 1970.

Schlaerth, J. B., et al. Prognostic characteristics of serum human chorionic gonadotropin titer regression following molar pregnancy. *Obstet. Gynecol.* 58:478, 1981.

32 The Puerperium

Helayne M. Silver and
Lloyd H. Smith

Complex adaptations of physiology and behavior occur in women during the six weeks following parturition, traditionally defined as the **puerperium.** Although usually a low-risk period, life-threatening emergencies or serious complications may occur that must be recognized and managed efficiently. For the majority, however, a minimum of interference is warranted. Those caring for women post partum should be sensitive to the initiation of **family bonding,** a special process not to be disturbed unless maternal or neonatal complications arise.

I. Postpartum maternal adaptations

A. Reproductive organs

1. **The uterus** begins to contract strongly immediately after delivery of the placenta, thus compressing the wide-open vessels supplying the placental site. Within minutes the uterus is hard and globular and can be palpated at or slightly below the level of the umbilicus. By two weeks post partum, the uterus is again a pelvic organ, and by four weeks post partum, the uterus returns to nonpregnant dimensions. Within days of delivery, the superficial decidua necroses and sloughs in the lochia. The basal layer is the source of the new endometrium and begins to regenerate. Within 7–10 days the surface endothelium is regenerated. With the exception of the placental site, the entire full thickness of the endometrium is regenerated by two to three weeks post partum. The placental site is slowly exfoliated by the undermining growth from the surrounding regenerating endometrium. This process may take up to six weeks and if faulty may result in delayed postpartum hemorrhage.
2. **The cervix** regains tone within two to three days after delivery. At this time the cervix will be dilated 2–3 cm. By one week post partum, the cervix will regain a nonpregnant appearance.
3. **The vagina** will remain edematous and enlarged for approximately three weeks. Involution is usually complete by six weeks post partum.
4. **Ovulation** occurs on the average at 10 weeks in the nonlactating woman [17]. The first menstrual cycle is frequently anovulatory, with a mean time to first menses 7 to 9 weeks in the nonlactating woman. Seventy percent of nonlactating women will menstruate by 12 weeks post partum [23]. The time to ovulation and menstruation is highly variable in the lactating woman and depends on the duration of breast-feeding.
5. **The breasts** are prepared for lactation during pregnancy by the high levels of estrogen, progesterone, cortisol, prolactin, placental lactogen, and insulin. Lactation is suppressed during pregnancy by the high levels of placental steroids. The rapid fall in these hormones post partum allows expression of the high prolactin levels and results in the initiation of lactation. The initial milk production consists mostly of colostrum, which is richer in proteins and immunoglobulins than mature milk.

B. Systemic changes

1. **Urinary tract.** The bladder frequently sustains injury during delivery. Overdistention and incomplete emptying are therefore common in the immediate postpartum period. This may be further aggravated by the use of conduction anesthesia. The immediate postpartum period is therefore a time of increased risk for urinary tract infection (see sec. **III.B.3.b**). Renal function decreases to nonpregnant levels by six weeks post partum, but the anatomic changes such as ureteral and calyceal dilatation may persist for several months.

2. **Cardiovascular system.** The normal blood loss at vaginal delivery is 500 ml, and at cesarean section is 1000 ml. Despite this blood loss, stroke volume is increased secondary to increased venous return due to loss of the placental shunt and mobilization of peripheral interstitial fluid. Cardiac output is usually unchanged or only slightly increased as a decrease in heart rate is concurrent with the increase in stroke volume. By two weeks post partum, cardiac output has decreased almost to baseline nonpregnant level.
3. **Gastrointestinal system.** The increased hepatic production of serum proteins induced by high levels of estrogen returns to normal levels within three weeks post partum.

II. Normal postpartum care

A. The immediate postpartum period requires close observation for potential complications such as abnormal bleeding and uterine atony. The patient may be recovering from an anesthetic. Ideally, the infant should be allowed to remain with the mother during this period to facilitate initial bonding.

B. Subsequent postpartum care

1. **Nursing care** will include vital signs every four hours, measurement of urine output, assessment of vaginal bleeding and uterine tone, assessment of maternal-infant interactions, aid with perineal care and with initiation of breastfeeding, assessment for and provision of adequate analgesia, and teaching basics of infant and self-care.
2. **Laboratory studies** should include a complete blood count on the first postpartum day, type and cross for RhoGAM in Rh-negative patients, and rubella titer if not previously known, to assess need for immunization.
3. **Daily rounds** by the physician staff should include the following assessments:
   a. **Uterus.** The uterine fundus should be palpated to evaluate for proper involution and tone. It should be slightly below the umbilicus and firm. If it is not, the patient may be experiencing significant bleeding, either concealed in the uterine cavity or per vaginum. The patient should be instructed to perform **uterine massage** every hour. Uterine tone can be increased with ecbolic agents such as oxytocin (20 units in 1 liter IV fluid at 100–200 ml/hour or 10 mg IM), methylergonovine maleate (0.2 mg PO q4–6h), or 15-methylprostaglandin $F_{2\alpha}$ (0.25 mg IM). Use of these agents will cause significant cramping and the patient should be offered a mild analgesic. Particularly in the postcesarean patient in whom the risk for endometritis is high, the uterus should be evaluated for an unusual degree of tenderness.
   b. **The abdomen** should be examined for distention, particularly in the postoperative patient. Following abdominal surgery, ileus is common, and bowel sounds should be evaluated. Bowel sounds are usually faint or absent on the first postoperative day. Most postcesarean patients experience return of coordinated bowel activity, as evidenced by passage of flatus by the second or third postoperative day. Patients with prolonged surgery or infection may experience prolonged ileus. Some physicians will begin the postcesarean patient on a clear-liquid diet when active bowel sounds return. Others prefer to await the passage of flatus. If the patient tolerates a clear-liquid diet without nausea and vomiting or abdominal distention, she may be rapidly advanced to a regular diet.
   c. **Lochia** should be assessed both in quantity and for unusual odor, suggesting infection. The lochia in the first several days consists mainly of blood and necrotic decidual tissue (**lochia rubra**). Generally, the quantity is similar to that of the menstrual flow. After several days the patient will note the lochia becoming lighter in color (**lochia serosa**) due to less content of blood. After several weeks only a **leukorrhea** remains (**lochia alba**).
   d. **The perineum** should be inspected for hematoma formation, signs of infection, or breakdown. Local perineal care consists of **gentle cleansing** and **warm sitz baths. Local anesthetics** such as witch hazel pads or benzocaine spray may be used. After a third- or fourth-degree laceration, **stool softeners** such as **docusate sodium** are frequently prescribed, and the patient is observed in the hospital until passage of her first bowel movement. **Hemor-**

rhoids may cause a great deal of discomfort, particularly after a prolonged second stage of labor. These may be treated with hydrocortisone-containing preparations, witch hazel pads, and warm sitz baths.

e. **Bladder function** may be abnormal, particularly following a traumatic delivery or epidural anesthesia. The patient may require catheterization. Generally a **Foley catheter** is left in place for 24 hours if the patient requires a second catheterization. A catheter may be left in place prophylactically for 24 hours at delivery if this difficulty is anticipated due to marked periurethral edema or repair.

f. **The breasts** should be examined for engorgement or signs of infection. If the patient is not planning to breast-feed, the breasts should be tightly bound to inhibit lactation. An alternative is to suppress lactation with bromocriptine, a dopamine agonist (2.5 mg PO bid for 14 days). **Rebound lactation** may occur in women after discontinuation of bromocriptine, and this is usually responsive to repeating a seven-day course of medication. Hypotension and hypertension, seizures, and strokes have been reported in postpartum women taking bromocriptine [6].

g. **The lungs** should be evaluated in all postcesarean section patients and in postvaginal delivery patients as indicated. As noted in sec. **III.B,** the lungs are an important source of postoperative fever, and postoperative patients should be encouraged and instructed in the proper use of incentive spirometry.

h. **The extremities.** As the postpartum patient is at increased risk for deep vein thrombosis, the extremities are evaluated for signs of developing thrombophlebitis.

III. Postpartum emergencies and complications

A. Hemorrhage

1. **Definition.** Although a total blood loss of greater than 500 ml at delivery and in the subsequent 24 hours has been used as a definition of abnormal postpartum hemorrhage, the average blood lost at normal vaginal delivery is probably close to this amount. Consequently, in clinical practice, experience and empiric estimates are important in the diagnosis of abnormal postpartum bleeding.

2. **Differential diagnosis.** The well-armed clinician has an understanding of the factors that predispose to postpartum hemorrhage, practices precautionary measures that minimize its occurrence, has a systematic method for evaluating such patients, and, once the diagnosis is established, moves efficiently to apply sometimes lifesaving, if not fertility-sparing, therapy. The differential diagnosis and predisposing factors for postpartum hemorrhage are listed in Table 32-1. Predelivery identification of such factors allows for preventive measures where appropriate (e.g., establishing intravenous access, obtaining blood products that might be needed, careful postdelivery evaluation) [13].

3. **Preliminary management.** Once excessive bleeding is observed, a prompt review of the clinical course, identification of predisposing factors, and physical examination should follow. If possible, premedication with parenteral analgesics is humane and allows a more thorough bimanual pelvic examination. Digital examination may reveal a poorly contracted uterus, vaginal lacerations, hematomas, and, occasionally, placental fragments. Intrauterine manual exploration and more thorough examination of the cervix and vagina may require return to the operating room and the possible use of general anesthesia. **Shock** is treated as described in Chap. 16; **coagulopathy** is identified and treated with blood, fresh-frozen plasma, or platelets, as appropriate [21]. When hemorrhage continues, early plans for operation should be made, including arrangements for an operating room and anesthesia personnel, and discussion should be initiated with the patient and family regarding the possible need for surgery and the patient's desire for future fertility. Those patients who refuse blood transfusion for religious reasons present a special problem; surgery should be performed when conservative measures do not quickly stem the bleeding.

Table 32-1. Differential diagnosis and predisposing factors for postpartum hemorrhage

Diagnosis	Predisposing factors
Uterine atony	Prolonged or precipitous labor, overdistention of the uterus (macrosomia, hydramnios, twins), grand multiparity, drugs (prolonged oxytocin, halothane, magnesium sulfate, tocolytics), amnionitis, previous postpartum hemorrhage, fetal demise, leiomyomas, amniotic fluid embolism
Lacerations, hematoma	Traumatic or instrumental delivery, breech extraction, pudendal anesthesia
Uterine rupture	Uterine scar, prolonged or precipitous labor, uterine overdistention, hyperstimulation with oxytocin, previous curettage, leiomyomas
Uterine inversion	Excessive cord traction or fundal pressure, adherent placenta, manual removal of placenta, fundal implantation, previous uterine inversion, congenital predisposition
Placenta accreta	Prior cesarean section, placenta previa, previous uterine curettage, multiparity, leiomyomas, adenomyosis, previous postpartum hemorrhage
Retained placenta	Early gestation, succenturiate lobe
Subinvolution	Retained placental fragments, endomyometritis, leiomyomas

4. Specific management

a. Uterine atony

(1) Bimanual uterine massage and expression of accumulated clots are all that are required to reverse many cases of uterine atony. Catheterization of a distended bladder may assist uterine contraction and descent.

(2) Medical management will be effective in the majority of cases of uterine atony and should be employed to prevent its recurrence. **Oxytocin** may be given intramuscularly (10 units), but the intravenous route may be more effective (20–40 units in 1000 ml of IV fluid infused at up to 200 ml/hour). Intravenous bolus administration of oxytocin may lead to transient but profound hypotension and could be fatal in patients with unrecognized cardiac disease.

(a) Methylergonovine maleate, 0.2 mg IM, is effective in causing prolonged tetanic contraction of the uterus. Especially when given as an intravenous bolus, methylergonovine can result in abrupt hypertension, and so **it should not be used in hypertensive patients.**

(b) Prostaglandins in the form of intravaginal suppositories (prostaglandin E_2, 20 mg), intramyometrial injection (prostaglandin $F_{2\alpha}$, 1 mg), and intramuscular injection of the 15-methyl analog of prostaglandin $F_{2\alpha}$ (Prostin 15/M, 0.25 mg) have all been used successfully in the setting of uterine atony unresponsive to other agents [13]. Of 51 patients with uterine atony studied by Hayashi and colleagues [11], 86% were controlled with Prostin 15/M given at intervals of 90 minutes or more for up to 5 doses. Four of seven failures had chorioamnionitis. Side effects including fever, vomiting, and diarrhea were common. Prostaglandins of the F series should be used with great caution in patients with bronchospastic or hypertensive disorders.

(3) Surgical intervention should not be delayed if the preceding measures fail to reverse uterine atony. Hot saline uterine lavage and uterine packing are temporizing measures that are often not effective. The use of the

military anti-shock trouser (MAST) suit or selective pelvic artery embolization may be appropriate and effective in some situations [9]. However, for most patients with intractable uterine atony, surgery is the treatment of choice. Conservative surgery is attempted when preservation of fertility is the goal. Ideally, the patient is prepared in the modified lithotomy position so that the effects of sequential surgical measures can be observed.

(a) **Bilateral uterine artery ligation,** as described by O'Leary [20], is safe, easily performed, often effective, and preserves fertility. The technique, designed for control of postcesarean hemorrhage, employs a single mass ligature of No. 1 chromic suture on a large atraumatic needle (Fig. 32-1). The ligature passes through the avascular space in the broad ligament and through the myometrium just inferior to the level of a cesarean myometrial incision, at a safe distance from the pelvic ureter. No attempt is made to dissect out the vessels being ligated, and thus the ascending branch of the uterine artery and adjacent veins are included. Though the uterus may remain soft, bleeding is often controlled. The vessels are not divided, and recanalization with subsequent normal pregnancy can be expected [19].

(b) **Bilateral hypogastric artery ligation** is performed after division of the round ligament and exposure of the pelvic side wall [22]. The pelvic ureter is moved medially with reflection of the pelvic peritoneum. The bifurcation of the common iliac artery is identified by blunt dissection, and the hypogastric artery is gently undermined using a **Mixter clamp. Care must be taken not to lacerate the very fragile underlying hypogastric vein.** Most authorities recommend double ligation with 0 silk suture proximal to the bifurcation of the anterior and posterior divisions (Fig. 32-1).

(c) **Bilateral ovarian artery ligation** may not add much to the preceding measures since more than 90% of the uterine blood flow in pregnancy

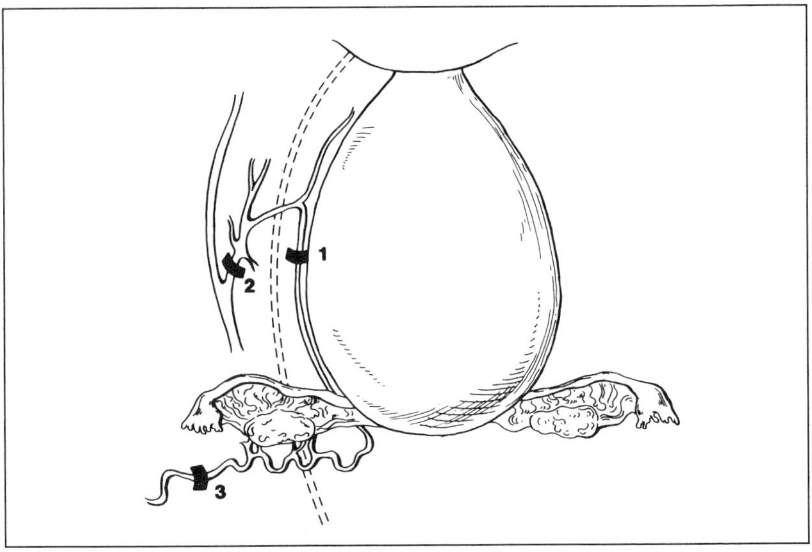

Fig. 32-1. Conservative surgical management for the intractable uterine artery. **1.** Uterine artery ligation (ascending branches). **2.** Hypogastric (internal iliac) artery ligation. **3.** Ovarian artery ligation.

passes through the uterine arteries. This procedure may, however, adversely affect subsequent fertility.

(d) Hysterectomy. Atony persisting despite conservative surgical measures should be managed with either total or supracervical hysterectomy. Clark and colleagues [4] reported an emergency hysterectomy rate of 0.7% following cesarean section and 0.02% following vaginal delivery. Among 70 such patients, uterine atony was the most common indication (43%), followed by placenta accreta (30%), uterine rupture (13%), extension of a low transverse incision (10%), and leiomyomas (4%). The average blood loss (approximately 3500 ml), mean operating time (more than three hours), and mean hospital stay (seven to eight days) may have been magnified by unsuccessful attempts of conservative surgical management.

b. Lacerations. Average blood loss from a median episiotomy is 200 ml, and consequently, loss from unrecognized cervical, vaginal, or perineal lacerations can be significant and should be suspected when bleeding continues despite a well-contracted uterus. Management consists of full-thickness mucosal repair, beginning above the apex of the laceration with continuous interlocking absorbable suture. Surgical assistants and general anesthesia are sometimes required.

c. Retained placental fragments should be suspected when bleeding persists in the absence of apparent lacerations or atony.

(1) The expelled placenta should be carefully inspected for completeness. When retained fragments are suspected, manual intrauterine exploration or curettage with a Hunter's curet is best performed under adequate anesthesia. Care must be taken to avoid uterine perforation, and when suspected, the patient must be observed closely and laparotomy performed if bleeding is excessive or hemodynamic criteria deteriorate. Late postpartum hemorrhage may also be caused by retained placental fragments. Ultrasonography is sometimes useful in confirming the diagnosis. Curettage at this time must be done with care to avoid creation of intrauterine synechiae (Asherman's syndrome).

d. Hematomas of the perineum, vagina, or subperitoneal (supralevator) space result from occasionally massive occult hemorrhage. Extreme perineal or pelvic pain, inability to void, or the presence of unexplained tachycardia, hypotension, or anemia should suggest the diagnosis, which is confirmed by inspection and palpation.

(1) Management consists of incision, removal of clots, ligation of bleeding vessels, and obliteration of the defect with interlocking absorbable sutures. Antibiotics and a vaginal pack may be beneficial for the 24 hours following evacuation of large vaginal hematomas. Subperitoneal hematomas are rare and may cause shock; when conservative measures fail to achieve improvement, laparotomy is indicated. Attempts to ligate bleeding vessels or perform bilateral hypogastric artery ligation may be difficult because of the distorted anatomy caused by the expanding hematoma. An alternative is selective arterial embolization.

e. Uterine rupture occurs once in 1000–1500 deliveries and can cause shock associated with minimal external blood loss. A defect in an old cesarean section scar in a stable patient with minimal bleeding may not require operative intervention. Defects associated with significant hemorrhage or worsening hemodynamic status require operation. For those patients who desire future childbearing, primary repair may be performed, though the risk of recurrent rupture is approximately 10% [12]. Hysterectomy is indicated when fertility is not desired or when the rupture is too extensive for repair.

f. Uterine inversion occurs once in 2000–20,000 deliveries and is associated with an average blood loss of 2000 ml.

(1) Presentation. Acute pain and profuse hemorrhage, often accompanied by shock, characterize its presentation. Uterine inversion may be complete or incomplete, and when incomplete may be recognizable only by pelvic examination.

(2) **Successful outcome** depends on rapid replacement by a variety of methods [10], as a cervical contraction ring may soon form, precluding replacement without general anesthesia, often including halothane. Tocolytic agents have been employed to facilitate uterine replacement [16], and prostaglandins have been used to prevent reinversion [14]. Uterine inversion refractory to manual replacement may require laparotomy and operative correction [10].

g. **Placenta accreta** occurs once in approximately 7000 deliveries and consists of relatively superficial attachment of the placenta to the myometrium. More invasive attachment (placenta increta and percreta) is less common. In the study by Clark and colleagues [4], 53% of all women presenting at term with both placenta previa and prior cesarean section required hysterectomy for placenta accreta. Significant placenta accreta is associated with a blood loss averaging nearly 4000 ml [13]. Treatment options consist of curettage, conservative surgical management, and hysterectomy.

h. **Subinvolution** of the uterus or placental site is associated with late-onset postpartum hemorrhage. The uterus is soft and has not undergone normal involution.

(1) **Treatment** consists of **methylergonovine maleate,** 0.2 mg PO q6h for 2 days, or **curettage,** or both. **Antibiotics** are given for associated endometritis. Gestational trophoblastic neoplasia should be considered when late postpartum hemorrhage is refractory to management.

B. Puerperal infections

1. **Epidemiology.** Puerperal febrile morbidity was defined by the U.S. Joint Committee on Maternal Welfare as "a temperature of 100.4°F (38°C), the temperature to occur in any two of the first ten days post partum, exclusive of the first 24 hours, and to be taken by mouth by a standard technique at least four times daily." Common infections in the postpartum period include endomyometritis, urinary tract infection, mastitis, and pneumonia. The overall rate of postpartum infection is difficult to ascertain as most patients are discharged from the hospital within days of delivery, but is estimated at 1–8%. Infection is the fourth most common cause of maternal death, with a rate of 1.2 in 100,000 live births in 1974–1978 [15]. Transient, low-grade fever is common in the postpartum period and will resolve spontaneously in the majority of patients delivered vaginally. These self-limited fevers may be secondary to dehydration, transient bacteremia, or a febrile response to exposure to foreign fetal proteins. In patients delivered by cesarean section, only 30% of fevers will resolve spontaneously, reflecting the greater risk for development of infection following an operative intervention.

2. **Evaluation of the febrile postpartum patient.** A thorough review of the patient's intrapartum and postpartum course will frequently reveal predisposing factors suggesting the source of infection. Further guidance comes from physical examination focusing particularly on the likely areas of concern.

a. **Minimum laboratory studies** should include a complete blood count with differential, a urinalysis and culture, two sets of blood cultures, and a chest x ray. Blood cultures will be positive in 10–20% of febrile postpartum patients. If respiratory infection is suspected, sputum should be obtained for a Gram's stain and culture.

b. If **endomyometritis** is suspected, endometrial cultures may be obtained. A simple swab of the endometrial cavity will result in the isolation of lower genital tract contaminants as well as the infecting organisms. Although of limited usefulness, this may be of some help in choosing a subsequent antibiotic regimen in a patient failing the initial treatment regimen. Less contaminated specimens may be obtained with use of a double-lumen catheter, but this may not be readily available.

3. **Specific diagnoses**

a. **Endometritis** is infection of the endometrium. **Endomyometritis** is infection of the endometrium and and myometrium. **Endoparametritis** includes infection of the parametrium. Clinically, these are difficult to distinguish, and most commonly the diagnosis is simply stated as endometritis.

(1) Diagnosis. The criteria for diagnosis usually include fever, uterine tenderness, foul or purulent lochia, elevated white blood cell count, and lack of other localizing symptoms. Symptoms generally appear within five days of delivery.

(2) Risk factors clearly correlated with development of endometritis include delivery by cesarean section, prolonged duration of ruptured membranes, prolonged labor, and lower socioeconomic status. The duration of internal fetal monitoring and the number of vaginal examinations do not appear to be independent risk factors in most studies [7]. The risk of developing postcesarean endometritis in laboring patients can be reduced by administration of prophylactic antibiotics such as cefazolin, 1 gm IV q6h for 3 doses.

(3) Microbiology. The infection is generally polymicrobial with mixed aerobic and anaerobic organisms. Commonly isolated pathogens include the aerobic gram-negative bacilli in 20–30% (*Escherichia coli, Klebsiella* sp., *Proteus* sp.), aerobic gram-positive streptococci in 10% (group B streptococcus, enterococcus), anaerobic gram-negative bacilli in 40–60% (*Bacteroides bivius, Bacteroides melaninogenicus, Bacteroides fragilis, Fusobacterium*), and anaerobic gram-positive cocci in 25–40% (*Peptostreptococcus, Peptococcus)* [5].

(4) Therapy. When endometritis develops after vaginal delivery, the response rate to a combination of penicillin and an aminoglycoside is 95%. Addition of anaerobic coverage such as clindamycin or metronidazole in primary treatment failures will increase the cure rate to 98% [8]. In patients with postcesarean endometritis, the combination of a penicillin and an aminoglycoside is clearly inferior, with reported response rates of 61–78% [5]. The antibiotic combination with the most consistently excellent cure rate (86–100%) in the therapy of postcesarean endometritis is that of **clindamycin** and an **aminoglycoside** [5]. The patient is treated with intravenous antibiotics until maintained afebrile for more than 48 hours. A course of oral antibiotics is not needed. **Treatment failures** with this regimen are usually due to inadequate aminoglycoside dosing (Table 32-2) or to a resistant organism such as enterococcus. In treatment failures with therapeutic aminoglycoside levels, ampicillin is generally added empirically to the regimen. Although use of third-generation cephalosporin agents is sometimes advocated for the simplicity of single-agent therapy, there is less experience with treatment of endometritis with these agents.

(5) Complications of refractory cases include septic pelvic thrombophlebitis, pelvic abscess, and septic shock. Uncomplicated endometritis is not associated with subsequent infertility.

Table 32-2. Antibiotic dosing in the postpartum patient

Antibiotic agent	Dose	Interval
Penicillin	5 million units	6 hr
Ampicillin	2 gm	4–6 hr
Cefazolin	1–2 gm	8 hr
Gentamicin	Loading: 2 mg/kg; maintenance: 1.5–1.75 mg/kg [2]	8 hr
Clindamycin	900 mg	8 hr

b. Urinary tract infection

(1) Diagnosis. Bacteriuria in the postpartum patient is usually asymptomatic. **Cystitis** may present with dysuria, urgency, and frequency, but these are common complaints in the postpartum patient. Bacteriuria and cystitis are established by the finding of a positive urine culture without signs suggesting pyelonephritis. **Pyelonephritis** is diagnosed in the patient with fever, flank pain, and a positive urine culture. Infection develops in the right kidney in the majority of pregnant patients with pyelonephritis.

(2) Risk factors for the development of pyelonephritis in the postpartum patient include the physiologic hydroureter of pregnancy, catheterization during labor or for cesarean section, and preexisting asymptomatic bacteriuria (occurs in 2–12% of pregnant women).

(3) Microbiology. The most commonly isolated organisms are the gram-negative bacilli *E. coli, Klebsiella enterobacter, Proteus* sp., and *Enterobacter* sp.; less commonly the gram-positive cocci, enterococcus, and group B streptococcus.

(4) Therapy. As many of the gram-negative bacilli are resistant to ampicillin, **initial therapy** should be a first-generation cephalosporin such as cefazolin, given intravenously. If the patient appears septic, an aminoglycoside should be added to the initial regimen. **Further therapy** is guided by results to culture sensitivities. **Intravenous therapy** should be continued until the patient remains afebrile for 48 hours. An oral antibiotic agent should be given to complete a 10- to 14-day course of therapy.

(5) Complications include septic shock and pulmonary capillary leak syndrome.

c. Mastitis is infection of the parenchyma of the mammary gland usually occurring two to three weeks post partum. Breast engorgement can cause low-grade fever in the early postpartum period, but other diagnoses must be carefully excluded before ascribing fever to this noninfectious etiology.

(1) Diagnosis. Usually a localized area of cellulitis, frequently V-shaped, delineates the infected lobule. The fever is usually higher than 102°F.

(2) Risk factors include breast-feeding, recent weaning, and fissures of the nipple.

(3) Microbiology. *Staphylococcus aureus* is the causative agent in 95% of cases. Other organisms include group A and B streptococci, *Haemophilus influenzae,* and *Haemophilus parainfluenzae.*

(4) Therapy. Local care includes continued breast-feeding or pumping from the affected side, ice packs, and support. The antibiotic chosen should be active against penicillinase-producing *S. aureus,* such as **dicloxacillin** (250–500 mg PO q6h) or a cephalosporin such as **cephalexin** (250–500 mg PO q6h). Antibiotic therapy should be prescribed for 7–10 days.

(5) Complications. Occasionally a breast **abscess** will develop. This requires incision and drainage. Breast-feeding should be stopped as long as purulent drainage continues.

d. Wound infections may involve an abdominal incision following cesarean section or, less commonly, an episiotomy incision following a vaginal delivery.

(1) Diagnosis. A wound infection is defined by the National Academy of Sciences–National Research Council [18] as "infected if pus discharges, and possibly infected if it develops the signs of inflammation or a serous discharge." Postcesarean wound infections usually become clinically apparent three to eight days postoperative. Temperature elevation is variable. The overlying skin is frequently erythematous and there may be tenderness and palpable fluctuance. **Drainage** of purulent material allows definitive diagnosis. **Postepisiotomy wound infection** is manifest as local edema and erythema with purulent exudate.

(2) Risk factors for postcesarean wound infection include chorioamnionitis, obesity, prolonged surgery, emergency surgery, diabetes, corticosteroid therapy, and malnutrition.

(3) **Microbiology.** The organisms isolated from a typical postcesarean wound infection are those found in the normal lower genital tract. Wound infection presenting with extensive cellulitis within the first 48 hours after surgery may be due to group A streptococci or *Clostridium perfringens.* In the latter case, a bronze discoloration of the skin with a watery discharge may be noted.

(4) **Therapy** for the usual **postcesarean wound infection** is local. The wound is opened and cleansed, and nonviable tissue is debrided. Generally, the wound is left open to heal by secondary intention. Antibiotic therapy is not necessary unless extensive overlying cellulitis is present. **Early-onset infection,** as described, should be treated with penicillin and extensive debridement. **Suspected episiotomy infection** are treated with sitz baths. If unsuccessful, the wound is opened and debrided and allowed to heal secondarily.

(5) **Complications** include superficial fascial necrosis, necrotizing fascitis, and myonecrosis. In the postcesarean wound, **superficial fascitis** involves Camper and Scarpa's fascia; necrotizing fascitis includes involvement of the deeper rectus sheath. In the episiotomy, superficial fascitis involves Colles' fascia; **necrotizing fascitis** involves the deeper inferior fascia of the urogenital diaphragm and leveator ani. **Myonecrosis** involves the underlying muscle. **Treatment** for all is high-dose antibiotic therapy including penicillin and extensive debridement.

e. **Pneumonia** may develop in the postcesarean patient, typically after 72 hours.

(1) **Atelectasis** is a frequent complication in the first 72 hours and may present with a low-grade fever and moist bibasilar rales. Atelectasis will resolve with deep breathing, encouraged with an incentive spirometer and ambulation. If not treated, bacterial infection leading to pneumonia may occur.

(2) **Diagnosis** is made by a combination of fever, tachypnea, localized coarse rales, and typical findings on chest x ray.

(3) **Risk factors** include obesity, chronic lung disease, smoking, and general anesthesia with intubation.

(4) **Microbiology.** Isolated organisms in nosocomial lower respiratory infections are usually found in the normal flora of the oral cavity.

(5) **Treatment.** Antibiotic choice should be guided by the results of a Gram's stain of the sputum, and subsequently results of culture. Usually the choice will be a penicillin or a first-generation cephalosporin. Local therapy should include incentive spirometry and chest physical therapy. Oxygen therapy should be guided by arterial blood gas and pulse oximetry, if available.

(6) **Complications** include empyema, septic shock, and pulmonary capillary leak syndrome.

f. **Septic pelvic thrombophlebitis** is the development of ovarian vein thrombosis in a patient with a preceding pelvic soft tissue infection.

(1) **Diagnosis.** The diagnosis is suspected in a patient responding poorly to appropriate antibiotic therapy for endometritis. A palpable mass may extend from the uterine cornua laterally and cephalad, usually on the right side. The diagnosis may be confirmed by ultrasound with duplex Doppler [1], computed tomography (CT) scan, or magnetic resonance imaging (MRI) [3].

(2) **Risk factors** include endometritis, traumatic delivery, major vulvovaginal hematomas, and lower socioeconomic status.

(3) **Microbiology.** The most commonly implicated organisms are aerobic and anaerobic streptococci, staphylococci, *Proteus* sp., and *Bacteroides* sp.

(4) **Therapy** includes broad-spectrum antibiotic coverage and therapeutic anticoagulation with heparin (see Chap. 15) for 7–10 days. Surgical therapy is reserved for medical failures.

(5) **Complications** include pelvic abscess and septic pulmonary thromboembolism.

g. **Pelvic abscess** may result from an infected hematoma, septic thrombophlebitis, or prior pelvic soft tissue infection such as endomyometritis or tuboovarian infection.

(1) **Diagnosis** is suspected in the patient with high spiking fevers unresponsive to broad-spectrum antibiotic therapy. A mass may be felt on pelvic examination. The diagnosis may be confirmed by ultrasound, CT scan, or MRI.

(2) **Risk factors** are the same as those for the development of endometritis.

(3) **Microbiology** is the same as for endometritis.

(4) **Therapy** is **surgical** following treatment failure with **broad-spectrum antibiotic therapy.** If the mass is pointing into the cul-de-sac, it may be drained vaginally by colpotomy incision.

(5) **Complications** include rupture with peritonitis and septic shock.

C. Other complications

1. **Amniotic fluid embolism** may occur immediately postdelivery. See Chap. 7.
2. **Thromboembolic disease.** As discussed in Chap. 15, pregnancy is a hypercoaguable state, with increased risk for the development of thromboembolic phenomena. This risk is even further increased in the puerperium with an incidence of 0.1–1.0%.
3. **Eclampsia** complicates approximately 0.5% of pregnancies, and one-third of seizures occur post partum. Treatment in the postpartum period is simplified by the absence of a fetus, allowing more aggressive antihypertensive and antiseizure therapy. See Chap. 19 for details.
4. **Postpartum depression.** Many patients experience some **mood swings** and depression in the immediate postpartum period. These are usually self-limited, and simple reassurance that these feelings are normal and a sympathetic attitude are usually sufficient therapy. Severe reactions ranging from clinical depression to frank psychosis may occur and should be evaluated by a psychiatrist for possible chemotherapy.
5. **Neurologic abnormalities** may develop after vaginal delivery. Pressure on branches of the sacral plexus by the fetal head may in rare cases lead to a temporary paralysis of the muscles supplied by the external popliteal nerve (the ankle flexors and the toe extensors). Improper positioning in stirrups may result in damage to the common peroneal nerve resulting in **footdrop.** Patients with **Pfannenstiel's incision** for cesarean section frequently will note **loss of sensation of the skin** surrounding the incision. The patient should be reassured this is normal and will resolve slowly, requiring up to six months for full recovery of sensation.

References

1. Baka, J. J., et al. Ovarian vein thrombosis with atypical presentation: Role of sonography and duplex Doppler. *Obstet. Gynecol.* 73:887, 1989.
2. Briggs, G. C., Ambrose, P., and Nageotte, M. P. Gentamicin dosing in postpartum women with endometritis. *Am. J. Obstet. Gynecol.* 160:309, 1989.
3. Brown, C. E., et al. Puerperal pelvic thrombophlebitis: Impact on diagnosis and treatment using x-ray computed tomography and magnetic resonance imaging. *Obstet. Gynecol.* 68:789, 1986.
4. Clark, S. L., et al. Emergency hysterectomy for obstetric hemorrhage. *Obstet. Gynecol.* 64:376, 1984.
5. Duff, P. Pathophysiology and management of postcesarean endomyometritis. *Obstet. Gynecol.* 67:269, 1986.
6. *F.D.A. Drug Bull.* 14:1, 1984.
7. Gibbs, R. S. Postpartum Infections. In R. L. Sweet and R. S. Gibbs (eds.), *Infectious Diseases of the Female Genital Tract.* Baltimore: Williams & Wilkins, 1985.
8. Gibbs, R. S., et al. Endometritis following vaginal delivery. *Obstet. Gynecol.* 56:55, 1980.

9. Glickman, M. G. Pelvic Artery Embolization. In R. L. Berkowitz (ed.), *Critical Care of the Obstetric Patient.* New York: Churchill-Livingstone, 1983.
10. Harris, B. A. Acute puerperal inversion of the uterus. *Clin. Obstet. Gynecol.* 23:134, 1984.
11. Hayashi, R. N., et al. Management of severe postpartum hemorrhage with a prostaglandin $F_{2\alpha}$ analogue. *Obstet. Gynecol.* 63:806, 1984.
12. Herbert, W. N. P. Complications of the immediate puerperium. *Clin. Obstet. Gynecol.* 25:219, 1982.
13. Herbert, W.N. P., and Cefalo, R. C. Management of postpartum hemorrhage. *Clin. Obstet. Gynecol.* 27:139, 1984.
14. Heyl, P. S., et al. Recurrent inversion of the puerperal uterus managed with 15(S)-15-methyl prostaglandin $F_{2\alpha}$ and uterine packing. *Obstet. Gynecol.* 63:263, 1984.
15. Kaunitz, A. M., et al. Causes of maternal morbidity in the United States. *Obstet. Gynecol.* 65:605, 1985.
16. Kovacs, B. W., and DeVore, G. R. Management of acute and subacute puerperal uterine inversion with terbutaline sulfate. *Am. J. Obstet. Gynecol.* 150:784, 1984.
17. Lyon, R. A., and Stamm, M. J. The onset of ovulation during the puerperium. *Cal. Med.* 65:99, 1946.
18. National Academy of Sciences–National Research Council, Division of Medical Sciences, Ad Hoc Committee on Trauma. Postoperative wound infections: The influence of ultraviolet irradiation of the operative and of various other factors. *Ann. Surg.* 160(Suppl. 2):1, 1964.
19. O'Leary, J. A. Pregnancy following uterine artery ligation. *Obstet. Gynecol.* 55:112, 1980.
20. O'Leary, J. L., and O'Leary, J. A. Uterine artery ligation for control of post-cesarean section hemorrhage. *Obstet. Gynecol.* 43:849, 1974.
21. Romero, R. The Management of Acquired Hemostatic Failure During Pregnancy. In R. L. Berkowitz (ed.), *Critical Care of the Obstetric Patient.* New York: Churchill-Livingstone, 1983.
22. Schwartz, P. E. The Surgical Approach to Severe Postpartum Hemorrhage. In R. L. Berkowitz (ed.)., *Critical Care of the Obstetric Patient.* New York: Churchill-Livingstone, 1983.
23. Sharman, A. Menstruation after childbirth. *J. Obstet. Gynaecol. Br. Emp.* 58:440, 1951.

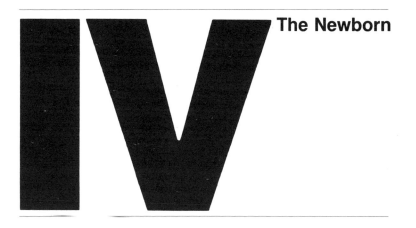

IV The Newborn

33 Resuscitation of the Newborn

Boyd W. Goetzman

Approximately 15% of all newborn infants have some degree of cardiorespiratory depression (heart rate < 100 beats/minute, hypotension, hypoventilation, or apnea) in the delivery room. These infants are at risk for loss of life or permanent central nervous system disability. Properly trained personnel in well-equipped delivery rooms are essential to the anticipation, recognition, and treatment of the depressed newborn child.

I. **Etiology of cardiorespiratory depression.** Although the cause of cardiorespiratory depression is often unknown, evidence for certain etiologies should be sought.

A. **Drugs.** With few exceptions, anesthetic and analgesic drugs used in obstetrics cross the placenta, with the potential for central respiratory depression in the fetus and newborn infant. However, this form of depression rarely is severe and may be treated effectively with assisted ventilation.

B. **Trauma.** Rapid labor, mid forceps or high forceps extraction, and breech delivery may be responsible for intracranial hemorrhage or injury. This form of depression has decreased in recent years, partly because of the more frequent use of cesarean section for breech presentations and the disappearance of the high forceps application.

C. **Hemorrhage.** Fetal blood loss into the mother, into a twin, or from umbilical cord or vessel rupture may be severe enough to require immediate resuscitation, including blood volume expansion.

D. **Intrinsic cardiac, pulmonary, or central nervous system disease.** Anomalies or fetal infection of the heart, lungs, or brain may produce infants with cardiorespiratory depression at great risk for mortality.

E. **Asphyxia.** One frequently considered cause of cardiorespiratory depression is asphyxia (decreased oxygen tension and pH and increased carbon dioxide tension). Some conditions associated with fetal asphyxia are predictable and potentially preventable prior to the infant's delivery. These include maternal conditions such as diabetes mellitus, toxemia, Rh isoimmunization, antepartum hemorrhage, and drug use; intrapartum conditions such as prolapsed cord, maternal hypotension, and breech delivery; and fetal conditions such as prematurity, meconium staining of amniotic fluid, and the second of twins. A common factor is marginal exchange of oxygen and carbon dioxide across the placenta, which becomes further compromised during labor.

1. **Physiology.** Acute total asphyxia of newborn animals for up to 15 minutes may be followed by successful resuscitation. Brain damage in survivors is rare and confined to the brainstem. Chronic partial asphyxia of nonhuman primate fetuses for periods of three to four hours followed by resuscitation can reproduce the clinical course and central nervous system damage observed in human infants following severe intrapartum asphyxia. Maintenance of brain perfusion and availability of glucose for conversion to lactate during asphyxia appear to be important factors in producing brain damage. Subsequent edema and decreased blood flow lead to necrosis.

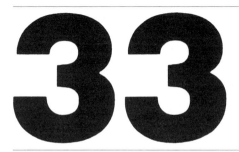

a. **Clinical course.** Following resuscitation, hypotonia persists. Myocardial dysfunction may lead to a prolonged period of low cardiac output. Cerebral edema begins in the first hours after birth, and seizures, if they occur, typically do so between 9 and 18 hours after birth. Ventilatory support usually is required from birth for shock lung or apnea. Oliguria secondary to acute tubular necrosis is almost routinely observed. Death may occur owing to cardiac, pulmonary, or brain injury. Recovery of neurologic function and normalization of the electroencephalogram by 1 week of age are predictive of normal outcome.

b. Pattern of central nervous system damage. In full-term infants, necrosis involves cortical gray matter, particularly in the postcentral gyrus and posterior parietal–anterior occipital regions, the underlying white matter, and the gray matter of the basal ganglia. Subsequently, ulegyria, cyst formation, and microcephaly occur. Preterm infants differ in that necrosis is primarily located in the deep white matter adjacent to the ventricles.

2. Management. Research is needed to confirm evidence that improved techniques for supporting the circulation, and pharmacologic management with barbiturates, prostaglandin antagonists, calcium antagonists, glutamate receptor antagonists, or antioxidants can prevent brain necrosis following asphyxia.

II. Resuscitation

A. Equipment. Only a modicum of resuscitation equipment, which must be well maintained, is required in the delivery room.

1. Overhead radiant warmer
2. Suction source (wall and bulb)
3. Suction catheters
4. Oxygen source
5. Infant resuscitation bag
6. Face masks (assorted sizes)
7. Laryngoscope (with 0 and 1 straight blades)
8. Endotracheal tubes (2.5, 3.0, and 3.5 mm)
9. Umbilical catheterization tray
10. Umbilical catheters (No. 3.5 and 5.0 French)
11. Drugs
12. Syringes and needles

B. Technique

1. Thermal protection. Rapidly wipe the infant dry and place him or her under the radiant warmer. Hypothermia is an unnecessary additional stress for an already depressed newborn infant. If resuscitative measures are required, the infant should remain under the warmer until transferred to the nursery.

2. Position for airway management. Place the infant in a left lateral, head-down tilt position (Fig. 33-1). The supine position is contraindicated since it promotes airway obstruction and aspiration.

3. Pharyngeal suctioning. Gently suction secretions from the pharynx with a bulb syringe or under direct vision (laryngoscope) with a whistle-tip catheter attached to wall suction. Some physicians prefer a catheter attached to a DeLee trap, employing mouth suction. Do not overdo suctioning. Avoid passing catheters through the nose and into the stomach for the first 5 minutes of life, as these maneuvers may induce bradycardia.

4. Airway suctioning. Thick secretions or meconium may require tracheal suctioning under direct vision (laryngoscope).

5. Positive pressure ventilation. Infants with heart rates of less than 100 beats/minute need immediate high-quality ventilation with oxygen-enriched gas, as do infants who remain apneic for 1 minute after birth. With effective ventilation, the heart rate should rise within 15–30 seconds. The first few insufflations may require pressures of 30–50 cm H_2O. Higher pressures may be necessary in premature infants. Thereafter, lower pressures should suffice. Therefore, a ventilating bag with a manometer to measure the delivered pressure is recommended (Fig. 33-2).

a. Bag and mask ventilation. Bag and mask ventilation is easily learned and usually effective.

(1) With the infant's head slightly extended, the mask is grasped with the thumb and first two fingers of the left hand and placed gently but firmly

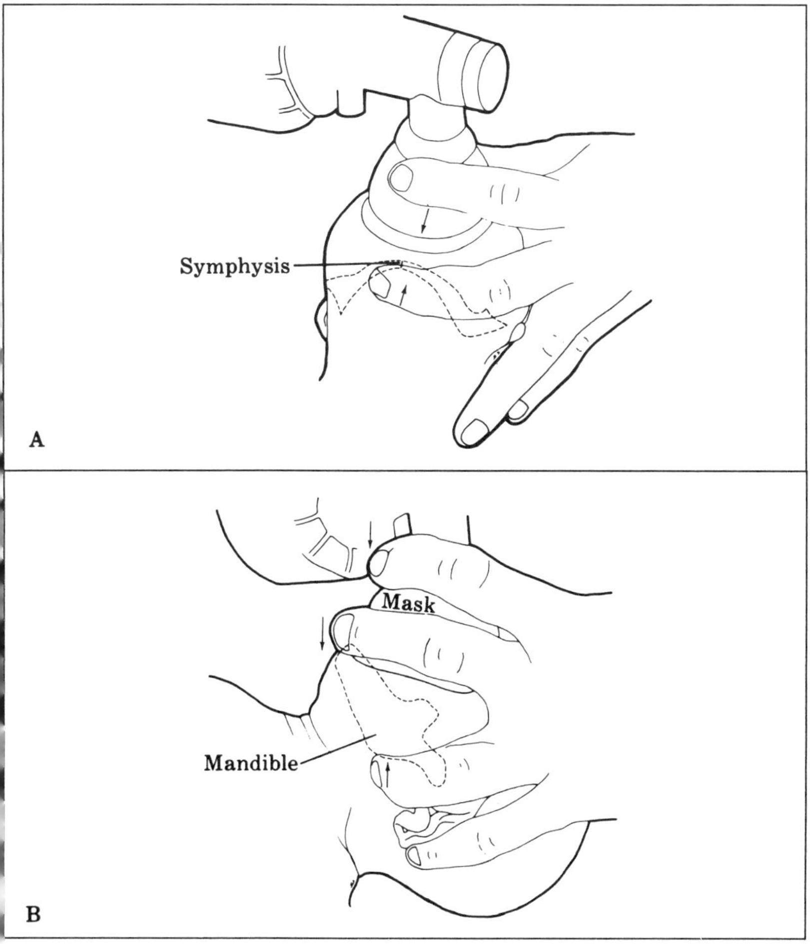

Fig. 33-1. Resuscitation of the neonate. The mask is applied firmly to the face, and counterpressure is exerted **(A)** with the middle finger against the symphysis menti or **(B)** with the ring finger behind the angle of the mandible. (From K. Niswander, *Obstetric and Gynecologic Disorders: A Practitioner's Guide*. Flushing, NY: Medical Examination, 1975.)

over the infant's mouth and nose. The other two fingers on the left hand are used to support the chin, as in Fig. 33-1.

(2) With oxygen-enriched gas running at 3–6 liters/minute, the tail of the anesthesia bag is partially obstructed with an adjustable clamp or the operator's right fifth finger. The bag is intermittently squeezed with the right hand to obtain the desired inflating pressure. The operator is best positioned at the patient's head.

(3) The effectiveness of ventilation is assessed by observation of chest motion and a prompt increase in heart rate. Auscultation of the chest should reveal air entry bilaterally.

(4) Gastric distention may be relieved by passing a nasogastric or orogastric tube.

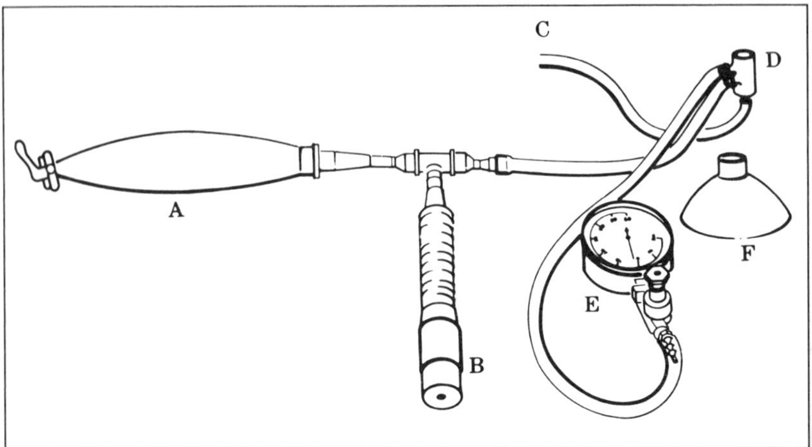

Fig. 33-2. Ventilating device for infant resuscitation. **A.** 500-ml anesthesia bag. **B.** Pressure relief valve. **C.** Oxygen line. **D.** Head (accepts mask or endotracheal tube). **E.** Pressure manometer. **F.** Infant ventilating mask.

b. Endotracheal intubation. The frequency of endotracheal intubation during resuscitation of newborn infants has largely been an artifact of the supine position. In this position, the large occiput and tongue and small posterior pharynx combine to produce airway obstruction. Proper positioning and airway management have decreased the need for endotracheal intubation; however, it may be required if bag and mask ventilation is ineffective (lack of thoracic movement and air exchange on auscultation or no increase in heart rate), if airway obstruction is suspected (goiter or micrognathia), if meconium aspiration or diaphragmatic hernia is suspected, or if external cardiac massage is necessary.

(1) Begin by choosing an appropriately sized endotracheal tube. Usually a 3.5-mm tube will suffice for a full-term newborn infant and a 3.0-mm tube for a premature infant.

(2) The infant should be properly positioned with the head slightly elevated and the neck slightly extended (sniff position).

(3) Advance the laryngoscope blade with the left hand (Fig. 33-3). Beginning at the right corner of the patient's mouth, as the laryngoscope blade is advanced, it is rotated to the midline, moving the tongue to the left. When the blade is in the space between the tongue and epiglottis, thus lifting the epiglottis, the glottis and vocal cords should be visible (Fig. 33-4).

(4) The endotracheal tube then is advanced beside the laryngoscope blade (**not** within its C-shaped opening, or your line of sight to the glottis will be obstructed).

(5) Insert the tip of the tube into the glottis, between the vocal cords, and advance 1.5–2 cm.

(6) For temporary fixation, grasp the endotracheal tube near the mouth with the thumb and finger of the right hand and rest the remainder of the fingers on the infant's cheek.

(7) Attach the ventilating device (see Fig. 33-2), and begin manual ventilation with oxygen-enriched gas.

(8) Auscultate the chest for evidence of air entry bilaterally and the expected response in heart rate.

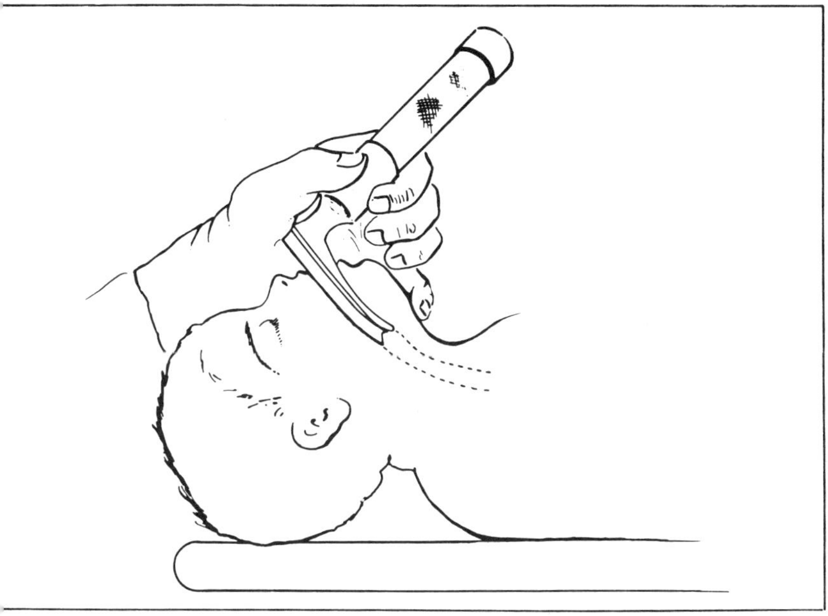

Fig. 33-3. Technique of endotracheal intubation. The head should be slightly elevated and the neck extended only slightly (sniff position).

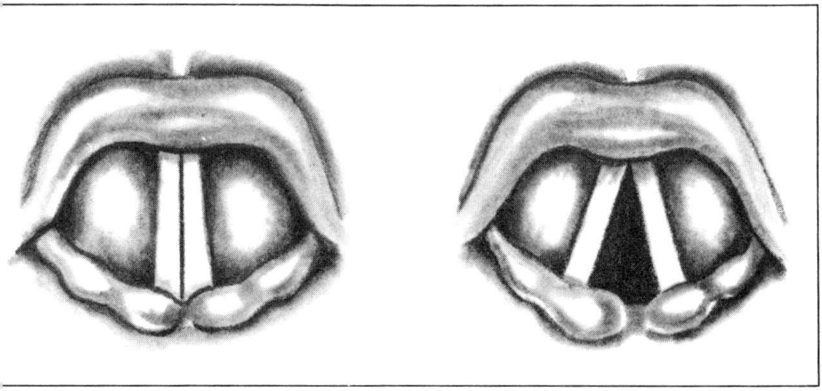

Fig. 33-4. View through laryngoscope: vocal cords closed *(left);* vocal cords open *(right),* revealing glottic opening.

6. **External cardiac message.** If the heart rate does not rise above 100 beats/minute within 30 seconds of beginning ventilation, external cardiac massage should be started. Compression, with two fingers, should be over the middle one-third of the sternum (Fig. 33-5). Lower positions are ineffective and may lacerate the liver. A frequency of 100–120 compressions/minute is adequate. No need to coordinate with ventilation has been documented.

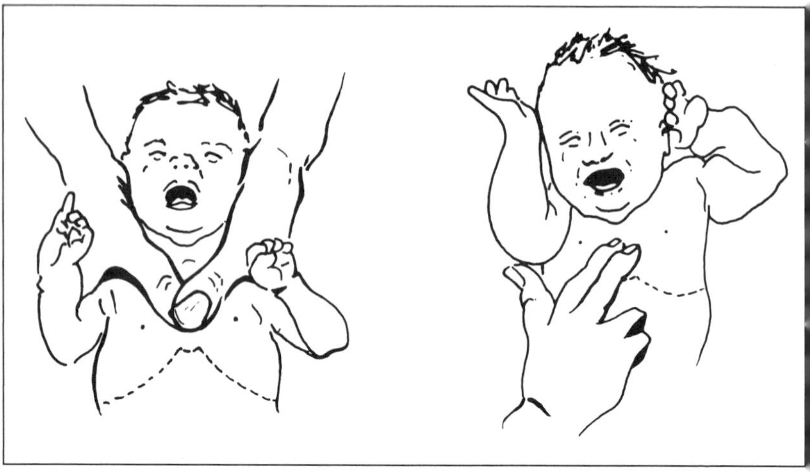

Fig. 33-5. External cardiac massage being performed on a newborn infant.

7. Pharmacologic therapy

a. Continued pallor and bradycardia. The infant who does not respond promptly to ventilation may benefit from the administration of pharmacologic agents.

(1) Catheterization of the umbilical vein with a No. 5 French catheter often provides the quickest route for emergency administration of drugs.

(2) Flush the drugs through the umbilical catheter with 3 ml isotonic saline.

(3) If the heart rate does not respond promptly, administer epinephrine 1 : 10,000 (0.1 ml/kg IV or 0.15 ml/kg down an endotracheal tube).

(4) If hypovolemia is suspected, volume expansion with Plasmanate 0.9% saline, type O Rh-negative blood, or heparinized placental blood in a volume of 10–20 ml/kg is indicated.

(5) Other drugs such as 10% calcium gluconate (0.5 mg/kg) to stimulate cardiac contractility or atropine (0.01 mg/kg) to inhibit vagal effects are rarely necessary.

b. Drug depression

(1) Narcotic antagonists, such as naloxone hydrochloride (Narcan), 0.1 mg/kg, should be administered for suspected drug depression only after appropriate initial resuscitation has taken place and the infant continues to hypoventilate. Too often, a narcotic antagonist is administered in lieu of assisting ventilation, and a wait-and-see attitude prevails, to the detriment of the patient.

(2) Knowledge of maternal heroin use is essential to avoid precipitation of acute narcotic withdrawal.

(3) Maternal general anesthesia may result in an anesthetized newborn who requires 10–15 minutes, occasionally longer, of manual ventilation to recover from the anesthetic.

(4) Magnesium sulfate, used as a tocolytic agent, may lead to hypotonia and hypoventilation necessitating 4–24 hours of mechanical ventilation.

c. Metabolic acidosis. The infant who remains pale and bradycardic for four to five minutes after beginning ventilation probably has metabolic acidosis and could benefit from the administration of sodium bicarbonate. Subsequent doses of sodium bicarbonate should be based on blood gas analysis. In general, metabolic acidosis with base deficits of 10 mEq/liter or greater should be corrected. A common practice is to correct one-half of the base requirement calculated from the following equation: base requirement =

base deficit (mEq/liter) × body weight (kg) × 0.6, where 0.6 is an estimate of the bicarbonate space as a fraction of the body weight. Blood gas analysis then is repeated to assess the acid-base status of the infant.

8. Aftercare. Successfully resuscitated infants require further observation and should not be assigned to well-baby nurseries. Sequelae to be anticipated include

a. Metabolic sequelae

(1) Lactic acidosis (blood pH < 7.3 and lactate > 3.0 mEq/liter) may persist, indicating low cardiac output or hepatic insufficiency. Alkali therapy, blood volume expansion, or cardiotonic agents may be indicated.

(2) Hypoglycemia (blood glucose < 40 mg/dl in full-term infants or 30 mg/dl in premature infants) is fairly common and responds well to glucose infusion at rates of 8 mg/kg/minute.

(3) Hypocalcemia (serum calcium < 8.0 mg/dl in full-term infants or 7.0 mg/dl in premature infants) frequently occurs during the second 24 hours of life in the asphyxiated infant. The indications for and risks of therapy for hypocalcemia are not well defined. Convulsions or heart failure caused by hypocalcemia should respond to infusion of 200 mg/kg of calcium gluconate over 10 minutes followed by 400–500 mg/kg/day.

b. Central nervous system sequelae

(1) Cerebral edema may lead to coma or convulsions. The syndrome of inappropriate antidiuretic hormone secretion also may occur. Assessment of fontanelle tension, cerebral suture width, and head circumference are helpful diagnostically. Fluid infusion in asphyxiated infants should be conservative initially, on the order of 50 ml/kg/day. The therapeutic use of glucocorticoids, barbiturates, and osmotic agents remains controversial.

(2) Cerebral hemorrhage, primarily intraventricular, may occur in premature infants, often with catastrophic results.

(3) Computed tomographic scans of the brain or ultrasonic examinations are useful diagnostic tools when cerebral edema or hemorrhage is suspected. The role of magnetic resonance imaging remains unclear.

c. Renal sequelae

(1) Acute renal failure, most commonly caused by acute tubular necrosis, may occur. Careful fluid and electrolyte management based on the patient's weight changes, serum sodium and potassium values, and urine output usually leads to recovery of renal function in three to five days. Occasionally, peritoneal dialysis is necessary before renal function returns.

(2) Renal cortical necrosis or renal vein thrombosis may be the etiology of the renal failure following asphyxia. Recovery of renal function is unusual in these entities.

d. Cardiac sequelae. The heart is often a target organ in asphyxia and may be damaged so severely that the infant dies. Myocardial damage that is less severe may produce hypotension, low cardiac output, and persistent metabolic acidosis. Radiographically, the heart is enlarged, and echocardiography reveals left ventricular dysfunction. Careful fluid and alkali therapy, along with the administration of oxygen, usually is necessary. Cardiotonic agents, such as dopamine hydrochloride, appear to be useful therapeutic adjuncts.

e. Pulmonary sequelae. A variety of pulmonary problems may be precipitated by asphyxia. Pulmonary vasospasm with right-to-left shunting of blood through the ductus arteriosus or foramen ovale (persistence of the fetal circulation) may lead to severe cyanosis refractory to oxygen and ventilatory therapy. Pulmonary vasodilator therapy with oxygen, alkalosis, and pharmacologic agents is useful in many of these infants. Cyanotic heart disease often is suspected. Asphyxia may lead to decreased surfactant production and result clinically and radiographically in the respiratory dis-

Table 33-1. Apgar scoring system

Sign	0	1	2
Heart rate	Absent	< 100 beats/min	> 100 beats/min
Respiratory effort	Absent	Slow, irregular	Good, crying
Muscle tone	Flaccid	Some flexion of extremities	Active motion; well-flexed extremities
Reflex irritability	No response	Grimace	Vigorous cry
Color	Blue; pale	Body pink; extremities blue	Completely pink

tress syndrome. Lung fluid clearance may also be disturbed. When seen together, the term **asphyxial** or **shock lung** often is applied. Monitoring of arterial blood gases is necessary to determine appropriate oxygen and ventilatory therapy.

9. **Apgar score.** The Apgar score has served to draw attention to the depressed newborn infant and provides a standard for comparing the condition of different populations of infants at birth. At 1 and 5 minutes after birth of the infant, five objective signs are evaluated (Table 33-1), and each is given a score of 0, 1, or 2. The sum of the five scores is the Apgar score. A score of 7–10 indicates an infant in excellent condition. A score of 3–6 indicates moderate depression, and a score of 0–2 indicates severe depression. These Apgar scores correlate best with survival. They are not sensitive prognosticators of subsequent neurologic damage. However, Apgar scores of 1–3 at 20 minutes predict a poor outcome, as evidenced by the presence of cerebral palsy in more than 50% of such cases. Additionally, it should be remembered that approximately 75% of children who are diagnosed as having cerebral palsy did not have birth asphyxia.

   Assessment of heart rate and respiratory effort, as discussed in secs. **5** and **6,** serve as indicators for beginning resuscitation and assessing its success.

10. **Outcome.** The mortality of severely asphyxiated human newborn infants (Apgar 0–3) is approximately 50%. Survivors have an increased risk for central nervous system damage; however, it must be remembered that more than 90% of these survivors develop normally. Thus, in the absence of serious congenital anomalies, it is prudent to begin resuscitation efforts in severely depressed infants. If an infant does not respond with a sustained increase in heart rate in 15–20 minutes, a decision to stop resuscitative efforts may be warranted.

    Laboratory investigations as adjuncts to the clinical examination for predicting long-term neurologic sequelae include brain scan, computed tomographic scan, electroencephalogram, and blood concentration of brain-type isoenzyme of creatine kinase. Although no test can predict outcome with certainty, some assurance can be provided when all these tests are normal.

Selected Readings

Committee on Drugs. Emergency drug doses for infants and children and naloxone use in newborns: Clarification. *Pediatrics* 83(5):803, 1989.

Freeman, J. M., and Nelson, K. B. Special articles: Intrapartum asphyxia and cerebral palsy. *Pediatrics* 82(2):240–249, 1988.

Montgomery, W. H., et al. Neonatal advanced life support. *J.A.M.A.* 255: 2969, 1986.

Rogers, M. C., and Kirsch, J. R. Current concepts in brain resuscitation. *J.A.M.A.* 261(21):3143–3147, 1989.

Sykes, G. S., et al. Do APGAR scores indicate asphyxia? *Lancet* 1:494–496, 1982.

34 Delivery Room Management of the Newborn

Boyd W. Goetzman

The evaluation and management of the newborn are begun in the delivery room. Optimal care requires preparation of the staff and a systematic approach. Thi chapter deals with those aspects of care applicable to all newborn infants, and i will specify all procedures that are necessary for the 80% of newborn infants wh are full-term, who have no malformations, and who make a normal transition t extrauterine existence. Resuscitation of the depressed newborn is discussed i Chap. 33.

I. Immediate clearing of the airway

A. The mouth and pharynx should be suctioned with a suction catheter or bul syringe (ear and ulcer syringe) after delivery of the infant's head and befor delivery of the body. Some may argue that this is difficult with the usual occipu anterior position. However, it has special significance if meconium was passe prior to delivery, since it may prevent aspiration of meconium on delivery of th chest.

B. Suction the mouth and pharynx again after complete delivery of the infant, wit the head in a dependent position at the level of the perineum.

II. Prevention of evaporative heat loss. Wipe the infant dry with a towel to preven undue cooling. Because of the newborn infant's large ratio of surface area to bod mass, the body temperature can quickly fall 2–3°C under delivery room conditions The infant's attempts at thermoregulation can double his or her caloric expenditur and oxygen consumption. The fact that the entirely normal newborn usually ca handle this degree of thermal stress is not justification for routinely imposing it o all infants.

III. Cord clamping

A. The optimal time for cord clamping still is controversial. Infants with late-clampe cords, three to five minutes after birth, have higher hematocrits at 2 days of ag and consequently higher iron stores later in infancy than do infants who hav immediate cord clamping. They also have a higher incidence of hyperbilirubi nemia, higher respiratory rates, lower pulmonary compliance, and higher carbo dioxide tension during the first days of life.

B. A middle-of-the-road approach is recommended. If the first 30–45 seconds afte delivery are spent clearing the airway and drying the infant, the cord can the be clamped and the one-minute Apgar score assigned. If the infant is asphyxiate these measures should be carried out with dispatch and resuscitation begun a discussed in Chap. 33. Stripping the umbilical cord and placing the infant on th mother's abdomen before clamping the cord are not recommended.

IV. Further thermal protection

A. Radiant heat source. Placing the newly delivered, dried infant under a radian heat source is effective in reducing further heat loss in the delivery room. Thi is especially useful when resuscitation or immediate observation is indicated.

B. Warm blanket. Information concerning heat loss in a nude infant placed imme diately on the mother's breast with skin-to-skin contact is not readily available However, thorough drying and wrapping in a warm blanket offer thermal pro tection near that of radiant warmers and provide for immediate contact with th new mother.

C. Bathing in the delivery room is not recommended.

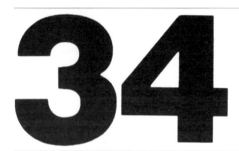

V. Apgar score. The Apgar score, which consists of an evaluation of five factors (heart rate, respiratory effort, muscle tone, responsiveness to noxious stimuli [reflex irritability], and skin color), is determined at one and five minutes after delivery (see Table 33-1). Most often a nurse is assigned to this task. The results of this evaluation are reproducible and allow comparison of the cardiopulmonary and neurologic status at birth of infants or groups of infants. This can be very useful in assessing obstetric technique. The one-minute Apgar score appears to correlate with the need for resuscitation.

A. Infants with Apgar scores of 7–10 rarely need any resuscitation. Proper airway management and oxygen by mask usually suffice for infants with scores of 3–6, whereas those scoring lower usually need some form of positive pressure ventilation.

B. The five-minute Apgar score provides information about the infant's adaptation to extrauterine life. It appears to correlate with survival and to some small degree with the subsequent neurologic status.

C. Approximately 50% of infants with Apgar score 0–3 at five minutes will die. Neurologic damage in the survivors is 4 times as common as in infants with Apgar scores of 7–10, but it must be remembered that more than 90% of the low Apgar score survivors will be neurologically normal at 4 years of age (Nelson and Ellenberg, 1981).

VI. Vitamin K administration. Vitamin K_1, 0.5–1.0 mg given parenterally in a single dose, is adequate to prevent hemorrhagic diatheses caused by deficiency of vitamin K–dependent coagulation factors. This is especially important for the premature infant, the ill infant who will be fed parentally, and the infant who will be breastfed.

VII. Eye care. The instillation of 0.5% erythromycin ointment or 1% silver nitrate solution is recommended for the prevention of gonococcal ophthalmia neonatorum. The former also prevents *Chlamydia* infections and is usually the preferred treatment when eye prophylaxis can be administered with the **first 30 minutes** of life. Otherwise, silver nitrate is recommended. There is a low incidence of failure with both of these methods, but conjunctival irritation is common with silver nitrate and unusual with erythromycin.

VIII. Hepatitis B prophylaxis. The transmission of hepatitis B virus to an infant from its O-positive mother with hepatitis B surface antigen (HBsAG) is well documented. Certain women are at high risk for being HBsAG-positive, including drug abusers, those of Asian descent, women who work in dialysis units or dental offices, and those with chronic liver disease. The infection rate of infants is high, as is the chronic carrier state. The latter puts the infants at risk for later cirrhosis or hepatic carcinoma. Thus, prophylaxis of all infants born to HBsAG-positive or suspect mothers is recommended. Currently, 0.5 ml hepatitis B immunoglobulin is recommended during the first 12 hours after birth, followed by hepatitis B vaccine (Heptavax) during the first week of life and one month later.

Obstetric and pediatric staff should take appropriate precautions to protect themselves from infectious blood and secretions. The infant should be bathed without delay and appropriate environmental cleaning then performed with a dilute hypochlorite solution.

IX. Physical examination. After the infant has been dried and Apgar scores have been assigned, a screening physical examination should be performed (see Chap. 35).

X. Circumcision should not be performed in the delivery room. It is not a medically indicated procedure, and if performed, it should be delayed for at least 12–24 hours to ensure that the infant's temperature remains stable and that he is without bleeding tendencies.

XI. Identification. Each newborn must be adequately identified before leaving the delivery area. This usually is accomplished by obtaining sole and palm prints of the infant and fingerprints of the mother, but these are not reliable. Therefore, wrist or ankle bracelets containing the mother's name and hospital number should also be attached.

XII. Continued observation. Infants need not be separated from their mothers if adequate trained staff are available for the observation of the mother-infant pair.

Selected Readings

AAP Committee on Fetus and Newborn/ACOG Committee on Obstetrics: Maternal and Fetal Medicine. *Guidelines for Perinatal Care* (2nd ed.). American Academy of Pediatrics/American College of Obstetricians and Gynecologists, 1988.

Centers for Disease Control. Postexposure prophylaxis of hepatitis B. *M.M.W.R.* 33(21):285, 1984.

Dahm, L. S., and James, L. S. Newborn temperature and calculated heat loss in the delivery room. *Pediatrics* 49:504, 1972.

Linder, N., et al. Need for endotracheal intubation and suction in meconium-stained neonates. *J. Pediatr.* 112:613–615, 1988.

Murphy, J. D., Vawter, G. F., and Reid, L. M. Pulmonary vascular disease in fetal meconium aspiration. *J. Pediatr.* 104:758–762, 1984.

Nelson, K. B., and Ellenberg, J. H. Apgar scores as predictors of chronic neurologic disability. *Pediatrics* 68:36, 1981.

Pelosi, M. A., and Apuzzio, J. Making circumcision a painless event. *Contemp. Pediatr.* January 1985. Pp. 85–88.

Shepherd, A. J., Richardson, J., and Brown, J. P. Nuchal cord as a cause of neonatal anemia. *Am. J. Dis. Child.* 139:71, 1985.

Yao, A. C., and Lind, J. Placental transfusion. *Am. J. Dis. Child.* 127:128, 1974.

35 Immediate Examination of the Newborn

Boyd W. Goetzman

All newborn infants should undergo an initial screening examination. Usually this is performed in the delivery room by the obstetrician or a nurse practitioner. However, when problems are anticipated, a pediatrician should be in the delivery room to manage and examine the infant. The goals of this examination are (1) to assess adaptation to extrauterine existence, (2) to detect obvious congenital anomalies, (3) to detect the effects of an adverse fetal environment, and (4) to detect evidence of birth trauma. The placenta, membranes, and umbilical cord should also be examined, for this may be the only opportunity to obtain information about them (see Chap. 31).

I. Technique. The infant should be protected from thermal stress during this examination, preferably by use of a radiant warming device. The examination should be performed rapidly, but gently, after respirations are sustained and resuscitation has been completed. Usually, this will occur after the five-minute Apgar score has been assigned.

The **order of examination** is usually (1) visual inspection (most of which has been completed during delivery, resuscitation, and assigning of Apgar scores); (2) auscultation of the chest; (3) palpation of head, clavicles, abdomen, and extremities; and (4) manipulation of the infant by passing catheters through various orifices. Organization according to systems is not efficient or practical.

A. Inspection. Visual inspection of the unclothed infant provides most of the useful information regarding the newborn.

1. Obvious malformations

a. Head. Characteristic facies occur in a number of syndromes:

(1) There may be Potter's facies in **renal agenesis.**

(2) Marked **microcephaly, anencephaly, cleft lip** or **palate, malformed ears,** and **micrognathia** may be observed as isolated entities or as part of a syndrome or chromosomal disorder. Severe micrognathia may produce respiratory obstruction and require an oral airway or tracheal intubation.

(3) Excessive, frothy oral secretions suggest the presence of **esophageal atresia,** which usually is accompanied by a **tracheoesophageal fistula.**

b. Neck. Goiters and **cystic lymphangiomas** may present as masses large enough to compromise the airway. Immediate tracheal intubation may be necessary.

c. Chest. Abnormalities such as **ectopia cordis** are extremely rare and require heroic surgical efforts.

d. Abdomen

(1) Omphalocele, an anomaly in which intestine and, sometimes, liver or spleen are present in a membrane-covered sac protruding through the base of the umbilicus, is immediately evident at birth. Large defects frequently rupture during the birth process and require immediate surgical attention.

(2) Gastroschisis, a right paramedian, anterior abdominal wall defect, may be initially mistaken for a ruptured omphalocele. However, unlike omphaloceles, gastroschisis is not associated with other congenital anomalies. In either case, the eviscerated organs should be covered with sterile gauze moistened with warm saline. Great care must be paid to maintaining the infant's body temperature and fluid balance.

(3) **Absent abdominal muscles** are readily apparent in the aptly named **prune-belly syndrome** and are associated with serious urologic disorders.

(4) Abdominal masses with distention of the flanks may indicate **tumors or cysts of the kidneys, liver, or other organs.**

e. **Extremities and back**

(1) **Absence and malformation of parts of extremities** are immediately obvious and may be associated with other defects or may occur as isolated defects, such as the phocomelia observed in the thalidomide tragedy or amputations caused by amniotic bands.

(2) **Meningomyelocele,** a defect in closure of the neural tube, presents with a fluid-filled sac usually on the thoracolumbar spine. Dislocated hips, anesthetic legs, and absent rectal sphincter tone usually are present also. Hydrocephalus often is present and progresses rapidly after surgical closure of the defect. Rupture of the sac during delivery often leads to meningitis.

f. **Anus.** Close inspection may reveal absence of an anal opening **(imperforate anus).** Pediatric surgical consultation is necessary.

g. **Genitalia.** Close inspection of the genitalia is required to assess the gender of the infant. Ambiguous genitalia may require endocrinologic evaluation before the sex is assigned.

2. **Skin**

a. **Vernix caseosa,** a white cheesy substance, normally is present on the skin of preterm infants after 24 weeks' gestation. At term, it is prominent only in the skin folds of the axillae and groin. It is absent in postterm infants.

b. **Cyanosis of the hands and feet** (acrocyanosis) normally may persist for some time after adequate respiration has been established. Focal cyanosis involving the scalp, scalp and face, and sometimes the thorax is really an ecchymotic lesion probably resulting from excessive pressures during delivery.

c. **Pallor of the skin** may indicate significant anemia, resulting from hemolysis or hemorrhage, or a state of shock with inadequate cardiac output. The latter state may persist for a number of hours in asphyxiated infants.

d. **Yellow or yellow-green staining of the skin**—predominantly the nails, umbilical cord, and vernix—by bile pigments from meconium-stained amniotic fluid suggests previous fetal distress. The pharynx and larynx should be visualized, and if meconium is present, endotracheal intubation and direct tracheal suction are recommended. Close observation for respiratory distress caused by meconium aspiration is indicated. Rarely is the skin jaundiced at birth. Even in severe erythroblastosis fetalis, usually only the umbilical cord is yellow, probably from amniotic fluid staining.

e. **Generalized petechiae and ecchymoses** may be present in congenital viral infections such as with rubella. Petechiae over the head and neck are common, especially in rapid or difficult deliveries. Premature infants bruise easily, and ecchymoses may appear in areas where they have been firmly grasped during delivery.

3. **Respiratory tract**

a. **Signs of respiratory distress** such as tachypnea, a rate higher than 50 breaths/minute, chest wall and sternal retractions, nasal flaring, and end-expiratory grunting indicate the need for close observation. Whereas many infants with these symptoms recover quickly and have a normal newborn course, others have potentially fatal problems such as hyaline membrane disease, meconium aspiration, pneumonia, or penumothorax. Radiographic evaluation almost always is indicated.

b. **Slow respiratory frequency** (rate < 30 breaths/minute), if shallow, suggests central nervous system depression. **Gasping respirations** suggest previous asphyxia.

4. **Urine and meconium.** The passage of urine and meconium from the appropriate orifices indicates patency of the urethra and anus and should be noted for the nursery staff who will be observing the function of these systems.

5. **Cry.** Most infants cry lustily after birth. Absence or weakness of the cry should

alert the observer to the possibility of central nervous system depression. A stridulous or hoarse cry may indicate obstruction in the glottic region. Immediate provision of an adequate airway may be necessary.

B. Auscultation of the chest

1. **Cardiovascular system.** The heart rate, rhythm, and presence of murmurs should be noted.
   a. **Tachycardia** (rates higher than 160 beats/minute) or **bradycardia** (rates lower than 120 beats/minute) are significant and usually indicate the need for rapid therapeutic and diagnostic intervention.
   b. **Heart murmurs** are common and usually are related to transient patency of the ductus arteriosus. Extrasystoles are common and usually transient. Heart sounds may be distant in the presence of pneumomediastinum or shifted to one side by a pneumothorax or a diaphragmatic hernia. It should be noted that **cyanotic congenital heart disease** may occur in the absence of a heart murmur.
2. **Respiratory system**
   a. **Coarse rales,** particularly at the lung bases, are common and normally disappear in the first few hours of life.
   b. **Unilateral absence of breath sounds** suggests a pneumothorax, diaphragmatic hernia, or lobar emphysema.
   c. The presence of **bowel sounds in the chest** is diagnostic of a diaphragmatic hernia.

C. Palpation

1. **Head**
   a. **The size and tenseness of fontanelles and cranial sutures** should be noted. Widely spread sutures and tense fontanelles suggest hydrocephalus or intracranial hemorrhage. Overlapping sutures may result from normal head molding.
   b. **Caput succedaneum** (edema of the presenting part of the head) is boggy and usually crosses suture lines. Cephalohematomas usually are slightly ballotable and do not cross suture lines.
2. **Clavicles. Crepitation over one of the clavicles** indicates a fracture and may confirm the suspicion of fracture when a snap is felt during delivery of the shoulder of a large infant.
3. **Abdomen.** The liver usually is palpable in the newborn. **Obvious hepatosplenomegaly** suggests congenital viral infection of severe hemolytic disease.
4. **Extremities. Crepitation and displacement of the humerus** should be carefully sought when a fracture during delivery is suspected.

D. Manipulation

1. **Moro's reflex**
   a. Moro's reflex is elicited by grasping the infant's hands and extending and abducting the arms with just enough force to almost raise the head from the surface on which the infant is lying. Sudden release normally is accompanied by an embrace response.
   b. Absence of this suggests intracranial pathology or marked prematurity.
   c. Asymmetry of the reflex suggests a fracture of a clavicle or humerus, or a brachial plexus injury.
   d. Brachial plexus injuries may be accompanied by phrenic nerve damage with respiratory distress caused by diaphragmatic paralysis.
2. **Muscle tone.** Assess muscle tone by suspending the infant prone and by passively flexing the extremities. If the infant is hypotonic (floppy), central nervous system depression, spinal cord damage, or muscle disease is present.
3. **Patency of nares.** Choanal atresia can be ruled out if the infant is able to breathe when his or her mouth is closed either spontaneously or by force. It is unnecessary and traumatic to pass rubber or plastic catheters through the nares routinely.
4. **Patency of the esophagus**
   a. If a catheter can be passed through the mouth and into the stomach, esophageal atresia is ruled out.

Table 35-1. Physical criteria for gestational age estimation in the delivery room

Physical finding	Weeks of gestation				
	< 30	32–34	36–38	40–42	> 42
Breast					
Areola	Inapparent	Apparent	Raised	Raised	Raised
Nodule	None	None	1–3 mm	7–10 mm	10 mm
Sole creases	None	One or two on anterior sole	Cover anterior two-thirds of sole	Heel also involved	Deep creases with desquamation
Skin	Thin, translucent, edematous	Smooth, ruddy, no edema	Pink, few vessels	Thick, pale pink, some desquamation	Thick, pale, desquamating
Lanugo	Covers entire body	Patches disappear from cheeks and flanks	Absent from face	Present on shoulders	Absent
Skull firmness	Bones soft	Soft within 1 in. from fontanelle	Soft at edges of fontanelle	Bones hard, sutures easy to displace	Bones hard, sutures difficult to displace

Source: Adapted from L. O. Lubchenco, Assessment of gestational age and development at birth. *Pediatr. Clin. North Am.* 17:125, 1970.

b. Aspiration of fluid from the stomach, if greater than 20–30 ml, especially if bile-stained, suggests a high intestinal obstruction.

c. Gastric fluid, essentially swallowed amniotic fluid, should be saved for analysis of bacteria and leukocytes or surfactant content when indicated.

5. Patency of the anus. Passage of a soft rubber or plastic catheter through the anus into the rectum and withdrawal of a meconium-stained catheter establishes anal-rectal patency.

6. Gestational age assessment. The obstetrician should have the ability to estimate the gestational age of the infants he or she delivers. This has special importance for elective deliveries. Classification as appropriate, small, or large for gestational age is covered in Chap. 36. Table 35-1 provides a guide for the estimation of gestational age in the delivery rom.

II. Placenta, cord, and membranes

A. Determination of the number of cord vessels is routine. A total of three vessels—two arteries and one vein—is normal. A single umbilical artery, occurring in 1% of singleton deliveries and 7% of twins, may be associated with other congenital anomalies, most of which are obvious.

B. The size of the placenta may correlate with the infant's condition (i.e., large in the affected infant born to a mother with diabetes mellitus and small in the infant who has suffered intrauterine growth retardation).

C. Placental infarctions and areas of premature separation (partial abruption) should be noted. (See Chap. 31 for a more complete discussion of placental pathology.)

D. The fetal surface of the placenta may have small yellow nodules (amnion nodosum), indicating renal agenesis. Oligohydramnios usually accompanies this condition.

E. Hydropic placentas and umbilical cords usually are seen in erythroblastosis fetalis.

F. In like-sex twin pregnancies, the placental membranes should be examined to determine whether the infants are identical.

III. Summary of findings. A summary of the findings of the screening examination, Apgar scores, and resuscitation measures, along with the maternal history and delivery room record, should be provided to the nursery personnel. The need for emergency treatment should be communicated verbally.

Selected Readings

Dubowitz, L. M. S., Dubowitz, V., and Goldberg, C. Clinical assessment of gestational age in the newborn infant. *J. Pediatr.* 77:1, 1970.

Lassau, J. P., et al. (eds.). *Atlas of Neonatal Anatomy, Correlation of Gross Anatomy, Computed Tomography and Ultrasonography.* Chicago: Year Book, 1982.

Seashore, J. H. Congenital abdominal wall defects. *Clin. Perinatol.* 5:61, 1978.

Smith, D. W. *Recognizable Patterns of Human Malformation* 2nd ed.). Philadelphia: Saunders, 1982.

Stern, L., and Vert, P. (eds.). *Neonatal Medicine.* New York: Masson, 1987.

36 Old Problems and New Solutions in the Neonate

Jay M. Milstein

Although some problems encountered by infants have been eliminated by advances in prenatal care, many have persisted. The approach to many of the unsolved, persistent problems has changed over the past decade. Some of these advances are highlighted in this chapter.

I. Classification of newborn infants

A. Current classification of newborn infants is based on **gestational age.**

1. Preterm refers to those neonates born before 38 weeks' gestation.

2. Term refers to those neonates born between 38 and 42 weeks' gestation.

3. Postterm refers to those neonates born after 42 weeks' gestation.

B. Further classification of neonates is based on their **birth weight.**

1. Those neonates whose weight falls between the tenth and ninetieth percentile are **appropriate for gestational age (AGA).**

2. Those neonates under the tenth percentile by weight are considered **small for gestational age (SGA).**

3. Those neonates whose weight falls over the ninetieth percentile are considered **large for gestational age (LGA).**

4. Those infants whose weight falls below 2500 or 1000 gm are considered **low birth weight or very low birth weight** infants, respectively.

II. Problems associated with abnormal size for gestational age

A. Small-for-gestational-age infants. The overall growth pattern of the neonate depends on when the etiologic "insult" took place. During the first trimester, weight, length, and head circumference are all affected; if, on the other hand, the insult occurred during the third trimester, the weight usually is markedly affected and the other two growth characteristics are less affected.

1. The possible factors responsible for neonates being SGA are numerous.

a. Chronic intrauterine infections such as toxoplasmosis, rubella, cytomegalovirus, herpes simplex, and syphilis.

b. Vascular problems in the mother such as those seen in preeclampsia, maternal hypertension, renal disease, or in advanced cases of diabetes mellitus (classes E and F) with significant vascular involvement.

c. Placental insufficiency of undetermined etiology.

d. Severe maternal malnutrition, which usually results in a decline in fertility and an increase in the stillbirth rate. The incidence of fetal growth retardation did increase in mothers whose prepregnancy body weight was low (<43.5 kg) and whose net pregnancy weight gain was low (<6 kg) [13].

e. Chromosomal abnormalities, such as trisomy 13 or trisomy 18.

f. Twins generally are AGA up to approximately 32 weeks' gestation; beyond that age, their weights generally drop to approximately the tenth percentile. Occasionally, when one is dealing with discordant twins, the smaller of the two may be SGA. To be discordant, the difference in the weights between the twins should be greater than or equal to 25%.

g. Maternal smoking has been implicated; however, data support the fact that infants of mothers who smoke are relatively small but not actually SGA (i.e., they do not fall below the tenth percentile unless other factors causing an infant to be SGA were present during the pregnancy) [6].

2. Problems encountered in the SGA neonate include the following:

a. Hypoglycemia, with blood glucose measurements of less than 20 mg/dl in the preterm neonate and 30 mg/dl in the term neonate, occurs frequently.

Impaired enzymes of gluconeogenesis are the major factor. This is supported by the finding of increased alanine in some of these infants. Diminished glycogen stores also may be a factor.

b. **Hypothermia** is another serious metabolic problem. Babies usually produce heat primarily by nonshivering thermogenesis; they metabolize brown fat, which is concentrated in the neck, between the scapula, behind the sternum, along the vertebral column, and around the kidneys and adrenal glands. These fat stores often are depleted in the SGA infant; therefore, heat production is impaired.

c. **Hyperviscosity syndrome** may occur. Hyperviscosity syndrome is caused by the polycythemia (central hematocrit >65%) that may be present in response to chronic intrauterine hypoxia. This may result in central nervous system dysfunction, and it also may rarely result in persistent pulmonary hypertension and persistent fetal circulation. In general, partial exchange transfusions are recommended when central hematocrits exceed 70% or 65% in the presence of associated symptoms. Unfortunately, the frequency of long-term central nervous system dysfunction is unaltered by the exchange transfusion, suggesting a prenatal basis for both the polycythemia and dysfunction.

d. **Meconium aspiration and intrapartum deaths** occur, since SGA infants often have hypoxic episodes during labor and delivery.

e. **Persistent pulmonary hypertension of the newborn** may be present. Intrauterine growth retardation is often associated with either chronic intrauterine hypoxia or intrauterine hypertension. Both forms of intrauterine stress have been associated with increased muscularization of the pulmonary vascular bed [18].

B. Large-for-gestational-age infants

1. The most frequent etiology is **diabetes mellitus** in the mother.
2. Uncommon causes may include the rare **Beckwith-Wiedemann syndrome.**
3. Problems that may occur with the LGA infant include **hypoglycemia, hypocalcemia, hyperviscosity, and hyperbilirubinemia** if the neonate is an infant of a diabetic mother.
4. **Birth trauma** also is seen more frequently.

III. Problems related to prematurity (< 38 weeks' gestation). These problems are primarily a result of the relative immaturity of the different organ or physiologic systems.

A. Respiratory system. The most common problems of the premature infant involve the respiratory system. These babies often develop **respiratory distress syndrome (RDS),** also commonly known as **hyaline membrane disease.** RDS occurs in approximately 15% of infants weighing less than 2500 gm, and the overall mortality from this disorder is between 20 and 30% of those affected.

1. **The underlying pathogenesis of RDS** is related to the relative pulmonary immaturity with respect to surfactant production. Surfactant is the material that provides stability to the air-breathing lung. It helps reduce the surface tension in the lung during expiration, which in turn prevents the lungs from completely collapsing or becoming atelectatic during expiration (i.e., allows the lung to retain functional residual capacity). At term, phosphatidylcholine (lecithin) is the principal surfactant phospholipid with phosphatidylglycerol and phosphatidylinositol comprising the second and third most abundant phospholipids, respectively.
2. **Assessment of fetal lung maturity,** including determination of the lecithin-sphingomyelin (L/S) ratio (with values > 2.0 indicating pulmonary maturity), as well as quantitative determination of the percentages of the various phospholipids, is helpful in the management of the high-risk pregnancy. The quality of the phospholipids may be more important than the quantity. Some babies with L/S ratios of less than 2.0 may have good-quality surfactant phospholipids and not have RDS. The relative lengths and saturations of the fatty acids in the phospholipids may be critical in terms of the qualitative differences.
3. Typically, neonates with RDS appear fairly healthy at birth but soon develop

abnormal patterns of respiration, including **forceful intercostal and suprasternal retractions, nasal flaring,** and **tachypnea,** as well as an audible **expiratory grunt.** The expiratory grunt, which may be caused by forced expiration past a partially closed glottis, may help to provide positive end-expiratory pressure (PEEP) at the alveolar level, which in turn may help prevent complete collapse of the lungs and maintain a functional residual capacity. This phenomenon has been used in therapy of neonatal RDS in the form of continuous positive airway pressure (CPAP) or in the form of PEEP when a baby is on intermittent mandatory ventilation (IMV).

4. Babies with RDS typically have an **increasing oxygen requirement** and may or may not require ventilatory support over the first 48–72 hours. They gradually show improvement following that time. Chest roentgenograms typically show a reticulogranular pattern with exaggeration of the normal bronchial air shadows (referred to as air bronchogram) as well as atelectasis [2].
5. Various states have been associated with **accelerated maturation of surfactant production,** including maternal vascular disease and prolonged rupture of membranes. Accelerated maturation has also been attained in mothers in premature labor who have been treated with betamethasone (see Chap. 28). This maturation has been shown to occur in babies whose mothers were treated between 28 and 32 weeks' gestation for more than 48 hours prior to delivery.
6. **Surfactant replacement** with various preparations including homologous or heterologous natural surfactant, artificial surfactant, and synthetic surfactant has been attempted [10]. A particularly impressive therapeutic trial with an artificial surfactant was reported by Fujiwara and colleagues [8]. Although the results of these studies are encouraging, controlled trials with long-term follow-up are essential before general usage of surfactant replacement can be recommended. Hallman and colleagues [9] utilized exogenous human surfactant in infants with severe RDS. The results were very encouraging; however, use of homologous human surfactant is unlikely in the future because of acquired immunodeficiency syndrome precautions. Recently, encouraging results were reported from a large randomized multicenter trial utilizing heterologous (from minced porcine lungs) surfactant [14]. Other large collaborative studies are currently underway.
7. **Respiratory complications** occur in RDS.
   a. **Air leak** often presents initially in the form of pulmonary interstitial emphysema in the neonate requiring ventilatory assistance and typically occurs as the interstitial fluid resorbs and as the lung compliance suddenly starts to improve. At this stage, alveoli may tear and air may dissect into the interstitial spaces. The interstitial air can then dissect into the mediastinal or pleural space, resulting in pneumomediastinum, pneumothorax, or pneumopericardium. Alternative modes of mechanical ventilation such as high-frequency oscillatory ventilation may have some applicability in the patient with severe **respiratory failure and air leaks** (see sec. **7.c.**).
   b. **Pneumothorax.** The reported incidence of pneumothorax in RDS ranges from 3.5% in those treated with no assisted ventilation, to 11% in those on CPAP only, to 24% in those treated with IMV and PEEP [3].
   c. **Bronchopulmonary dysplasia,** a form of chronic lung disease, occurs in neonates treated primarily with elevated oxygen concentration, positive pressure ventilation, and endotracheal intubation. The incidence may be as high as 30% in those surviving RDS and treated with IMV. Mortality is as high as 38%. Prevention may depend on how quickly one can decrease the supplemental oxygen and ventilatory pressures.

      Pharmacologic agents have been used to prevent bronchopulmonary dysplasia. Although an initial evaluation of one antioxidant, vitamin E, showed beneficial effects, subsequent studies did not confirm such effects [15]. This recent preliminary study showed that the radiologic and clinical manifestations of bronchopulmonary dysplasia can be significantly reduced with exogenous superoxide dismutase [15]. Clinical trials with other agents that are not specifically antioxidants, such as vitamin A, are currently underway. Further study is still necessary, however.

Alternative modes of mechanical ventilation are also being employed in some infants with RDS. In short trials, high-frequency oscillatory ventilation has been shown to permit use of lower inspired oxygen fractions than conventional ventilation. Although phasic pressure swings are reduced, mean airway pressure could not be lowered without compromising oxygenation [12]. High-frequency jet ventilation has also been shown to permit use of lower inspired oxygen fractions as well as lower mean airway pressure than with conventional ventilation [4]. In a multicenter randomized clinical trial comparing the efficacy and safety of high-frequency oscillatory versus conventional mechanical ventilation for the treatment of respiratory failure in premature infants, the severity and frequency of bronchopulmonary dysplasia and mortality are similar. Therefore, widespread use of this technique is unwarranted for severe RDS [17].

8. **Nonrespiratory complications** occur in RDS.

a. **Retinopathy of prematurity,** sometimes referred to as **retrolental fibroplasia,** is a major complication. Although multiple factors have been implicated in its pathogenesis, hyperoxia and ischemia are considered the most important factors. The growing retinal vessels in the premature infant are adversely affected by hyperoxia. During the active phase of growth, excess oxygen causes the immature retinal vessels to vasoconstrict, particularly on the temporal side. This is followed by vasoobliteration and then vasoproliferation after the oxygen tension has been normalized. The incidence of this complication depends on the birth weight, with as many as 35% of cases occurring in infants weighing less than 1500 gm and less than 17% in those weighing more than 1500 gm. Because of the increased incidence of infants weighing less than 1500 gm at birth who receive supplemental oxygen, the American Academy of Pediatrics recommends an ophthalmologic evaluation prior to discharge and at least one follow-up during the first 6 months of life [1]. The long-term effects, manifest in the cicatricial phase, may include myopia or late retinal detachment. While the disease persists, some therapeutic progress is being made. In a multicenter trial of cryotherapy for retinopathy of prematurity, unfavorable outcomes were significantly reduced in frequency [5].

b. **Intracranial hemorrhage,** especially intraventricular hemorrhage, is another major complication. The exact etiology is not clear but may be related to periods of asphyxia, infusions of hypertonic solutions, sudden changes in arterial carbon dioxide tensions, or changes in central venous or arterial pressure. These hemorrhages may originate in the area of the choroid plexus, and because of the relative immaturity of the surrounding brain substance, particularly between 28 and 32 weeks' gestation, the hemorrhage may either rupture into the ventricles or extend into the subependymal area.

c. **Patent ductus arteriosus** is another major complication. The overall incidence in infants with RDS is approximately 18%, with the incidence approaching 75% in those born at very early gestational ages. Although the ductus arteriosus often manifests itself in neonates of very early gestational ages, it usually appears in the neonate recovering from RDS.

(1) As such an infant is improving and being weaned from a ventilator, **left-to-right ductus arteriosus shunting** frequently manifests itself. Common findings include

(a) Increased precordial activity

(b) Murmurs, which are usually systolic but occasionally continuous

(c) Widened pulse pressures

(d) Bounding pulses

(2) These babies may not be successfully weaned from the ventilator because of **progressive shunting and cardiac failure.** Owing to increasing blood flow across the ductus arteriosus into the lungs, there is increasing ven-

ous return to the left atrium and, in turn, to the left ventricle, which may decompensate in the face of this increasing blood volume.

(3) Many of these neonates require either **medical ligation of the ductus** using prostaglandin synthetase inhibitors or **surgical ligation** prior to successful weaning from the ventilator.

(4) These babies also may have **fluid or calorie intolerance** and thus fail to thrive.

B. **Gastrointestinal system.** Premature neonates may have several problems related to their gastrointestinal immaturity.

1. **Necrotizing enterocolitis** is one of the most serious problems. The exact etiology of this disorder is not understood thoroughly. It may be related to the relatively poor perfusion of the bowel, the osmotic loads presented to the bowel, or the bacterial colonization of the bowel, particularly with gas-forming organisms. The disorder may manifest itself with abdominal distention, reducing substance-positive and guaiac-positive stools, sepsis, acidosis, and shock or death. Radiographically, it may be characterized by distended loops of bowel, pneumatosis intestinalis, or intestinal perforation with free air.

2. **Feeding.** The most frequently encountered gastrointestinal problem in the premature infant is the feeding problem related to the relatively small stomach volume, the short gastric emptying time, and, possibly, the relative immaturity of exocrine enzymes necessary for digestion of the formulas fed to the infant.

3. **Hepatic function** in the premature neonate is also somewhat immature. This may result in delayed metabolism of various agents. The most frequently encountered endogenous agent is bilirubin, which is formed as fetal erythrocytes are destroyed and which undergoes conjugation in the liver. Because the responsible enzyme is somewhat deficient, the bilirubin does not undergo conjugation as quickly as it is formed, and the baby will become jaundiced. If the unconjugated bilirubin reaches high enough levels, the infant is at risk for kernicterus (bilirubin encephalopathy). Some exogenous agents also are metabolized by the liver, and their dosage schedules must be adjusted accordingly.

   a. **Hyperbilirubinemia** represents one of the oldest problems in neonatology. Finally, new controversial approaches are being evaluated. Sn-protoporphyrin, an inhibitor of heme oxygenase, which catabolizes heme to bilirubin, moderates the postnatal rate of increase of plasma bilirubin as well as the intensity of hyperbilirubinemia [11]. Further evaluation is necessary before use of this or other heme analogs as treatment modalities.

C. **The genitourinary system** of the premature neonate also is relatively immature. The neonate has its full complement of glomeruli by approximately 36 weeks' gestation, and the anatomic tubular development follows. Because of the relative immaturity of the genitourinary system at the earlier gestational ages, premature neonates usually cannot concentrate their urine as well as the term neonate and older infant. The rate of excretion of certain endogenous agents, including various antibiotics such as the penicillin derivatives or aminoglycosides, or other drugs such as digitalis, may be delayed; drug schedules must therefore be adjusted accordingly.

D. **Neurologic system.** Problems related to the neurologic immaturity of the premature neonate are as follows:

1. **Feeding.** The most common problem in the otherwise healthy premature neonate is related to feeding. After 28–29 weeks' gestation, the neonate usually has a suck, but it is not coordinated with swallowing until the baby is approximately 32 or 33 weeks' gestation. Consequently, such babies have to be fed by gavage tube feeding or other routes.

2. **Intracranial hemorrhage.** Another major problem that premature neonates may encounter is intracranial hemorrhage secondary to perinatal asphyxia. These hemorrhages usually are periventricular or intraventricular. Although these central nervous system defects frequently are seen in neonates surviving ventilation, they probably are not caused by the ventilation per se but by the hypoxia occurring before or during the ventilation.

3. **The central nervous system defects** include spastic diplegia, hemiplegia, sen-

sorineural hearing loss, epilepsy, cerebral palsy, or hydrocephalus. The frequency of these neurologic defects in premature infants with birth weights of less than 1500 gm, and particularly in those surviving ventilatory assistance, has declined over the past few years. In four different follow-up studies, an average of 21% of the survivors had neurologic defects. In one of the centers that had reported 29% defects, a later study performed in 1974 revealed a decrease to 11% defects in their survivors [7].

Major centers have been reporting improved survival of infants whose birth weights are less than 1000 gm. In one large review of infants weighing between 501 and 1000 gm at birth, 46% survived. Of the survivors, 24% had neurosensory handicaps. Within 100-gm birth weight groups from 501–1000 gm, survival improved significantly with increasing birth weight whereas the handicap rates remained fairly constant [16].

E. The defense mechanisms of the premature neonate also are immature.

1. These babies have **decreased opsonic activity, decreased complement, and suboptimal phagocytosis.** Immunoglobulins in the baby are primarily of the IgG variety, which passively cross from the mother. The only antibodies the baby forms are of the IgM class; IgM may be increased in the presence of intrauterine infection.
2. In addition to the immature defense mechanisms in the premature neonate, other **factors predispose to infection:**
   - **a. Physical** factors may include thin, immature skin or the umbilical stump.
   - **b. Environmental** factors may include prolonged rupture of the membranes (>24 hours), difficult labor, or obstetric manipulations, among others.
3. **Infections** acquired early in gestation usually are acquired **transplacentally.** The infections commonly known to affect the fetus early in gestation include those designated by the abbreviation **TORCH: *T*oxoplasmosis, *r*ubella, *c*ytomegalovirus,** and ***h*erpes simplex.** Other causative agents include *Treponema pallidum* and *Listeria monocytogenes.*
4. **Other infections** may be acquired through the **birth canal** at the time of delivery or shortly before delivery. Gram-negative bacilli or group B beta-hemolytic streptococci frequently are involved. Other organisms, such as *L. monocytogenes,* gonococci, and staphylococci, may also be involved.
5. **Some infections,** such as herpes simplex, group B beta-hemolytic streptococci, and *L. monocytogenes,* may be acquired by **either the transplacental or ascending route.** Many of these infections may occur and manifest themselves after birth in the form of septicemia, meningitis, pneumonia, or pyelonephritis. The group B streptococci may have an early presentation with sepsis and pneumonia, but occasionally they will present in a late-onset form, which may appear at approximately 2 weeks of age as meningitis. This latter form may be acquired nosocomially.
6. Although the defense mechanisms are more immature in the premature neonate than in the term neonate, the term neonate also is vulnerable to infections by the same spectrum of organisms.

IV. The term neonate (38–42 weeks' gestation)

A. Congenital birth defects. Because the organ systems are relatively more mature in the full-term neonate, he or she may be slightly less predisposed to some of the problems that occur in the premature neonate, and congenital birth defects have a relatively greater importance. Such defects may include

1. Cardiac defects
2. Anterior abdominal wall defects
3. Diaphragmatic hernias
4. Tracheoesophageal fistulas
5. Chromosomal abnormalities

B. Problems in the term neonate typically occur in certain **organ or physiologic systems.**

1. **Transient tachypnea of the newborn, or RDS type 2.** These babies often are products of cesarean sections. They often have grunting respirations as well as tachypnea and retractions. They tend to have some hyperventilation with

low carbon dioxide tensions and may require supplemental oxygen for the first 24 hours of life. Chest roentgenograms in these babies usually reveal hyperinflation as well as some retained fluid.

2. **Abnormal cardiopulmonary adaptation with persistent fetal circulation.** Many of these babies have either acute birth asphyxia, chronic asphyxia, pneumonia, meconium aspiration, or undetermined underlying pulmonary disease. They often have hypoxemia that exceeds the severity of the radiographic findings. They have a persistently elevated pulmonary vascular resistance, which results in right-to-left shunting across the ductus arteriosus or the foramen ovale (or both) as well. Hypoglycemia, hypocalcemia, and hyperviscosity may all predispose to persistent elevation of the pulmonary vascular resistance and persistent fetal circulation. Therapeutic approaches to persistent pulmonary hypertension of the newborn, a problem that continues to plague infants and intrigue neonatologists, have continually evolved over the past decade. Both pharmacologic and mechanical approaches have been utilized with variable success. Extracorporeal membrane oxygenation, although the subject of controversy, has been one of the most successful technologic advances, whereas high-frequency ventilation has been less effective.
3. **The defense mechanisms** are somewhat immature in the term neonate. Consequently, the term neonate also is subject to the risk of intrauterine infection. These infections may be either transplacental or ascending infections. Additionally, the babies are at risk for nosocomial infections.
4. **The hepatic function** of the term neonate is also somewhat immature, manifested primarily in the form of physiologic hyperbilirubinemia.

V. The postterm neonate (>42 weeks' gestation)

A. Postmaturity syndrome. The most common problem encountered by the postterm neonate is what has been referred to as the postmaturity syndrome. With the postmaturity syndrome, the baby may have been subjected to placental insufficiency, usually exhibiting loss of subcutaneous tissue as well as loose, thin skin and a decreased muscle mass. Often, there is no decrease in the length or head circumference but only in the weight.

B. Acute hypoxemia and meconium aspiration. Because of the placental dysfunction, postterm babies may have acute hypoxemia. Consequently, they may pass meconium in utero and be predisposed to meconium aspiration when they gasp. Studies over the last several years have demonstrated that many of these babies who aspirate meconium go on to develop persistent fetal circulation and persistent pulmonary hypertension. The overall mortality for this condition has probably been reduced by early tracheal lavage at the time of birth.

C. Anencephaly. Occasionally, the fetus with anencephaly will gestate beyond term.

VI. Birth injuries that are not specific for any given gestational age

A. Various injuries that usually are not of great significance may be associated with a difficult delivery.

1. **Soft-tissue injury** may lead to subcutaneous fat necrosis, usually a benign entity.
2. **Fractures** can occur in several locations.
    a. **The clavicle and humerus** may be fractured in difficult delivery and are easily treated with minor immobilization. Examination for a concurrent **brachial plexus injury** is imperative.
    b. **The skull** may also be fractured during a difficult delivery. If the skull fracture is depressed significantly, it should be elevated. Frequently, cephalhematomas will be present overlying occult skull fractures and may represent a fairly sizable collection of blood. They resolve on their own and should not be aspirated because of the risk of introducing infection. They may be a source of increased bilirubin levels.

B. More significant injuries may occur during a difficult delivery, particularly during difficult breech deliveries when the upper abdomen may be held tightly during delivery of the body.

1. **Rupture of either a solid organ or a hollow viscus** may occur.

2. Difficult deliveries have also been associated with **neurologic injuries** of minor and major significance.
   a. The **facial nerve** can be injured as a result of forceps application.
   b. Various **spinal roots** in the brachial plexus may be involved in a difficult delivery.
      (1) In **Erb's palsy,** the upper arm, which is served by nerve root C5 and C6, is involved.
      (2) In **Klumpke's paralysis,** the lower portion of the arm and intrinsic muscles of the hand that are innervated by nerve roots C8 and T1 may be involved.
   c. If extensive flexion of the head or stretching and tension of the neck occur, **spinal cord injury** may result.
   d. In the rapid uncontrolled delivery, the term neonate may develop a **subdural hematoma** or **subtentorial and subarachnoid hemorrhages.**
3. The baby delivered in the breech presentation occasionally may exhibit a **congenitally dislocated hip,** often manifested by a limitation in the range of motion of the hip (particularly during abduction), abnormal skin folds, differential leg length, or palpable and audible hip clicks using the Ortolani maneuver.

References

1. AAP Committee on Fetus and Newborn and ACOG Committee on Obstetrics: Maternal and Fetal Medicine. *Guidelines for Perinatal Care.* American Academy of Pediatrics/American College of Obstetricians and Gynecologists, 1988.
2. Avery, M. E., Fletcher, B. D., and Williams, R. G. The lung and its disorders in the newborn infant. Philadelphia: Saunders, 1981. Pp. 233–234.
3. Boyle, R. J., and Oh, W. Respiratory distress syndrome. *Clin. Perinatol.* 5:283, 1978.
4. Carlo, W. A., et al. Decrease in airway pressure during high-frequency jet ventilation in infants with respiratory distress syndrome. *J. Pediatr.* 104:101, 1984.
5. CRYO-ROP Cooperative Group. Multicenter trial of cryotherapy for retinopathy of prematurity: Preliminary results. *Pediatrics* 81:697, 1988.
6. Davies, D. P., et al. Cigarette smoking in pregnancy: Association with maternal weight gain and fetal growth. *Lancet* 1:385, 1976.
7. Fitzhardinge, P. M. Follow-up studies in infants treated by mechanical ventilation. *Clin. Perinatol.* 5:451, 1978.
8. Fujiwara, T., et al. Artificial surfactant therapy in hyaline membrane disease. *Lancet* 1:55, 1980.
9. Hallman, M., et al. Exogenous human surfactant for treatment of severe respiratory distress syndrome: A randomized, prospective clinical trial. *J. Pediatrics* 106:963–969, 1985.
10. Hallman, M., and Gluck, L. Respiratory distress syndrome—update 1982. *Pediatr. Clin. North Am.* 29:1067, 1982.
11. Kappas, A., et al. Sn-Protoporphyrin use in the management of hyperbilirubinemia in term newborns with direct Coombs-positive ABO incompatibility. *Pediatrics* 81:485, 1988.
12. Marchak, B. E., et al. Treatment of RDS by high-frequency oscillatory ventilation: A preliminary report. *J. Pediatr.* 99:287, 1981.
13. Naeye, R. L. Effects of Maternal Nutrition on the Outcome of Pregnancy. In I. H. Porter and E. B. Hook (eds.), *Human Embryonic and Fetal Death.* New York: Academic, 1980.
14. Robertson, B. Surfactant replacement therapy for severe neonatal respiratory distress syndrome: An international randomized clinical trial. *Pediatrics* 82:683, 1988.
15. Rosenfeld, W., et al. Prevention of bronchopulmonary dysplasia by administration of bovine superoxide dismutase in preterm infants with respiratory distress syndrome. *J. Pediatr.* 105:781, 1984.

16. Saigal, S., et al. Outcome in infants 501 to 1000 gm birthweight delivered to residents of the McMaster Health Region. *J. Pediatr.* 105:969, 1984.
17. Sinnett, E. High frequency oscillatory ventilation compared with conventional mechanical ventilation in the treatment of respiratory failure in preterm infants. *N. Engl. J. Med.* 320:88, 1989.
18. Stenmark, K. R., Abman, S. H., and Accurso, F. J. Etiologic Mechanisms in Persistent Pulmonary Hypertension of the Newborn. In E. K. Weir and J. T. Reeves (eds.), *Pulmonary Vascular Physiology and Pathophysiology*. New York: Dekker, 1988.

Selected Readings

Avery, G. B. *Neonatology: Pathophysiology and Management of the Newborn* (3rd ed.). Philadelphia: Lippincott, 1987.

Purohit, D. M., and Levkoff, A. H. Common Neonatal Problems. In K. R. Niswander (ed.), *Obstetrics: Essentials of Clinical Practice* (2nd ed.). Boston: Little, Brown, 1981.

Saunders, B. S., Kulovich, M. V., and Gluck, L. Antenatal assessment of pulmonary maturation. *Clin. Perinatol.* 5:231, 1978.

Schaffer, A. J., and Avery, M. E. *Diseases of the Newborn*. Philadelphia: Saunders, 1977.

37 Sexually and Socially Transmitted Diseases of the Newborn

Jay M. Milstein

As the population grows, problems more commonly identified in major cities have made their appearance in smaller communities. These problems include **maternal substance abuse** and, in turn, **fetal drug exposure** with their associated congenital and perinatal manifestations as well as **sexually** (and often **socially) transmitted diseases** including **human immunodeficiency virus** (HIV) infection and hepatitis. Most disease entities have been approached by research, development, and education in order to eliminate or decrease their clinical significance. In contrast, these entities represent both major medical and social challenges requiring far more educational approaches in order to be effective.

I. Fetal drug exposure

A. Prescribed medications should be kept to a minimum during pregnancy, particularly if their reduction or elimination will not compromise maternal health and if their continued use either is teratogenic or has other adverse clinical manifestations in the fetus or neonate (see Chap. 25).

B. Unprescribed substances that have a variety of fetal and neonatal manifestions, including congenital anomalies, addiction, and withdrawal, should be avoided. These substances include several classes of drugs:

1. Alcohol
2. Barbiturates
3. Cocaine and amphetamines
4. Opiates (codeine, heroin, methadone, morphine)
5. Tranquilizers and others

C. Nonwithdrawal manifestations of fetal substance exposure depend on the agent.

1. **Alcohol** may result in dysmorphogenesis with prenatal and persistent postnatal growth retardation; facial, cardiac, and limb abnormalities; as well as delayed development [3, 5, 6].
2. **Cocaine** exposure may result in intrauterine growth retardation, microcephaly, cerebral infarction, prematurity, abruptio placentae, and spontaneous abortions [3, 5, 6].
3. **Barbiturates and opiates** are generally not associated with congenital anomalies.

D. Neonatal abstinence or withdrawal syndrome

1. **General characteristics** are central nervous system hyperirritability; gastrointestinal dysfunction; metabolic, vasomotor, and respiratory disturbances; and vague autonomic symptoms such as hyperthermia [1].
2. **Symptoms** depend on duration of addiction, daily maternal dose, time of last maternal dose, and half-life of addictive substance [3].
3. **Diagnosis** is made based on clinical course and physical exam of the infant, which includes signs and symptoms outlined in Finnegan's Neonatal Abstinence Scoring System [1]; maternal history of substance abuse; and presence of toxic substances in urine of infant and mother (withdrawal may be present in absence of positive urine screen).
4. **General management of infants undergoing withdrawal should be supportive.** This may include placement in a quiet, darkened environment where the infant is swaddled and handled less often. Frequent, small feedings may be preferable in the presence of gastrointestinal symptomatology. Finally, administration of hepatitis B immunoglobulin (HBIG) and hepatitis vaccination may be appropriate.

5. **Pharmacologic treatment** depends on the severity of withdrawal signs and symptoms as well as the responsible agent. If an opiate is the sole substance involved, paregoric is preferable. If multiple substances are responsible, phenobarbital is preferable. Duration of treatment depends on the rate of improvement of withdrawal symptoms and their continual decline as treatment is tapered [1].
6. **Discharge planning** is often very difficult because of the multitude of social and medical problems, but it is **essential.**

E. **Neurodevelopmental** and general follow-up evaluation are indicated. Because the incidence of sexually transmitted diseases and other diseases are more frequent in these infants, additional specific medical follow-up may be indicated (see next section).

II. **Sexually and socially transmitted diseases**

A. **Incidence.** Sexually and socially transmitted diseases have become more frequent in infants. Although the risks are greater in infants born to drug-abusing mothers, the risks to infants in the general population are increased as well, since the incidence of sexually transmitted diseases is now at alarming levels in the general adolescent and young adult population.

B. **Numerous infectious diseases due to bacterial and nonbacterial organisms are often venereal in transmission.**

1. **Major bacterial infections** are caused by group B beta-hemolytic streptococci, *Neisseria gonorrhoeae, Treponema pallidum,* and *Chlamydia trachomatis.* Numerous other bacteria cause sexually transmitted diseases in addition to the traditional venereal diseases (for a more complete description of manifestations and management, see the *Red Book*) [4].
2. **Major sexually transmitted viral infections** are due to herpes simplex virus (HSV), human cytomegalovirus, HIV, and hepatitis B virus (HBV). The latter two are transmitted both sexually and by other social habits, particularly by intravenous drug abuse. (For more complete information regarding manifestations, transmission, and management, see the *Red Book* [4].)

C. **HIV and HBV**

1. Both viruses are transmitted through sexual or blood-to-blood contact [2].
2. **Prenatal screening for HBV.** Screening of all pregnant women, not just those most likely to be hepatitis B surface antigen (HBsAg) carriers, is currently recommended by the American Academy of Pediatrics [4]. Such identification and surveillance of HBsAg-positive pregnant women is critical to prevent perinatal transmission of HBV. In general, infants of positive mothers should be carefully bathed to remove any maternal blood and secretions. Personnel should be gloved. HBIG (0.5 ml) should be given to infants. In addition, HBV vaccine (0.5 ml) should be given at the time of HBIG at a different site. Two additional doses of HBV vaccine should be given at 1 and 6 months of age [4].
3. **Perinatal screening for HIV.** Screening for HIV infection is recommended for all mothers in high-risk groups, including those with a history of intravenous drug use, those who have bisexual partners or multiple sexual partners, women who received a transfusion between 1977 and 1985, and women from high-risk immigrant groups, such as Haitians. If the HIV antibody screen is negative for the mother, counseling and repeat testing may be warranted. If the HIV antibody screen is positive (and confirmed), HIV antibody testing of the infant (with screening and confirmatory tests) is indicated. If the infant's antibody screen is negative, further counseling regarding transmission is indicated. Breast-feeding should be discouraged. If the infant's screen is positive, further evaluation and follow-up beyond the scope of this chapter are indicated [4].

D. The magnitude of this group of sexually and socially transmitted diseases and their consequences for infants is overwhelming. Major educational programs are essential to help control these public-health threats. Regional AIDS foundations and the U.S. Public Health Service have educational materials available.

References

1. Finnegan, L. P. Neonatal Abstinence. In N. Nelson (ed.), *Current Therapy in Neonatal-Perinatal Medicine*. Ontario: Decker, 1984.
2. Flynn, N. HIV Infection. In T. W. Hudson et al. (eds.), *Clinical Preventive Medicine*. Boston: Little, Brown, 1988.
3. Narcotic Addiction and Withdrawal. In R. E. Behrman, V. C. Vaughan, and W. E. Nelson (eds.), *Nelson Textbook of Pediatrics*. Philadelphia: Saunders, 1987. Pp. 417–419.
4. Peter, G. (ed.). Red Book: Report of the Committee on Infectious Diseases. Elk Grove Village, IL: American Academy of Pediatrics, 1988.
5. Rosen, T. S. Infants of Addicted Mothers. In A. A. Fanaroff and R. J. Martin (eds.), *Neonatal-Perinatal Medicine*. St. Louis: Mosby, 1987.
6. Ryan, L., Ehrlich, S., and Finnegan, L. Cocaine abuse in pregnancy: Effects on the fetus and newborn. *Neurotoxicol. Teratol.* 9:295–299, 1987.

Index

Index

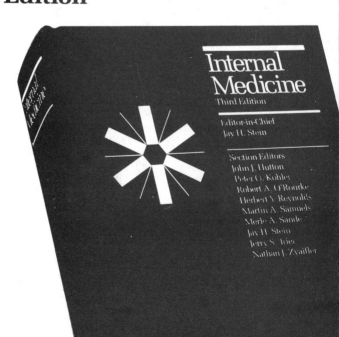

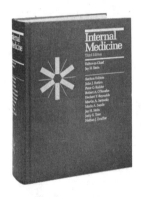